The Lippincott Manual of
Primary Eye Care

The Lippincott Manual of Primary Eye Care

Edited by

Kevin L. Alexander, OD, PhD

Retina Vitreous Associates, Inc.
St. Vincent Medical Center
Toledo, Ohio
Clinical Associate Professor
The Ohio State University
College of Optometry
Columbus, Ohio

With 13 contributors

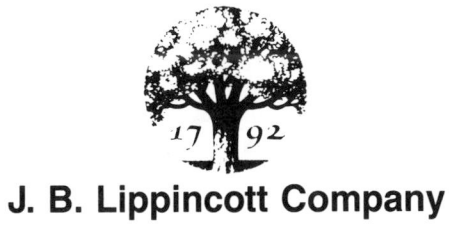

J. B. Lippincott Company

Philadelphia

Acquisitions Editor: Mary K. Smith
Sponsoring Editor: Anne Geyer
Production Editor: Mary Kinsella
Indexer: Melanie Belkin
Cover Designer: Anne R. Bullen
Production Manager: Janet Greenwood
Production Service: Chernow Editorial Services, Inc.
Compositor: The Composing Room of Michigan, Inc.
Printer/Binder: Quebecor/Kingsport

6 5 4 3 2 1

    Library of Congress Cataloging-in-Publication Data
    The Lippincott manual of primary eye care / edited by Kevin L. Alexander
      : with 11 contributors.
        p. cm.
    Includes bibliographical references and index.
    ISBN 0-397-51109-4
    1. Optometry. 2. Eye—Care and hygiene. I. Alexander, Kevin
Lee, 1941–
    [DNLM: 1. Vision disorders—therapy. 2. Primary Health Care. WW
140 L765 1995]
    RE951.L56 1995
    617.7—dc20
    DNLM/DLC
    for Library of Congress   94-24472
                                                              CIP

The authors and publisher have exerted every effort to ensure that drug selection and dosage set forth
in this text are in accord with current recommendations and practice at the time of publication.
However, in view of ongoing research, changes in government regulations, and the constant flow of
information relating to drug therapy and drug reactions, the reader is urged to check the package
insert for each drug for any change in indications and dosage and for added warnings and precautions. This is particularly important when the recommended agent is a new or infrequently employed
drug.

To my family—Carol, Nick, and Lindsay
the reason for love, pride, and accomplishment

And to my parents—Betty and Nelson
for the opportunity of education and
instilling the value of keeping busy

Contributors

Kevin L. Alexander, OD, PhD
Retina Vitreous Associates, Inc.
St. Vincent Medical Center
Toledo, Ohio
Clinical Associate Professor
The Ohio State University
College of Optometry
Columbus, Ohio

Edward S. Bennett, OD, MSEd
Associate Professor and Director of Contact Lens Service
University of Missouri–St. Louis
School of Optometry
Adjunct Assistant Professor
St. Louis University Hospital
Department of Ophthalmology
St. Louis, Missouri

William L. Brown, OD, PhD
Associate Professor of Optometry
Illinois College of Optometry
Chicago, Illinois
Low Vision Specialist
La Porte Hospital
La Porte, Indiana

Elise Ciner, OD
Director
Infants Vision Service
Associate Professor
Pennsylvania College of Optometry
Philadelphia, Pennsylvania

Graham B. Erickson, OD
Assistant Professor
Southern California College of Optometry
Fullerton, California

John R. Griffin, MOpt, OD, MSEd
Professor
Southern California College of Optometry
Fullerton, California

Vinita Allee Henry, OD
Clinical Associate Professor
University of Missouri–St. Louis
School of Optometry
St. Louis, Missouri

Chaya Herzberg, BS, OD
Pennsylvania College of Optometry
Philadelphia, Pennsylvania

Jeffrey L. Kegarise, OD
Vice President and Regional Director
Omega Health Systems Inc.
Center Director, VisionAmerica
Nashville, Tennessee

Robert D. Newcomb, OD, MPH
Clinical Associate Professor
The Ohio State University
College of Optometry
Chief of Optometry Service
Veterans Affairs Outpatient Clinic
Columbus, Ohio

Maria L. Parisi, OD
Pennsylvania College of Optometry
Philadelphia, Pennsylvania

Michael Polasky, BS, OD
Assistant Professor
Assistant Dean
The Ohio State University
College of Optometry
Columbus, Ohio

Rick E. Ricer, MD
Associate Professor
Department of Family Medicine
University of Cincinnati
Active Staff
University of Cincinnati Hospital
Cincinnati, Ohio

J. James Thimons, OD
Associate Professor
State University of New York
College of Optometry
University Optometric Center
Chairman, Department of Clinical Sciences
New York, New York

Editorial Consultants

Foreword

Occasionally in the development of such a profession as optometry, a constellation of events puts a unique person in the position of designing a classic book. *The Lippincott Manual of Primary Eye Care* is such a book, and Kevin Alexander is the editor.

The Lippincott Manual of Primary Eye Care describes the real patient care that optometrists provide, and does it in a no-nonsense fashion. The approach is both refreshingly honest and tempered with the values of superb clinicians. Dr. Alexander tells it like it is, not like someone would like it to be. Having insisted on a style that gets right to the heart of patient care issues, the book does not bother the reader with superfluous details related to once-in-a-lifetime occurrences.

It is not surprising that Dr. Alexander has been able to put this book together. He has been there; private practice, group practice, academic health care centers, co-management centers. At the present time and for the last 18 years he has practiced optometry and cared for patients in some of the most productive settings. As the Optometric Director of The Eye Center of Toledo, he has fostered the cooperative spirit between optometrists and ophthalmologists so essential to comprehensive eye and vision care, and worked for the integration of the optometrist into the health care system through the provision of outstanding patient care and appropriate consultations with other health care providers.

Within the structure of the book, other essential patient care is provided to patients of optometrists by other notable specialists. Dr. Alexander fully advocates and demonstrates how the protocols for integration of the patient into this network of care providers works. Optometrists are part of the health care team; they may not do everything, but they do provide primary eye and vision care better than any other group.

The contributors to *The Lippincott Manual of Primary Eye Care* are all steeped in practice traditions. All regularly care for patients. All are well grounded in academic optometry while at the same time maintaining a practice perspective for what works and what is regularly used by optometrists. All of the contributors follow the traditions of Dr. Alexander as outstanding educators in this advancing field.

If you want to know what clinical optometric care is and how it should be delivered, if you want to know about the range of primary health care optometrists provide, if you want a true guide to patient care decision making that is both practical and contemporary—this book is for you. The evolution and events that have changed optometric patient care during the last decade have made this book essential. *The Lippincott Manual of Primary Eye Care* shows the way for the best primary eye and vision care available—optometric care.

Arol R. Augsburger, MS, OD
Dean
University of Alabama
School of Optometry
Birmingham, Alabama

Preface

The growth and development of optometry in the past twenty years has been phenomenal. In addition to the expanded scope of practice, a central feature of optometry's growth has been the recognition of optometrists as primary care providers. For some, the term "primary eye care" has come to mean the treatment of eye disease. This is unfortunate, because primary eye care really means much more.

Primary eye care practitioners take care of most of the problems of most patients most of the time. Primary eye care may include the management of problems with vision/refraction, contact lenses, fitting glasses, binocular vision, low vision, and pediatric problems, as well as the treatment of eye disease. Primary eye care practitioners also recognize eye signs of systemic disease and consult and co-manage with practitioners of other disciplines in the health care system to provide the best patient care.

The Lippincott Manual of Primary Eye Care was written to aid the primary eye care practitioner achieve the goal of taking care of most of the problems of most patients most of the time.

The original concept of this text was to produce a one-volume, comprehensive guide to the practice of optometry. It was a noble idea, but given the enormity of the profession, it was a totally unrealistic task. Still, there seemed to be a need for a single-volume textbook that the "front-line" primary eye care practitioner could consult for guidance. *The Lippincott Manual of Primary Eye Care* is our best attempt to fill that need with a straightforward, concise format based on the "spend a day with the expert" approach.

Rather than write the "definitive treatise" in a specialty area, each contributor was asked to write a chapter as if the reader were "spending the day" with an expert. Using this concept as a guide, each contributor has distilled his or her area to the essential information the primary care practitioner needs to know for daily practice.

The Lippincott Manual of Primary Eye Care is not everything you wanted to know about optometry. It is what you already learned but may have forgotten, and a quick reference is all that is needed to bring it to mind. It is new information that reflects the new scope of the practice of optometry. This text is what you need to know to take care of most of the problems of most patients most of the time.

Kevin L. Alexander, OD, PhD

Acknowledgments

The production of a comprehensive text such as this requires the skills, suggestions, insights, and cooperation of many people. I wish to thank the following whose contributions made this book a reality:

The contributors who stayed with us through many changes in text format to cheerfully produce manuscripts on time. You were each a pleasure to work with.

The editorial consultants who helped mold the initial concept into a workable textbook for clinicians and devoted many hours to manuscript review.

The doctors, staff, and patients at The Eye Center of Toledo. My appreciation for the support and encouragement to complete the task.

The Ohio State University College of Optometry, especially Dean Richard M. Hill who supported the project, and Wendy Clark who produced many of the graphics used in the book.

Lippincott medical editor Mary K. Smith who took the time to get to know optometry and helped bring the text to a successful conclusion.

Dean Arol Augsburger who encouraged me to take on the project and who was always ready with a helpful suggestion or idea.

All my love and appreciation to Carol L. Brown, OD, my colleague, wife, and best friend. Thanks for all the times we put things off and for listening.

Contents

CHAPTER **1**

Optometry Is Primary Eye and Vision Care

Kevin L. Alexander
Robert D. Newcomb

Before exploring the various areas of primary eye care covered in this manual, it is worthwhile to review the general concept of primary health care and how optometrists fulfill the role of primary eye care providers. Referral of patients with health problems beyond the scope of optometric practice is reviewed along with the definitions of commonly utilized medical consultants.

I. Primary Care Defined

A. *Primary care*

Doctors of optometry have always provided general eye and vision care services on an ambulatory, "first contact" basis, treating most of the patients' basic eye problems most of the time. When indicated, optometrists recommend consultation or referral for patients with more complex conditions.

With the advent of health care reform in the United States, the concept of primary care has gained additional importance. The fundamental basis for primary care practice continues to be caring for most of the problems that patients have most of the time. Several important features of primary care practitioners are consistent regardless of the discipline.[1] The primary care practitioner:

1. Is the first contact of the patient with the health care system and practices within an ambulatory (as opposed to a hospital) setting;
2. Provides comprehensive service in his or her discipline, taking care of 90% of patient needs;
3. Coordinates care with other providers while continuing to be responsible for the long-term care of the patient; in patients with multiple health problems, this may be a shared responsibility;
4. Embraces long-term responsibility for patient care, not just acute or episodic care; and
5. Educates patients to help them understand their health care problems and needs; this always includes a strong component of preventive as well as therapeutic health education.

B. *Definition of an optometrist*

The American Optometric Association defines doctors of optometry as:

independent primary health care providers who examine, diagnose, treat and manage disease and disorders of the visual system, the eye and associated structures as well as diagnose related systemic conditions.*

---

*Definition adopted by The American Optometric Association Board of Trustees, September 1993.

The optometrist fulfills the role of the primary eye care provider in several ways. Problems of the human visual system are the second most common chronic health problems in our society (dental caries are first).

1. The need for vision care is frequently the impetus for patients seeking entry into the health care system.
2. Acute eye problems such as a corneal foreign body or red eye prompt entry into the health care system.
3. With therapeutic eye treatment by optometrists available in the majority of states today, optometrists now provide even more services for most patients than previously.
4. When indicated, optometrists refer patients directly to specialists for care and often comanage or help coordinate care for such patients.
5. The optometrist cares for the long-term needs of patients whether they be functional, organic, or both.
6. Compassion and understanding are required by the optometrist whether a patient is adapting to new glasses, or coming to grips with permanent vision loss as the result of disease or trauma.
7. Optometrists are experts in eye safety and vision performance. Therefore, advice regarding preventive eye and vision care is routinely included as part of a comprehensive optometric examination.

In summary, the primary eye care optometrist serves as the best point of entry into the health delivery system for eye and vision problems and is able to efficiently treat most of his or her patients most of the time in a highly cost-effective manner.

II. Optometrists and Other Health Professionals

A. Referral and consultation

In the course of patient care, the primary care optometrist may refer patients to other practitioners for an opinion, procedure, or continuing care. Such circumstances arise when the patient's needs are beyond the scope of optometric practice or a second opinion is desired. It is helpful to understand the difference between a referral and a consultation when sending a patient to another practitioner for services.

1. A *referral* is appropriate when the optometrist wishes to place a patient under someone else's care. Services will be rendered by that provider, following which the patient may be returned to the original provider for ongoing care. It is also possible that the new provider will provide all future care, for example, when a patient moves to a new location or has a chronic disease such as neovascular glaucoma or proliferative diabetic retinopathy.

   Generally there are three types of referrals:

   a. *Routine referrals* are made without regard to time. The patient may be seen in a few days or weeks. Delay in being seen will have no adverse effect on the patient's welfare or outcome. Referral for cataract surgery represents a routine eye referral.

   b. *Urgent referrals* are usually seen by the specialist within 12 to 24 hours. Additional delay may affect outcome. Referral for probable subretinal neovascular membrane is an example of an urgent referral.

   c. *Emergency referral* is made immediately. Any delay in referring the patient may result in a worsening of the condition. Examples of ocular conditions requiring emergency referrals are central retinal artery occlusion, acute angle closure glaucoma, and intraocular foreign bodies.

2. A *consultation* occurs when a patient is referred for an opinion regarding a condition or need for treatment. In a consultation, after an opinion is rendered, the patient is returned for treatment and monitoring to the referring practitioner. A consultation becomes a referral when the consultant provides care to the patient.

It is important to note that the terms *referral* and *consultation* have specific meanings. What occurs when a patient is sent to another practitioner may depend on the terminology used when arranging the visit.

B. *Referring the patient*

When referring the patient to another practitioner for an opinion or procedure, some guidelines are helpful.

1. Clearly explain the need for referral to the patient.
2. The primary care practitioner should make the appointment. Rarely should patients be given a name and phone number and asked to make the appointment on their own.
3. Tell the patient what to expect. Inform the patient as to what type of examination will occur and how long they may expect to be at the specialist's office. Such information decreases the patient's anxiety and increases the patient's confidence in the referring practitioner.
4. Communicate with the specialist or new provider. Explain why the patient is being referred and provide any pertinent information that may aid in the care of the patient.
5. Accurately document the need for the referral, as well as the date and time of the appointment on the optometric examination record.
6. Many health plans require approval by the "gatekeeper" primary physician prior to referral to a specialist. Irrespective of health coverage, referral courtesy dictates that the patient's primary physician be consulted prior to referral for nonocular conditions (for example, for neurology, imaging studies, dermatology).

III. Specialties and Services Frequently Utilized by Optometry

The following are some specialties and services frequently used by optometrists in the course of patient care. Following each description are examples of patient problems that might be referred to that specialist.

A. *Cardiovascular medicine*

Cardiologists subspecialize in diseases of the heart, lungs, and blood vessels and manage complex cardiac conditions such as heart attacks and life-threatening abnormal heartbeat rhythms. They often perform complicated diagnostic procedures such as cardiac catheterization and consult with surgeons on heart surgery.

Examples of Problems Referred to Cardiologists

1. Hollenhorst plaques or other embolic phenomena observed in the retina (rule out possible carotid artery or heart disease)
2. Marfan's syndrome (subluxated lens)
3. Suspected carotid artery disease

B. *Dermatology*

A dermatologist is a physician who has expertise in the diagnosis and treatment of patients with benign and malignant disorders of the skin, mouth, external genitalia, hair, and nails. Dermatologists have training and experience in the diagnosis and treatment of skin cancers and other tumors of the skin, contact dermatitis, and other allergic and nonallergic disorders, and in the recognition of the skin manifestations of systemic (including internal malignancy) and infectious disease.

Examples of Problems Referred to Dermatologists

1. Acne rosacea
2. Skin tumors (e.g., basal cell carcinoma)
3. Herpes zoster
4. Molluscum contagiosum
5. Stevens-Johnson syndrome

C. *Endocrinology*

The endocrinologist concentrates on disorders of the internal (endocrine) glands such as the thyroid, adrenal, and pancreas. Endocrinology is the specialty that deals with disorders of metabolism and nutrition, such as diabetes, pituitary diseases, thyroid diseases, and menstrual and sexual problems.

Examples of Problems Referred to Endocrinologists
1. Diabetes
2. Thyroid dysfunction
3. Pituitary problems (suspected pituitary tumors may be evaluated by the endocrinologist for possible medical management)

D. *Family practice and internal medicine*
1. Family Practice
Family physicians are trained to prevent, diagnose, and treat a wide variety of ailments in patients of all ages. They have received a broad range of training that includes surgery, psychiatry, internal medicine, obstetrics and gynecology, pediatrics, and geriatrics. They place special emphasis on care of families on a continuing basis, utilizing consultations and community resources when appropriate.
2. Internal Medicine
The general internist is a personal physician who provides long-term, comprehensive care in the office and the hospital, managing both common illnesses and complex problems for adolescents, adults, and the elderly. General internists are trained in the essentials of primary care internal medicine, which incorporates an understanding of disease prevention, wellness, substance abuse, mental health, and effective treatment of common health problems. All internists are trained in the subspecialty areas of internal medicine including emergency internal medicine and critical care.
3. Examples of Problems Referred to Family Physicians and Internists
   A. Initial evaluation for suspected systemic disease
   B. Hypertension
   C. Diabetes
   D. Thyroid disease
   E. Rheumatologic problems
   F. Evidence of other systemic disease (infections, trauma, etc.)
   Note: There is considerable overlap in the scope of practice between family physicians and internists.

E. *Neurology*

The specialty of neurology is concerned with the diagnosis and treatment of all categories of disease or impaired function of the brain, spinal cord, peripheral nerves, muscles, and autonomic nervous system, as well as the blood vessels that relate to these structures. The neurologist serves as a consultant to other physicians but also is often the principal or primary physician and may render all levels of care commensurate with his or her training. This may include continuing care of outpatients or inpatients.

Examples of Problems Referred to Neurologists
1. Headache
2. Suspected intracranial lesions
3. Optic nerve problems
4. Suspected demyelinating disease
5. Myasthenia gravis
6. Temporal arteritis and other vascular phenomena.

F. *Nursing*

Nurses provide a valuable support service to physicians and other direct patient care providers in ambulatory, hospital, schools, rehabilitative, and long-term care facilities.

Nurses specialize in a variety of areas depending upon individual interests and requirements of employment.

Examples of Problems Referred to Nurses
1. Health education
2. Monitoring of stabilized medical conditions
3. Interaction with family and community health resources
4. Triage of patient symptoms

G. *Ophthalmology*

An ophthalmologist is a physician who has satisfactorily completed three or more years of postgraduate medical and surgical training in an accredited ophthalmology residency program. Upon completion of this training, board-certified ophthalmologists have passed the written and oral examinations of the American Board of Ophthalmology.

Examples of Problems Referred to Ophthalmologists
1. *Eye surgeries:* cataract, glaucoma, retinal detachment
2. *Laser procedures:* argon laser trabeculoplasty (ALT), iridotomies, YAG laser capsulotomies
3. Secondary and tertiary care medical eye problems
4. Orbital problems

H. *Pharmacy*

Registered pharmacists are health care providers who fill requests for pharmaceutical agents as well as providing counseling for the proper use of these agents. Pharmacists serve as a valuable resource to providers as well as patients because they are knowledgeable about how drugs work and how certain drugs may adversely affect beneficial results of other drugs.

Examples of Problems Referred to Pharmacists
1. Unusual side effects of medications
2. Polypharmacy (patients taking an unusually high number of drugs)
3. Drug education

I. *Psychiatry*

Psychiatrists are medical doctors who specialize in the mental aspects of health care. They can counsel patients, prescribe medications, and recommend a variety of psychiatric treatment plans to help patients cope with everyday living.

Examples of Problems Referred to Psychiatrists
1. Depression
2. Suicidal tendencies
3. Substance abuse (alcohol, tobacco, drugs, etc.)
4. Hysterical blindness

J. *Radiology*

Diagnostic radiology is that branch of medicine which deals with the utilization of all modalities of radiant energy in disease diagnoses and therapeutic procedures utilizing radiologic guidance. This includes, but is not restricted to, imaging techniques and methodologies utilizing radiations emitted by x-ray tubes, radionuclides, ultrasonographic devices, and the radio frequency electromagnetic radiation emitted by atoms.

Examples of Problems Referred to Radiologists for Imaging Studies
1. Suspected intracranial or optic nerve lesions
2. Eye and/or facial trauma
3. Papilledema/papillitis
4. Unexplained loss of vision or visual field loss
5. Headache

K. *Rheumatology*

The rheumatologist is a physician concerned with diseases of the joints, muscles, bones, and tendons. The rheumatologist diagnoses and treats arthritis, back pain, muscle strains, common athletic injuries, and collagen diseases. The rheumatologist may work closely with other specialists such as physical therapists and orthopedic surgeons.

Examples of Problems Referred to Rheumatologists

1. Juvenile rheumatoid arthritis
2. Rheumatoid arthritis
3. Sarcoidosis
4. Ankylosis spondylitis
5. Sjogren's syndrome

Note: Iritis and episcleritis/scleritis are frequently associated with many diseases of the joints and connective tissue.

L. *Social work*

Social workers usually work in institutional settings such as hospitals and nursing homes. Some work for governmental agencies. They are important to patient care because they can provide a special insight into the patient's need for health care services beyond the traditional ones. They can also arrange for various support systems to help with the control of chronic illnesses.

Examples of Problems Referred to Social Workers

1. Homelessness
2. Poverty
3. Suspected child or elder abuse
4. Eligibility for special programs

Although the above list represents some of the practitioners commonly referred to by optometrists, it is important to recognize that optometrists work with virtually all types of other health care providers in the course of caring for patients. Optometrists must be knowledgeable about the availability of these other practitioners in their communities as well as keeping the patient's primary medical care provider informed during any referral process.

Reference

1. Catania LJ. Primary care. In: Newcomb RD, Marshall EC, eds. *Public Health and Community Optometry.* 2nd ed. Stoneham, MA: Butterworth; 1990:296–297.

Kevin L. Alexander. *The Lippincott Manual of Primary Eye Care*. Copyright © 1995 by J.B. Lippincott Company.

CHAPTER **2**

Data Collection and Record Keeping for Optometrists

Robert D. Newcomb

I. **The optometric record serves a variety of purposes and should not be viewed simply as a substitute for poor long-term memory skills. The written account of an optometrist–patient encounter documents facts and professional judgments that:**

   A. *Chronicle the patient's presenting signs and symptoms at a particular point in time, as well as his or her past history;*

   B. *Record what testing was performed and what results were obtained from that testing;*

   C. *Establish a diagnosis, treatment plan, and follow-up recommendations that are acceptable to both the doctor and the patient;*

   D. *Create baseline data for comparison by the same or another doctor at a future point in time;*

   E. *Integrate ocular and visual clinical data with medical, surgical, psychiatric, and/or socioeconomic information obtained from other health care providers;*

   F. *Allow for the formulation of correspondence with other health care providers, insurance companies, social welfare agencies, employers, school systems, governmental entities, etc.;*

   G. *Substantiate the doctor's diagnostic logic in a reproducible, scientific manner for personal (e.g., educational or research) or other (e.g., quality assurance, utilization reviews, reimbursement mechanisms) purposes;*

   H. *Control health care costs by not duplicating tests unnecessarily during future visits to the same or another doctor;*

   I. *Prove certain tests were performed and generated data for which payments may be received from third party sources; and*

   J. *Defend the doctor against threatened or actual charges of inferior practice standards.*

   The optometric record is a sacred bond between the doctor and the patient, and it must be kept confidential. It is important to remember, however, that although the physical record belongs to the doctor, the patient has a right to know all of the information contained within it.

II. **Guidelines for Record Keeping**

   A. *General principles*

      1. Record data immediately to prevent inadvertent loss or distortion of factual information.

      2. Organize data in a logical fashion so it tells a story accurately yet concisely.

      3. Use only standardized abbreviations that are easily recognizable by professional colleagues.

      4. Always remember that the optometric record is a *legal document* and must be produced and maintained like any other record which is subject to a court summons.

Erasures and use of typewriter correction fluid are forbidden. Recording errors should have a single line drawn through them and the doctor's initials entered close by. All information must be kept confidential, and release to *anyone other than the patient* must be preceded by a signed consent statement. All entries must be dated and all examiners (doctors and technicians) should sign the record.

B. *Format*
 1. Record signs and symptoms in chronological order.
 2. Use probing questions to establish onset, duration, severity, and predisposing factors.
 3. Document pertinent clinical findings as well as absences of potential or expected conditions (e.g., no background diabetic retinopathy in known insulin-dependent diabetic for 10 years; or no cells or flare in arthritic patient with conjunctivitis).
 4. Avoid notations such as No Apparent Pathology (NAP) and Within Normal Limits (WNL).
 5. Use a blank piece of paper to accommodate unusually long case histories or testing procedures. Never let the exam form limit or complicate the exam function.
 6. Before examining a patient for the second time, recapitulate the previous findings and recommendations. Verify if previous treatment plans have been accomplished. Ascertain if current symptoms are acute or chronic.
 7. Patient records must be finished immediately following the examination and case discussion. Avoid holding the record until the end of the day to finish writing your diagnosis and treatment plans: this will cause an increase in verbiage and a decrease in accuracy and relevance.
 8. A separate listing of all identified problems (like a table of contents) at the front of the patient's chart helps to organize conditions diagnosed at different visits over many years.

III. History of the Problem-Oriented Approach

A. *In 1964 Weed[1,2] proposed radical new changes in the way physicians should annotate their hospital records:*
 1. Patient histories should be obtained by interviews that elicit chief complaints as well as general health problems in the patient and family members.
 2. Patient expectations (now termed "outcomes") should be documented.
 3. Physical examinations should be conducted to corroborate histories as well as to uncover latent disease processes.
 4. Laboratory tests and other data should be ordered for a specific reason to confirm or rule out the examiner's provisional diagnoses (also known as working or tentative diagnoses).
 5. Treatment plans should be formulated with the patient's concurrence; a recall date should be established to evaluate improvement, stability, or deterioration of the patient's condition.

B. *The problem-oriented optometric record (POOR) was developed by Sloan,[3] Dunsky,[4] Barresi,[5] and others from 1978 through 1987. Classe[6,7] has eloquently stated its purpose and usefulness for practicing doctors of optometry:*

> The problem-oriented record system is solution oriented and enables the practitioner to manage patients in a logical and efficient manner by helping to define problems, plan for their resolution, and properly monitor their progress. When used appropriately, the problem-oriented record system also provides the documentation that is essential for clinicolegal purposes while requiring a minimum of time for recording and interpretation.

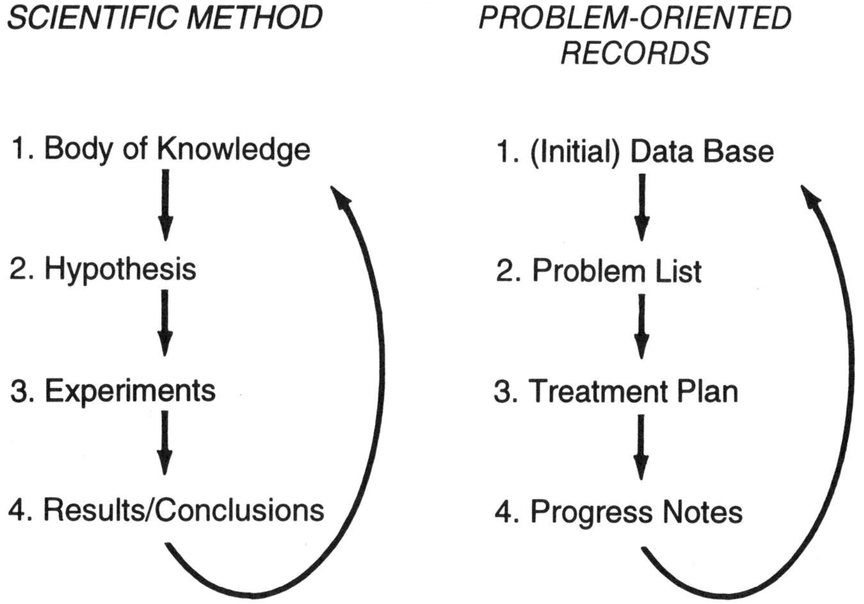

SCIENTIFIC METHOD   PROBLEM-ORIENTED
                              RECORDS

1. Body of Knowledge   1. (Initial) Data Base

2. Hypothesis   2. Problem List

3. Experiments   3. Treatment Plan

4. Results/Conclusions   4. Progress Notes

Figure 2-1.   The logical sequence of events in the scientific method and the problem-oriented approach to optometric record keeping.

C. *The POOR is based upon the time-honored scientific method of basic research, as illustrated in Figure 2-1:*
    1. Hypotheses are derived from a known body of information.
    2. Carefully designed experimental studies are conducted.
    3. Results are analyzed, and hypotheses are confirmed or rejected.
    4. All work is documented to allow another researcher to replicate the process.

IV. **Components of the System**[8]

    A. *Initial data base*
        1. Generated and maintained for two purposes:
            a. To solve the patient's problems and document the chronological sequence of events;
            b. To establish baseline and normative information for use in future eye examinations.
        2. It is a list of questions and routine tests asked of and performed for every new patient.
        3. It is determined by the examining optometrist *a priori* (i.e., before meeting the patient) so as not to omit any important elements.
        4. Data may be collected on a preprinted form by an office assistant, or they may be written or dictated by the doctor.
        5. Typical case history questions and basic eye and vision testing procedures are listed in Table 2-1; depending upon the education, experience, and preferences of the doctor, other questions and/or tests may be added.

    B. *Problem list*
        1. A list of actual or potential problems identified from the initial data base.
        2. They may be labeled as diagnoses, assessments, or impressions if well defined and fully understood.

Table 2-1. Suggested Questioning and Testing for All New Patients in an Optometric Office

Minimum Case History Questions	Minimum Data Base Examination
Demographics	Habitual visual acuities at distance and near
Name, address, phone number?	Lensometry
Age, sex, race?	Keratometry
Chief complaint(s)	Retinoscopy
When did this begin?	Subjective refraction at distance and near
Is it all of the time or just sometime?	Cover test at distance and near
Have any other doctors evaluated this?	External exam (pupils, versions, ductions)
Last eye exam	Color vision testing
When, by whom, where?	Stereoacuity
What was recommended?	Sphygmomanometry
Medical history	Biomicroscopy
Any past hospitalizations or surgery?	Tonometry
Current medications?	Dilated fundus examination
Name of family physician?	Visual fields
Genetics	Ocular photography
Any relatives who are blind?	
Any relatives who have eye disease?	
Ocular history	
Ever had any eye disease, injury or surgery, or used eyedrops?	
Visual history	
Ever have glasses prescribed for your eyes?	
Is vision clear or blurred? At distance or near? Some or all of the time?	
Is your symptom acute or chronic?	
Allergies	
Any food or drug allergies?	
Occupation/avocation	
Visual requirements?	
Safety considerations?	

3. They may be simply written as unusual clinical signs or symptoms if not well defined and fully understood.

4. NEVER WRITE ANY INFORMATION OR CONCLUSION THAT IS NOT ACCURATE ENOUGH TO BE SWORN TO IN A COURT OF LAW (Do not over-diagnose).

5. Use modifying adjectives such as "suspected," "possible," "questionable," or "likely" to record clinical uncertainties. Then formulate a management plan to further clarify the patient's problems.

6. Each patient problem is assigned a unique numerical identifier. This number should be used consistently throughout all subsequent problem-oriented optometric records. Problems are numbered from 1 to *n,* where *n* is the total number of actual or potential problems discovered by the doctor for any individual patient.

7. Problem number 1 is not necessarily the most important condition. Numbers are used only to indicate that a condition does now (or may later) exist.

8. If a condition ever completely resolves, such as an allergic conjunctivitis, then that condition need not be listed in future problem lists, and its number can be reassigned to a new problem.

C. *Treatment plan*

1. This is where the doctor recommends interventions that are believed to be helpful in ameliorating the patient's problem.

2. Examples of treatment plans would be the prescribing of eyeglasses, contact lenses, low vision devices, vision training, ophthalmic pharmaceutical agents, reassurance, patient health education, consultation with another health professional, referral for surgery, etc.

3. The number of the treatment plan corresponds with the number of the problem. *Be consistent!*

4. Discuss all reasonable treatment options with the patient before recording the one that is best for him or her. Annotating a treatment plan on the patient's record implies the patient understands and agrees with it, can afford it, and will comply with it.

D. *Progress notes*

1. The fourth and final phase of the POOR occurs when the patient contacts the doctor's office for a follow-up visit. This may be in the form of a telephone call, a written communication, or an office visit.

2. Now a tentative or working diagnosis can be advanced to a definitive diagnosis if the treatment plan has cured the patient's problem. Uncertainties from previous visits should now be better understood, and modified treatment plans can be suggested.

3. Progress notes should be recorded in the SOAP format: Subjective, Objective, Assessment, and Plan:

   a. *Subjective.* Begin by reviewing the previous clinical record(s). Ask the patient if symptoms are better, worse, or unchanged after complying with the recommended treatment plan. Address each numbered problem separately and record what the patient says.

   b. *Objective.* Repeat pertinent clinical tests to evaluate changes in ocular structure and/or function. Record findings that would enable another optometrist to follow the course of the condition. Diagrams, charts (Amsler grids, visual fields, etc.) or photographs may be useful during this portion of the progress note visit if baseline diagrams, charts, or photographs are available from previous visits.

   c. *Assessment.* With the additional information gained during the intervening time period, a redefinition of the condition(s) may now be appropriate. Keep the numbering system consistent, but describe the problem more precisely if you can. Indicate if it is better, worse, or stable in relationship to the previous visit.

   d. *Plan.* Continue, modify, or cease the original treatment plan, depending upon the information documented in the subjective, objective, and assessment sections of the progress note visit.

   Bartlett[9] reminded optometrists that the "P" is also for "management," and in an editorial published in the *Journal of the American Optometric Association*, he stated:

   > This whole (S-O-A-P) process has helped optometry evolve as a primary care profession as we think and communicate with each other in terms of these four crucial steps.

   In addition to the above, a recommended recall date is also advised and documented in this section. This reminds the patient to regard optometric care as continuous and not episodic; it also helps defend the optometrist from charges of abandonment or negligence if the patient suffers a permanent vision loss during subsequent months or years.

   Most optometrists advise their patients to return "PRN," which is the abbreviated form of the Latin words *pro re nata,* which mean "according to circumstances." This places the responsibility for continuous monitoring of eye health and visual performance upon the patient, who should return for further care whenever changes in or around the eyes are first noticed.

   e. A sample progress note in the SOAP format is shown in Figure 2-2.

Ⓢ 68 yowf was last seen by me on October 20 when transient blur was reported. She was advised to have a repeat MVA today and DFE ⊕ MED Hx for IDDM x 14 yrs — say vision is blurred at far and near s̄ Rx but is now stable. Dr. Smith changed insulin Rx last month and pt reports better BS control now

Ⓞ Old Rx lost

MVA   OD −1.50 −0.25 x 085   20/20−   TA 19
      OS −1.25 −0.50 x 100   20/30=   17

SLE − clear corneae except for arcus senilis ou
    − quiet ext eyes − angles are grade II ou
    − 1 + PSC lens Δ's
T gt 1% M ou @ 9:25A
DFE − clear media ou c̄ 0.2 cups and mild BDR ou in
        temporal quadrants — possible macular edema OS
Amsler − wl OD − distorted centrally OS (see attached)

Ⓐ 1) Myopic astigmatism or c̄ presbyopia — now stable
  2) BDR ou (mild) c̄ possible macular edema OS
  3) 1+ PSC lenses or
Ⓟ 1) Rx MVA in ST-25 plastic lenses
  2) Photos today − RTC Nov. 19 for FA and probable laser OS
  3) No Rx needed now − recheck in 1 yr or prn

Robert Newcomb OD
November 13, 1991

Figure 2-2.   Sample progress note for a patient with insulin-dependent diabetes mellitus.

V. Record Reviews and Quality Assurance

Now that an increasing number of optometric patients have third-party payment plans, it is reasonable to assume the payer of services will want to assure quality by reviewing patient records on a periodic basis. The record should:

A.   *Document what procedures were performed (and not performed!);*
B.   *Support the diagnoses (and diagnostic logic) of the doctor;*
C.   *Be legible and be signed and dated at every visit;*

D. *Be understandable by another optometrist;*

E. *Be maintained in a safe and confidential manner;*

F. *Include ALL information about a patient (visual fields, letters to and from other practitioners, photographs, specifications of glasses, contact lenses, and low vision devices, reports of telephone calls, etc.). Multiple patient visits should be consolidated into one file for each patient, and this one document should be easily retrievable yet safeguarded against unauthorized use.*

Remember, optometrists are part of the multibillion dollar health care system in the United States, and good record keeping skills help control health care costs by minimizing duplication and overutilization of health care services.

VI. Summary

A. *The Problem Oriented Optometric Record (POOR) is the best format for all types of optometric services because it requires the doctor to perform tests and analyze data with respect to the patient's problems (actual or potential).*

B. *It can be used to refer patients for consultation of a particular symptom or finding, or to transfer care to an optometrist in another city.*

C. *The POOR can be used for optometric education and/or research, since it is arranged in a logical and consistent format from one eye examination to another (even if they are performed by different doctors).*

D. *It improves office efficiency by requiring the doctor to perform relevant tests but not extraneous ones.*

E. *It is the document that protects the doctor against liability claims because it establishes what was done, when it was done, and why it was done. If data are not properly recorded and filed for future reference, there is no proof that a quality eye examination was performed.*

F. *Multiple problems can be appropriately managed concurrently by assigning a unique number to each problem and then consistently using this number throughout all subsequent examinations.*

References

1. Weed LL. Medical records, patient care and medical education. *Ir J Med Sci* 1964;57:271–282.

2. Weed LL. Medical records that guide and teach. *N Engl J Med* 1968;278:593–600, 652–657.

3. Sloan PG. A problem oriented optometric record? *Am J Optom Physiol Optics* 1978;55:352–357.

4. Dunsky IL. Optometry and the problem oriented record. *South J Optom* 1979;21:10–19.

5. Barresi BJ. Problem orientation. In: Baressi BJ, ed. *Ocular Assessment: The Manual of Diagnosis for Office Practice.* Boston: Butterworth; 1984:3–10 (Chapter 1).

6. Classe JG. Record-keeping and documentation in clinical practice. *South J Optom* 1987;5:11–25.

7. Classe JG. *Legal Aspects of Optometry.* Boston: Butterworth; 1989:215–233.

8. Ruskiewicz JP. Quality assurance. In: Newcomb RD, Marshall EC, eds. *Public Health and Community Optometry.* 2nd ed. Boston: Butterworth; 1990:240–246 (Chapter 14).

9. Bartlett JD. The p is for management. *J Am Optom Assoc* 1987;58:82–83.

CHAPTER **3**

Physical Examination for Optometrists

Rick E. Ricer

I. General Principles

A. *The physical examination begins at the first meeting with the patient.*

B. *Observe during the walk to the examining office and during the history for:*

1. Gait
2. Response
3. Appropriateness of behavior
4. Mood
5. Facial appearance
6. Obvious deformities
7. Posture
8. Symmetry
9. Nutritional status
10. Grooming
11. Abnormal movements
12. Tremor
13. Speech pattern
14. Body habitus
15. Dress
16. Alertness
17. Signs of distress
18. Awareness

C. *This observation will yield a gestalt or overall impression of the patient and give a clue to the state of health of the patient (acutely ill vs. chronically ill, ill vs. healthy).*

Clinical Alert

Many times just the overall observation of a patient walking to the examining office or during the history will give clues to diagnoses such as cerebral palsy, a stroke with residual hemiparesis; Down's syndrome with the classic stature and facial features; Marfan's syndrome with the classic tall, thin features; or depression suggested by the affect and mood of the patient. This overall observation can give clues to whether a patient has an acute illness such as Graves' disease with its attendant weight loss versus the weight loss of a chronic illness like rheumatoid arthritis.

D. *The history guides the physical exam because most diagnoses are made by listening to the history and then confirmed by the physical exam.*

    E. It should be rare to discover a physical finding that wasn't expected from a good history.

    F. Being comprehensive in all areas of the physical exam will increase the yield of unexpected and expected physical findings.

    G. In systemic diseases, changes seen in the eye are happening elsewhere in the body as well.

II. Approach to the Patient

    A. The physical exam should be conducted in a quiet room with great attention to the patient's comfort and privacy.

    B. Be aware of the patient's feelings and anxieties at all times.

    C. Always be appropriate and professional during the exam, explaining why each area is being examined and the mechanism of each procedure.

    D. A systematic approach is used for completeness and comprehensibility.

    E. Remember the structure and function of the tissues in each area examined and match the findings with what is expected from the history or diagnosis.

    F. Since most of the body is bilaterally symmetrical, compare findings to the opposing side of the body or to yourself.

    G. Be organized and have all needed equipment ready and available.

III. Techniques of Examination

    A. Principles

        1. THINK during the examination; the history and physical exam should match if the diagnosis is correct.

Clinical Alert

A history of symptoms of hyperthyroidism such as acute weight loss even though the patient is eating well, palpitations, shakiness, thinning of the hair and skin, and a feeling of fullness in the neck leads the practitioner to the diagnosis of hyperthyroidism and alerts that person to the physical findings that should be present. Without the physical findings of fine tremor, an enlarged thyroid, tachycardia, lateral thinning of the eyebrows, and documented weight loss, however, the practitioner must question the diagnosis of hyperthyroidism.

---

        2. Progress from distal to proximal and from head to toe.

        3. The socially acceptable first touch of a person is a handshake; therefore begin the exam with the hands.

        4. An organ systems approach to the physical exam is simple to learn but results in returning to the same area of the body multiple times.

        5. The regional approach described in this chapter examines all systems in that area of the body, can be more complete, and is usually more time efficient.

Clinical Alert

During the organ systems approach to the physical examination, the cardio-vascular system is examined, including pulses, carotid arteries and jugular veins in the neck, heart sounds in the chest, etc. Then the musculoskeletal system is examined, going back to the extremities, head, neck, chest, etc. Then the neurological system is checked again, going back to the extremities, head, neck, chest, etc. Then the skin is examined, going back to the extremities, head, neck, chest, etc. The regional exam, however, looks at all of these organ systems at the same time while concentrating on that specific region of the body. This requires a higher order of thinking process during the examination.

---

6. The four techniques most often used during a physical exam are inspection, palpation, percussion, and auscultation.

B. *Inspection*
1. Inspection is an organized scrutiny of each area's visual clues and may be the most important of all techniques.
2. Inspection is always the first technique used in each area.

Clinical Alert

If an optometrist notices that the sclerae are jaundiced or yellowed, then inspecting the conjunctiva, the skin, and the under surface of the tongue for jaundice would confirm a total picture of jaundice and point toward a diagnosis of hepatitis or hepatic malfunction.

C. *Palpation*
1. Palpation is using the sense of feel or touch to examine a body part.
2. It is not necessarily used for every body part.
3. Different techniques are used for different areas of the body.
4. Use the most sensitive part of the hands:
   a. *Tactile:* tips of the fingers
   b. *Temperature:* dorsum of the hand
   c. *Vibration:* palmar aspects of the metacarpophalangeal joints or hypothenar eminences

---

Clinical Alert

Tactile sensations are used when palpating the growths of neurofibromatosis or the subcutaneous nodules of rheumatoid arthritis. *Temperature* sensation is used when examining specific areas of the body for local heat of inflammation, such as over the sinuses in sinusitis. *Vibratory* sensation is used mostly during the cardiac examination when feeling for a heart murmur. Vibratory sensation would rarely be used by optometrists.

D. *Percussion*
1. *Percussion* is a technique of setting underlying tissues in motion, since different sounds will emanate from hollow and solid structures.
2. A hollow area will produce a resonant sound while a solid structure should sound dull.
3. Percussion can also elicit pain over an inflamed structure.
4. There are three techniques for percussion (Figure 3-1):
   a. Press the distal portion of the middle finger firmly against the surface of the structure and strike just behind the nail portion of this finger with the tip of the opposite middle finger.
   b. Strike the structure directly with the tip of the middle finger or a tongue blade.
   c. Strike the structure with the hypothenar eminence of a closed fist.
   d. Practice by trying to find the studs in a wall.

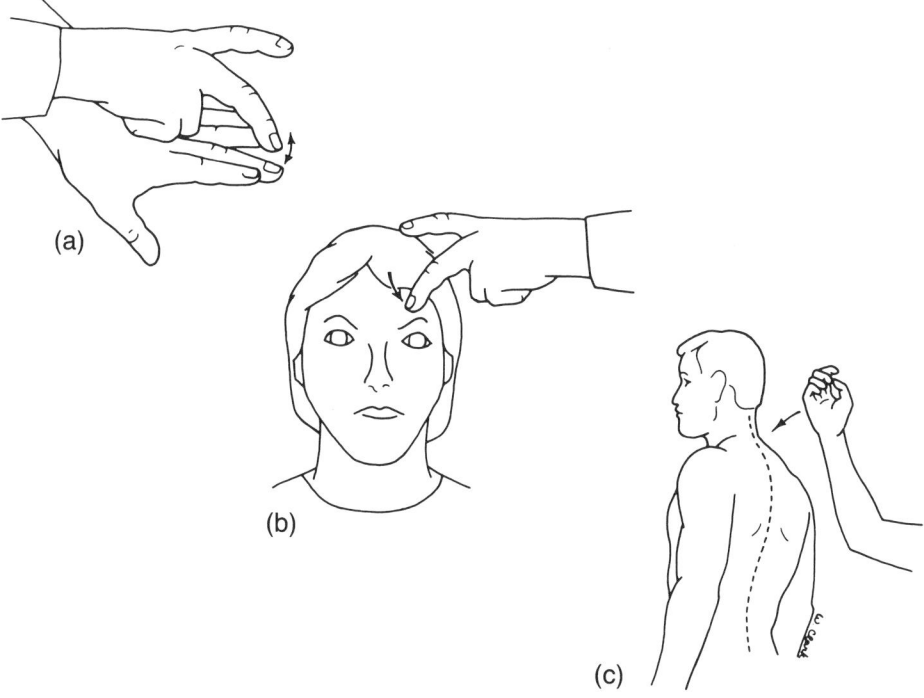

Figure 3-1. Three techniques of percussion.

Clinical Alert

The first technique of percussion is usually used to find the edge of the liver, determine if consolidation of the lung exists, determine the edge of the heart, and determine structures in the abdomen. This technique would rarely be used by optometrists. The second technique of percussion is used to determine local tenderness such as percussing the sinuses during acute sinusitis for pain or using a tongue blade to percuss the teeth to determine if a dental abscess is present. The third technique of percussion can be used when percussing the spine to see if any local area of tenderness exists; again, this would rarely be used by optometrists.

E. *Auscultation*
1. *Auscultation* is the art of listening to an area with a stethoscope.
2. The stethoscope is usually equipped with a bell and a diaphragm head (Fig. 3-2).
3. The bell is used for low-pitched sounds and the diaphragm is used for high-pitched sounds.
4. The bell should touch the skin lightly just to ensure occlusion whereas the diaphragm should be pressed firmly into the skin.
5. Pressing the bell into the skin tightens the skin and transforms the bell into a diaphragm.
6. Movement of the stethoscope across skin, hair, or clothing will produce extraneous sounds.

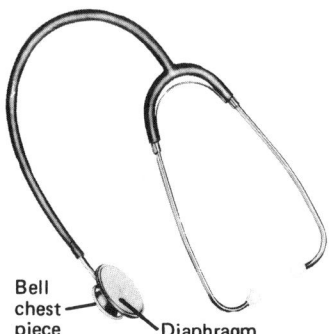

Bell
chest
piece   Diaphragm

Figure 3-2. Stethoscope. From *Lippincott Manual of Nursing Practice*. Philadelphia, PA: J.B. Lippincott Company, 1991: 19, with permission.

Clinical Alert

The diaphragm of the stethoscope is used to hear high-pitched sounds such as the Korotkoff sounds of blood pressure or carotid bruits. The bell is used for low-pitched sounds and is usually used when listening to the heart for extra heart sounds and certain murmurs. The bell would rarely be used by an optometrist.

    F. Other senses
       1. Although rarely used in an organized procedure, taste and smell can give diagnostic information.
       2. Smell can be used to help diagnose certain disorders by characteristic odors of pus, breath, or feces.
       3. Taste was used in the past to help diagnose the urine of diabetes. (This is, however, not recommended now).

IV. Equipment (Fig. 3-3)

    A. Stethoscope
    B. Thermometer
    C. Tuning forks
    D. Light source
    E. Oto-ophthalmoscope
    F. Tongue depressors
    G. Nasal speculum
    H. Reflex hammer
    I. Cotton sticks
    J. Gloves
    K. Sphygmomanometer

V. Vital Signs (Temperature, Pulse, Respiration, Blood Pressure)

    A. General
       1. All vital signs are not always necessary for every patient but should be included if this information could be helpful.
       2. Vital signs can be incorporated into the physical exam during the appropriate regional exam.
       3. Blood pressure determination in every patient can help screen for silent hypertension.

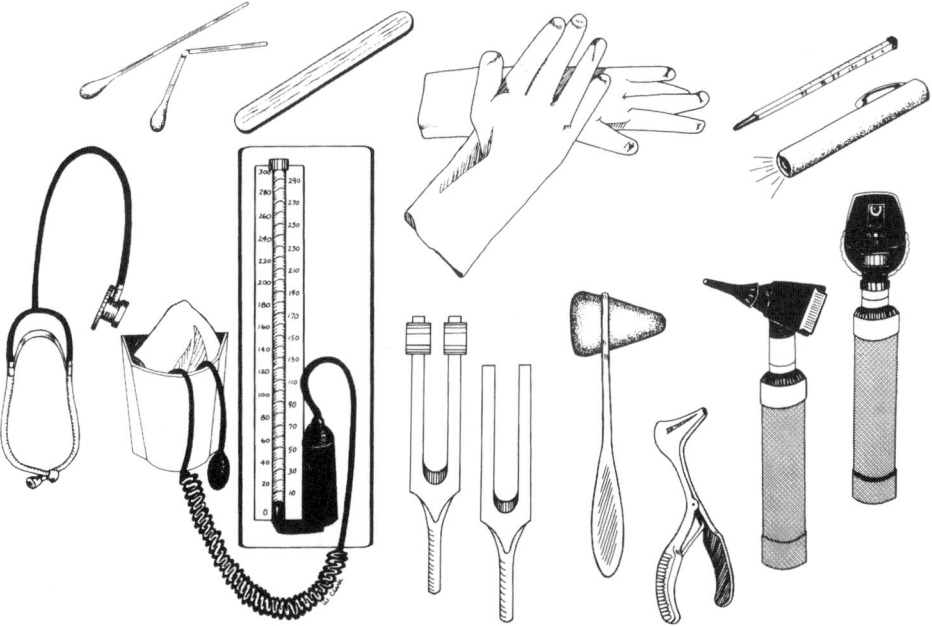

Figure 3-3.   Equipment needed when performing a physical exam.

Clinical Alert

There are many clinical situations that will alter the normal pattern of vital signs. Fever, the hallmark of most infections, will increase the temperature, pulse, and respiratory rate. Graves' disease can increase all of the vital signs. A well-conditioned athlete will actually have a lowered blood pressure and pulse rate. Medications can change the vital signs. Beta blockers decrease pulse and blood pressure.

B. *Temperature*
1.   An oral reading is usually sufficient.
2.   Feeling the skin provides an inexact estimate.
3.   98.6°F (37°C) is only an average of normal people, so that few patients will register this number exactly.
4.   The temperature of an individual patient will vary at different times of the day.
5.   Normal can vary from 96.4°F to 99.1°F (35.8°C to 37.3°C).

Clinical Alert

An increased temperature is usually associated with an infection, although this is not always the case. Hyperthyroidism can increase the temperature and hypothyroidism can decrease the temperature. Hot flashes associated with menopause can increase the temperature of the skin but not necessarily the oral temperature. A person just coming in from cold weather can have a falsely lowered temperature, just as a person drinking warm beverages can have a falsely elevated temperature.

C. *Pulse*
1. Pulse usually can be determined by palpating any artery.
2. Count the number of beats for 15 seconds and multiply by 4 to get beats per minute.
3. Note the rate, rhythm, strength, and symmetry.
4. Normal is usually between 60 and 100 beats per minute in a resting adult.

Clinical Alert

Anxiety is one of the causes of an increased pulse rate that can be benign. There are myriad pathologic causes for elevation of the pulse rate, including anemia, hyperthyroidism, medications, and pheochromocytoma. Arrhythmias of the heart can give tachycardia, bradycardia, or an irregular pulse.

D. *Respiration*
1. Count while the patient is distracted (e.g., counting respiratory rate while checking a distal pulse).
2. Note the rate, rhythm, depth, and muscles used.
3. Normal is usually 14–20 per minute in a resting adult.

Clinical Alert

Chronic obstructive pulmonary disease certainly can change the respiratory rate as well as being correlated with the use of accessory muscles for breathing, increased diameter of the chest, or audible wheezing. Anxiety or hyperventilation syndrome can give a variety of symptoms, such as tingling of the fingers and toes, tingling around the mouth, frontal headache, feeling of suffocation, fast heartbeat, dizziness, and blurred vision. One of the physical signs of anxiety or hyperventilation is increased rate or depth of respiration measured when the patient is unaware that the practitioner is measuring respiratory rate.

E. *Blood pressure (Fig. 3-4)*
1. Measure with the patient sitting with the arm at the level of the heart.
2. Always use an appropriate-sized cuff or a spurious reading will result.

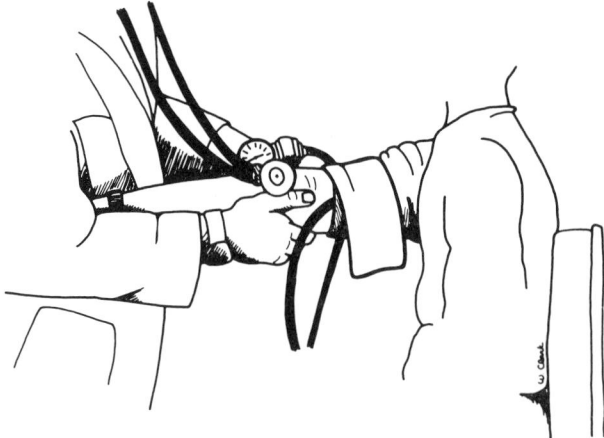

Figure 3-4. Measuring blood pressure of a sitting patient.

3. The bladder of the cuff should encircle two-thirds of the arm.
4. The bladder should be directly over the brachial artery and should be 1 inch above the antecubital fossa.
5. The brachial pulse at the antecubital fossa is palpated on the medial aspect when the patient's palm is facing upward.
6. Palpate the brachial pulse and pump the blood pressure cuff 30–50 mm Hg above the point at which the pulse can no longer be felt.
7. Place the diaphragm of the stethoscope lightly over the brachial artery while supporting the patient's arm.
8. Pressing the diaphragm too firmly over the artery will compress the artery and produce Korotkoff sounds.
9. Deflate the cuff at a rate of 2–4 mm/s and listen for all five Korotkoff sounds to avoid missing an auscultatory gap (absent second sound).
    a. The first Korotkoff sound is a loud tapping noise.
    b. The second Korotkoff sound is a tap-murmur.
    c. The third Korotkoff sound is a tapping noise again.
    d. The fourth Korotkoff sound is a diminished tapping noise.
    e. The fifth Korotkoff sound is the disappearance of the diminished tapping.
10. Record the first sound (systolic) and when sounds disappear (diastolic).
11. The normal range of blood pressure is 90–140 mm Hg systolic and 60–90 mm Hg diastolic.
12. High blood pressure (hypertension) is a chronic, long-term problem and unless the blood pressure is exceedingly high, it has few short-term problems.

Clinical Alert

Routine screening of the blood pressure for silent hypertension is one way to identify this process. However, if the optometrist notices retinal hemorrhages suggestive of hypertension, retinal branch vein occlusion, or hyperviscosity syndrome changes of the eye, the practitioner would certainly want to examine that patient for hypertension.

F. *Height and weight*
    1. Ideal body weight is the range of weight for a specific height where the patient has the greatest chance of living the maximal number of years.
    2. Medically, ideal body weight is usually determined by life insurance tables and not by movie and magazine standards.
    3. Determine height and weight using standard scales.
    4. Observation will give an estimate of appropriate weight for height.
    5. Determine appropriate weight for height more specifically using standard tables.
    6. A rough estimate for women of medium build can be obtained using 100 lb for 5 feet and adding 5 lb for every inch over 5 feet as the lower range and adding 10% of this figure for the higher range.
    7. A rough estimate for men of medium build can be obtained using 107 lb for 5 feet and adding 6 lb for every inch over 5 feet as the lower range and 106 lb for 5 feet plus 7 lb for every inch over 5 feet as the higher range.

Clinical Alert

The causes of weight loss are many, including hyperthyroidism, diabetes mellitus, cancer, anorexia nervosa, and malabsorption syndromes. Weight gain can be attributed to hypothyroidism, Cushing's disease, and overeating. A very tall, thin person suggests Marfan's syndrome and a very short person suggests endocrine disorders.

VI. Getting Started

   A. *Wash your hands in full view of the patient.*
   B. *Specifically take time to view the general appearance of the patient noting:*

1.	Race	9.	Distress
2.	Sex	10.	Alertness
3.	Dress	11.	Hygiene
4.	Anxiety	12.	Muscle wasting
5.	Edema	13.	Nutritional status
6.	Body type	14.	Appropriateness of behavior
7.	Face	15.	Obvious deformities
8.	Eye contact	16.	Appearance appropriate to stated age

VII. Skin

   A. *A skin examination should be part of every regional exam.*
   B. *Inspection and palpation are the two most important techniques of examining the skin.*
   C. *Natural light is best for skin examination, but if it is not available, at least a good artificial light source is a must.*
   D. *Specifically note:*

1.	Pigment	10.	Breaks
2.	Jaundice	11.	Rash
3.	Cyanosis	12.	Moisture
4.	Paleness	13.	Ulcerations
5.	Turgor	14.	Texture
6.	Edema	15.	Temperature
7.	Color	16.	Bleeding
8.	Hair pattern	17.	Bruises
9.	Scars	18.	Petechiae

   E. *Describe lesions as to:*

1.	Distribution	6.	Pain
2.	Size	7.	Mobility
3.	Fluctuance	8.	Uniformity
4.	Local heat	9.	Blanching
5.	Color		

Clinical Alert

If an optometrist sees evidence of a bleeding disorder in the eye grounds, then that practitioner would want to check the skin for confirmation of a bleeding disorder (e.g., petechiae, purpura, or hemorrhages). If the optometrist sees Roth's spots in the eye grounds, which may be due to subacute bacterial endocarditis, then that practitioner would want to check the skin for subcutaneous nodules and splinter hemorrhages. If the practitioner noted atopic keratoconjunctivitis, then confirmation of atopic dermatitis might be helped by the characteristic skin changes behind the knees, on the cheeks, and in the antecubital fossa. If the optometrist noticed ultraviolet exposure keratopathy, then the skin would need to be checked for evidence of basal cell carcinoma.

VIII. Upper Extremity (Fig. 3-5)

   A. *This is a socially acceptable place to start with a handshake.*
   B. *The equipment needed will be a light source, reflex hammer, blood pressure cuff, and stethoscope.*

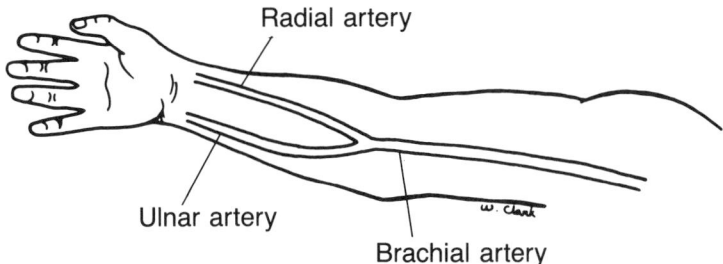

Figure 3-5.   Ventral view of right upper arm extremity.

C. *Inspect both hands for edema.*
D. *Inspect for signs of anemia such as pale nails or pale palmar lines.*
E. *Check adequacy of capillary refill by pressing pulp of fingertip to produce blanching, then release and observe for normal color return within 2 seconds.*
F. *Inspect the fingertips for clubbing.*
G. *Inspect the nails for pitting, spooning, dystrophic changes, bands, and petechiae (Fig. 3-6).*
H. *Inspect the hands for tremor or contractures.*
I. *Examine range of motion of joints of all fingers.*
J. *Test the strength of all muscle groups of the hands.*
K. *Palpate both radial and ulnar pulses.*

Clinical Alert

Many conditions in the eye would lead the optometrist to check the upper extremities and the hands. Upward displacement of the lens might suggest Marfan's syndrome and the hands might show arachnodactyly. Scleral nodules might suggest rheumatoid arthritis and the joints might need to be examined. Changes of the fingers, skin, and lid consistent with psoriasis might correlate with pitted nails. Exophthalmos might be correlated with the tremor of the hands of Graves' disease. Calcium emboli in the eye grounds may suggest a calcific heart valve which could release emboli to other small vessels of the body such as the fingers.

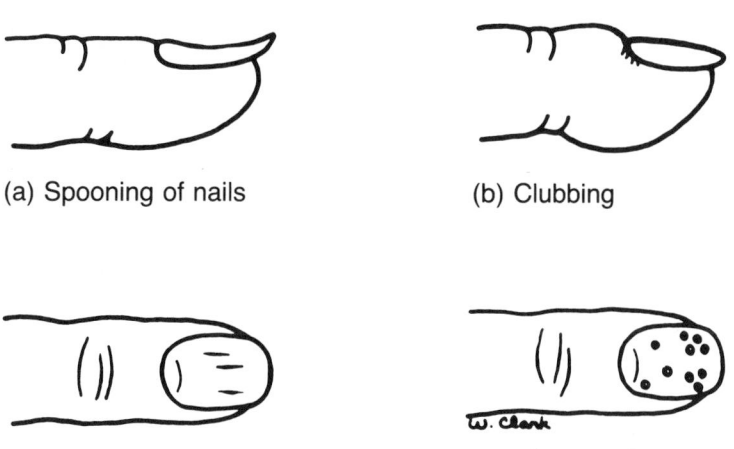

(a) Spooning of nails   (b) Clubbing

(c) Splinter hemorrhages   (d) Pitted nails of psoriasis

Figure 3-6.   Examples of fingernails.

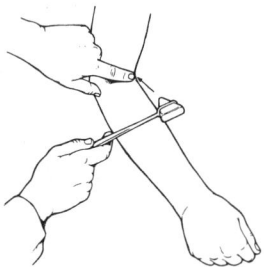

Figure 3-7.   Testing reflexes of the upper extremity. From *Lippincott Manual of Nursing Practice*. Philadelphia, PA: J.B. Lippincott Company, 1991: 47, with permission.

L. *Examine range of motion of wrists.*
M. *Inspect wrists for ganglion cysts.*
N. *Test the strength of the forearm muscles.*
O. *Test the brachial, brachioradialis, and triceps reflexes (Fig. 3-7).*
P. *Examine the range of motion of the elbows.*
Q. *Palpate for epitrochlear nodes.*
R. *Check blood pressure in both arms.*
S. *Test the strength of the muscles of the upper arms and shoulders (Fig. 3-8).*
T. *Examine the range of motion of the shoulders.*
U. *Palpate for enlarged axillary nodes supporting the patient's arm hanging loosely and relaxed at the shoulder (Fig. 3-9).*
V. *Remember to examine the skin of this region.*

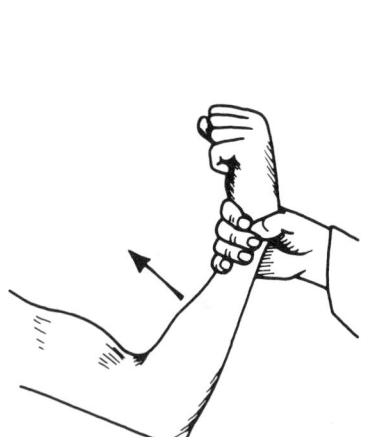

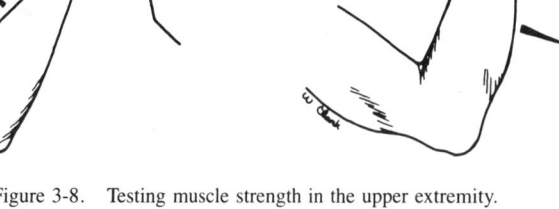

Figure 3-8.   Testing muscle strength in the upper extremity.

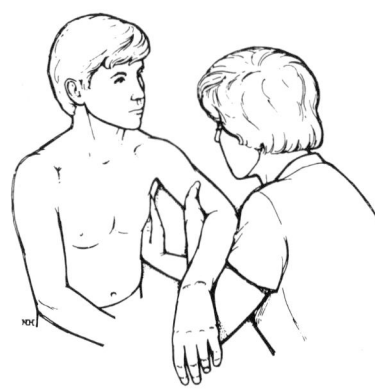

Figure 3-9.   Technique of examining the axillary nodes. From *Lippincott Manual of Nursing Practice*. Philadelphia, PA: J.B. Lippincott Company, 1991: 28, with permission.

Clinical Alert

Optic neuritis might suggest multiple sclerosis, which could correlate with increased reflexes and spasticity of the upper extremities (which could vary from one office visit to the next). Sky-blue sclera might suggest osteogenesis imperfecta, which could correlate with multiple old fractures of the upper extremities.

IX. **Head, Eyes, Ears, Nose, and Throat (HEENT)**

    A. *The equipment needed will be a light source, oto-ophthalmoscope, thermometer, tuning forks, nasal speculum, gloves, and tongue depressors.*

    B. *Inspect and palpate the scalp and hair for lumps or deformities.*

    C. *Note hair pattern, baldness, dandruff, and lesions.*

    D. *Observe the face for expression, symmetry, masses, edema, and abnormal movements.*

    E. *Perform complete eye examination.*

    F. *Inspect and palpate the external ear for shape and lesions (Fig. 3-10).*

    G. *Properly perform an otoscopic examination (Fig. 3-11):*

        1. Pull the pinna upward and away from the head to straighten the adult ear canal.

        2. Hold the inverted otoscope like a pencil, grasping the handle just below the junction of the handle with the head and resting your hypothenar eminence against the patient's temple so that if the patient's head moves, the otoscope will automatically move with it and not drive the ear speculum into the canal.

        3. Introduce the ear speculum just inside the external canal without causing pain.

        4. Inspect the canal for erythema, pus, swelling, exudate, abrasion, foreign body, and cerumen.

        5. Inspect the drum for perforation, erythema, bulging, retraction, growths, fluid level, and landmarks (Fig. 3-12).

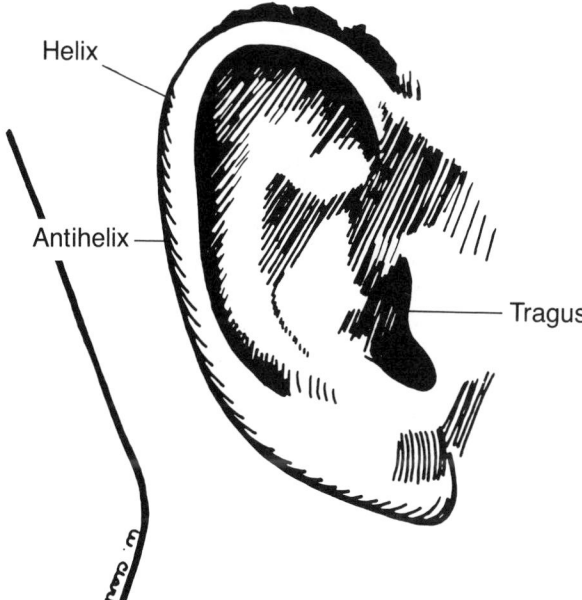

Figure 3-10. External ear.

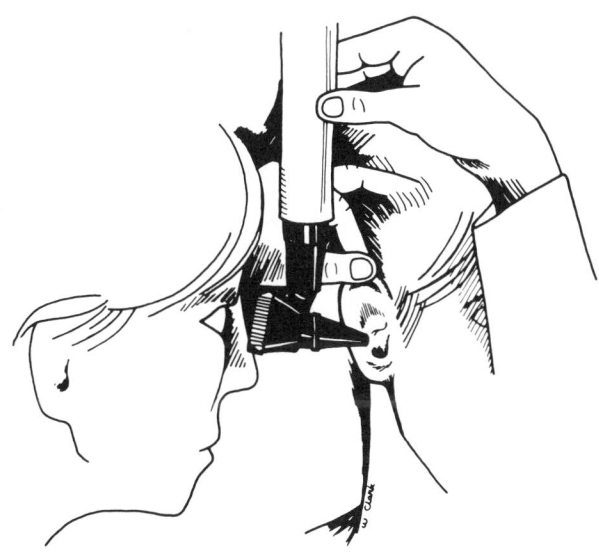

Figure 3-11. Proper use of the otoscope when examining the ear canal and tympanic membrane.

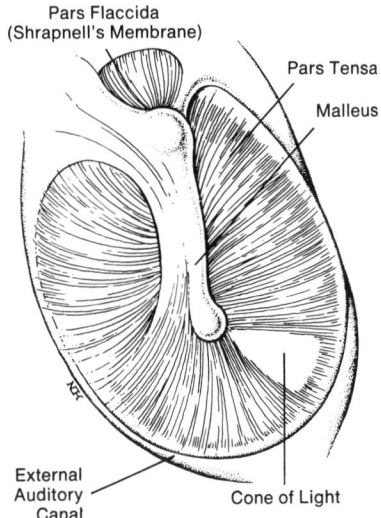

Figure 3-12.   Tympanic membrane. From *Lippincott Manual of Nursing Practice*. Philadelphia, PA: J.B. Lippincott Company, 1991: 24, with permission.

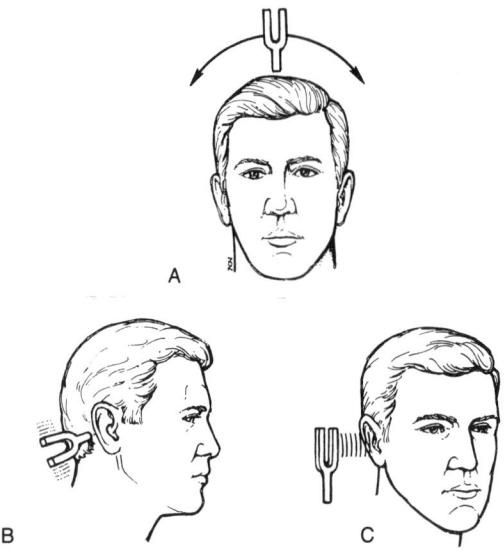

Figure 3-13.   Rinne test. From *Lippincott Manual of Nursing Practice*. Philadelphia, PA: J.B. Lippincott Company, 1991: 24, with permission.

H. *Grossly test auditory acuity by whispering or lightly rubbing fingers together at the entrance of the external canal.*

I. *Use the other ear or your own hearing as a standard.*

J. *Perform a Rinne test to compare air and bone conduction (Fig. 3-13):*
   1. Use a 512-Hz tuning fork.
   2. Lightly set the tuning fork into vibration by pinching the ends of the fork between the thumb and forefinger or striking the hypothenar eminence of your hand.
   3. Place the base of the vibrating tuning fork on the mastoid process behind the ear and check if the patient can feel or hear the vibration.
   4. If the patient can hear or feel the vibration, quickly move the vibrating tines close to the ear canal and ask if the sound is louder or softer.
   5. Normally, air conduction is better than bone conduction so the patient should be able to hear the vibrations better beside the ear than on the mastoid.

K. *Perform a Weber test to check for lateralization of the vibration (Fig. 3-14):*
   1. Begin vibration of the tuning fork as previously described.
   2. Imagine a W (for Weber) written across the forehead with the beginning and end of the W at the temporal balding areas and the center peak of the W at the center of the forehead.
   3. Place the vibrating tuning fork over the center peak of the imagined W.
   4. Ask the patient in which ear the vibration is loudest.
   5. Normally, both ears sense the vibrations equally.

Clinical Alert

Vertigo and nystagmus could correlate with labyrinthitis or fluid in the middle ear. Changes in the eye grounds from arteriosclerotic disease could correlate with a crease in the ear lobe, which may be associated with a higher risk of heart attack. Decreased hearing could be associated with a process involving the cranial nerves or simply fluid in the middle ear. Headaches can be associated with allergies and again fluid in the middle ear (called serous otitis media).

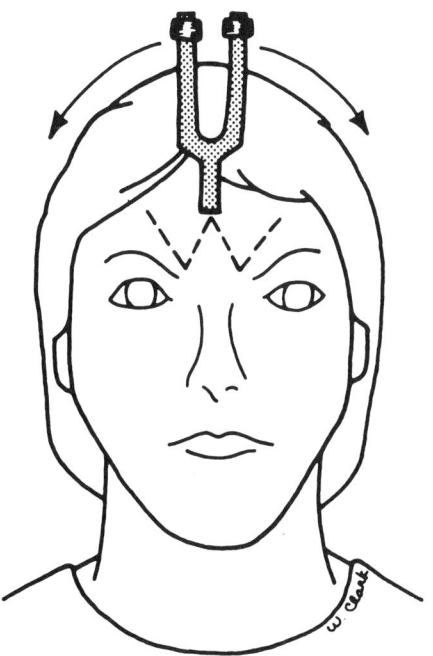

Figure 3-14. Weber test.

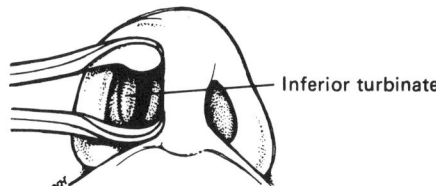

Inferior turbinate

Figure 3-15. Inside of the nose. From *Lippincott Manual of Nursing Practice*. Philadelphia, PA: J.B. Lippincott Company, 1991: 25, with permission.

L. *Inspect the nasal vaults by inserting the nasal speculum just inside one naris and opening the speculum (Fig. 3-15).*
M. *Using a good light source, inspect for septal deviation, cyanosis, swelling of the turbinates, exudate, bleeding sites, polyps, lesions, and perforations.*
N. *Inspect and palpate the sinuses for tenderness, erythema, and local heat (Fig. 3-16).*
O. *Percuss the sinuses for tenderness.*

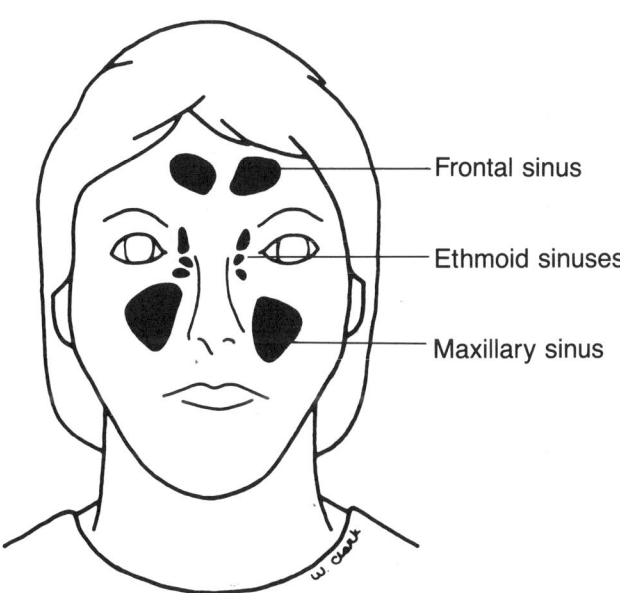

Frontal sinus

Ethmoid sinuses

Maxillary sinus

Figure 3-16. Sinuses of the face.

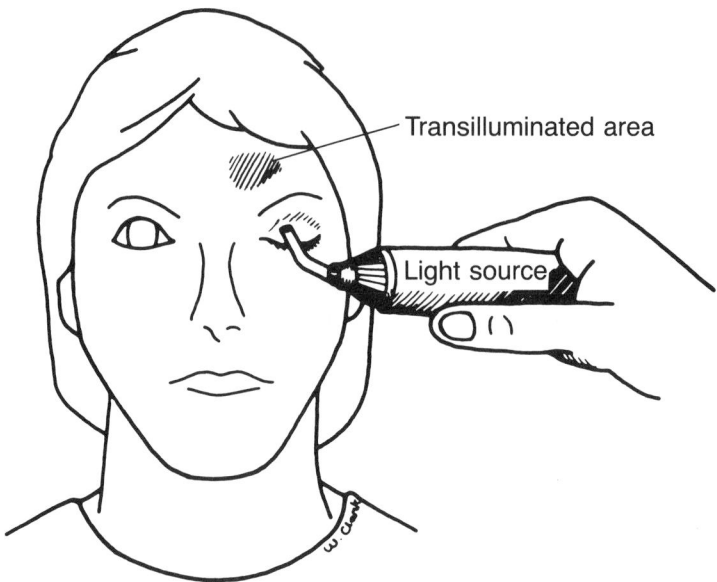

Figure 3-17.   Transillumination of left frontal sinus.

P. *Transilluminate the sinuses for opacification and fluid levels (Fig. 3-17):*
   1. The room must be very dark and you need a powerful, small-tipped light source.
   2. The frontal sinuses are transilluminated by firmly placing the tip of the light source against the inner aspect of the supraorbital ridge above the eye and directing the light toward the top of the forehead.
   3. Normally, this sinus is outlined by a faint glow of light.
   4. Compare the size and transparency of the sinuses.
   5. The maxillary sinuses are transilluminated by placing the light tip inside the mouth against either side of the hard palate and observing the sinus glow on the corresponding cheek (or placing the light source against the cheek and observing the glow through the palate).
   6. Compare both maxillary sinuses.

Clinical Alert

Many people with headaches attribute their symptoms to sinusitis and may need to have the sinuses examined. Chemosis and conjunctivitis of hay fever would correlate with similar changes in the nose and sinuses.

Q. *Inspect and palpate the lips for color, cyanosis, nodules, trauma, swelling, or crevices.*
R. *Inspect and palpate the gums for color, lesions, bleeding, swelling, hypertrophy, atrophy, tenderness, or a line of discoloration.*
S. *Always use gloves when palpating the oral area.*
T. *Inspect the teeth and percuss using the tongue blade.*
U. *Observe the occlusion or bite of the teeth.*
V. *Inspect and palpate the tongue, floor of the mouth, and base of the tongue for lesions, swelling, color, and ulcerations (Fig. 3-18).*
W. *Inspect the throat, tonsils, palate, pharynx, and uvula for ulcerations, petechiae, discharge, exudate, erythema, swelling, hypertrophy, and lesions.*

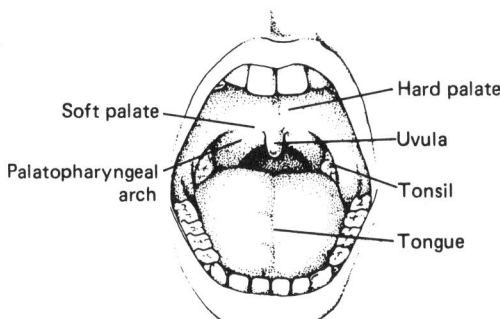

Soft palate — Hard palate
— Uvula
Palatopharyngeal — — Tonsil
arch — Tongue

Figure 3-18.   Inside of the mouth. From *Lippincott Manual of Nursing Practice*. Philadelphia, PA: J.B. Lippincott Company, 1991: 25, with permission.

X.   *If a tongue blade is needed for viewing the posterior pharynx, press the free end of one or two stacked tongue blades firmly down on the tongue two-thirds of the way back of the length of the tongue.*

Y.   *Usually, having the patient stick out the tongue and say "ahhh" will give a sufficient view.*

Z.   *Palpate the temporomandibular joints while the patient opens and closes the mouth.*

Clinical Alert

The differential diagnosis of headaches includes malocclusion of the teeth, temporomandibular joint syndrome, and dental abscesses. The keratoconus of Marfan's syndrome might be related to the high arched palate of Marfan's. Necrotizing granulomatous retinitis suggestive of candida may correlate with the milky white patches of candida in the mouth. Keratoconjunctivitis sicca suggestive of Sjogren's syndrome could correlate with a very dry mouth.

A'.   *Examine the cranial nerves:*
   1.   I (olfactory): usually not examined.
   2.   II (optic): visual acuity.
   3.   III (oculomotor), IV (trochlear), and VI (abducens): extraocular muscles.
   4.   V (trigeminal): have patient clench teeth.
   5.   VII (facial): have patient smile and raise eyebrows.
   6.   VIII (acoustic): auditory acuity.
   7.   IX (glossopharyngeal) and X (vagus): have patient say "ahhh."
   8.   XI (spinal accessory): have patient shrug shoulders.
   9.   XII (hypoglossal): have patient stick tongue out.

Clinical Alert

Examination of the cranial nerves might differentiate a cerebral vascular accident from Bell's palsy or even a brain tumor.

B'.   *Remember to examine the skin of each region.*

X.   Neck

A.   *The equipment needed will be a light source and a stethoscope.*

B.   *Inspect the neck for muscle symmetry, torticollis, and tracheal deviation.*

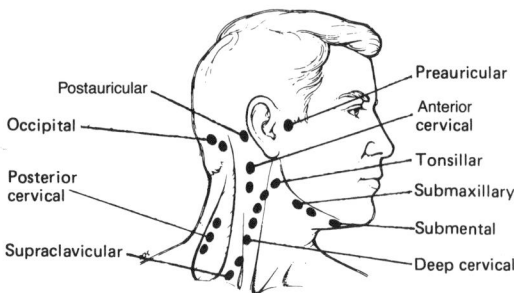

Figure 3-19. Lymph nodes of the head and neck. From *Lippincott Manual of Nursing Practice*. Philadelphia, PA: J.B. Lippincott Company, 1991: 27, with permission.

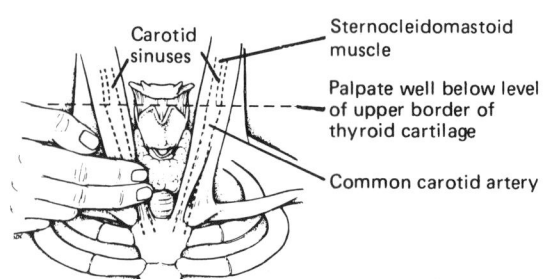

Figure 3-20. Thyroid, carotid arteries, and other structures of the neck. From *Lippincott Manual of Nursing Practice*. Philadelphia, PA: J.B. Lippincott Company, 1991: 28, with permission.

C. *Inspect and palpate the nine lymph node areas (Fig. 3-19):*
 1. Preauricular
 2. Postauricular
 3. Occipital
 4. Tonsillar
 5. Submaxillary
 6. Submental
 7. Anterior cervical
 8. Posterior cervical
 9. Supraclavicular

Clinical Alert

Changes of sarcoidosis in and around the eye might be correlated with enlarged lymph nodes in the neck area. Koplik's spots in the conjunctiva could be correlated not only with the skin changes of measles but also with Koplik's spots in the mouth and enlarged postauricular and cervical lymph nodes. Nongranulomatous uveitis and scleritis suggestive of mononucleosis might be correlated with the very large lymph nodes, especially in the anterior cervical chain.

D. *Palpate both carotid arteries, avoiding too vigorous an examination, which can stimulate the vagus nerve, reduce the blood pressure and pulse, and cause the patient to faint.*
E. *Auscultate the carotids for bruits, placing the diaphragm of the stethoscope lightly over the carotid just below the angle of the jaw.*

Clinical Alert

If a Hollenhorst plaque is noticed in the eye grounds, this could be due to arteriosclerotic changes in the carotid arteries. Bruits over the carotids may be heard. A stroke also suggests disease in the carotids and a bruit may be heard.

F. *Palpate the thyroid gland (Fig. 3-20):*
    1. Stand behind the seated patient and flex the neck slightly forward.
    2. Use the fingertips to lightly palpate the thyroid.
    3. Locate the thyroid-surrounded cartilage by finding the larynx or voice box (most prominent ring in the anterior trachea), moving the finger down the trachea to the V of the cricoid cartilage just below the larynx, then moving the finger down the trachea to the next ring, which is the cartilage surrounded by the thyroid.
    4. The thyroid can be palpated on both sides of this cartilage ring and medial to the sternocleidomastoid muscles.
    5. If the patient swallows some water, the thyroid will slide up under the examining fingers and can be more easily palpated.
    6. Check for symmetry, nodules, enlargement, and tenderness.

Clinical Alert

Exophthalmos, lid retraction, and lateral thinning of the eyebrows are suggestive of Graves' disease and should correlate with a diffusely enlarged thyroid gland.

G. *Examine the skin of this region.*

XI. Lower Extremity

   A. *The equipment needed will be a light source and a reflex hammer.*
   B. *Examine range of motion of the hips.*
   C. *Test the strength of the muscles of the hips and upper legs.*
   D. *Examine the range of motion of the knees.*
   E. *Test the strength of the muscles of the lower legs and feet.*
   F. *Observe for varicosities.*
   G. *Test the knee-jerk and ankle-jerk reflexes (Fig. 3-21).*

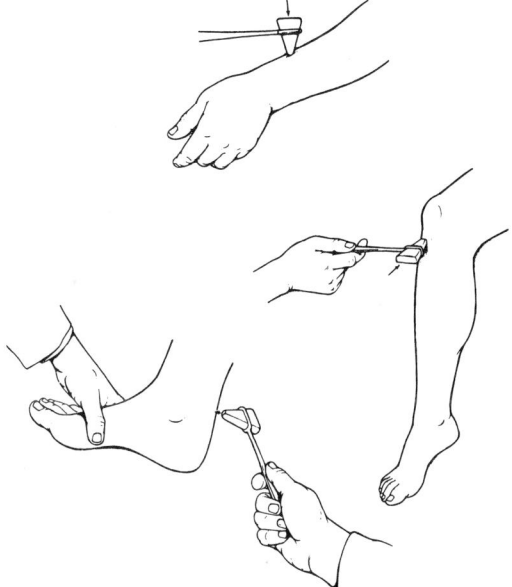

Figure 3-21. Reflexes of the lower extremity. From *Lippincott Manual of Nursing Practice*. Philadelphia, PA: J.B. Lippincott Company, 1991: 48

H. *Examine the range of motion of the ankles.*
I. *Palpate the pulses of the feet:*
    1. The dorsalis pedis artery can be found between the dorsiflexor tendons of the great and third toes.
    2. The posterior tibial artery can be found behind and below the medial malleolus.

J. *Inspect the ankles and feet for edema.*
K. *Inspect and palpate the toes, feet, and arches for deformities.*
L. *Inspect the toes for hair growth, clubbing, and capillary refill.*
M. *Inspect the toenails in the same manner as the fingernails.*
N. *Inspect the skin of the region.*

Clinical Alert

Inflammatory changes in the eye may suggest gout, and the joints of the lower extremity (especially the great toe) might provide clues to this diagnosis. Arteriosclerotic changes of the eye would suggest these same changes throughout the body and may be correlated with decreased distal pulses. Arthritic changes seen in the eye might suggest rheumatoid arthritis, systemic lupus erythematosus, or osteoarthritis, and examination of the joints of the lower extremity might prove helpful. Dilatation of the arteries and veins, retinal hemorrhages, microaneurysms, and areas of capillary closure might suggest hyperviscosity syndromes, which are correlated with ulcerations of the lower extremity, especially around the ankles.

XII. Neurological Examination

A. *Cranial nerves, muscle strength, gait, reflexes, and much of the mental status has already been accomplished during the history and regional exams.*
B. *The equipment needed for the rest of the neurological exam will be a 256-Hz tuning fork and cotton sticks.*
C. *The components of the neurological exam are:*
    1. Cerebral function (mental status)
    2. Cranial nerves
    3. Cerebellar functioning
    4. Deep tendon reflexes
    5. Motor function (muscle strength)
    6. Sensory function (touch, pain, vibration, pressure, proprioception)

D. *The mental status is tested by asking specific questions:*
    1. Orientation to time, place, and person
    2. Recent and remote memory
    3. Concentration
    4. Alertness
    5. Speech
    6. Object recognition

E. *Light touch can be tested by fluffing the cotton tip of an applicator and lightly touching the skin of any region with the patient's eyes closed and questioning the patient to determine whether or not the patient can feel this in each region.*
F. *Pain can be tested in the same fashion using a cotton-tipped applicator broken to create a sharp point.*
G. *Vibratory sense is tested using a low-frequency tuning fork.*
H. *Set the tuning fork vibrating in the fashion previously described and place the base of the tuning fork firmly over a joint to determine if the patient can feel the vibration.*

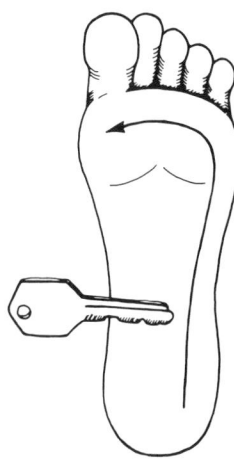 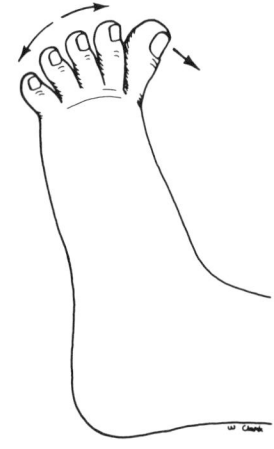

Figure 3-22. Babinski response.

I. *Discrimination can be tested by placing an object in the patient's hand with eyes closed and having the patient identify the object.*

J. *Two-point discrimination is tested by placing two sharp points on the skin to determine if the patient feels one or two points.*

K. *Temperature discrimination can be tested using warm or cool water in test tubes or on a cotton-tipped applicator.*

L. *Proprioception or position sense can be tested by moving a finger or toe up or down with eyes closed and asking the patient which direction it was moved.*

M. *Cerebellar or coordination function is tested in multiple ways:*
   1. *Romberg test:* observe for loss of balance when the patient stands unsupported with feet close together and eyes closed.
   2. Observe gait when the patient walks a straight line.
   3. Observe for loss of balance when the patient stands on one leg and runs the heel up the opposite shin.
   4. Observe for incoordination when the patient uses the forefinger to touch his or her nose and then the examiner's outheld forefinger.
   5. Observe for slowness when the patient rapidly touches the thumb to each finger of the same hand.

N. *The Babinski or plantar response is elicited when a hard object is stroked along the lateral aspect of the sole of the foot from the heel to the ball of the foot (Fig. 3-22).*

O. *An abnormal plantar response is present when the great toe dorsiflexes and the other toes fan out, indicating upper motor neuron disease.*

Clinical Alert

A pale conjunctiva suggestive of anemia might be due to vitamin B_{12} deficiency, which also causes loss of vibratory sensation. Optic neuritis may be due to multiple sclerosis, which also causes ataxia, paresthesias, paralysis of position sensation, and changes in mental status. A Hollenhorst plaque might be suggestive of an impending or old cerebral vascular accident and could be associated with a hemiparesis. Neurofibromatosis of the lids could be associated with these changes anywhere in the body, giving almost any neurological deficit. Changes in the eye grounds from diabetes might be correlated with a loss of sensation of the feet and hands. Decreased strength of the muscles of blinking might be due to myasthenia gravis which could decrease the strength of other muscles in the body.

XIII. Ending Comments

A. *The pediatric physical examination differs significantly in many of the regional examinations and has not been discussed in this chapter.*

B. *If an organ-specific examination is indicated, parts of each regional examination may need to be incorporated in order to be complete.*

C. *The breast, heart, thorax, lung, abdomen, and genital exams have not been discussed in this chapter.*

D. *This chapter is not meant to be a substitute for formal training in physical examination techniques.*

E. *This chapter is not meant to replace a physical examination done by a physician.*

F. *The clinical examples offered in this chapter are not all-inclusive.*

Acknowledgment

The author wishes to thank Wendy Clark of the Instructional Media Center of The Ohio State University College of Optometry for preparation of many of the illustrations in this chapter.

Suggested Readings

Bates B. *A Guide to Physical Examination and History Taking.* 5th ed. Philadelphia: JB Lippincott; 1991.

Brunner LS. *The Lippincott Manual of Nursing Practice.* 4th ed. Philadelphia: JB Lippincott; 1986.

Clain A. *Hamilton Bailey's Demonstration of Physical Signs in Clinical Surgery.* 17th ed. Bristol: John Wright; 1986.

Classe JG. A review of 50 malpractice claims. *J Am Optom Assoc* 1989;60:694–706.

DeGowin EL, DeGowin RL. *Bedside Diagnostic Examination.* 4th ed. New York: Macmillan; 1981.

Executive Summary of the American Optometric Association Strategic Long-Range Plan. AOA Long-Range Planning Task Force, September, 1984.

Good GW, Augsburger AR. Role of optometrists in combating high blood pressure. *J Am Optom Assoc* 1989;60:352–355.

Prior JA, Silberstein JS, Stang JM. *Physical Diagnosis.* 6th ed. St. Louis: CV Mosby; 1981.

Rakel RE. *Textbook of Family Practice.* 4th ed. Philadelphia: WB Saunders Co.; 1990.

Silverman MW. Optometry and its expanded role in health care delivery systems (1600–1987). *J Am Optom Assoc* 1989;60:52–55.

Smith SK. Child abuse and neglect: a diagnostic guide for the optometrist. *J Am Optom Assoc* 1988;59:760–765.

Swartz MH. *Textbook of Physical Diagnosis History and Examination.* Philadelphia: WB Saunders Co.; 1989.

Vaughan D, Asbury T. *General Ophthalmology.* 12th ed. Los Altos: Lange Medical Publications; 1989.

Walker HK, Hall WD, Hurst JW. *Clinical Methods: The History, Physical, and Laboratory Examinations.* 3rd ed. Boston: Butterworth Publishers; 1990.

Weiner WJ, Goetz CG. *Neurology for the Non-Neurologist.* 2nd ed. Philadelphia: JP Lippincott; 1989.

Wilson JD, Braunwald E, Isselbacher KJ, et al. *Harrison's Principles of Internal Medicine.* 12th ed. New York: McGraw-Hill; 1991.

CHAPTER **4**

Ocular Pharmacology

Jeffrey L. Kegarise

I. Topical Ophthalmic Therapy

   A. General principles

      1. Suspensions, solutions, ointments

         a. Demonstrate the importance of shaking suspensions to patients. Recommend shake 20×. Percentage of drug can vary tremendously otherwise.

         b. Inform patients suspension drops should look milky.

         c. Suspensions increase contact time versus solutions.

         d. Ointments prolong contact time, which can also result in increased incidence of contact dermatitis.

         e. Avoid ointments immediately after radial keratotomy or clear corneal cataract incisions.

      2. Drug delivery and systems

Clinical Alert

Currently available dropper volumes exceed cul-de-sac capacity. Expect overflow—when patient complains of overflow of topical medications, consider:
   Patient missing the eye
   Patient squeezing the bottle
   Washout from reflex tearing
   Patient lid position—ectropion?
   Normal—due to limited cul-de-sac capacity

---

         a. Nasolacrimal duct occlusion. "Punctal occlusion" increases drug contact time and may decrease potential for systemic absorption.

         b. Soft contact lenses and soaked collagen shields may serve as drug delivery vehicles. Difficult to quantify concentration delivered.

         c. Consider one-eye trials with certain medications and ocular diseases (e.g., β-blocker in chronic open angle glaucoma (COAG).

Clinical Rule of Thumb Estimate for Patient Drug Use

Bottle Volume	Dosage i gtt bid	i gtt qid
5 cc	4 weeks	2 weeks
10 cc	8 weeks	4 weeks
15 cc	12 weeks	6 weeks

Note that this is far less than estimates based on capacity of bottle and drop size. Will vary among patients due to experience using eye drops, male vs female, physical factors (arthritis?), and compliance.

3. Clinical properties
   a. Expect drug effect less in inflamed eyes (e.g., uveitis).
   b. Use minimum dosage necessary to obtain therapeutic benefit. Possible exception: corticosteroid use in uveitis should be at frequency levels to ensure adequate treatment.
   c. Drops tend to sting more in patients with dry eye conditions—particularly aqueous deficiency (less buffering).
   d. If unexpected worsening of condition, always physically examine drug dispensed for accuracy and question patient compliance.

B. *In-office administration*
   1. Samples
      a. Always provide written instructions to patients—even with samples.
      b. Small "zip-lock bags" with peel-off labels work well for sample use.
      c. Check expiration dates before handing out.
   2. Exam room
      a. Avoid contamination by avoiding dropper tip contact with patient's lashes.
      b. Precede mydriatic and cycloplegics with anesthetic agents for improved patient comfort, better penetration.
      c. Perform all tests necessary prior to pharmacologic administration. E.g.:
         (1) Visual acuity prior to proparacaine/fluorescein for tonometry.
         (2) Motility, muscle balance prior to cycloplegic agents.
      d. Always wipe first squeeze of gonioscopic solution into tissue to avoid bubbles in lens or store solution upside down.
      e. Store all diagnostic drugs, therapeutic agents, samples, etc. fully capped and out of reach of inquisitive children's hands.

C. *Patient instructions and compliance*
   1. Write all prescriptions legibly.
   2. Spell out dosage, number of pills, and refill number in all narcotic prescriptions (see XV. E).
   3. Encourage punctal occlusion to patients.
   4. Separate multiple drop instillations by 3–5 minutes.
   5. Written instructions help compliance. Include diagnosis, drug, possible side effects. Emergency phone number should be clearly indicated.
   6. Use pupil size and reactivity as indicator of compliance.
   7. Ask "how often" patient misses drop instillation, rather than "if."
   8. Refrigerator storage of medications may aid instillation success, lessen contamination risk, and keep drop visible as reminder.
   9. Inform family members of medication side effects. Certain side effects ("depression" via β-blockers) may be noticed by those who accompany patient.
   10. Assume cost of medication *is* an issue for all patients.

II. Prescription Writing

A. *Accurate prescriptions should:*
    1. Be legible
       The possibility of misinterpretation of data compromises quality patient care.
    2. Include
       a. Patient's name.
       b. Date.
       c. Chemical name of medication (trade name used if desire specificity).
       d. Concentration of medication (%, mg).
       e. Instructions for use (see Table 4-1).

Table 4-1. Latin Abbreviations

Abbreviation	Latin	English Meaning
ac	ante cibum	before meals
bid	bis in die	twice a day
c	cum	with
caps	capsula	capsule
d	dies	day
gtt	gutta	drop
h	hora	hour
hs	hora somni	at bedtime
od	oculus dexter	right eye
oh	omni hora	every hour
os	oculus sinister	left eye
ou	oculus uterque	each eye
p	post	after
pc	post cibum	after meals
po	per os	by mouth
prn	pro re nata	as needed
q	quaque	each, every
qd	quaque die	every day
qh	quaque hora	every hour
qid	quater in die	four times a day
s	sine	without
sig	signa	label
sol	solutio	solution
tab	tabella	tablet
tid	ter in die	three times a day
ung	unguentum	ointment
ut dict	ut dictum	as directed

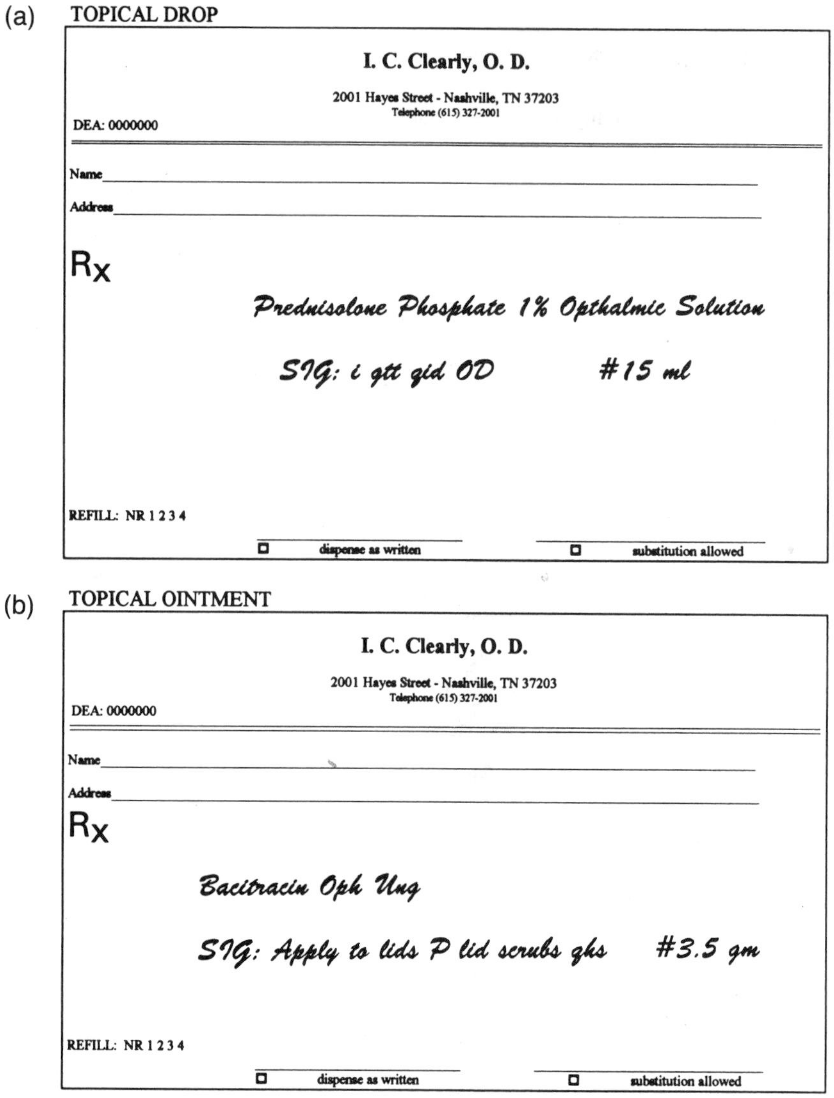

(a) TOPICAL DROP

I. C. Clearly, O. D.

2001 Hayes Street - Nashville, TN 37203
Telephone (615) 327-2001

DEA: 0000000

Name_____

Address_____

R_x

Prednisolone Phosphate 1% Opthalmic Solution

SIG: i gtt qid OD   #15 ml

REFILL: NR 1 2 3 4

☐   dispense as written   ☐   substitution allowed

(b) TOPICAL OINTMENT

I. C. Clearly, O. D.

2001 Hayes Street - Nashville, TN 37203
Telephone (615) 327-2001

DEA: 0000000

Name_____

Address_____

R_x

Bacitracin Oph Ung

SIG: Apply to lids P lid scrubs qhs   #3.5 gm

REFILL: NR 1 2 3 4

☐   dispense as written   ☐   substitution allowed

Figure 4-1. Examples of prescriptions for (a) topical drops, (b) topical ointments, (c) oral medication.

>   f. Size of bottle (number of pills if oral).
>   g. Doctor's signature—personally signed, not stamped.
>   h. Number of refills (Fig. 4-1).
>
> B. *Prescriptions for over the counter (OTC) medication may be written as legend drug format but should have "OTC" designated on the prescriptions.*
>
> C. *Preprinted prescription pads save time. However, do not allow a stamped doctor's signature.*
>
> D. *Ophthalmic assistants who help the doctor by writing prescriptions or responding to pharmacists' calls should be trained and follow strict written protocol.*
>
> E. *In general, prescriptions should not be provided for patient symptoms discussed over the phone. Refills on medication requested by patients should be authorized by the doctor and recorded on the clinic chart.*

(c)   ORAL

I. C. Clearly, O. D.

2001 Hayes Street - Nashville, TN 37203
Telephone (615) 327-2001

DEA: 0000000

Name_____

Address_____

R_X *Tetracycline 250 mg.*

#84 (eight-four)

SIG: 1 cap P.O. qid x 21d

REFILL: NR 1 2 3 4

☐ dispense as written   ☐ substitution allowed

Figure 4-1   *Continued.*

III.   **Topical Anesthetics**

A.   *Clinical uses*

1.   Ameliorate symptoms of pain related to corneal and conjunctival disorders, thus enhancing ocular examination.
2.   Allow applanation of cornea for diagnostic tests (e.g., A-scan, Goldmann tonometry, gonioscopy).
3.   Precursor to corneal foreign body removal and other minor surgical procedures of cornea and conjunctiva.
4.   Enhance adaptation to rigid contact lenses during clinical fitting evaluation.

B.   *Method of action*

1.   Reversible blockage of nerve impulses through effects on cell membrane (decreased sodium permeability).
2.   The primary route of administration used for anesthetics in ophthalmic practice is topical.
3.   Onset of action: within 20–30 seconds.
4.   Duration of action: 15–20 minutes.

C.   *Side effects and adverse reactions*

1.   Vasovagal and/or psychosomatic reactions can occur but are rare with topically applied anesthetics.
2.   Stinging or burning upon instillation. Decreasing intensity: tetracaine, proparacaine, benoxinate.
3.   Corneal epithelial disruption. Decreasing intensity: tetracaine, proparacaine, benoxinate.

D.   *Specific ocular anesthetic agents (Table 4-2)*

1.   Benoxinate 0.4%
   a.   Bacteriostatic.
   b.   Less corneal toxicity and fewer side effects than other topical anesthetics.
   c.   Combined with 0.25% sodium fluorescein (Fluress) for diagnostic use.
   d.   Drug of choice for routine applanation tonometry.

Table 4-2.   Topical Anesthetics[a]

Generic Name (commercial)	Pharmacologic Derivation	Drug Forms	Specific Notes
Benoxinate HCI (Fluress)	*para*-Aminobenzoic acid	0.4% benoxinate in solution with 0.25% Na fluorescein	Bacteriostatic
Proparacaine HCI (AK-Taine, Al-caine, Fluorcaine, I-Paracaine, Kainaire, Ophthaine, Ophthetic)	*meta*-Aminobenzoic acid	0.5% solution	Good general purpose
Tetracaine HCI (Pontocaine, others)	*para*-Aminobenzoic acid	0.5% solution 0.5% ointment	Stings more Increased depth of anesthesia

[a]All are ester linked and, therefore potentially sensitizing.

Reprinted from Pavan Langston, M.D. *Handbook of Ocular Drug Therapy and Ocular Side Effects of Systemic Drugs.* 1991:220.

    e. Least likely of fluorescein anesthetic combinations to allow *Pseudomonas* growth in solution.
2. Proparacaine 0.5%
    a. Available in solution singly or in combination with 0.25% sodium fluorescein (Fluorocaine).
    b. Slightly greater toxicity to cornea and more frequent hypersensitivity reaction than benoxinate, though both are rare.
    c. More cost-effective than benoxinate and fluorescein; however, proparacaine is not bacteriostatic.
    d. Can also be combined with fluorescein strips (e.g., Fluor-I-Strips) for tonometry and corneal evaluations.
3. Tetracaine 0.5%
    a. Not available in combination with sodium fluorescein. Must use in conjunction with fluorescein strips for corneal evaluation.
    b. Increased stinging upon instillation as compared to other anesthetic choices.
    c. Clinically provides somewhat deeper anesthesia (penetrates cornea better).

Clinical Alert

The prolonged use of topical anesthetics delays mitotic activity and corneal wound healing, and can lead to ulceration. Topical anesthetic agents should not be given or prescribed for patient use as "at home" therapy.

---

4. Drug of choice
    a. Tonometry: benoxinate + fluorescein (Fluress).
    b. Corneal evaluation (patient in pain): proparacaine + fluorescein.
    c. Foreign body removal: proparacaine (tetracaine if limbal).
    d. General ophthalmic use: proparacaine.

Clinical Alert

Most ophthalmic offices use proparacaine as standard topical anesthetic agent. Benoxinate + fluorescein (Fluress) should be available in clinic as an alternative for patients who have proparacaine sensitivity.

Table 4-3.   Method to Fortify Antibiotics (gentamicin)

Use TB syringe to draw up 2.0 ml of parenteral gentamicin preparation.

Remove cap from previously unopened bottle of 5cc gentamicin ophthalmic solution and inject parenteral solution.

Dosage frequency q 30 minutes (Note: if only sample size 0.3-ml bottle available, use 1.2 ml of parenteral preparation.

Adapted from *PDR for Ophthalmology,* 18th ed. Oradell, N.J.: Medical Economics Company, 1990:4

IV.   Anti-Infective/Antibacterial Agents

A.   *General principles (see also Tables 4-3 and 4-4)*
   1.   Anti-infective treatment is an elaboration of the diagnostic process: the more accurate the diagnosis, the more effective will be the treatment.
   2.   When choosing an antibiotic, it is important to consider the drug's activity spectrum, mechanism of action, and potential for side effects.
   3.   A good understanding of a pathogen's characteristics allows more specific and more effective treatment.
   4.   Drug resistance and toxicity to surrounding ocular structures is minimized with more specific treatment.
   5.   The most common route for antibacterial treatment of eye disease is topical.
   6.   It is important to rule out noninfectious causes prior to initiating therapy for suspected infectious problems.
   7.   Practical drug treatment consists of having a primary and secondary drug of choice.
   8.   Bacterial scrapings and cultures are considered essential in cases of central corneal ulcerations, and highly recommended in cases unresponsive to treatment.
   9.   Soft contact lenses and collagen shields may be used as drug delivery vehicles to aid the treatment and healing process, but variable quantities of drug delivered can increase potential toxicity.
   10.   Systemic complications from the use of topical antibiotics are rare.

B.   *Aminoglycosides*
   Table 4-5 lists common ophthalmic drugs in this category. See individual drug for specific discussion and summary.
   1.   Bactericidal—inhibits synthesis.
   2.   Broad spectrum of activity against gram-positive and gram-negative organisms.

Table 4-4.   Factors to Consider When Inadequate Response to Antibacterial Therapy

Incorrect diagnosis

Incorrect drug spectrum

Improper dosage

Ineffective route

Poor patient compliance

Resistant organisms

Noninfectious cause of problem

Side effects of therapy (e.g., toxicity) masking benefits of treatment

Culture-sensitivity

Table 4-5. Common Topical Ophthalmic Aminoglycoside Solutions

Gentamicin 3 mg sulfate/1 ml
  Genoptic (Allergan)
  Garamycin (Schering)
  Gentacidin (Iolab)
  Gentak (Akorn)
  Gentrasul (Bausch & Lomb)
  Gentamicin Ophthalmic (multiple suppliers)

Neomycin 3.5 mg/ml with polymyxin B sulfate and
  gramicidin solution (multiple suppliers)

Tobramycin 3 mg/ml
  Tobrex (Alcon)

Adapted from *Ophthalmic Drug Facts*, 1993.

3. Especially effective against *Pseudomonas* sp.
4. Not effective—certain strains of *Streptococcus*.
5. Available in solution and ointment.
6. Tend to have higher incidence of microbial resistance when compared to other antibacterial drugs (microbial enzyme production responsible).
7. Watch for superficial punctate keratitis as indicator of toxicity with all drugs in this category.
8. Neomycin is most likely of the aminoglycosides to cause allergic reactions (contact dermatitis, erythema, conjunctival injection, preseptal cellulitis).
9. Due to higher incidence of microbial resistance and less effectiveness versus streptococcus, aminoglycosides are *not* good drugs of first choice in children (prefer sulfacetamide + trimethoprim [Polytrim] or erythromycin).
10. Ototoxicity and nephrotoxicity occur but are more likely with systemic administration (discontinue if onset of vertigo, tinnitis, or dizziness occurs).

C. *Bacitracin*
1. Bactericidal—inhibits cell wall synthesis.
2. Especially effective against gram-positive organisms.
3. Available only in ointment form.
4. Very low incidence of hypersensitivity reaction.
5. Used frequently in treatment of blepharitis or other ocular disease where gram-positive organisms are suspected.

D. *Cephalosporins*
1. Bactericidal—inhibit cell wall synthesis (see Table 4-6).
2. Spectrum of activity depends on generation:
   a. In general, 1st generation = broad spectrum with more effectiveness against gram-positive.
   b. 2nd and 3rd generation = narrower spectrum with better effectiveness against gram-negative.
3. Oral, topical (by formulation).
4. Actions are similar to those of penicillin.
5. Fortified cephalosporin may be made soluble for treatment of corneal ulcers where gram-positive organisms are suspected or identified (e.g., cefazolin 50 mg/ml [Ancef]). Topical Ancef must be refrigerated and shaken, and is only sterile ×7 days.
6. Cephalosporins can be enzymatically inactivated.
7. Low toxicity topically and orally.

Table 4-6.   Cephalosporins

Drug	Route of Administration	Clinically Useful Spectrum of Activity
First generation		
Cephalothin	iv	Gram-positive except enterococci, *Escherichia coli,*
Cefazolin	iv,im	*Klebsiella, Proteus mirabilis*
Cephapirin	iv,im	
Cephradine	po,iv,im	
Cephalexin	po	
Cefadroxil	po	
Cephaloridine	iv,im	
Second generation		
Cefamandole	iv,im	Gram-positive cocci, *Haemophilus influenzae,*
Cefoxitin	iv,im	*Enterobacter, Proteus mirabilis, Escherichia coli,*
Cefaclor	po	*Klebsiella,* anaerobes especially *Bacteroides*
Ceforanide	iv,im	
Cefuroxime	iv,im	
Third generation		
Ceftriaxone	iv,im	*Escherichia coli, Klebsiella, Proteus, Haemophilus*
Ceftizoxime	iv,im	*influenzae, Enterobacter, Serratia*
Cefotaxime	iv,im	
Cefoperazone	iv,im	All of the above plus *Pseudomonas*
Ceftazidime	iv,im	

From Bartlett JD, Jannus SD. *Clinical Ocular Pharmacology.* 2nd ed. Stoneham, Mass: Butterworth, 1989, p. 208.

8. Must monitor oral administration if on concomitant aminoglycoside or other potentially nephrotoxic agents.
9. Use cautiously in patients with known penicillin sensitivity.
10. Useful in treatment of preseptal cellulitis (e.g., cefaclor [Ceclor] 250 mg q 8 hours, Cephalexin [Keflex] 500 mg tid).

E. *Chloramphenicol*
1. Bacteriostatic—inhibits protein synthesis.
2. Broad spectrum—however, limited activity: *Staphylococcus, Pseudomonas aeruginosa,* and *Serratia marcescens.*
3. Available as solution or ointment.
4. Resistance to this drug is increasing, particularly among staphylococci.
5. Adverse side effects reported with the use of this drug topically (aplastic anemia, bone marrow suppression, pancytopenia, leukopenia, agranulocytosis—some leading to death), though rare, make this drug *NOT* recommended for first-line therapy.
6. Use of this drug should be limited to specific indications for effectiveness—especially if longer-term therapy is anticipated.

F. *Ciprofloxacin*
1. Fluoroquinolone—for general discussion of this class of drugs see IV. I.
2. Bactericidal—inhibits DNA synthesis (DNA gyrase).
3. Broad spectrum (gram-positive and gram-negative) including *Pseudomonas aeruginosa.*
4. Solution.
5. Low bacterial resistance due to two mutations necessary for resistance.
6. Indicated for treatment of keratitis, including corneal ulcer and conjunctivitis.
7. May be used topically in children over 12.

8. Very low frequency of adverse reactions.
9. White precipitates may occur with prolonged and frequent treatment but do not generally indicate reason for cessation.

Recommended Treatment Regimen

Conjunctivitis
    1–2 drops qid ×7 days
Keratitis (e.g., coneal ulcer)
    Day 1
        2 drops q 15 minutes ×6 hours
        2 drops q 30 minutes ×18 hours
    Day 2
        2 drops q 1 hour
    Day 3–14
        2 drops q 4 hours
    Day 14
        Continued treatment if no corneal reepithelization

G. *Clindamycin*
    1. Inhibits protein synthesis.
    2. Bacteriostatic.
    3. Useful in treatment of certain anaerobic bacilli and *Toxoplasma gondii*—see VI.C.
    4. Due to the potential for psuedomembranous colitis to occur, this drug should be discontinued if patients develop diarrhea.
    5. SIG: 300 mg po × 4 weeks qid.

H. *Erythromycin*
    1. Bacteriostatic—inhibits protein synthesis.
    2. Most effective against gram-positive.
    3. Ointment, tablets, or capsule.
    4. Low toxicity.
    5. GI upset is common, but less likely with ethylsuccinate form E.E.S.
    6. When prescribing 250 stearate filmtabs q 6 hours = 400 mg ethylsuccinate filmtabs q 6 hours.

Clinical Alert

Due to increased staphylococcal resistance developing with extended topical use of erythromycin, patients treated for blepharitis or other disorders requiring long-term therapy should use alternating treatment regimens (e.g., bacitracin).

---

    7. Oral preparation useful for treatment of resistant hordeola and mild preseptal cellulitis.
    8. Allergic reactions are rare.
    9. SIG: 250 mg po qid.

I. *Fluoroquinolones (newest class of antibiotic drugs)*
    1. Inhibition of DNA (specifically enzyme DNA gyrase).
    2. Broad spectrum of activity against gram-positive and gram-negative organisms.
    3. Solution.
    4. Requires two bacterial mutations to develop microbial resistance.

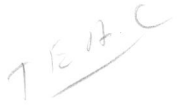

5. Indicated for treatment of conjunctivitis and keratitis. (See individual discussion of ciprofloxacin and norfloxacin (IV. F and IV. M). Though there are limited reports of norfloxacin effectiveness in treatment of corneal ulcer, only ciprofloxacin is approved for use in keratitis)

J. *Gentamicin*
   1. Aminoglycoside—for discussion of this general category, see IV. B.
   2. Bactericidal—inhibits protein synthesis.
   3. Effective against many gram-positive and most gram-negative organisms.
   4. Solution and ointment.
   5. Particularly effective against *Pseudomonas*.
   6. Can be fortified for use in treatment of corneal ulcers (see Table 4-3).

Clinical Alert

Gentamicin (with cefazolin) has been a mainstay of nonspecific corneal ulcer therapy. An alternative now exists with ciprofloxacin (Ciloxan) which has a broader spectrum, can be used without fortification, and has less microbial resistance potential.

---

   7. Toxic effects (superficial punctate keratitis, conjunctivitis [some pseudomembranous] dermatologic) are seen in association with gentamicin therapy. Any superficial punctate keratitis noted does not necessarily indicate gentamacin toxicity, but should be monitored appropriately.
   8. Cross resistance and hypersensitivity can occur with other aminoglycosides.

K. *Gramicidin*
   1. Bactericidal—inhibits cell wall permeability.
   2. Effective against gram-positive organisms primarily.
   3. Solution—combination with neomycin and polymyxin B as in neosporin ophthalmic solution.

L. *Neomycin*
   1. Aminoglycoside—for discussion of this general category, see IV. B.
   2. Bactericidal—inhibits protein synthesis.
   3. Effective against most gram-positive and gram-negative organisms, but NOT *Pseudomonas*.
   4. Solution and ointment in combination with polymyxin B, bacitracin, and/or gramicidin.
   5. Hypersensitivity reactions (6%–8%) characteristically consist of conjunctival injection, lid edema, and erythema of the lids. This is reversible with discontinuation of the drug with or without topical steroid preparations and cold compresses.
   6. Since the advent of other topical combination antibiotics and single broader-spectrum antibiotics, neomycin is no longer considered the drug of first choice for the routine treatment of conjunctivitis.

M. *Norfloxacin*
   1. Fluoroquinolone—for discussion of this general category of drug, see IV. I.
   2. Bactericidal—inhibits DNA synthesis (DNA gyrase).
   3. Broad spectrum against gram-positive and gram-negative organisms.
   4. May not have concentration topically to treat keratitis associated with *Pseudomonas aeruginosa*.
   5. Bactericidal—inhibits DNA synthesis (DNA gyrase).
   6. Low microbial resistance—similar to ciprofloxacin.
   7. Solution.

8. Indicated for treatment of conjunctivitis.
9. May be used in children over 1 year.
10. ·Low incidence of adverse reactions.

Recommended Treatment Regimen

1–2 drops qid ×7 days. May be used q 2 hours ×2 days in severe conjunctivitis.

N. *Penicillin*
1. Bactericidal—inhibits microbial cell wall.
2. Broad spectrum—mostly gram-positive.
3. *There are no topical solutions or ointments in the penicillin family.*
4. Penicillin G, amoxicillin (extended gram-negative) may be drugs of choice for certain periorbital ocular disorders (e.g., preseptal cellulitis).
5. Cross sensitivity can occur with patients allergic to cephalosporins (5%–20%).
6. Approximately 1 in 20 to 1 in 10 patients develop an allergy to penicillin.
7. If allergic to one type of penicillin, then patient assumed allergic to all penicillin.
8. Alternative treatment: gram-positive infections—erythromycin, vancomycin. Gram-negative infections—gentamicin.

O *Polymyxin B*
1. Bactericidal—disrupt cell membrane structure.
2. Spectrum limited to gram-negative.
3. Ointment and solution—in conjunction with other agents (e.g., bacitracin, neomycin, or trimethoprim).
4. Good broad spectrum coverage when used in combination with drug with gram-positive coverage (e.g., bacitracin).
5. Very low toxicity and seldom seen allergic reactions.

P. *Sulfonamides*
1. Bacteriostatic—disrupt bacterial metabolism through folic acid inhibition.
2. Broad spectrum but *Staphylococcus, Neisseria,* and *Pseudomonas* are likely resistant.
3. Solutions and ointment.
4. Inactivated in presence of pus—therefore limited use in mucopurulent conjunctivitis.
5. Hypersensitivity reactions in 5% of patients.
6. Available in solution with vasoconstrictive agent phenylephrine HCl 0.125% (Vasosulf) Iolab.
7. Sulfacetamide
   a. Sulamyd 10% (30% seldom used and not recommended due to stinging).
   b. Bleph 10 (10%).
   c. Cetamide (10%).
   d. Isopto Cetamide (15%).
8. Sulfisoxazole
   a. Gantrisin (4%).
9. Dosage
   a. Solution 1–2 drops q 1–3 hours.
   b. Ointment one-half inch 1–4×/daily.

Q. *Tetracyclines*
1. Bacteriostatic—inhibit protein synthesis.
2. Broad spectrum
   a. Gram-positive shows high resistance (e.g., *Staphylococcus* sp).
   b. Gram-negative are well inhibited except *Pseudomonas.*

3. Suspension, ointment, and oral.
4. Topical ointment—available in combination with polymyxin B (Terramycin).
5. Orally effective in treatment of acne rosacea, meibomianitis, chlamydial infections, and Lyme disease (*Borrelia burgdorferi*).
6. Discoloration of teeth may occur and therefore those drugs should be avoided in children.
7. Toxic effects characterized by superficial punctate keratitis, conjunctival irritation with topical drug therapy.
8. Tetracyclines are inhibited in presence of milk products and antacids. Exception: doxycycline, which can be administered with milk products.
9. Oral administration can frequently cause:
   a. GI upset.
   b. photosensitivity.
10. Oral dosage:
   a. Tetracycline 250 mg i cap po qid.
   b. Doxycyline 100 mg i cap po bid.

Clinical Alert

Patients being treated with oral tetracycline (e.g., for acne rosacea) should be advised to avoid prolonged UV exposure due to increased photosensitivity from melanocytic stimulation.

---

11. Tetracycline should *not* be used in patients who are pregnant, attempting to become pregnant, or lactating.

R. *Tobramycin*
1. Aminoglycoside—for discussion of this general category, see IV. B.
2. Bactericidal—inhibits protein synthesis.
3. Effective against many gram-positive and most gram-negative organisms.
4. Very effective against *Pseudomonas*.
5. Solution and ointment.
6. Can be fortified for use in treatment of corneal ulcers (see Table 4-3) similar to gentamicin.
7. Some microbes are becoming increasingly resistant to the use of Tobramycin due to its popularity and frequent administration as first-line drug for conjunctivitis and keratitis.
8. Dosage: 1–2 drops hourly (possibly more frequent and with parenteral fortification) in severe infections.

S. *Trimethoprim*
1. Bacteriostatic—inhibits protein synthesis.
2. Broad spectrum—gram-positive and gram-negative except *Pseudomonas aeruginosa*.
3. Solution in combination with polymyxin B (Polytrim).
4. Very well tolerated—low incidence of side effects, hypersensitivity, or resistance.
5. Polytrim is commonly prescribed for conjunctivitis in children due to trimethoprim effectiveness against *Streptococcus pneumoniae* and *Haemophilus influenzae*.

T. *Vancomycin*
1. Bactericidal—inhibits cell wall synthesis.
2. Spectrum—primarily gram-positive.
3. Particularly useful against methicillin-resistant staphylococci.
4. Also may be indicated for use against other gram-positive organisms in patients with known penicillin allergies.
5. Topical (fortified) or oral.

Table 4-7. Antibacterial Drugs for Topical Ocular Therapy

Generic Name	Trade Name (manufacturer)	Formulation	Spectrum of Activity	Adverse Reactions
Single Drugs				
Bacitracin	Bacitracin (various) AK-Tracin (Akorn)	Ointment	Staphylococci, streptococci, *Neisseria, Haemophilus*	Very rare hypersensitivity reactions
Chloramphenicol	Chloramphenicol (various) Chloroptic (Allergan) Ophthochlor (Parke-Davis) Ak-Chlor (Akorn)	Solution and ointment	Staphylococci,* streptococci, *Neisseria, Hemophulus,** gram-negative enterics*	Bone marrow depression, aplastic anemia
Chlortetracycline	Achromycin (Storz)	Ointment	Staphylococci,* streptococci,* *Haemophilus,** *Neisseria,* gram-negative enterics*	Extremely rare toxic reaction—punctate keratitis, conjunctival hyperemia, phototoxicity
Erythromycin	Erythromycin (various) AK-Mycin (Akorn)	Ointment	Staphylococci,* streptococci,* *Neisseria*	Extremely rare toxic or allergic reaction
Gentamicin	Erythromycin (various) Gentak-AK (Akorn) Genoptic (Allergan) Gentacidin (Iolab) Gentafair (Pharmafair) Garamycin (Schering)	Solution and ointment	Staphylococci,* streptococci,* *Haemophilus, Neisseria,* gram-negative enterics,* *Pseudomonas*	Transient irritation, burning, stinging superficial punctate keratitis/conjunctivitis; pseudomembranous conjunctivitis
Sulfacetamide	Sulfacetamide (various) AK-Sulf (Akorn) Bleph-10 Sulf-10 (Iolab) Sulten-10 (Bausch & Lomb)	Solution and ointment	Staphylococci,* streptococci,* *Haemophilus, Neisseria,** gram-negative enterics*	Hypersensitivity reactions—itching, hyperemia, lid edema; may include Stevens-Johnson syndrome; sulfite sensitivity, headache, blurry vision, burning sensation
Sulfisoxazole	Gantrisin (Roche)	Solution and ointment	Staphylococci,* streptococci,* *Haemophilus, Neisseria,** gram-negative enterics*	Hypersensitivity reactions—itching, hyperemia, lid edema; may include Stevens-Johnson syndrome, headache, blurry vision, burning sensation
Tetracycline	Achromycin (Lederle)	Suspension and ointment	Staphylococci,* streptococci,* *Haemophilus, Neisseria,* gram-negative enterics*	Extremely rare toxic reactions—punctate keratitis conjunctival hyperemia, phototoxicity
Tobramycin	Tobrex (Alcon)	Solution and ointment	Staphylococci,* streptococci,* *Haemophilus, Neisseria,* gram-negative enterics,* *Pseudomonas**	Transient irritation, burning, stinging, superficial punctate keratitis/conjunctivitis
Combination Drugs				
Polymyxin B/neomycin/ gramicidin	(various) Neosporin (Burroughs Wellcome) AK-Spore (Akorn) Neocidin (Major)	Solution	Broad spectrum (neomycin*)	Hypersensitivity reactions to neomycin—skin rashes, hyperemia, punctate keratitis

(continued)

Table 4-7. *Continued.*

Generic Name	Trade Name (manufacturer)	Formulation	Spectrum of Activity	Adverse Reactions
Combination Drugs				
Polymyxin B/neomycin	Statrol (Alcon)	Solution and ointment	Broad spectrum (neomycin*)	Hypersensitivity reactions to neomycin—skin rashes, hyperemia, punctate keratitis
Polymyxin B/neomycin/ bacitracin	(various) Neotricin (Bausch & Kinb) Neosporin (Burroughs Wellcome) AK-Spore (Akorn)	Ointment	Broad spectrum (neomycin*)	Hypersensitivity reactions to neomycin—skin rashes, hyperemia, punctate keratitis
Polymyxin B/bacitracin	AK-Poly-Bac (Akorn) Polysporin (Burroughs Wellcome)	Ointment	Broad spectrum	Very rare reactions
Polymyxin B/oxytetracycline	Terramycin w/Polymyxin B (Roerig)	Ointment	Broad spectrum	Very rare reactions
Trimethoprim/polymyxin B	Polytrim (Allergan)	Solution	Staphylococci, streptococci, *Haemophilus, Pseudomonas,* gram-negative enterics	Transient burning, stinging, itching, hyperemia, hypersensitivity reactions

*Significant bacterial resistance

Reprinted with permission of the author *Optometry Clinics* Vol 2:59–72.

V. **Antifungals**

    A. *General principles*

        1. Fungi are generally opportunistic infections.

        2. Therapy for fungal infections is indicated most in chronically ill or immunosuppressed patients.

        3. Generally, increased side effects due to toxicity of medications to host tissue.

        4. Most drugs need to be formulated by pharmacist.

        5. Comanagement with other health professionals (e.g., internist) is recommended when oral antifungal agents are used.

        6. Of antifungal categories, polyenes have better potency but are more toxic than imidazoles.

        7. No effect in bacterial or viral disease.

        8. Ocular penetration of topical agents is poor.

Clinical Alert

Antifungal agents have generally poor penetration topically. Debridement and/or removal of surface obstructions may be necessary to enhance the therapeutic effect of these agents.

    B. *Antifungal agents*

        1. Polyenes

           a. Amphotericin B

              (1) Alters fungal cell membrane permeability.

          (2)   0.075–0.3% solution (formulated from suspension).

          (3)   SIG: i gtt q 1 hour.

          (4)   *Side effects:* local tissue irritation, hyperemia, chemosis, keratitis, discoloration of ocular structures with prolonged use.

      b. Natamycin

          (1)   Alters fungal cell membrane permeability.

          (2)   5% suspension (commercially available as Natacyn).

          (3)   ***This is currently the only topical ophthalmic antifungal agent available commercially.***

          (4)   SIG: i gtt q 1 hour ×3 days; then i gtt q 2 hours ×4 days.

          (5)   *Side effects:* similar to amphotericin.

   2. Imidazoles

      a. Miconazole

          (1)   Alters cell membrane permeability.

          (2)   SIG: 10 mg/ml formulated.

               10 mg subconjunctival injection.

               i gtt q 1 hour topically.

      b. Ketoconazole

          (1)   Alters cell membrane permeability.

          (2)   SIG: 400 mg po.

          (3)   May be used for long-term therapy in chronic ocular infection.

          (4)   Antacids and H_2-blockers (e.g., Pepcid) reduce drug absorption.

VI. Antiparasitics

   A. *General principles*

      1. Posterior ocular infections (e.g., nematodes, protozoa) require oral therapy.

      2. Adnexal ocular infection (e.g., lice, mites) susceptible to topical therapy.

      3. Certain parasitic ocular diseases (e.g., toxoplasmosis) increasing in clinical presentation in immunosuppressed (i.e., AIDS) patients.

      4. Oral agents are quite toxic, have many potentially deleterious side effects, and should therefore be used with prudence and in conjunction with patient's general physician.

      5. Patients suspected of parasitic disease should be questioned regarding country of origin, previous travel to foreign locations, HIV risk factors.

   B. *Antiparasitic agents*

      1. Bland lubricating ointment (Lacrilube, Refresh PM)

          a. Applied liberally to lids and lashes, these agents smother parasites and inhibit reproductive cycles (e.g., use in *Demodex* and phthiriasis infection).

          b. Side effects limited to those generally associated with ocular ointment.

      2. Physostigmine (Eserine)

          a. Traditional treatment for phthiriasis.

          b. 0.25% ung SIG: Apply to lids bid ×21 days.

          c. Effectiveness thought to be related to ointment as vehicle as opposed to drug itself.

          d. Anticholinesterase—therefore side effects of miosis, accommodative spasm, hyperemia may be associated.

          e. Myokymia has also been reported in conjunction with longer-term use of this drug.

      3. Pyrimethamine (Daraprim)

          a. Inhibits essential enzyme for cell growth.

          b. Inhibition is greater for parasitic than for human cells.

          c. Synergistic effect with sulfonamides.

          d. Treatment indications—toxoplasmosis retinochoroiditis involving macula, optic nerve, or threat to vision.

e. 25 mg tablet.
f. SIG: i tab po qd-bid ×21 days.
g. Side effects
   (1) Bone marrow suppression.
   (2) Should not be used in pregnant or lactating women.

Clinical Alert

Use of pyrimethamine presents a significant risk of anemia and requires con-comitant use of folic acid to minimize the possibility of bone marrow suppres-sion. Weekly CBC and platelet counts should be obtained during therapy.

  C. *Additional drugs useful in parasitic disease*
    1. Clindamycin
      See discussion in IV. G.
    2. A discussion of antiparasitic treatment for worldwide or domestic, yet infrequently encountered, ocular parasites is outside the scope of this text's succinct format. For additional information on the diagnosis and therapeutic intervention of ocular parasites, the reader is referred to the accompanying suggested readings.

VII. Antivirals

  A. *General principles*
    Topical agents share common characteristics:
    1. Expensive.
    2. Efficacy limited to certain viral diseases (i.e., herpes simplex [HSV], varicella zoster).
    3. Can be toxic to ocular structures and therefore used only on a short-term basis.
    4. Common side effects
      a. Superficial punctate keratitis.
      b. Follicular conjunctivitis.
      c. Punctal stenosis.
      d. Hypersensitivity reactions, lid edema, redness, itching.
    5. Useful in treatment of primary epithelial keratitis where tissue damage is due to active insult by viral agents.

  B. *Antiviral agents*
    1. Topical
      a. Idoxuridine (IDU)
        (1) Drop (0.1%) and ointment (0.5%).
        (2) Least effective of topical antivirals.
        (3) Poor corneal penetration.
        (4) Less effective in presence of topical steroids.
        (5) Trade names: Herplex, Stoxil.
        (6) SIG: i gtt q 2 hours or 1/4-inch ung ribbon 5×/day for HSV keratitis.
      b. Vidarabine
        (1) Ointment only (3%).
        (2) Good choice for use after debridement.
        (3) Trade name: Vira-A.
        (4) SIG: 1/4-inch ung ribbon 5×/day for HSV keratitis.
      c. Trifluridine
        (1) Drop only (1%).
        (2) Most effective of available topical antivirals in treatment of HSV keratitis.

        (3)   Retains effective antiviral properties in presence of corticosteroids.

        (4)   Limited response, non reepithelization within 1 week suggests:

             (a)   Viral resistance.

             (b)   Misdiagnosis.

             (c)   Toxicity > therapeutic benefit.

             (d)   Questionable patient compliance.

        (5)   Trade name: Viroptic.

        (6)   SIG: i gtt q 2 hours ×7–10 days for HSV keratitis.

   2.   Oral

      a.   Acyclovir (Zovirax)

        (1)   Useful in treatment of varicella zoster ophthalmic infections.

        (2)   HSV infections?—effectiveness not yet proven.

        (3)   Relatively low toxicity.

        (4)   Side effects

             (a)   Nausea (most common).

             (b)   Other GI disturbance.

             (c)   Rash.

        (5)   Initiate within 72 hours of onset of disease for maximum effectiveness.

        (6)   SIG: 800 mg po, 5×/daily ×1 week.

      b.   Ganciclovir

        (1)   IV only.

        (2)   Treatment of cytomegalovirus retinitis (CMV).

        (3)   Side effects

             (a)   GI.

             (b)   Kidney.

             (c)   Bone marrow suppression.

        (4)   Strongly consider HIV infection in patients being treated for cyto-megalovirus infections.

      C.   3-Azidothymidine (AZT)

        (1)   Oral.

        (2)   Treatment of human immunodeficiency virus (HIV).

        (3)   Inhibits HIV ability to infect host.

        (4)   SIG: 100–200 mg po qid.

        (5)   Side effects

             (a)   GI, kidney.

             (b)   Anemia.

             (c)   Fatigue.

             (d)   Bone marrow suppression.

VIII.   Anti-Inflammatory Agents

   A.   *Nonsteroidal anti-inflammatory drugs (NSAIDs)*

      1.   General principles

        a.   Work by inhibiting prostaglandins.

        b.   Intraoperative and external ocular disease use primarily.

        c.   Topical agents—very well tolerated.

        d.   Oral agents—used as adjunct in more intense inflammatory processes.

        e.   Oral agents—GI side effects most common. Avoid or use short term and with caution in patients with GI disease or history of salicylate sensitivity. Better tolerated after meals.

        f.   Drugs (topical and oral) may only impact one of many mechanisms of inflammatory process.

        g.   Examples of NSAID use in ocular disease

             (1)   Allergic conjunctivitis (Vernal, etc.).

             (2)   Giant papillary conjunctivitis.

        (3)   Cystoid macular edema.

        (4)   Postoperative refractive surgery (e.g., radial keratotomy [RK] or photo-refractive keratotomy [PRK]).

        (5)   Uveitis as adjunctive agents.

Clinical Alert

Patients on oral nonsteroidal anti-inflammatory agents for more than 1 week should have baseline creatinine and blood urea nitrogen (BUN) to rule out rare complication of renal failure.

---

  2. Nonsteroidal agents

     a. Diclofenac (0.1%) (Voltaren)

        (1)   Solution

        (2)   Uses

            (a)   Decrease postoperative inflammation.

            (b)   Decrease pain, light sensitivity, and inflammation post-PRK.

            (c)   Adjunctive agent in treatment of cystoid macular edema (CME).

     b. Flurbiprofen (0.03%) (Ocufen)

        (1)   Solution

        (2)   Uses

            (a)   Maintain intraoperative mydriasis.

            (b)   Decrease postcataract surgery cystoid macular edema?

     c. Ketorolac (0.5%) (Acular)

        (1)   Solution

        (2)   Uses

            (a)   Decrease itching in allergic conjunctivitis (GPC?).

            (b)   Topical use for CME?

            (c)   Expense-benefit ratio?

            (d)   Stings upon instillation.

     d. Suprofen (1%) (Profenal)

        (1)   Solution

        (2)   Uses

            (a)   Inhibits intraoperative miosis

            (b)   Allergic and giant papillary conjunctivitis

 B. *Corticosteroids*

  1. General principles

     a. Corticosteroid agents inhibit inflammation in a nonspecific manner.

     b. Decrease of inflammatory reaction may mask persistent infectious process in patients on steroid therapy.

     c. To avoid "rebound effect," steroids should be tapered upon discontinuation.

     d. Tapering allows body's own circulating corticosteroids to achieve homeostatic level.

     e. Oral steroids should be used with knowledge of patient's general physician.

     f. Most common ocular side effects:

        (1)   Topical

            (a)   Increased IOP (duration, potency of drug related). Higher incidence of "steroid responders" in glaucoma patients.

        (2)   Oral

            (a)   Posterior subcapsular cataract (long term therapy).

     g. Contraindicated in HSV, fungal disease during active infection.

      h. Beneficial in infectious processes where damage to ocular structures from inflammatory process may exceed morbidity associated with the infectious agent.

      i. Selection of drug depends on many factors:

        (1) Cause of inflammation.

        (2) Intensity of inflammation.

        (3) Location of insult.

        (4) Expected treatment time course.

        (5) Patient's concomitant ocular and systemic health.

Clinical Alert

Options to consider when patients on topical corticosteroid therapy present with increased IOP:

Rule out	Secondary to underlying disease
	Other glaucomatous cause (check IOP and evaluate fellow eye)
Monitor	Without change of medication (if higher IOP is able to be sufficiently tolerated)
Add	β-Blocker ± carbonic anhydrase inhibitor
Decrease	Frequency of steroid use (taper)
Change to	Alternate steroid with less IOP-raising tendency (e.g., fluorometholone)
NOTE:	If IOP is increased, avoid pilocarpine and other cholinergic agents in presence of active inflammation.

Status of a patient's optic nerve and thus its predicted ability to withstand increased IOP may influence clinical choice of above options.

---

  2. Topical corticosteroids (in order of increasing potency)

    a. Hydrocortisone

      Weak corticosteroid best used for external ocular inflammation (e.g., dermatologic and lid disorders)

      (1) Available in suspension combinations

        (a) 0.5% hydrocortisone + 0.25% chloramphenicol suspension.

        (b) 1% hydrocortisone + 0.35% neomycin + 10,000 units polymyxin B suspension (e.g., Cortisporin).

        (c) 1.5% hydrocortisone + 0.35% neomycin suspension (e.g., Ak-Neo-Cort).

        (d) 1.5% hydrocortisone + 0.5% oxytetracycline suspension (e.g., terracortril).

      (2) Available in combination ointments

        (a) 0.5% hydrocortisone + 1% chloramphenicol + 10,000 units polymyxin B B/sulfate (e.g., Ophthocort).

        (b) 1% hydrocortisone + 0.5% neomycin sulfate + 400 units bacitracin zinc + 10,000 units polymyxin B sulfate (e.g., Coracin).

      (3) Available over the counter:

        0.5% and 1% hydrocortisone cream (Cortaid).

    b. Medrysone 1% (e.g., HMS)

      (1) Suspension.

      (2) Weak anti-inflammatory properties.

      (3) Best used for mild external eye disorders (e.g., pingueculitis).

      (4) Less potency and penetration increase safety and decrease potential risks associated with topical use of other agents.

c.   Prednisolone (0.12%–1%)
    (1)   Solution—phosphate base (e.g., Inflamase Forte).
    (2)   Suspension—acetate base (e.g., Pred Forte).
    (3)   Moderate anti-inflammatory property with excellent penetration (acetate).
    (4)   Drug of choice for active anterior uveitis and many other intraocular inflammatory conditions.
    (5)   Available in combinations. Combination corticosteroid-antibiotic formulations clinically efficacious when inflammation exists and there is risk of concomitant bacterial infection.
        (a)   0.2%–0.25% prednisolone acetate + 10% sodium sulfacetamide
            i.   Suspension (e.g., "Blephamide" or "Cetapred").
            ii.   Ointment (e.g., "Blephamide" or "Cetapred").
        (b)   0.5% prednisolone acetate + 10% sodium sulfactamide
            i.   Suspension (e.g., Ak-cide).
            ii.   Ointment (e.g., Metimyd).
        (c)   0.25%–0.5% prednisolone phosphate + 10% sodium sulfacetamide
            Solution and ointment (e.g., Vasocidin).
        (d)   1% prednisolone acetate + 0.30% gentamicin sulfate
            Suspension (e.g., Pred G).
        (e)   0.6% prednisolone acetate + 0.3% gentamicine sulfate
            Ointment (e.g., Pred G).
        (f)   0.5% prednisolone acetate + neomycin sulfate + 10,000 units polymyxin B sulfate
            i.   Suspension (Poly-Pred).
        (g)   Other combination drugs
            0.25% prednisolone acetate + 1% atropine (e.g., Mydraped)
            i.   Limited use due to low concentration of corticosteroid with strong cycloplegic agent.
            ii.   Alternative choices may be more appropriate for treatment of anterior segment inflammation.

d.   Dexamethasone
    (1)   Suspension 0.1% (e.g., Maxidex).
    (2)   Solution 0.1% (e.g., Ak-Dex).
    (3)   Ointment 0.05% (e.g., dexamethasone phosphate [Decadron]).
    (4)   More potent than prednisolone in equal amounts.
    (5)   Available in much lower concentrations ophthalmically.
    (6)   Increased risk of IOP elevation.
    (7)   Best concentration depends on site and extent of inflammation.
    (8)   Available combinations
        (a)   0.1% dexamethasone phosphate + neomycin sulfate
            Solution and ointment (e.g., Neo-decadron).
        (b)   0.1% dexamethasone + neomycin sulfate + 10,000 units polmyxin B sulfate
            Suspension and ointment (e.g., Dexacidin).
        (c)   0.1% dexamethasone + 0.3% tobramycin
            Suspension and ointment (e.g., Tobradex).

6.   Fluorometholone (0.1%, 0.25%)
    a.   Most potent anti-inflammatory ophthalmic corticosteroid.
    b.   Poor penetration.
    c.   Good for external ocular inflammation not requiring good corneal drug penetration.
    d.   Higher concentration recommended for intraocular treatment.
    e.   Good choice for ocular disease requiring chronic therapy.

  f. Less likely to induce IOP rise.

   (1) Suspension

    (a) Fluorometholone alcohol.

    (b) 0.1% (Fluor-OP).

    (c) 0.25% (FML-Forte).

   (2) Ointment

    0.1% FML S.O.P.

   (3) Solution

    (a) 0.1% fluorometholone acetate (e.g., Flarex).

    (b) Better penetration than alcohol base (IOP risk?).

  g. Available in combination

   (1) Suspension

    (a) 0.1% fluorometholone alcohol + 10% sodium sulfacetamide (e.g., FML-S).

Clinical Alert

Factors affecting clinical anti-inflammatory effectiveness of topical steroids
Potency of corticosteroid
Concentration of corticosteroid
Penetration characteristics
 Acetate (best)
 Alcohol
 Phosphate (worst)
Rate of drug elimination
High concentration of high-potency corticosteroid with acetate base and slow body elimination should have most effective anti-inflammatory properties.

IX. Drugs That Affect Intraocular Pressure

 A. *General principles*

  1. Drugs (topical and oral) that lower intraocular pressure (IOP) have generally been thought to be synonymous with glaucoma therapy. Although treatment of elevated IOP associated with glaucoma remains the most common indication for these agents, there are other clinical indications in which the effects of IOP-reducing agents may be beneficial. For example:

   a. Corneal edema associated with Fuchs' dystrophy.

   b. Wound leaks.

   c. Post cataract surgery IOP elevation.

   d. Post laser (Yag, ALT) IOP elevation.

   e. Retinal venous occlusive disease.

   f. Cystoid macular edema.

  2. IOP is maintained by a delicate balance between inflow (production in the ciliary processes of the ciliary body) and outflow (filtration through trabecular meshwork). Topical and oral agents that lower IOP act predominantly on one of these systems. The most significant IOP lowering is experienced when an aqueous inhibitor is combined with an outflow facilitator.

  3. Drugs in this category have more common ocular and systemic side effects than any other frequently prescribed ophthalmic medications. The combination of high cost, increased side effects, and less patient benefit recognition can pose compliance problems in patients, particularly observable in ocular diseases such as glaucoma.

B. *Ocular agents: Nonselective β-blockers*
  1. Action
     Blockage of β_1 (heart) and β_2 (lung) receptors. Reduce aqueous production.
  2. Side effects
     a. Lowering of IOP.
     b. Bronchospasm.
     c. Localized allergic hypersensitivity characterized by dermatitis, blepharoconjunctivitis.
     d. Superficial punctate keratitis.
     e. Bradycardia, hypotension.
     f. Mental confusion, hallucinations.
     g. Dizziness, headache.
     h. Depression (probably underdiagnosed).
     i. Chronic sinusitis.
     j. Fatigue, malaise.
     k. Loss of libido, impotence in males.
     l. Blurred vision.
     m. GI effects.
  3. Agents
     a. Timolol maleate (Timoptic).
        (1) 0.25% solution: powder blue cap.
        (2) 0.50% solution: yellow cap.
        (3) 0.25%, 0.50% preservative free, single vials Ocudose.
        (4) 0.25%, 0.50% once a day therapy Timoptic XE.
        (5) SIG: i gtt q 12 hours.
        (6) Most clinically evaluated of β-blockers due to being first approved.
        (7) Avoid in pregnant or lactating women.
        (8) Commercially available dropper yields less oversupply to cul-de-sac.

Clinical Alert

Topical β-blockers can cause significant and potentially life-threatening cardiovascular complications. It is prudent to check pulse and blood pressure prior to initiating these medications. A pretreatment pulse of <60 beats/min should suggest alternative therapy.

---

     b. Levobunolol (Betagan)
        (1) 0.25% solution: powder blue cap.
        (2) 0.50% solution: yellow cap.
        (3) SIG: i gtt qd or q 12 hours.
        (4) Available with compliance C-cap.
        (5) Longer half-life allows some use on once-a-day therapy.
        (6) IOP reduction comparable to Timolol when used q 12 hours.
     c. Carteolol (Ocupress)
        (1) 1% solution: clear cap.
        (2) SIG: i gtt q 12 hours.
        (3) Fewer cardiovascular side effects due to intrinsic sympathomimetic activity?
     d. Metipranolol (OptiPranolol)
        (1) 0.3% solution.
        (2) SIG: i gtt q 12 hours.
        (3) IOP reduction comparable to other nonselective β-blockers?
        (4) Most cost-friendly to patients (improved compliance?)

C. *Ocular agents: Selective β-blockers*
1. Action
    Block β_1 receptors (heart) selectively with little or no affinity for β_2 receptors (lungs). Reduce aqueous production.
2. Side effects
    Same as non-selective β-blockers, but much safer and better tolerated by patients with a history of asthma or chronic obstructive pulmonary disease (COPD).
3. Betaxolol (Betoptic, Betoptic-S)
    a. 0.25% suspension (Betoptic-S): powder blue cap.
    b. 0.5% solution (Betoptic): navy blue cap.
    c. SIG: i gtt q 12 hours.
    d. Both formulations are clinically equal in IOP lowering effect.
    e. Betoptic-S stings less and requires less drug chemically to maintain therapeutic effect.
    f. Safer for patients with lung disease, but risk *not* completely eliminated.
    g. Less effective in black patients.
    h. Less IOP reduction than nonselective β-blockers.
    i. β_1-selective, but less cardiovascular effect due to less potency, i.e., receptor affinity.

D. *Ocular agents: Adrenergic agents*
1. Action
    Predominantly increase facility of outflow. Very limited effect on aqueous production.
2. Side effects
    Dilate pupil and vasoconstrict blood vessels.
    a. Reduction of IOP.
    b. Stinging, burning upon instillation.
    c. Local allergy characterized by dermatitis; blepharoconjunctivitis.
    d. Adrenochrome conjunctival deposits.
    e. Discoloration of contact lenses.
    f. Tachycardia, arrythmias.
    g. Hypertension.
    h. Irritability.
    i. Rebound conjunctival hyperemia (vasodilation usually observed at midpoint of day between therapy).
    j. Follicular conjunctivitis.
    k. Aphakic/pseudophakic can get epinephrine maculopathy (CME)—90% resolution with discontinuation.
    l. Angle closure glaucoma.
    m. Blurred vision.
    n. Halos, photophobia.
    o. Xerostomia (dry mouth).
3. Agents
    a. Epinephrine
        (1) Bitartrate 2% solution (Epitrate).
        (2) Borate (0.5%, 1.2%) solution (Eppy N).
        (3) Hydrochloride solution (0.1%, 0.25%, 0.5%, 1%, 2%) (Glaucon).
        (4) SIG: i gtt q 12 hours.
        (5) Also available in combination with pilocarpine, e.g., E-Pilo 1 (see discussion under IX.F.2.).
        (6) To minimize side effects and enhance effectiveness, prodrug Dipivalyl is preferred agent.
        (7) Relatively low cost compared to prodrug Propine.
    b. Dipivalyl epinephrine (Propine)
        (1) 0.1% solution.

(2) SIG: i gtt q 12 hours.
    (a) Improved corneal permeability.
    (b) Inactive until reaches anterior chamber.
    (c) Primary IOP effect—increases outflow.
    (d) Most frequent side effects are local (stinging, burning, glare, halos—from mild pupillary dilation).
    (e) Long-term therapy can result in midday conjunctival vasodilation.
    (f) Follicular conjunctivitis (toxic).
    (g) As with all drops, use punctual occlusion or 1–2 minute eyelid closure in patients at risk for systemic effects or substitute alternate therapy.
    (h) Avoid or use with caution: patients on tricyclic antidepressants and/or monamine oxidase inhibitors.
    (i) IOP decreases less than with cholinergics or β-blockers. Best used as additive with other glaucoma therapy, although gives better IOP reduction alone than in combination.
    (j) Epinephrine maculopathy—reversible in most cases. Observed particularly in aphakes or pseudophakes with defect in posterior capsule.

Clinical Alert

"My eyes are red . . . ."
Long-term epinephrine users may develop a dependency on the vasoconstrictive action of epinephrine. Chronic redness should be evaluated by the clinician. It is essential to ask *when* the eyes become red.
    Transient injection (accompanying, or seconds after instillation).
        Associated with local irritation = normal.
    Injection (lasting minutes after instillation).
        Allergic = discontinue.
    Injection (hours after instillation).
        Rebound effect: vasodilation will usually be eliminated by therapy at end of day—may indicate need to discontinue drug. Watch for other toxic-associated effects.

Clinical Alert

"But Doctor, it says I can't use this if I have glaucoma. . . ."
Over-the-counter sympathomimetic agents for mild ocular irritation or nasal congestion warn patients of contraindications in the presence of glaucoma. Patients with open angles are not at elevated risk with these agents. Adrenergic mydriasis and iris-angle blockage could, in rare cases, precipitate angle closure, which is the reason for the cautionary message. Most patients should be reassured, yet those potentially at risk should have gonioscopy performed and cautioned appropriately.

---

c. α-Agonists: apraclonidine HCl (Iopidine)
    (1) 1% ml units preservative free.
    (2) 0.05% SIG: i gtt tid.
    (3) Inhibits aqueous formation to lower IOP.
    (4) Side effects
        (a) Conjunctival blanching.
        (b) Mydriasis.

               (c) Lid retraction.

               (d) tachyphylaxis.

(5) Uses

      (a) Pre/post argon laser trabeculoplasty and peripheral iridotomy.

      (b) Primary open angle glaucoma.

      (c) Adjunctive in treatment of acute angle closure glaucoma.

(6) For chronic open angle glaucoma, may be best used to decrease IOP short term in preparation for trabeculectomy.

(7) Tolerance to this drug develops after short-term use.

(8) Very expensive.

(9) Approved in open angle glaucoma treatment on short-term (90-day) basis.

E. *Ocular agents: Cholinergic agents*

1. Actions

    a. Increase outflow through pull on scleral spur via longitudinal muscle fibers of ciliary body.

    b. Net effect: widens trabecular meshwork.

    c. Constricts pupil (miosis) through pupillary sphincter receptors.

    d. Stimulates accommodative spasm via ciliary body.

2. Side effects

    a. Ocular pain/asthenopia/headache. Usually transient and improves with time.

    b. Blurred vision due to spasm of accommodation (especially problematic in young patients).

    c. Miosis which restricts vision at night or in poor contrast situations (rain, fog, etc.).

    d. Deleterious vision effects occur particularly when patients have central posterior subcapsular or nuclear sclerotic cataracts.

    e. Stinging, burning upon instillation.

    f. Conjunctival injection and congestion.

    g. GI upset—cholinergic effects increase gastric motility, may cause nausea and vomiting.

    h. Sweating.

    i. Increased salivation.

    j. Other ocular: retinal detachment, cataract.

3. Topical cholinergic agents

    a. Pilocarpine topical (1/4%, 1/2%, 1–6%, 8%, 10%) solution; 4% gel (ointment), P-20, P-40 timed release Ocusert.

      (1) SIG: i gtt qid (may have efficacy bid with punctal occlusion).

      (2) Treatment of open angle glaucoma.

      (3) Recommended starting dose:

          (a) 1% qid (blue irides patients).

          (b) 2% qid (brown irides patients).

          (c) Concentrations above 4% are seldom useful clinically except in black patients.

      (4) All patients initiating this drug should be warned of side effects and their alleviation with time. Headache, ocular pain worse within first 5–7 days. Consider short-term concomitant oral pain medications for patients contemplating pilocarpine discontinuation due to ocular pain and headache; e.g.:

          (a) Ibuprofen 400 mg q 6 hours (Motrin).

          (b) Ketorolac 10 mg tid (Toradol).

      (5) Hypotensive effect less predictable in angle recession patients.

      (6) Use with caution in:

          (a) Myopes: pilocarpine may precipitate retinal detachment especially in presence of peripheral retinal breaks.

          (b) Narrow angle patients: miotic effect can increase chance of relative or absolute pupillary block.

        (c)   Active inflammation: cholinergics exacerbate inflammation and worsen patient comfort.

b.   Pilocarpine 4% gel (Pilopine)
   (1)   SIG: 1/4-inch ribbon qhs.
   (2)   Better tolerated by younger patients —less intense side effects.
   (3)   Diurnal control?

c.   Ocusert (Pilo-20, Pilo-40)
   (1)   SIG: i membrane q 5–7 days.
   (2)   P-20 equivalent to Pilocarpine 1%–2%.
   (3)   P-40 equivalent to Pilocarpine 4%.
   (4)   Better tolerated by younger patients—less intense cholinergic side effects.
   (5)   Must be refrigerated.
   (6)   Other side effects and factors to consider:
        (a)   Cost: more expensive.
        (b)   Retention: more difficult at night.
        (c)   Foreign body sensation—adaptation period similar to contact lenses.
        (d)   Patient dexterity?
        (e)   Better compliance if successfully inserted/tolerated.

Clinical Alert

Patients on pilocarpine therapy can develop pupillary seclusion in the presence of anterior uveitis. Whether iritis exists post argon laser treatment or from other causes of uveitis, the miotic pupil can become bound down to the anterior lens surface (posterior synechiae). Patients, in these situations, who are poorly compliant with topical corticosteroid use are particularly at risk for the development of pupillary block glaucoma.

---

d.   Carbachol (0.75%, 1.5%, 2.25%, 3% solution)
   (1)   SIG: i gtt tid-qid.
   (2)   Direct- and indirect-acting miotic.
   (3)   Longer acting than pilocarpine, thus tid dosage.
   (4)   Available as intraoperative agent (Miostat by Alcon) to close pupil and lower IOP after cataract surgery.

e.   Echothiophate iodide (0.03%, 0.06%, 0.125%, 0.25%) solution (phospholine iodide)
   (1)   SIG: i gtt qhs-bid.
   (2)   Indirect-acting cholinergic agent.
   (3)   Inhibits cholinesterase action, thus potentiating acetylcholine effects. Results in miosis, IOP reduction through increased aqueous outflow.
   (4)   Used when pilocarpine 4% or carbachol 3% not effective.
   (5)   Other side effects: similar to pilocarpine yet more frequent and generally more severe.
   (6)   Additional side effects
        (a)   Iris cysts—reversible upon discontinuation of therapy. Greater in children than adults.
        (b)   Cataracts—greater in adults than children.
        (c)   Vitreoretinal disease—increased risk of tractional detachment or vitropathies.
        (d)   Systemic—GI, respiratory, and glandular (alert anesthesia before any general anesthetic is used).
        (e)   Avoid use in patients with active anterior uveitis—exacerbation of inflammation and patient discomfort.
        (f)   Myasthenia gravis—potential drug interactions and summation.

Clinical Alert

2.5% phenylephrine used concomitantly with anticholinergic agents (echo-thiophage iodide) is effective in retarding iris cyst development.

F. *Other clinical indications for cholinergic agents*
1. Accommodative esotropia—cholinergic agents decrease accommodation/convergence (AC/A) ratios. Can be used diagnostically or therapeutically. Typically long-acting indirect agent (e.g., echothiophate iodide 0.125% qd) is preferred.
2. Anisocoria—diluted pilocarpine used to demonstrate denervation hypersensitivity diagnostically. Pilocarpine 1/2% may be used in affected eye to minimize anisocoric visual or cosmetic side effects in patients with Adie's pupil.
3. Post refractive surgery
    a. Patients with small diameter optic zones with complaints of star burst or glare from radial keratotomy incisions.
    b. Occasionally used to lower IOP in an attempt to decrease effect in overcorrected patients.
    c. Low % pilocarpine may assist visual functioning of overcorrected patients in selected situations.

G. *Oral agents: Carbonic anhydrase inhibitors*
1. Action
    Reduce aqueous production in ciliary processes.
2. Side effects
    a. Numerous clinically observable.
        (1) 30–50% of patients are intolerant to CAIs and will need to discontinue therapy.
    b. Frequent
        (1) CNS—depression, confusion.
        (2) Gastrointestinal—cramping, nausea, diarrhea.
        (3) Increased urination.
        (4) Numbness (paresthesia) in fingers and toes.
        (5) Decreased libido.
        (6) Weight loss.
        (7) Transient myopia—acetazolamide.
        (8) Renal stones—especially acetazolamide.
        (9) Aplastic anemia and other blood dyscrasias—can result in death.
        (10) Most frequent side effects due to electrolyte depletion and acidosis as result of bicarbonate. All patients on carbonic anhydrase inhibitors should increase intake of potassium (bananas, diet cola).

Clinical Alert

Avoid the use of carbonic anhydrase inhibiting agents in patients with sulfa sensitivities (allergic history, previous side effects, etc.). Both Diamox and Neptazane are sulfonamides.

---

3. Cautions
    a. Do not use if:
        (1) Pregnant or nursing mother.
        (2) Allergy to sulfa.
        (3) History of kidney stones.
        (4) Severe lung problems.
        (5) Liver disease (e.g., cirrhosis).

b. Use with caution if:
   (1) Hypertensive medications include diuretics.
   (2) Diabetic.
4. Drug interactions
  Digitalis.

Clinical Alert

Due to the potential risk of blood dyscrasias, including aplastic anemia, patients must be questioned appropriately for suggestive signs or symptoms (e.g., ecchymosis, weight loss, diarrhea, fever, malaise). A CBC and consultation with the patient's general physician is indicated if the history or physical signs are suggestive.

---

5. Agents
  a. Acetazolamide (Diamox) 125, 250 mg tabs, 500 mg sequel
    (1) SIG: i tab po qd-qid OR 1 sequel qd-bid.
    (2) Maximum effective dosage—1 g/day.
    (3) Side effects increase at greater doses.
    (4) Most potent ocular hypotensive carbonic anhydrase inhibitor.
    (5) More frequent side effects than methazolamide (Neptazane)
      (a) Kidney stones.
      (b) Paresthesia of extremities.
      (c) Mental confusion.
      (d) Malaise.
    (6) Uses
      (a) Chronic open angle glaucoma.
      (b) Acute angle closure glaucoma.
      (c) Decrease IOP associated with hyphema.
      (d) Cystoid macular edema.
      (e) Postsurgical elevated IOP.
    (7) Start therapy 250 mg bid and adjust accordingly to a maximum of 1 g/day.
    (8) Side effects are dose related.
    (9) IOP reduction usually occurs early.
    (10) Side effects may present early or late.
    (11) Monitor CBC, electrolytes depending on area standard of care.
  b. Methazolamide (Neptazane) 25, 50 mg tabs
    (1) SIG: 1 tab po bid-tid.
    (2) Maximum clinical dose 150 mg/day.
    (3) Safer for patients with kidney stones.
    (4) Fewer side effects than acetazolamide (see IX.G.2 and IX.G.5.a).
    (5) Slightly less hypotensive effect clinically.

Clinical Alert

Management options if side effects occur with carbonic anhydrase inhibitors.
Discontinue therapy—try alternate class of IOP-lowering drug, laser, or filter.
Reduce dosage (e.g., Diamox 250 mg po bid—reduce to 125 mg tab po bid).
Switch to other carbonic anhydrase inhibitor (acetazolamide to methazolamide or visa versa).
Use concomitant therapy (e.g., oral potassium supplements).
No change in medication—monitor side effects. Some side effects improve with time (e.g., mild paresthesia, frequent urination).

X.   Hyperosmotic Agents

A.   *General principles*

1. Reduce corneal edema by creating osmolarity gradient which draws water from cornea into the tear film.
2. Topically, an adjunct in the treatment of anterior corneal edema in ocular problems such as:
   a. Fuchs' endothelial dystrophy.
   b. Recurrent corneal erosion.
   c. Pseudophakic bullous keratopathy.
3. Show limited therapeutic benefit in the management of posterior stromal or (deep corneal) edema.
4. Some agents are helpful in the medical and diagnostic management of corneal edema and elevated IOP secondary to acute angle closure glaucoma.

B.   *Hyperosmotic agents for topical management of ocular diseases causing mild to moderate corneal edema. (These are available over the counter)*

1. 2% sodium chloride (NaCl) solution
   Adsorbonac or Muro 128. SIG: i gtt qid/prn.
2. 5% sodium chloride (NaCl) solution.
   Adsorbonac or Muro 128. SIG: i gtt qid/prn.
3. 5% sodium chloride ointment.
   AK-NaCl or Muro 128. SIG: instill qhs.

C.   *Agents for topical management of corneal edema to allow adequate visualization of internal structures of the eye.*

1. Glycerin solution

Clinical Alert

Topical glycerin causes significant ocular irritation upon instillation and should be preceded by topical anesthesia.

---

2. Action: osmolarity difference induces short-term resolution of corneal edema. Clinically helpful in gonioscopic evaluation. E.g., differentiation of acute angle closure versus neovascular glaucoma also allows internal evaluation of ocular structures.

D.   *Agents for oral management of acutely elevated IOP*

1. Glycerin (Osmoglyn). Dosage 2–3 ml/kg.
2. Isosorbide (Ismotic). Dosage 1–3 g/kg.
3. Isosorbide is nonmetabolized and therefore is the drug of choice for diabetic patients.

Practical Clinical Rule of Thumb for Administration of Oral Hyperosmotics for All Diabetics and Whenever Possible in All Patients—Use Isosorbide

Patient Weight (lb)	Dosage
<100	³/₄ bottle over ice
150	1 bottle over ice
250	1¹/₂ bottles over ice
300+	2 bottles over ice

Note: One bottle contains 220 ml of 40% solution isosorbide or 50% solution glycerin.

4. Actions
   a. Reduction of IOP as a result of creating an osmolar gradient in the blood-stream. Clinical reductions of IOP are evident, on average, within 30–60 minutes.
   b. Both of these agents should be swallowed within a short time period. A "cocktail" over crushed ice sipped alone or through a straw helps palatability.
5. Side effects: nausea and vomiting, which may inhibit successful action of the agent. Both agents should be used cautiously or avoided in patients suffering from dehydration. Due to the displeasing taste and high incidence of nausea associated with these agents, some practitioners may pretreat patients with antiemetic orals or suppositories. E.g., promethazine (Phenergan) 25 mg po; prochlorperazine (Compazine) 5 mg po.

E. *Intravenous management of elevated IOP*
   1. Mannitol 5%, 10%, 15%, 20%, 25%. Various suppliers.
   2. Action: Essentially nonmetabolized agent which creates osmolar gradient and subsequent diuresis.
   3. Side effects: Same as prescribed for oral hyperosmotic agents, plus possibility of adverse effect in patients with known cardiovascular, cerebral, or kidney disease.

XI. Ocular Lubricants

A. *Clinical uses*
   1. Reduce symptomatic discomfort associated with ocular surface irritation.
   2. Stabilize, or enhance, precorneal tear film.
   3. Protect, or prevent, ocular surface damage (as in recurrent corneal erosion).
   4. Adjunct to ocular defense mechanism through washout or dilution of surface antigens.

B. *General principles*
   1. Whenever possible, use nonpreserved solutions.
   2. Match severity of ocular problem with appropriate choice of ocular lubricant (Table 4-8).

Table 4-8 Considerations in Clinical Use of Ocular Lubrication

Sign	Symptoms	Staining Pattern	Recommended Agents
Conjunctival dryness/ irritation	Mild/transient— situational	+Fl stain	Low-viscosity lubricants qid/prn (e.g., polyvinyl alcohol)
Mild corneal disruption (superficial punctate keratitis; SPK)	Mild/occasional— exacerbated in certain situations	+Fl	Low-moderate viscosity lubricants qid/prn preferably without preservatives (e.g., hydroxy propyl or low % carboxyl methyl cellulose)
Moderate/severe corneal disruption (SPK-confluent SPK patches)	Mild/moderate Chronic	+Fl +RB	Higher-viscosity agents (e.g., carboxymethyl cellulose) q 2 hours prn + punctal occlusion
Severe corneal disruption (geographic epithelial breakdown)	Severe/chronic	Heavy sodium fluorescein (Fl) and rose bengal (RB)	High-viscosity agents q 30 minutes prn + punctal occlusion + ocular ointment preparations + adjunctive agent considerations

3. Identify "root cause" of ocular problem. Lubricants are an adjunct once the root cause or causes have been identified and, whenever possible, eliminated.

C. *Effective selective adjuncts to be used in combination with ocular lubricants for ocular surface disorders*
1. Elimination of contributing problems! E.g.:
    a. Blepharitis: lid scrubs ± antibiotic ointment.
    b. Meibomianitis: tetracycline 250 mg po qid ×21 days.
    c. Exposure (e.g., thyroid eye disease): lateral tarsal sling or tarsorrhaphy or appropriate oculoplastics procedure.
2. Also consider when efficacious:
    a. Mucomyst—5%–10% acetylcysteine.
    b. Alternative systemic medications.
    c. Permanent punctal occlusion.
    d. Sodium hyaluronidase (Healon).
    e. Homeopathic agents (Similasan).
    f. Lacriserts.
    g. Spectacle side shields/goggles—moisture chamber.
    h. Environmental modifications—humidifiers.
    i. Vitamin A?

D. *Selected ocular lubricant agents*
1. With preservative
   Hypotears: polyvinyl alcohol 1% (PVA) + polyethylene glycol 400.
   Tears Naturale II: hydroxypropyl methyl cellulose 0.3% + dextran 70 0.1%.
2. Without preservative
   Dry Eye Therapy: glycerin 0.3%.
   Hypotears PF: polyvinyl alcohol 1% + polyethylene glycol 400.
   Refresh Plus (Cellufresh): caboxymethyl cellulose 0.5%.
   AquaSite: polyethylene glycol 400 0.2% + dextran 70 0.1%.
   Celluvisc: carboxymethyl cellulose 1.0%.
   BION Tears: hydroxypropyl methyl cellulose 0.3% + dextran 70 0.1%.
3. Ointments
    a. With preservative
       Lacrilube S.O.P.: 42.5% mineral oil, 55% white petrolatum, lanolin alcohol and chlorobutanol.
    b. Without Preservative
       Refresh PM: 41.4% mineral oil, 55% white petrolatum, petrolatum, lanolin alcohol.

E. *Clinical considerations when utilizing lubricants*
1. Identify root cause or causes (eliminate or modify whenever possible).
2. Select *proper* lubricating agent.
3. Select appropriate instillation *frequency.*
4. Add/consider other effective adjuncts.
5. Work with patient to tailor therapy (modify agents/treatment until best agent or combination is found).
6. Stress control, not cure.
7. Follow-up visits to ensure maintenance.

XII. Anti-Allergy

A. *General principles*
1. Body mounts immune response that exceeds the damage potential of the offending (usually innocuous) antigen. Requires sensitization event.
2. Hallmark symptoms of allergy = itching.

3. Other signs of ocular allergy:
   a. Conjunctival infection = usually pink.
   b. Conjunctival chemosis.
   c. Lid swelling—lacrimation and mucoid discharge.
4. Asthma, rhinitis may also be present as systemic indicators of allergy.
5. Prevalence of systemic allergy in general population is high, with ocular involvement most prevalent in teenagers.
6. Course of disease generally exhibits remissions and exacerbations—often seasonal.
7. Mast cell degranulation accounts for release of mediators of inflammation, specifically histamine, serotonin, leukotrienes, and prostaglandins.
8. Mast cells found in large numbers in lid conjunctiva, limbal and episcleral vasculature, and uvea.
9. Giemsa smear shows presence of eosinophils.
10. Immune response reactions of importance in ocular allergy.
    a. Type I immediate—response well to antihistamine or mast cell stabilization therapy, e.g., vernal conjunctivitis.
    b. Type IV cell-mediated or delayed, e.g., contact dermatitis. Onset of symptoms 12–24 hours; responds well to elimination of offending antigen plus nonspecific anti-inflammatory treatment.

B. *Pharmacologic management of ocular allergy*
   1. Avoidance
      Treatment of symptoms associated with ocular allergy should be preceded by determination of antigen and, whenever possible, elimination of contact with antigenic substance.
   2. Supportive
      a. Cold compress: local vasoconstriction decreases permeability. Coolness also contributes to reducing symptoms of itching and controls edema.
   3. Topical
      a. Artificial tear or lubricant solutions assist washout of antigenic substance.
      b. Should use preservative-free lubricants, e.g., HypoTears P.F., Cellufresh, to avoid a complicating preservative hypersensitivity.
   4. Astringents
      Rose petal extract Estivin available over the counter for relief of mild allergic symptoms.
   5. Vasoconstrictive agents
      Local blood vessel constriction decreases permeability of vasculature to products of mass cell degranulation. Symptomatic relief through decongestants, phenylephrine, oxymetazoline, tetrahydrozoline, naphazoline. Available in many over-the-counter solutions.
      a. Naphazoline (0.012% to 0.02%)
         (1) Allerest.
         (2) Degest 2.
         (3) Vasoclear.
      b. Oxymetazoline (0.25%)
         (1) Ocuclear.
      c. Tetrahydrozoline (0.05%)
         (1) Murine Plus.
         (2) Visine.
      d. Phenylephrine (0.12%)
         (1) Relief.
         (2) Prefrin.
      e. Longest-lasting over-the-counter: Ocuclear (oxymetazoline 0.25%).

Table 4-9. Antihistamine-Decongestant Combinations

Trade Name (manufacturer)	Composition	Concentration (%)
Albalon-A (Allergan)	Antazoline phosphate Naphazoline HCl	0.5 0.05
Vasocon-A (Iolab)	Antazoline phosphate Naphazoline HCl	0.5 0.05
Naphcon-A (Alcon)	Pheniramine maleate Naphazoline HCl	0.3 0.025
Prefrin-A (Allergan)	Pyrilamine maleate Phenylephrine HCl	0.1 0.12
AK-Vernacon (Akorn)	Pheniramine maleate Phenylephrine HCl	0.5 0.125
AK-Con-A (Akorn)	Pheniramine maleate Naphazoline HCl	0.3 0.025
Muro's Opcon-A (Bausch & Lomb)	Pheniramine maleate Naphazoline HCl	0.3 0.025

Recommended dosage for all these preparations is 1–2 drops/eye q 3–4 hours or less to relieve discomfort. From Bartlett & Jannus. *Clinical Ocular Pharmacology,* 2nd ed. Stoneham, Mass: Butterworth, 1989:319.

6. Vasoconstrictive agents + zinc sulfate
    a. Vasoclear A: naphazoline 0.02% + $ZnSO_4$ 0.25.
    b. Zincfrin: phenylephrine 0.12% + $ZnSO_4$ 0.25.
    c. These over-the-counter agents combine vasoconstrictive benefits of sympathomimetics with astringent affects of zinc as an adjunct to lessen itching and mucus production.
7. Vasoconstrictive agents + antihistamines
    a. Enhanced symptomatic relief is afforded with addition of antihistamines to ocular decongestants (Table 4-9):
        (1) Pheniramine maleate (0.3%) (Naphcon-A Ophthalmic Solution).
        (2) Antazoline phosphate (0.5%) (Vasocon-A).
        (3) Pyrilamine maleate (0.1%) (Prefrin-A).
        (4) SIG: i gtt q 3–4 hours.
    b. Topical ocular antihistamines are H_1-blockers that competitively block histamine effects by binding to receptor sites, blood vessels, and nerves. H_1-receptor sites cause itching when stimulated. H_2-receptor sites when stimulated result in vasodilation. There are no ocular preparations available which are H_2-blockers.

Clinical Alert

Vasoconstrictive agents are α-agonists and therefore may also mildly dilate the pupil. The risk of precipitating angle closure is small, yet patients at risk should have gonioscopy performed prior to prescribing these agents.

---

8. Topical antihistamines
    a. H_1-blocker with additional benefit of vasoconstrictive properties.
    b. Levocabastine (0.05%) (Livostin)
        (1) Approved for use for signs and symptoms of allergic conjunctivitis.

      (2) Suspension.

      (3) Not to be used with contact lenses.

      (4) Pediatric safety not yet established.

9.   Mast cell stabilizers

   a. Prevent mast cell degranulation via reduction of cell membrane permeability to calcium.

   b. Stabilization prevents release of mediators of inflammation. May take days or weeks to observe clinical symptomatic effectiveness.

   c. Cromolyn sodium 4% (Opticrom) SIG: i gtt 4–6 ×/day.

   d. NOTE: Opticrom is not commercially available currently in the United States. The chemical can be formulated, however, in the following manner:

Nasalcrom

Filter cromolyn sodium nasal solution through 0.22-ml filter under aseptic conditions into sterile dropper bottle. Solution may be retained for up to 1 month and stored in the refrigerator.

---

   e. Lodoxamide tromethamine 0.1% (Alomide). SIG: i gtt 4×/day.

      (1) For use in vernal keratoconjunctivitis.

      (2) Decreases itching.

      (3) Solution.

10. Topical nonsteroidal anti-inflammatory agents

   a. Reduce prostaglandin effects through interfering with cyclooxygenase pathway.

   b. Ketorolac Tromethamine 0.5% (Acular). SIG: i gtt q 4 hours.

      (1) For use in seasonal allergic conjunctivitis.

      (2) Possible adjunctive therapy for cystoid macular edema (CME)?

      (3) Solution.

   c. For additional discussion of topical nonsteroidal drugs, see VIII.

11. Topical corticosteroids

   a. Inhibit inflammation nonspecifically

      (1) Reduce formation of prostaglandins.

      (2) Decrease capillary permeability.

      (3) Reduce release of inflammatory mediators through mast cell stabilization.

      (4) Block exudative phase of inflammatory response.

   b. For treatment of mild allergic conjunctivitis of the conjunctiva and lids when low ocular penetration is desired:

      (1) Fluorometholone suspension

         (a) FML 0.1%.

         (b) FML-Forte 0.25%.

      (2) Prednisolone phosphate solution

         (a) Inflamase 0.125%.

         (b) Inflamase Forte 1%.

      (3) Prednisolone acetate suspension

         (a) Pred Mild 0.125%.

         (b) Econopred.

   c. For treatment of more severe signs and symptoms:

      (1) Prednisolone acetate suspension 1% (Pred Forte).

      (2) Fluorometholone acetate suspension 0.1% (Flarex).

   d. For more information on topical corticosteroids, see VIII.

Clinical Alert

Patients undergoing treatment with topical corticosteroid drugs should be monitored for possible IOP elevations. Cataracts and glaucoma have been associated with the use of steroids on a chronic basis, particularly with increased frequency and duration of drug use.

---

12. Oral analgesics
    a. Salicylates OR nonsteroidal anti-inflammatory agents.
    b. Adjunctive relief for some individuals when combined with topical and supportive therapy. Prostaglandin inhibition with analgesia.
        (1) ASA—650 mg po tid.
        (2) Ibuprofen (Motrin)—400 mg po qid.
        (3) Indomethacin (Indocin)—25 mg po tid.
13. Oral antihistamines
    a. Combination of H_1-blockers, sedation, and anticholinergic properties.
    b. Over the counter.
        (1) Diphenyhdramine (Benadryl). SIG: 25–50 mg po q 6–8 hours.
        (2) Chlorpheniramine (Chlortrimeton). SIG: 4 mg po q 4–6 hours.
    c. Prescription
        (1) Terfenadine (Seldane). SIG: 60 mg po q 12 hours.
        (2) Astemizole (Hismanal). SIG: 10 mg po qd.

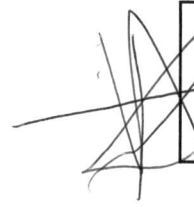

Clinical Alert

Concomitant use of Seldane plus erythromycin has resulted in cardiac arrest and death in rare cases. The combination should be absolutely avoided. Seldane should also be avoided in patients with liver disease.

Clinical Alert

Relief for the symptoms accompanying allergic conjunctivitis and rhinitis should be adequate with over-the-counter antihistamines. Chlorpheniramine causes less sedation and may therefore be better tolerated. Both legend drugs listed do not cross the blood-brain barrier and therefore sedative effects are minimized.

---

    d. H_2-blockers (e.g., Tagamet), although effective for peptic ulcer disease, are not approved, and have not shown effectiveness, in the treatment of ocular allergy.
    e. Action
        (1) Prevent histamine binding to H_1-receptor sites on blood vessels and nerves. H_1-receptors plentiful in ocular vasculature.
        (2) H_1-blocker actions
            (a) Anticholinergic.
            (b) Antiemetic.
            (c) CNS sedation.
            (d) Local anesthesia, i.e., relief from itching.
    f. Other uses
        (1) Lid myokymia (twitching).
        (2) Motion sickness.

         (3)   Counteract surgical miosis.

         (4)   Sleeping aid.

    g. Additive effects with:

         (1)   CNS depressants, e.g., alcohol.

         (2)   Antianxiety agents, e.g., Valium.

         (3)   Narcotic analgesics, e.g., codeine.

    h. Avoid or use extreme caution:

         (1)   Pregnant or nursing mothers.

         (2)   Patients with stomach ulcer.

         (3)   Alcohol or barbiturate users.

         (4)   Patients with occupational contraindications, e.g., pilots, crane operators, truck drivers.

         (5)   Patients with liver disease.

         (6)   NOTE: Seldane should not be used in patients taking erythromycin.

    i. Side effects—eye

         (1)   Decreased tear production.

         (2)   Decreased accommodation.

         (3)   Slight mydriasis.

         (4)   Hypersensitivity allergic reactions.

    j. Toxicity indicated by convulsions in children and adults

XIII. "Nutritional" Vitamin Supplements

    A. *General principles*

      1. Pharmaceutical companies claim supplements of value in treating age-related macular degeneration.

      2. Clinically represents "might help, can't hurt" treatment.

      3. Philosophies among practitioners regarding when to (if at all) initiate therapy vary widely.

      4. Most supportive data are anecdotal.

      5. Psychologically helpful to patients facing no treatment options other than low-vision aids.

      6. Supplemental trace metallic elements plus vitamins.

      7. Should be used in combination with close monitorization via Amsler or Diamond grid for changes in macular status.

      8. Review all currently used drugs (legend + over-the-counter + vitamin supplements) with patients prior to initiation.

      9. Current agents all contain vitamins A, C, E, plus trace amounts of copper, selenium, and zinc.

     10. All of these drugs are available over the counter (Table 4-10).

     11. Dosage for all is: SIG: i po qd–bid.

Table 4-10. Range of Vitamin and Mineral Quantities in Commercially Available Supplements

Vitamin A	5,000–6,000 IU
Vitamin C	60–400 mg
Vitamin E	30–200 IU
Copper (Cu)	1.5–2.0 mg
Selenium (Se)	30–40 μg
Zinc (Zn)	30–40 mg

B. *Agents*
1. Icaps (vitamin A, C, E; Cu, Se, Zn)
   a. Higher in vitamin A.
   b. Contains trace manganese.
2. Lipotriad (vitamin A, C, E; Cu, Se, Zn)
   a. B complex also included.
   b. Cautions against use in children and pregnant women.
3. Ocucaps (vitamin A, C, E; Cu, Se, Zn)
   a. Higher in vitamin C and E than other formulations.
   b. Also contains trace amount manganese.
4. Ocuvite
   Similar to Lipotriad, but with slightly more zinc.
5. Spectro-Antioxidants
   Similar to Ocucaps but does not include manganese.

XIV. Mydriatic/Cycloplegic Agents

A. *General principles*
1. Mydriatic/cycloplegic agents are denoted by red caps.
2. Moderate "stinging" associated with these agents.
3. Enhanced effect and better tolerated by patient if preceded with topical anesthetic.
4. Pupil size affected by cholinergic action on pupil sphincter muscle vs adrenergic action on iris dilator muscle (maximal dilation accomplished through cholinergic blockage plus adrenergic stimulation).
5. Clinical situation may dictate one mechanism of action preferred over another.
6. Other factors, such as color of iris (amount of melanin), age, concomitant drug therapy, patient's systemic health status, may also determine drug effect.
7. These agents may be used diagnostically and therapeutically (Table 4-11).
8. Routine clinical dilation goal = provide quick onset of adequate dilation with minimal duration of effect.

Table 4-11. Clinical Use of Mydriatic/Cycloplegic Agents

Indications	Agent
Routine dilation	1% tropicamide + 2.5% phenylephrine
Dilation with little to no accommodative interruption	2.5% phenylephrine (2 drops) or Paremyd
Dilation in narrow angles	1/2% tropicamide
Dilation in neonates	1/2% tropicamide
Routine cycloplegic refraction in child	1% cyclopentolate
Cycloplegic refraction in association with accommodative esotropia in child	1% atropine
Acute anterior uveitis	5% homatropine
Chronic anterior uveitis (prevention of posterior synechiae)	1% cyclopentolate
Enhance visual acuity with central media opacity (i.e., cataract)	2.5% phylephrine
Pseudophakic anterior and posterior chamber implants	Same as routine dilation *Do not dilate iris fixated intra ocular lenses*

9. Patients at risk for angle closure should have gonioscopy performed and be warned of symptoms: mid dilation = greatest risk.

B. *Uses*
1. Routine pupillary dilation to enhance clinical examination.
2. Cycloplegic refraction.
3. Uveitis therapy
    a. Prevent posterior synechia.
    b. Break posterior synechia.
    c. Reduce pain associated with spasm of ciliary muscle.
4. Amblyopia therapy to blur good eye.
5. Enhance visual acuity in cataract patients as alternative to surgery.

C. *Agents*
1. Dilation/cycloplegic through cholinergic blockage.
    a. Actions
        (1) Relax iris sphincter.
        (2) Paralyze accommodation.
    b. Side effects
        (1) Blurred vision—especially at near.
        (2) Photophobia.
        (3) Potential for angle closure in at risk patients—rare.
        (4) Intraocular pressure rise—most common in glaucoma patients.
        (5) Stinging upon instillation.
    c. Tropicamide
        (1) $\frac{1}{2}$% and 1% solution.
        (2) Quick onset—15–30 minutes.
        (3) Short duration.
        (4) Best for routine pupillary dilation.
        (5) Better dilator than cycloplegic agent.
    d. Cyclopentolate
        (1) $\frac{1}{2}$%, 1%, and 2% solution (1% most common).
        (2) Quick onset—15–30 minutes.
        (3) Duration—8 hours.
        (4) Better cycloplegic agent than Tropicamide.
        (5) 2% contraindicated in children due to psychosis and other CNS effects.
        (6) Increased stinging upon instillation.
        (7) Drug of choice when cycloplegia greater than tropicamide desired (e.g., evaluation of latent hyperopia, accommodative spasm, esotropia).
    e. Homatropine
        (1) 2% and 5% solution.
        (2) Onset—15–30 minutes.
        (3) Duration—12–24 hours.
        (4) Good agent for treatment of anterior uveitis (used bid–qid).
    f. Scopolamine
        (1) 0.25% solution.
        (2) Onset—15–30 minutes.
        (3) Duration—5–7 days.
        (4) Used when longer duration mydriasis/cycloplegia are desired.
        (5) Also available as transdermal patch for treatment of motion sickness.
    g. Atropine
        (1) 0.5%, 1%, 2%, 3% solution.
        (2) 0.5%, 1% ointment.
        (3) Onset—30 minutes.
        (4) Duration—1–2 weeks.

        (5)   Best cycloplegic agent, but impractical for routine diagnostic ophthalmic use. Has particular value when longer-term cycloplegia is desired in treatment of ocular disorders.

        (6)   Recommended agent for evaluation of accommodative esotropia in children.

2.   Dilation by adrenergic agonism
  a.   Action
      Stimulates iris dilator muscle.
  b.   Side effects
      (1)   Halos, photophobia.
      (2)   Blurred vision.
      (3)   Conjunctival vasoconstriction.
      (4)   Potential for angle closure in at-risk patients.
  c.   Phenylephrine
      (1)   2.5%, 10% solution.
      (2)   Onset—15–30 minutes.
      (3)   Duration—2–4 hours.
      (4)   Multiple instillations can afford adequate mydriasis with minimal light reaction and cycloplegia.
      (6)   Minimized ptosis in Horner's patients (Mueller's muscle).
  d.   Hydroxyamphetamine
      (1)   1% solution.
      (2)   Onset—45 minutes.
      (3)   Duration—2–4 hours.
      (4)   No longer commercially available (Paradrene).
      (5)   Also used in evaluation of postganglionic Horner's syndrome.

3.   Combination anticholinergic/adrenergic agonist agents
  a.   Cyclopentolate 0.2%/phenylephrine (Cyclomydril)
      Cycloplegia greater than 1% tropicamide.
  b.   Scopolamine 0.3%/phenylephrine (Murocoll)
      Long duration limits clinical applications.
  c.   Tropicamide 0.25%/hydroxyamphetamine 1% (Paremyd)
      (1)   Less cycloplegia and mydriasis.
      (2)   Quicker return to normal pupil size and accommodative state.
      (3)   Recently approved, may not be suitable for all dilation indications (e.g., peripheral retinal disease).

Clinical Alert

Because certain dyes, chemicals, and drugs may contain atropine-like substances, pharmacologic mydriasis characterized by a dilated, poorly (or non) reactive pupil with absent accommodation must be considered in patients presenting with anisocoria.

---

4.   Reversal of mydriasis by adrenergic blockers
  a.   Action
      Reverse dilation by preventing iris dilator muscle stimulation.
  b.   Side effects
      (1)   Stinging upon instillation.
      (2)   Conjunctival hyperemia.
      (3)   No effect on anterior chamber depth.
      (4)   No significant effect on accommodative amplitude.
      (5)   Binds melanin—less timely effect in dark irides.

     c. Dapiprazole (Rev-eyes)
       (1) 0.5% solution.
       (2) SIG: following dilation ii gtts q 5 minutes ×2.
       (3) May also reduce IOP but not approved for this use.
     d. Thymoxamine hydrochloride (Thymoxid)—not currently FDA approved
       (1) 0.5% solution.
       (2) SIG: i gtt postdilation.
       (3) Treatment—pigmentary glaucoma?
       (4) No effect on IOP, but may decrease iris-zonular rubbing.

**Formulation of Mydriatic Spray
for Use with Uncooperative Children**

Mix
  3.75 ml 2% cyclopentolate
  7.5 ml 1% tropicamide
  3.75 ml 10% phenylephrine
Place resultant mixture in commercially available atomizer (e.g., empty, unused perfume sprayer). Can be used with children and closed eyelids. Resultant spray equals:
  0.5% cyclopentolate
  0.5% tropicamide
  2.5% phenylephrine

XV. Ophthalmic Pain Relief

  A. General principles
    1. Most ophthalmic conditions can be managed with over-the-counter analgesics.
    2. Goal of therapy is to maintain patient comfort during therapeutic process.
    3. Identification of underlying ocular disease most important step in initiating pain relief (e.g., recurrent corneal erosion, anterior uveitis).
    4. Some agents have significant potential for drug abuse and must be used with prudence (Fig. 4-2).

  B. Agents used to decrease pain in ophthalmic care
    1. Pressure patching: immobilize lid over corneal wound.
    2. Lubricants: gtts and ung "cushion" superficially irritated areas of the eye (cornea).
    3. Bandage or soft contact lens: prevent persistent irritation as in trichiasis.
    4. Collagen shield: improves healing while preventing lid interaction. Alternative drug delivery system.
    5. Topical anesthetics: used only in office to facilitate examination.
    6. Cycloplegic agents: decreases pain from ciliary spasm and reduces photophobia.
    7. Topical steroids: nonspecific anti-inflammatory properties.
    8. Topical nonsteroidal agents: block pain through cyclo-oxygenase pathway.

  C. Oral—over the counter nonsteroidal anti-inflammatory agents (NSAIDs)
    1. Salicylate
     a. Aspirin (ASA) 325 mg
       (1) SIG: i–ii q 4–6 hours.
       (2) Prostaglandin inhibitor not to be used in patients with coagulopathies (e.g., hemophilia or GI bleeding).
     b. Ibuprofen 200 mg (Nuprin, Advil)
       (1) 400, 600, 800 mg Rx (Motrin).

NARCOTIC AGENTS RX

```
┌─────────────────────────────────────────────────────────────┐
│ DEA #MK0000000         I. C. FINE, O. D.                      │
│                        2001 Hayes Street                      │
│                        Nashville, TN 37203                    │
│                                          Date:_____        │
│ ─────────────────────────────────────────────────────────     │
│ Name:_____         │
│ Address:_____         │
│                                                                │
│              Mepergan Fortis                                   │
│                                                                │
│       SIG: 1 capsule q 4-6h /pm for severe pain #12            │
│                                      (twelve)                  │
│                                                                │
│       REFILL: 0 1 2 3 4                                        │
│       (zero refill)                                            │
│                                      _____ OD     │
│                              □  dispense as written            │
│                                      _____ OD     │
│                              □  substitution allowed           │
└─────────────────────────────────────────────────────────────┘
```

Figure 4-2.   To prevent patient modification of prescription, always *write* the number of refills (zero) and the number of pills to be dispensed. DO NOT phone in narcotic prescriptions.

      (2)   Prostaglandin inhibitor.
      (3)   400 mg = best analgesic.
      (4)   600 mg + added anti-inflammatory, but no additional analgesia.
      (5)   Peripheral acting.
      (6)   GI upset common.
  2.   Para-aminophenol: acetaminophen (APAP) 325 mg (Tylenol)
      (1)   500 mg (Extra Strength Tylenol).
      (2)   Non-prostaglandin-inhibiting agent.
      (3)   Mode of analgesia unclear.
      (4)   Good GI tolerance.
      (5)   Liver toxicity potential in high doses. Use with caution or consider alternative drug in patients with cirrhosis or other known liver disease.

D.   *Oral—legend (Rx) selected agents: Ketorolac (Toradol). SIG: 20 mg loading dose then 10 mg q 4–6 hours/prn for pain*
  1.   Contraindicated in active peptic ulcer disease.
  2.   GI side effects.

E.   *Oral—narcotic (Rx). Requires DEA Number. Selected agents.*
  1.   Propoxyphene—good pain relief with less addictive potential
    a.   Darvocet N-100: propoxyphene + tylenol.
    b.   Darvon: propoxyphene + aspirin.
  2.   Butorphanol (Stadol)
    a.   Nasal inhalant for pain relief.
    b.   Quick onset.
    c.   SIG: 1 puff in each nostril or 2 puffs in one nostril q 4–6 hours/prn pain relief.
  3.   Codeine
    a.   Better pain relief with additional benefit of euphoria.
    b.   GI upset common.

c. NOTE: most people who claim "allergy" to codeine have had adverse side effects (e.g., GI upset/nausea) rather than true hypersensitivity.
d. Also is excellent cough suppressant.
e. Acetaminophen + codeine 30 mg (example: Tylenol 3).
f. Acetaminophen + codeine 60 mg (example: Tylenol 4).
g. Hydrocodone + acetaminophen (example: Lorcet). Less nausea than codeine with somewhat greater analgesia.
h. Oxycodone + acetaminophen (example: Tylox). Similar to hydrocodone but better analgesia and less GI upset.
i. Meperidine HCl 50 mg + phenergan 25 mg (example: Mepergan Fortis). Due to potential for nausea it is combined with antiemetic.

Recommendations for Pain Relief (States Allowing Narcotic Use)

Mild (e.g., pseudomembranous keratoconjunctivitis)
400–600 mg ibuprofen po q 4–6 hours/pain
Motrin

OR

20 mg ketorolac loading then 10 mg po tid/prn pain

Moderate (e.g., corneal abrasion)
Ketorolac—as described above

OR

Darvocet N-100
SIG: i–ii po q 4–6 hours/pain

OR

Tylenol 3
SIG: i–ii po q 4–6 hours/pain

Severe (e.g., corneal debridement)
Tylox
SIG: i–ii caps po q 4–6 hours/prn severe pain

OR

Mepergan Fortis (Meperidine HCl + promethazine)
SIG: i–ii caps po q 4–6 hours/prn pain

Suggested Readings

Bartlett JD. Pitfalls encountered in the clinical utilization of mydriatic drugs. *South J Optom* 1980;22:8–14.

Bartlett JD, Jaanus SD. *Clinical Ocular Pharmacology.* Stoneham, MA: Butterworth, 1989.

Bartlett JD, Wesson MD, Swiatocha J, Woolley T. Efficacy of a pediatric cycloplegic administered as a spray. *J Am Optom Assoc* 1993;64:617–621.

Becker B. Intraocular pressure response to topical corticosteroids. *Invest Ophthalmol* 1965;4:198–205.

Brown SI, Shahinian L. Diagnosis and treatment of ocular rosacea. *Ophthalmology* 1978;85:779–786.

Bryant JA. Local and topical anesthetics in ophthalmology. *Surv Ophthalmol* 1969;13:262–283.

Caldwell DR, Verin P, Hartwich-Young R, Meyer SM, Drake MM. Efficacy and safety of lodoxamide 0.1% vs cromolyn sodium 4% in patients with vernal keratoconjunctivitis. *Am J Ophthalmol* 1992;113:632–637.

Classe JG. *Optometry Clinics.* Ocular Pharmacology Update. Norwalk, CT: Appleton and Lange, Vol 2, No. 4, 1992;59–72.

Ellis PP. *Ocular Therapeutics and Pharmacology.* St. Louis: C.V. Mosby Co., 1980.

Geeting DG, Bakar SR. In vivo comparison of ocular lubricants in patients having reduced tear film break-up times. *J Am Optom Assoc* 1980;8:757–780.

Gigliotti F, Williams WT, Hayden FG, et al. Etiology of acute conjunctivitis in children. *J Pediatr* 1981;98:531–536.

Jones DB. Decision making in the management of microbial keratitis. *Ophthalmology* 1981;88:814–820.

Kaila T, Huupponen R, Salminen L. Effects of eyelid closure and nasolacrimal duct occlusion on the systemic absorption of ocular timolol in human subjects. *J Ocul Pharmacol* 1986;2:365–369.

Leibowitz HM. Clinical evaluation of ciprofloxacin 0.3% ophthalmic solution for treatment of bacterial keratitis. *Am J Ophthalmol* 1991;112:34S–47S.

Leibowitz HM, Hyndiuk RA, Lindsey C, Rosenthal AL. Fluorometholone acetate: Clinical evaluation in the treatment of external ocular inflammation. *Ann Ophthalmol* 1984;16:1110–1115.

Lemp MA, Hamill JR. Factors affecting tear film breakup in normal eyes. *Arch Ophthalmol* 1973;89:103–105.

Melton R, Thomas R. 2nd annual practical guide to therapeutic drugs. *Optometric Management*, May 1993 (suppl).

Mogk LG, Cyrlin MN. Blood dyscrasias and carbonic anhydrase inhibitors. *Ophthalmology* 1988;95:768–771.

Ophthalmic Drug Facts. St. Louis: J.B. Lippincott Co., 1993.

Pavan-Langston D, Dunkel EC. *Handbook of Ocular Drug Therapy and Ocular Side Effects of Systemic Drugs.* Boston: Little, Brown and Co., 1991.

Physicians Desk Reference for Ophthalmology. 21st ed. Montvale, NJ: Medical Economics Data, 1993.

Schlaeger TF. Toxoplasmosis. In: Fraunfelder FT, Roy FH, eds. *Current Ocular Therapy.* 2nd ed. Philadelphia: W.B. Saunders Co., 1985:80–82.

Smith RE, Nozik RA. *Uveitis: A Clinical Approach to Diagnosis and Management.* Baltimore: Williams and Wilkins, 1983.

Stuart JC, Linn JG. Dilute sodium hyaluronate (Healon) in the treatment of ocular surface disorders. *Ann Ophthalmol* 1985;17:190–192.

Zimmerman TJ. Topical ophthalmic beta blockers: A comparative review. *J Ocul Pharmacol.* 1993;9:373–384.

Zimmerman TJ, Kooner KS, Kandarakis AS, et al. Improving the therapeutic index of topically applied ocular drugs. *Arch Ophthalmol* 1984;102:551–553.

CHAPTER **5**

Ocular Disease

Kevin L. Alexander

I. **Eyelids and Lacrimal System**

  A. *Features of the eyelids and lacrimal system*

   1. The eyelids serve to protect the eye by preventing foreign objects and excessive light from entering the eye and helping retain corneal and conjunctival moisture.
   2. Lid action promotes tear flow across the eye and through the upper and lower canaliculi.
   3. The opening between the two lids is termed the palpebral fissure and is symmetrical except in diseased states.
   4. Eye lashes (cilia) line the lid margin and help keep foreign material from entering the eye.
   5. Three layers in tear "anatomy" produced by glands in lids are:
       a. Oil—secreted by meibomian glands and glands of Zeis.
       b. Aqueous—secreted by lacrimal gland and glands of Krause and Wolfring.
       c. Mucin—secreted by goblet cells of conjunctiva.
   6. The average tear volume is 6 µl with turnover of 1.2 µl/min.
   7. Gamma globulins IgA (most common), IgG, and IgE are present in tears.
   8. Upper excretory system consists of punctum and canaliculus leading to the lacrimal sac.
   9. Lower excretory system consists of punctum and canaliculus leading to the lacrimal sac.
   10. Nasolacrimal duct leads to inferior meatus.

  B. *General assessment of eyelids*

   1. Note position of eyelids—does ptosis or blepharochalasis exist?
   2. Observe a blink—is closure complete?
   3. Note direction of cilia and lid margin. Is there good apposition of the lid margins? Do any cilia turn in?
   4. Note any in-turning (entropion) or out-turning (ectropion) of lid margin.
   5. Observe the upper and lower puncta—are they open and in good apposition with the globe?
   6. Observe lid margin for evidence of redness, ulceration, or discharge.

  C. *Pathophysiology of symptoms—eyelids*

   1. Lid problems are among the most common of all eye problems encountered by primary eye care practitioners.
   2. Hordeola (stye), chalazia, and blepharitis are common.
   3. Common patient complaints related to the lids:
       a. Pain—due to swelling of tissue near pain receptors.
       b. Itching (pruritus)—due to hypersensitivity to allergens or toxins produced by bacteria.

     c. Red rimmed lids—due to localized hyperemia.

     d. Foreign body sensation—related to entropion, inturned lashes (trichiasis), or corneal exposure from poor lid closure.

     e. Tearing (epiphora)—due to ectropion, blocked excretory system, or irritation.

D. *Inflammatory diseases of the eyelids*

  1. Blepharitis

     a. Generalized inflammation of lid margin.

     b. Symptoms. Itching, foreign body sensation, burning, mattering of eye lashes, eyelids stuck together upon awakening.

     c. Clinical signs

       (1) Redness, thickened lid margin, crusty matter along lid margin and lashes, conjunctival redness.

       (2) May have corneal involvement—usually punctate staining of lower one-third of cornea.

     d. Etiology

       (1) May be differentiated into subtypes

       Staphylococcal blepharitis

         Infection caused by *Staphylococcus aureus* resulting in redness and ulceration at base of cilia.

       Seborrheic blepharitis

         Blepharitis associated with seborrhea of scalp and eyebrows. Causative agent, usually *Pityrosporum ovale,* results in "speared" dandruff flakes along cilia. Marked itching.

       (2) Blepharitis is usually a mix of both types.

       (3) May be associated with dermatologic problem such as acne rosacea.

     e. Diagnostic evaluation

       (1) Differential diagnosis includes hordeola, diffuse chalazia, meibomianitis.

       (2) It is difficult to differentiate between staphylococcal blepharitis and seborrheic blepharitis, as they frequently occur together. Be sure to rule out conjunctival and corneal problems; may be associated with dry eye.

     f. Treatment

       (1) Lid scrubs (see Clinical Procedure) twice daily with baby shampoo or commercial eye scrub preparation.

       (2) Severe forms benefit by lid scrub with antibiotic/steroid ointment (Blephamide).

       (3) Warm compresses 10–15 minutes daily.

       (4) If severe, treat with erythromycin or bacitracin ointment at bedtime.

       (5) Associated conjunctivitis or keratitis may be treated with combination antibiotic–steroid drops tid or qid depending on severity.

     g. Follow-up

       (1) Follow-up in 3–4 weeks or sooner if needed. Discontinue steroid preparations as soon as possible.

       (2) Continue lid scrubs and warm compresses indefinitely.

Clinical Procedure—Lid Scrubs

Description/ Purpose	Technique of cleansing the lid margin to remove debris or microbial pathogens.
Equipment	Baby shampoo or commercial eye scrub. Cotton-tipped applicator.
Procedure	Moisten cotton-tipped applicator with baby shampoo and apply along lid margins from inner canthus to outer canthus. Rinse eyelids with warm water.

Clinical Alert

Long-term use of steroid ointments may result in cataract formation or glaucoma due to inadvertent application into the conjunctival cul-de-sac.

---

2. External hordeolum
    a. Acute, localized infection of the glands of Zeis or Moll.
    b. Symptoms. Acute onset of tenderness, itching, and occasional pain, localized redness and swelling.
    c. Clinical signs
        (1) Localized redness and swelling in the area of infected glands.
        (2) Generalized lid redness and swelling if associated with blepharitis.
        (3) Pus pointing occurs as the lesion resolves.
    d. Etiology
        (1) Usually *Staphylococcus*
        (2) May be associated with blepharitis.
    e. Diagnostic evaluation
        (1) Differential diagnosis includes marginal blepharitis and chalazia.
        (2) One must rule out associated conjunctivitis or keratitis.
    f. Treatment
        (1) Warm compresses hasten pus pointing and resolution.
        (2) Epilation (removal of cilia) facilitates draining of the localized abscess.
        (3) Topical broad-spectrum antibiotics are of little use in treating the lid lesion; however, they may be used prophylactically for associated conjunctivitis or keratitis and may be used on a tid or qid basis depending on severity.
        (4) Severe cases may be treated with systemic antibiotics such as erythromycin or tetracycline 250 mg po qid ×10 days.
        (5) Occasionally a stab incision is necessary to relieve abscess.
    g. Follow-up. Follow-up in 7–10 days to be certain abscess has resolved. Practitioners should be alert to the possible development of lid cellulitis.

Clinical Procedure—Epilation

Description/ Purpose	Technique utilized to remove cilia to aid in draining external hordeola or to relieve corneal irritation due to trichiasis.
Equipment	Zeigler or other epilating forceps.
Procedure	Position patient at biomicroscope and explain procedure. Apply topical anesthetic such as proparacaine if needed. Direct patient to specific point of fixation. Grasp cilia to be epilated near the skin and remove with quick, brisk pull.

---

3. Internal hordeolum
    a. Acute localized infection of the meibomian gland.
    b. Symptoms. Pain, swelling, and tenderness of affected lid.
    c. Clinical signs
        (1) Generalized lid swelling.
        (2) On lid eversion, redness noted in area of the meibomian gland.
        (3) Occasional mucopurulent discharge may be expressed from the meibomian gland by gentle pressure.
    d. Etiology
        (1) Acute, localized infection (usually *Staphylococcus*) of the meibomian gland.
        (2) May be associated with staphylococcal blepharitis.

  e. Diagnostic evaluation
      (1) Differential diagnosis includes external hordeolum.
      (2) Internal hordeolum may be differentiated from chalazion by the presence of pain and tenderness.
  f. Treatment
      (1) Hot compresses will hasten resolution.
      (2) Topical antibiotics are ineffective due to poor penetration.
      (3) Oral antibiotics (erythromycin or tetracycline 250 mg qid × 10 days) may be of value in difficult cases.
      (4) Daily expression of the meibomian gland is recommended.
  g. Follow-up. Ten days following initiation of treatment. Internal hordeola frequently lead to chalazia development.

4. Chalazion
  a. Chronic, sterile granulomatous inflammation of the meibomian gland.
  b. Symptoms. Patient complains of a painless lump of the affected lid generally developing over several days or weeks.
  c. Clinical signs
      (1) Localized lump which is immobile.
      (2) Rarely painful, although in acute phase there may be some discomfort.
      (3) In the acute phase, lid swelling may be diffuse but localizes quickly forming hard, immobile lump.
  d. Etiology
      (1) Chalazion is a granulomatous inflammation of the meibomian gland, generally due to a blocked opening of the gland.
      (2) May be associated with internal and/or external hordeola.
      (3) May be associated with blepharitis.
  e. Diagnostic evaluation
      (1) Differential diagnosis includes external hordeolum, internal hordeolum, meibomianitis, and blepharitis.
      (2) Important to the differential diagnosis is consideration of possible malignancy—recurrent chalazia should be biopsied.
      (3) Chalazia are easily identified by drawing examiner's finger lightly across the affected lid from inner canthus to outer canthus and palpating a hard lump.
  f. Treatment
      (1) In the acute phase, hot compresses hasten localization of the inflammation.
      (2) Digital massage helps relieve blockage at the opening the meibomian gland.
      (3) Surgical drainage is accomplished by incision and curettage.
      (4) Intralesional injection of steroids (0.2–1.0 ml of triamcinolone 40 mg/ml) may be of value.
      (5) Topical and oral antibiotics are ineffective.
  g. Follow-up. Follow-up should be 7–10 days after initiating mechanical or medical treatment. If chalazion has not resolved, may proceed with surgical drainage.

Clinical Alert

Recurrent chalazia should be biopsied to rule out malignancy (sebaceous cell carcinoma).

5. Meibomianitis
  a. Stagnation of meibomian secretions resulting in chronic inflammation.

    b. Symptoms. Irritation, burning, and stinging of affected lid.

    c. Clinical Signs

       (1) Lids appear thickened and openings of meibomian glands may be blocked.

       (2) Thick, toothpaste-like discharge may be expressed from meibomian glands.

       (3) May be associated with mild keratoconjunctivitis.

    d. Etiology. Poor meibomian secretion and chronic blockage of the openings of the meibomian glands result in chronic inflammation of the meibomian gland.

    e. Diagnostic evaluation

       (1) Careful slit lamp evaluation while applying gentle pressure to lid margin.

       (2) Differential diagnosis includes blepharitis, hordeolum, and chalazion.

    f. Treatment

       (1) Digital massage to express discharge combined with hot compresses.

       (2) Topical antibiotics such as sulfacetamide or garamycin tid or qid may be useful in treating associated keratoconjunctivitis.

    g. Follow-up. Follow-up should be in 2–3 weeks. Mechanical expression is frequently necessary long term as this condition is a chronic problem.

6. Angular blepharitis

    a. Lid inflammation limited to inner and outer canthus.

    b. Symptoms. Irritation, tenderness, scaling, and flaking at the inner or outer canthus.

    c. Clinical signs.

       (1) Redness at the inner or outer canthus.

       (2) Scaling and flaking skin in the affected area.

       (3) Associated conjunctivitis may be present at the inner or outer canthus.

    d. Etiology. Inflammation of the inner or outer canthus typically due to *Moraxella lacunata.*

    e. Diagnostic evaluation. Differential diagnosis includes ulcerative blepharitis.

    f. Treatment

       (1) Zinc sulfate or sulfacetamide drops qid ×10–14 days.

       (2) Occasionally erythromycin ointment applied at bedtime is helpful.

    g. Follow-up. Follow-up in 2–3 weeks.

7. Preseptal cellulitis

    a. Inflammation of lid structures anterior to the orbital septum of the upper lid.

    b. Symptoms. Patients complain of pain, swelling, and redness of the upper lid. There may be mild fever.

    c. Clinical signs. Eyelid redness, swelling, tenderness. There is no restriction of extraocular muscle motility nor is there proptosis. There is no pain with eye movement.

    d. Etiology

       (1) Inflammation and swelling may be secondary to primary lid infection.

       (2) Occasionally a history of trauma—especially a puncture wound or laceration—will be present.

       (3) Causative organisms usually are *Staphylococcus aureus,* streptococci, and *Haemophilus influenzae* (in children).

    e. Diagnostic evaluation

       (1) Complete eye examination with special emphasis on extraocular muscle movements and assessment for proptosis.

       (2) Careful history for preexisting trauma and any pain with eye movements.

       (3) Computed tomographic (CT) scan of brain and orbits is mandatory if there is a concern about intraocular foreign body or orbital mass.

       (4) Differential diagnosis includes:

          (a) Orbital cellulitis.

          (b) Hordeola.

          (c) Chalazia.

          (d) Meibomianitis.

          (e) Viral conjunctivitis or allergic conjunctivitis with severe eyelid swelling.

          (f) Insect bite of upper or lower lid.

    f. Treatment

        (1) Mild preseptal cellulitis may be treated with oral antibiotics such as cephalexin or erythromycin 250 mg qid combined with hot compresses.

        (2) If preseptal cellulitis is moderate to severe or if there is no improvement, patient should be referred for more aggressive treatment and possible surgical drainage.

Clinical Alert

Treatment of preseptal cellulitis should be aggressive, as this can represent a life-threatening situation.

---

   8. Herpes simplex dermatitis

     a. Dermatitis of the lid resulting in redness and blister formation due to herpes simplex I virus.

     b. Symptoms. Itching, pain, and irritation of affected lids. Patients may complain of redness and swelling of the upper and lower lid.

     c. Etiology. Herpes simplex infection of the lids is typically due to HSV I virus.

     d. Diagnostic evaluation

        (1) Careful evaluation with slit lamp biomicroscope to identify clear, fluid-filled vesicles on lid.

        (2) Evaluate conjunctiva and cornea for evidence of conjunctivitis or dendritic keratitis.

        (3) Differential diagnosis includes ulcerative and squamous blepharitis.

     e. Treatment

        (1) Herpes simplex dermatitis is frequently self-limiting.

        (2) Topical antibiotics and drying agents are useful in minimizing symptoms.

        (3) Antivirals may be indicated if the cornea is affected. Antivirals should be avoided if the cornea is clear.

        (4) Steroids should be avoided

     f. Follow-up. See patient in 5–7 days. Watch for corneal involvement.

Clinical Alert

The use of topical steroids in the treatment of any herpetic condition in the early stages may result in exacerbation of the condition and should be avoided.

---

   9. Varicella zoster (herpes zoster) dermatitis

     a. Inflammation, redness, and vesicle formation along the course of the fifth cranial nerve of the lid. Commonly referred to as "shingles."

     b. Symptoms. Headache, malaise, fever, pain, and numbness.

     c. Etiology. Varicella zoster represents chickenpox virus along the course of the fifth cranial nerve.

     d. Diagnostic evaluation

        (1) Careful external evaluation as well as biomicroscopy to determine extent of corneal involvement as well as rule out uveitis.

        (2) Note that skin lesions extend to the midline only.

   (3) Differential diagnosis includes contact dermatitis.

   (4) If tip of the nose is affected, herpes zoster uveitis should be assumed.

  e. Treatment

   (1) Herpes zoster is frequently self-limiting.

   (2) Analgesics and antibiotics are helpful in a supportive role to reduce pain and prevent secondary infection.

   (3) Associated keratitis may be treated with antibiotic or antiviral.

   (4) Associated uveitis may be treated with cycloplegic and anti-inflammatory drugs.

   (5) Acyclovir 600–800 mg 5× (adults)/day for 7–10 days is helpful in the acute phase.

   (6) A dermatology consult is indicated if lid lesions are extensive.

  f. Follow-up. 3–5 days until resolved.

Clinical Alert

As herpes zoster usually affects older patients, young patients presenting with herpes zoster should be carefully screened for other evidence of acquired immune deficiency syndrome (AIDS).

 E. *Infestations of the eyelids: Phthiriasis palpebrum*

  1. Lid infestation by crab or body louse.

  2. Symptoms. Itching, stinging, and redness of the lid.

  3. Clinical signs. Redness and itching of the affected lid. Adult lice and nits (eggs) may be noted along lid margin with the biomicroscope. May be associated with blepharitis.

  4. Etiology

   a. Infestation of the lid by crab or body louse.

   b. Generally associated with poor hygiene.

   c. Found frequently in settings where numerous children are in close contact.

   d. May be transmitted sexually.

  5. Diagnostic evaluation

   a. Careful evaluation of the lid with biomicroscope is indicated.

   b. Adult lice may be seen or observed best in a dark room.

   c. Differential diagnosis includes blepharitis.

  6. Treatment

   a. Mechanical removal of adult lice and nits may be accomplished with jeweler's forceps.

   b. Ointments applied along lid margin will suffocate lice.

   c. Eserine ointment may be applied to lid margin to paralyze the parasite (may cause spasm of accommodation if gets in cul-de-sac).

   d. The head may be cleansed with pediculocides such as Kwell or Rid.

Clinical Alert

Infestation of the lid by crab lice or body lice represents a public health problem.
For children, the school nurse should be advised.
For adults, sexual partners should be notified.

 F. *Allergic disease of the eyelids: Contact dermatitis*

  1. Redness of the lids in periorbital area as the result of sensitivity to one or more allergens.

2. Symptoms. Sudden onset of redness or eyelid swelling. Patient may complain of itching or watery discharge.
3. Clinical signs
    a. Periorbital edema, redness (erythema).
    b. Conjunctival redness and/or watery discharge.
    c. Secondary lid infection.
4. Etiology
    a. Usually medication, eyeglass frame, or eye makeup.
    b. May be due to environmental allergen such as soaps, shampoos, perfume, detergents, or fabric softeners.
5. Diagnostic evaluation. Differential diagnosis includes blepharitis, acute chalazion, lid cellulitis.
6. Treatment
    a. Avoid offending allergen.
    b. Cold compresses several times a day.
    c. Topical steroid cream bid or tid 3–5 days.
    d. Oral antihistamine for several days until resolved.
7. Follow-up. 7–10 days.

Clinical Procedure—Skin Patch Test

Description/ Purpose:	Skin patch test is useful in helping to identify the cause of a contact dermatitis.
Equipment	Suspected allergen.
Procedure	Suspected allergen such as a frame temple or makeup is placed in contact with the skin elsewhere in the body (usually the arm) for a period of 24 hours.
	Makeup or eye solutions may be tested by soaking a gauze pad with substance and taping pad to skin.
	If redness and swelling result, allergen is identified.

G. *Abnormalities of motility or position of eyelids*
    1. Ptosis
        a. Congenital or progressive droopy lid.
        b. Symptoms. Patients complain of cosmetic appearance of lowered lids and blurred vision.
        c. Clinical signs. Narrowed palpebral aperture. Subjectively one lid frequently appears lower than the other.
        d. Etiology. May be congenital or acquired.
        e. Diagnostic evaluation
            (1) Assessment of ptosis involves measurement of the palpebral aperture as well as levator function.
            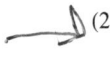(2) Application of 2½% phenylephrine will result in a widening of the palpebral aperture in patients with senile acquired ptosis.
            (3) If ptosis is severe or worse at end of day, a Tensilon test may be indicated to rule out myasthenia gravis (refer to neurologist or internist).
            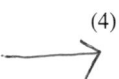(4) Ptosis associated with Horner's syndrome may be identified by application of 0.12% phenylephrine which will cause a rather marked elevation of the lid.
            (5) Ptosis of sudden onset should raise suspicion of Horner's syndrome. Further studies including chest x-ray to rule out aortic aneurysm are indicated.

    f.   Treatment
- (1)   An oculoplastic consult is indicated if no systemic cause found.
- (2)   Mild ptosis may be managed with ptosis crutch or tape.

    g.   Follow-up. If no evidence of neurologic problem, routine exam every 1–2 years.

Clinical Procedure—Palpebral Aperture/Levator Function

Description/ Purpose	The purpose of lid motility testing is to evaluate the extent of ptosis by measurement of the palpebral fissure as well as the evaluation of levator function.
Equipment	PD rule and good illumination.
Procedure	MEASURING PALPEBRAL APERTURE.
	Patient looks straight ahead.
	Place zero mark of PD rule on lower lid margin.
	Measure distance to upper lid margin.
	Normal range 9–12 mm.
	MEASURING LEVATOR FUNCTION
	Stabilize frontalis muscle by placing fingers on forehead.
	Have patient look down, place zero mark of PD rule on upper lid margin.
	Holding PD rule steady, have patient look up.
	Distance upper lid margins move is measure of levator function.
	Normal levator function is 5–8 mm or more.

---

2.   Myokymia
- a.   Twitching of the upper or lower lid.
- b.   Symptoms. Patients complain of lid "quivering" or "twitching," especially when fatigued.
- c.   Clinical signs. Few; occasionally a slight lid quiver can be observed directly or with the biomicroscope.
- d.   Etiology. Myokymia represents lid twitching due to a spasm of the orbicularis muscle. It is associated with a history of fatigue, stress, or poor nutrition.
- e.   Diagnostic evaluation. Rule out other anterior segment problem, especially conjunctival or corneal foreign body.
- f.   Treatment
  - (1)   Management is essentially supportive.
  - (2)   Patients are reassured that there is no pathologic problem and are encouraged to get proper rest and nutrition.
  - (3)   Occasionally topical antihistamines (Vasocon-A or Naphcon-A) may lessen lid twitching.
  - (4)   Oral antihistamines may be helpful.
- g.   Follow-up. 4–6 weeks following initial examination or initiation of treatment.

3.   Essential blepharospasm
- a.   Involuntary contracture of the orbicularis or facial muscles.
- b.   Symptoms. Chronic spasm of the facial muscles on affected side.
- c.   Clinical signs. Updrawn face. Blepharospasm may be so severe that one cannot examine the eye.
- d.   Etiology. Essential blepharospasm is the result of a chronic irritative lesion of the seventh cranial nerve.
- e.   Diagnostic evaluation
  - (1)   Careful history reveals chronic nature of the disease.
  - (2)   One should rule out all other ocular or systemic causes.

f. Treatment
    (1) Management is essentially supportive.
    (2) Surgical denervation or alcohol block may result in permanent repair.
    (3) Botulinum injections give temporary relief up to 3–6 months.
g. Follow-up. Depending upon treatment selected, anywhere from 3 to 9 months.

4. Lagophthalmos
    a. Incomplete blink or incomplete closure during sleep or related to disease.
    b. Symptoms. Patients frequently complain of redness and irritation of the cornea or conjunctiva due to exposure.
    c. Clinical signs
        (1) Incomplete closure observed.
        (2) Punctate staining or evidence of conjunctivitis.
        (3) Possible history of thyroid disease.
    d. Etiology
        (1) Lagophthalmos may be associated with exophthalmos in thyroid disease.
        (2) Incomplete closure during sleep.
    e. Diagnostic evaluation
        (1) Careful evaluation with biomicroscope reveals punctate staining of the cornea or dryness of the conjunctiva—especially inferiorly.
        (2) Exposure of the cornea may be observed when patient is asked to voluntarily close eyes.
    f. Treatment
        (1) Identify possible systemic cause such as thyroid disease.
        (2) Corneal disease and/or conjunctival problems treated with lubricants or appropriate antibiotics.
        (3) Eyelid can be taped shut at bedtime.
        (4) Consider surgical correction in severe cases.
    g. Follow-up. Follow-up should be within the first few weeks, as chronic corneal exposure can lead to corneal ulceration and permanent scarring.

Clinical Procedure—Identifying Incomplete Lid Closure

Description/Purpose   Purpose is to identify incomplete lid closure, especially during sleep.
Equipment   Pen light.
Procedure   Have patient voluntarily, but not forcefully, close eyes and tip head backwards.
Cornea will be in the area of the palpebral aperture.
-Direct pen light to the palpebral aperture.
If incomplete closure is present, corneal reflex will be observed.

---

5. Ectropion
    a. Out-turning of the lid margin resulting in epiphora (excessive tearing).
    b. Symptoms
        (1) Excessive tearing.
        (2) Possible redness of the lid margin.
    c. Clinical signs
        (1) Epiphora.
        (2) Punctum is generally not in good apposition to the lacrimal lake.
        (3) Lid margin may be thickened and reddened similar to blepharitis.
    d. Etiology
        (1) Senile ectropion is due to aging and loss of elasticity of the lid muscles.

        (2) Cicatricial ectropion is due to scarring of the conjunctiva.

        (3) Paralytic ectropion is due to seventh cranial nerve paralysis.

    e. Diagnostic evaluation

        (1) Careful evaluation of the anterior segment to rule out other disease.

        (2) "Pinch test" will identify laxity of the lower lid (see Clinical Procedures).

        (3) Differential diagnosis includes blepharitis, conjunctivitis, and punctal stenosis.

    f. Treatment

        (1) Management includes lubricants to protect the eye

        (2) Surgical repair affords permanent correction.

    g. Follow-up. Follow-up is indicated if surgical repair is not required. Patients should be monitored every few months due to exposure of the cornea and high probability of developing corneal ulceration.

Clinical Procedure—Pinch Test

Description/Purpose   To identify clinical or subclinical ectropion.

Equipment   Good illumination of the area.

Procedure   Take the lower lid between the thumb and forefinger and squeeze, pulling the lid and conjunctival fornix outward.
With normal lid laxity, the lid will retract to good apposition with the globe.
With clinically significant ectropion, the lower lid will remain away from the globe.

---

  6. Entropion

    a. In-turning of the lid margin.

    b. Symptoms. Foreign body sensation, conjunctival redness.

    c. Clinical signs

        (1) In-turned lid with trichiasis (in-turned lashes).

        (2) Possible corneal abrasion due to trichiasis or chronic conjunctivitis.

    d. Etiology. Entropion may be congenital, senile, cicatricial, or spastic.

    e. Diagnostic evaluation

        (1) Intermittent entropion may be identified by asking patients to squeeze lids together, resulting in obvious entropion.

        (2) Differential diagnosis includes trichiasis not associated with entropion.

        (3) Careful examination of the anterior segment to rule out foreign body.

    f. Treatment

        (1) Protect cornea from trichiasis with lubricants, contact lens, or epilation.

        (2) Surgical procedure affords permanent repair.

        (3) Occasionally Zeigler cautery can be helpful.

    g. Follow-up

        (1) Every 3–4 months.

        (2) After surgical repair follow every 6–12 months.

 H. *Benign eyelid tumors*

  1. Verruca (papilloma)

    a. Wart of upper or lower lid.

    b. Symptoms. Complaint of "growth" on the upper or lower lid.

    c. Clinical signs. Flat-topped or raised lesion which is not vascularized.

    d. Diagnostic evaluation

        (1) Evaluate size, color, vascularity.

        (2)   Differential diagnosis includes malignant lid lesions.

        (3)   Lack of change, vascularity, or bleeding is associated with a benign lesion.

   e. Etiology. Viral.

   f. Treatment

        (1)   Verrucae are generally self-limiting.

        (2)   Surgical removal is indicated if cosmetic problem is pronounced.

   g. Follow-up. Monitor every 6–12 months if no treatment.

2. Sudoriferous cysts

   a. Clear cysts forming at the opening of the Moll gland.

   b. Symptoms. Patient complains of a bump at the lid margin.

   c. Clinical signs. Clear, cystic formation at lid margin.

   d. Etiology. Cystic formation at the opening of the Moll gland due to stagnant flow.

   e. Diagnostic evaluation. May be differentiated from malignant tumors by lack of change or vascularization.

   f. Treatment. May be eliminated by a stab incision with hypodermic needle followed by antibiotic ointment tid for 2–3 days.

   g. Follow-up. Follow-up in 1–2 weeks.

3. Xanthelasma

   a. Yellow, flat lesions of the upper or lower lid.

   b. Symptoms. Patients complain of cosmetic problem related to the appearance of yellow lesions.

   c. Clinical signs. Yellow, flat lesions most often noted toward the inner canthus of the upper and lower lid.

   d. Etiology. Xanthelasma are frequently associated with elevated blood lipids.

   e. Diagnostic evaluation. Differential diagnosis includes basal cell or squamous cell carcinoma.

   f. Treatment

        (1)   Frequently best left alone.

        (2)   May be surgically removed.

   g. Follow-up. Annual examination if no treatment instituted.

4. Nevi

   a. Elevated pigmented lesions.

   b. Symptoms. Patient complains of a "dark spot" along the upper or lower lid.

   c. Clinical signs. Dark, pigmented lesion noted on upper or lower lid. Generally not vascularized.

   d. Etiology. Accumulation of melanin pigment within the skin.

   e. Diagnostic evaluation

        (1)   Careful monitoring, looking for change or vascularization.

        (2)   Differential diagnosis includes malignant melanoma of the skin.

   f. Treatment. No treatment is indicated unless a cosmetic problem exists. If suspicious of tumor or lesion presents cosmetic problem, refer to oculoplastic surgeon.

   g. Follow-up

        (1)   Annual examination.

        (2)   Photography may be helpful.

I. Malignant tumors

1. Basal cell carcinoma

   a. Rapidly growing elevated skin lesions.

   b. Most common malignant tumor of the eyelids.

   c. Symptoms

        (1)   Patients complain of a "growth" in affected areas of the lid.

        (2)   Elevated lesions are frequently irritating to the patient.

     d. Clinical signs
       (1) A nodular or flat lesion along the lids.
       (2) Frequently a history of change or bleeding is associated with basal cell carcinoma.
       (3) Lesion frequently becomes indolent, bleeding in the center.
     e. Diagnostic evaluation. Differential diagnosis includes benign papilloma, xanthelasma, and squamous cell carcinoma.
     f. Treatment
       (1) Surgical removal is indicated.
       (2) Pathology evaluation is mandatory.
     g. Follow-up. If uncertain of diagnosis, follow patient every 2–3 months; otherwise referral to oculoplastic ophthalmologist or plastic surgeon is indicated.

2. Squamous cell carcinoma
     a. Common in older patients who exhibit precancerous keratoses.
     b. Symptoms. Patients complain of change of preexisting lid lesion.
     c. Clinical signs. An elevated, somewhat vascularized lesion may be noted.
     d. Etiology. Squamous cell carcinoma arises from senile keratosis.
     e. Diagnostic evaluation. Diagnosis is often difficult because change of the lesion is very subtle.
     f. Treatment
       (1) Surgical removal is indicated.
       (2) Lesion should be removed completely as metastases can occur.
     g. Follow-up. Observe every 6–12 months.

3. Malignant melanoma
     a. Dark, malignant lesion along lid margin.
     b. Symptoms. Patients complain of a "mole" along the lid margin at the junction between the conjunctiva and lid tissue.
     c. Clinical signs. Dark, elevated lesion.
     d. Etiology. Malignant melanoma generally arises from pigmented skin lesion.
     e. Diagnostic evaluation. Careful history to ascertain the preexisting quality of the lesion.
     f. Treatment
       (1) Surgical removal is indicated.
       (2) High mortality rate is associated with these lesions.
     g. Follow-up. Every 6–12 months if uncertain as to the etiology of the lid lesion.

4. Sebaceous cell carcinoma
     a. Chronic "lump" of the upper lid.
     b. Symptoms. Patients complain of lump of the upper lid.
     c. Clinical signs. A lump similar to a chalazion in the upper tarsus.
     d. Etiology. Sebaceous cell carcinomas arise from the meibomian glands.
     e. Diagnostic evaluation
       (1) Differential diagnosis includes chalazia, which tend to have a rather acute onset.
       (2) Lesions tend to be highly malignant.
       (3) Clinicians should be alert for recurrent chalazia in the affected area.
     f. Treatment. Surgical removal is mandatory with pathologic evaluation.
     g. Follow-up. Every 2–3 months if uncertain as to the etiology of the lid lesion.

J. *Disease of the lacrimal system*
1. Dry eye
     a. Tear insufficiency associated with aging and a variety of systemic diseases. One of the most common causes of low-grade irritation of the eyes.
     b. Symptoms
       (1) Scratchiness or foreign body sensation, particularly upon awakening.
       (2) Excessive tearing due to reflex tearing.

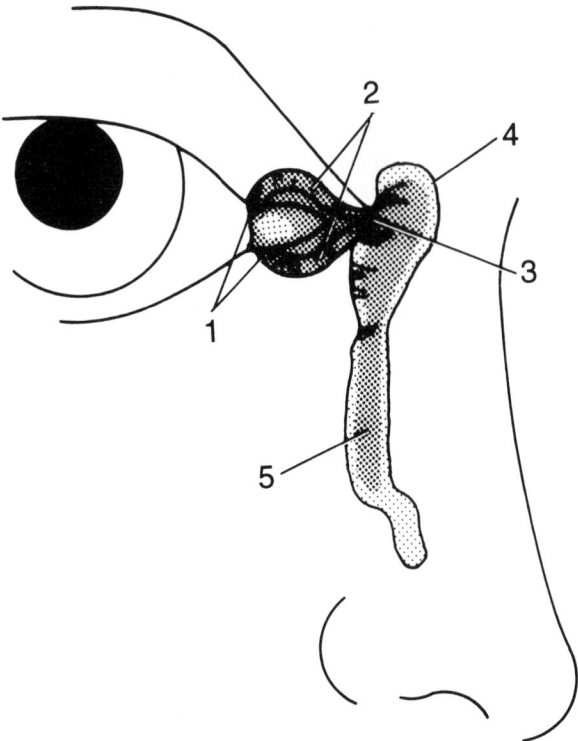

Figure 5-1. Structures of the lacrimal drainage system. (1) Upper and lower puncta, (2) upper and lower canaliculi, (3) common canaliculus, (4) lacrimal sac, (5) nasolacrimal duct.

     (3) Air conditioning, low humidity, and exposure to elements may worsen complaints.

     (4) Usually bilateral.

     (5) Symptoms may be worse than clinical presentation.

  c. Clinical signs

     (1) Mild conjunctival hyperemia/chemosis.

     (2) Mild punctate keratitis.

     (3) Corneal and/or conjunctival staining with rose bengal.

     (4) Decreased tear breakup time (<10 seconds)

     (5) Reduced Schirmer tear test (<5 mm in 5 minutes with anesthetic). See Clinical Procedures.

  d. Etiology

     (1) Idiopathic—no associated systemic disease. May be drug-induced (such as oral contraceptives, phenothiazines, antihistamines, anticholinergics, tricyclic antidepressants).

     (2) Sjögren's syndrome (keratitis sicca, xerostomia, arthritis). These patients also have arthritic joints and dry mouths. (Asking a Sjögren's patient if they can eat a soda cracker will result in a resounding NO!)

     (3) Other systemic diseases such as lupus erythematosus, pemphigoid, Stevens-Johnson syndrome, and sarcoid.

     (4) Status post-trauma or following radiation of lacrimal gland.

     (5) Vitamin A deficiency.

e. Diagnostic evaluation
   (1) Careful examination to rule out other causes of irritation.
   (2) Differential diagnosis includes blepharokeratoconjunctivitis of other causes, abnormal lid position, VII nerve palsy, and lagophthalmos.
   (3) Schirmer testing.
   (4) Tear breakup time measurement.
f. Treatment
   (1) *Mild.* Best treated with drops several times during the day (Tears Naturale, Hypotears, Refresh).
   (2) *Moderate*
       (a) Use artificial tears more frequently (q 1–2 hours).
       (b) Use more viscous preparations such as Cell-U-Visc.
       (c) Lubricating ointment (Lacri-Lube, Refresh P.M.) at bedtime.
   (3) *Severe*
       (a) Lubricating ointment 3–4 times per day.
       (b) Viscous artificial tears q 1 hour.
       (c) Punctal occlusion—temporary collagen plugs first to identify candidates for more permanent occlusion. (See Clinical Procedures.)
       (d) Thermal punctoplasty or silicone plugs if collagen plugs improve condition. (Author prefers Herrick silicone plugs.)
       (e) Refer for tarsorrhaphy if above measures do not protect cornea.
g. Follow-up
   (1) Depends on severity. If mild, may see in weeks to months.
   (2) Severe dry eye should be monitored closely as it may lead to corneal ulceration and blindness.

Clinical Procedure—Schirmer Test

Description/ Purpose	Purpose of Schirmer testing is to identify those patients with reduced tear production.
Equipment	Topical anesthetic such as proparacaine. Schirmer strips.
Procedure	Schirmer test measuring total reflex and basic tear secretion (topical anesthetic not used). Schirmer strips are folded approximately 5 mm from the end. Schirmer strips are placed in the lower cul-de-sac at the outer canthus. Patient is instructed to close his or her eyes and the test runs for 5 minutes. Remove strip and measure using millimeter rule. Interpretation—between 10 and 30 mm of wetting is considered normal. Schirmer test for basic secretion only (with anesthetic). This test is run exactly the same as the Schirmer test for total secretion except that anesthetic drops are instilled in the cul-de-sac prior to placing the strips. It is important to note that the anesthetic drops should be dabbed from the eye with a cotton-tipped applicator once anesthesia takes place, to remove any residual moisture. Test results—less than 5 mm of wetting is indicative of a problem with basic tear secretion.

Clinical Procedure—Temporary Canalicular Collagen Implant

Description/ Purpose:	Purpose of a temporary canalicular collagen implant is to help identify those patients who may benefit by permanent punctal occlusion.
Equipment:	Collagen implants available in diameters of 0.2, 0.3, and 0.4 mm. Jeweler's forceps. Topical anesthetic. Biomicroscope.
Procedure:	Topical anesthetic drops are placed in the lower cul-de-sac. Patient is placed at the slit lamp. Collagen implant is grasped using a jeweler's forceps and removed from the foam package (0.3- and 0.4-mm plugs work in most cases). With free hand, pull the lower lid outward so that the punctum is exposed and place the implant into the opening of the punctum. Once the plug is seated, gently push implant into the punctum until it is flush with the lid margin. With one pointed end of the jeweler's forceps, implant may be pushed into the canaliculus until it cannot be seen from the punctum. Repeat the procedure for all other puncta. Patients are asked to return to the office in a few days and report any subjective improvement. Subjective or objective improvement is an indication for more permanent punctal occlusion with a silicone plug or thermal cautery.

Clinical Procedure—Silicone Canalicular Implant

Description/ Purpose	Purpose is to effect semipermanent closure of upper or lower canaliculus with silicone implant.
Equipment	Herrick silicone plugs (0.3 or 0.5 mm) available from Lacrimedics, Inc. Plug serves as dilator and comes on stainless steel inserter. Topical anesthetic. Biomicroscope.
Procedure	Topical anesthetic drops placed in lower cul-de-sac. Patient placed at the slit lamp. Patient looks up and silicone plug is placed in lower punctum. Gently push plug into canaliculus (5 mm) and remove inserter. Repeat for other puncta if desired. Suggest occlude lower first then upper at later date. If patient experiences epiphora, may remove by irrigation.

---

2. Epiphora (wet eye)
   a. Patients with true epiphora generally require the use of a handkerchief at all times.
   b. Symptoms
      (1) Excessive tearing.
      (2) History of previous anterior segment disease.

c. Clinical signs
  (1) Excessive tearing.
  (2) Signs of stenotic punctum.
  (3) Signs of associated anterior segment disease.
d. Etiology
  (1) Associated with anterior segment disease such as keratoconjunctivitis or foreign body.
  (2) Blockage of lacrimal system.
  (3) Associated with poor lid apposition.
e. Diagnostic evaluation
  (1) Differential diagnosis includes: anterior segment causes such as foreign body or keratoconjunctivitis, lacrimal stenosis or blockage, dacryocystitis (infection of lacrimal sac).
  (2) Careful slit lamp examination.
  (3) Jones dye test (see Clinical Procedures).
  (4) Lacrimal dilation and irrigation (see Clinical Procedures).
  (5) Lacrimal probing.
  (6) Evaluation for regurgitation (gentle pressure on lacrimal sac—watch for mucopurulent discharge from punctum).
f. Treatment
  (1) Treat primary eye condition—conjunctivitis or keratitis should be treated appropriately.
  (2) Lacrimal stenosis—may be treated by dilation and irrigation. If unable to irrigate, lacrimal probing or dacryocystorhinostomy (DCR) may be indicated.
  (3) If epiphora due to dacryocystitis
    (a) Do not attempt to irrigate!
    (b) Prescribe dicloxacillin 500 mg po q 6 hours ×10 days.
    (c) Topical antibiotics if associated conjunctivitis.
    (d) Warm compresses bid or tid.
g. Follow-up
  (1) Reexamine patient in 7–10 days.
  (2) Refer if patient does not improve.
  (3) Consider DCR if chronic or if epiphora persists.

Clinical Procedure—Jones Dye Test

Description/Purpose: Purpose of Jones dye test is to determine the patency of the nasolacrimal system. It is indicated when patients complain of epiphora.

Equipment: Sodium fluorescein strips. Cotton-tipped applicators. Lacrimal dilation and irrigation set.

Procedure: Jones dye test I
Place sodium fluorescein in the inferior cul-de-sac of the affected side.
After 5 minutes ask patient to blow nose into white tissue and inspect tissue for evidence of fluorescein.
If no fluorescein is found, insert a cotton-tipped applicator into the inferior turbinate on the nostril of the affected side for 5–10 seconds.

(continued)

Clinical Procedure (*continued*)

Cotton-tipped applicator is then removed and examined for evidence of fluorescein.

If dye is not seen, then proceed with Jones dye test II.

Jones dye test II

After Jones dye test I is completed and dye fails to show up in the nostril on the affected side, a Jones dye test II may be performed.

The inferior canaliculus on the affected side is irrigated with saline solution and some of the saline is recovered in a basin. The saline solution is examined with cobalt light to identify fluorescein.

If fluorescein is found following a Jones II test, then a functional blockage exists which requires further evaluation.

Clinical Procedure—Lacrimal Dilation and Irrigation

Description/ Purpose	Lacrimal dilation and irrigation is useful in the evaluation and treatment of epiphora. It will identify a blocked nasolacrimal system and may clear out minor blockages in the process of the test.
Equipment	Lacrimal dilator. Lacrimal cannula. Sterile syringe. Topical anesthetic. Cotton-tipped applicator. Sterile solution.
Procedure	Topical anesthetic is placed in the lower cul-de-sac of the eye which is to be dilated and irrigated. Additional anesthesia may be obtained by placing a soaked cotton-tipped applicator over the punctum and allowing it to remain in position for 2 minutes. Fill syringe with 3–5 cc of saline and place cannula onto syringe. Gently pull lower lid down to expose the inferior punctum and allow lacrimal dilator to descend vertically into canaliculus approximately 2 mm. Lacrimal dilator is then rotated outward so that the tapered tip points toward the nose and the dilator is gently rotated between the fingers to enlarge the punctum. Care is taken not to force the dilator deep into the canaliculus or tear the punctal opening. Remove the dilator and insert the lacrimal cannula perpendicular to the lid margin, sliding it downward for approximately 2 mm. Cannula is then rotated so that the tip points toward the nose and the cannula is inserted 2–4 mm further. A syringe is gently depressed to inject saline into the canaliculus. Enough saline is injected when the patient coughs or reports a salty taste in the back of the throat. Cannula is removed once saline passes through system.

II. **Disease of the Conjunctiva**

   A. *Features of the conjunctiva*

      1. The conjunctiva overlies the sclera and lines the lid.

      2. The anatomic divisions of the conjunctiva consist of the palpebral conjunctiva, which lines the lids; the fornix, which is the junction of the palpebral and bulbar conjunctiva; and the bulbar conjunctiva, which overlies the sclera.

      3. Various glands are present in the conjunctiva which contribute to production of tears as well as mucin observed in diseased states.

   B. *General assessment of conjunctiva*

      1. Note color and thickness of the conjunctiva.

      2. Note the presence of redness.

      3. Note the presence or absence of discharge.

   C. *Pathophysiology of symptoms—conjunctiva.*

      1. Inflammation of the conjunctiva (conjunctivitis) is one of the most common anterior segment problems seen by primary care practitioners.

      2. Patient complaints related to the conjunctiva:

         a. Redness—may be localized or diffuse.

         b. Itching—due to histamine released from mast cells of conjunctiva.

         c. Lid swelling—due to chemosis or swelling of underlying conjunctiva.

         d. Discharge—may be watery, mucoid, or mucopurulent.

   D. *Inflammatory disease of the conjunctiva*

      1. Signs of inflammation include:

         a. Papillae—areas of vascularized tissue hypertrophy in response to long-term chronic irritation.

         b. Follicles—bumps on the palpebral conjunctiva which represent hypertrophied lymphoid tissue.

         c. Hyperemia—may be observed in both the bulbar and the palpebral conjunctiva as dilation of conjunctival vessels.

         d. Chemosis—edema of the conjunctiva.

      2. Bacterial conjunctivitis

         a. Acute, usually mucopurulent inflammation of the conjunctiva.

         b. Symptoms

            (1) Red eye and purulent discharge.

            (2) Frequently eyelids are stuck together in the morning.

         c. Clinical signs

            (1) Diffuse redness, usually bilateral.

            (2) Preauricular node swelling in severe forms.

            (3) Papillary hypertrophy of the bulbar conjunctiva.

         d. Etiology

            (1) Most common microbial pathogens include *Staphylococcus aureus*, *Streptococcus pneumoniae*, and *Haemophilus influenzae*.

            (2) Easily transmitted by contact.

         e. Diagnostic evaluation

            (1) Differential diagnosis includes viral, chlamydial, and allergic forms of conjunctivitis.

            (2) Conjunctival culture (see Clinical Procedures)

         f. Treatment

            (1) Topical antibiotics (erythromycin ointment qid, Trimethoprim/polymyxin (e.g., Polytrim) or gentamicin drops qid).

            (2) Lid scrubs may be helpful if there is associated blepharitis.

         g. Follow-up

            (1) Usually self-limiting.

            (2) Follow-up if not resolved within 7–10 days.

Clinical Procedure—Conjunctival Culture

Description/ Purpose	To aid in identification of microorganisms responsible for infection and help in the selection of appropriate antibiotic therapy through sensitivity testing.
Equipment	Culturette tube containing transport medium (Stuart's) and rayon-tipped applicator.
Procedure	Wash hands and wear gloves.
	Do culture prior to use of any drops.
	Evert lower lid exposing conjunctiva.
	Gently roll applicator along conjunctiva several times collecting material.
	Place applicator in culturette tube.
	Squeeze ampule activating transport medium.
	Label and ship to laboratory.

---

3. Simple allergic conjunctivitis
   a. Allergic conjunctivitis represents one of the most commonly seen conjunctivitides.
   b. Symptoms
      (1) Itching, tearing, and redness.
      (2) There may be a history of topical drug use.
   c. Clinical signs
      (1) Chemosis and hyperemia.
      (2) Papillary hypertrophy is sometimes observed.
   d. Etiology
      (1) Hypersensitivity reaction may be of immediate or delayed type.
      (2) May be associated with contact lens wear or solutions.
      (3) May be associated with eye makeup.
      (4) May be associated with hay fever or seasonal allergy.
   e. Diagnostic evaluation
      (1) Differential diagnosis includes bacterial or viral conjunctivitis as well as episcleritis.
      (2) Hyperemia associated with allergic conjunctivitis usually blanches with 0.12% phenylephrine within a few minutes following instillation.
   f. Treatment
      (1) Mild forms of allergic conjunctivitis may be treated with the use of vasoconstrictors and topical antihistamines 3–4 ×/day.
      (2) Moderate presentations of allergic conjunctivitis may be treated with antihistamines, mast cell stabilizers (Alomide .1%) or non-steroidal anti-inflammatory agents such as ketorolac (Acular 0.5%) used 3–4 ×/day.
      (3) Severe cases of allergic conjunctivitis may be treated with topical steroids (0.12% or 1% prednisolone or fluorometholone) used 3–4 ×/day on a short-term basis.
      (4) Severe forms may benefit from oral antihistamine use (Benadryl, Seldane, or Hismanal) in addition to topical therapy.
   g. Follow-up. Monitor IOP on patients using steroids every 4–6 weeks.
4. Giant papillary conjunctivitis
   a. Commonly encountered inflammatory disease associated with soft contact lens wear.
   b. Symptoms. Subjectively patients complain of itching, tearing, discomfort, and multiple lens problems including lens deposits.

c. Clinical signs
   (1) Papillary hypertrophy is noted, especially on upper palpebral conjunctiva.
   (2) Poor fitting and coated lens surfaces may be observed.
   (3) Occasionally corneal vascularization at the 12:00 meridian may be noted.
d. Etiology. Type IV hypersensitivity reaction to tear proteins found on soft lenses.
e. Diagnostic evaluation
   (1) Differential diagnosis includes simple allergic conjunctivitis and seasonal conjunctivitis.
   (2) Evert upper lid and look for papillae.
f. Treatment
   (1) Discontinuation of soft contact lens wear.
   (2) Refitting with alternative contact lens material.
   (3) Mast cell stabilizer or topical antihistamine several times per day on an ongoing basis.
   (4) Severe cases may be treated with 0.25% fluorometholone or 0.12% prednisolone 3–4 ×/day for a few weeks (observe usual precautions when using topical steroids).
g. Follow-up. Recheck every 3–4 weeks.

Clinical Procedure—Lid Eversion

Description/ Purpose	To evert the upper lid for examination to determine the presence of papillae or conjunctival foreign body.
Equipment	Cotton-tipped applicator. Slit lamp.
Procedure	Place patient at slit lamp. Have patient look down. Gently pull the upper lid away from the globe grasping the cilia at the lid margin. While patient continues to look down, fold the upper lid back over the cotton-tipped applicator and hold against the superior orbital bone. Examine upper palpebral conjunctiva for tissue change or foreign body.

---

5. Vernal conjunctivitis
   a. Seasonal allergy of the eye.
   b. Affects males more often than females.
   c. Usually a history of atopic disease is present.
   d. Symptoms
      (1) Itching, burning, and tearing, typically in the spring and fall.
      (2) May be associated with a history of hay fever or atopy.
   e. Clinical signs
      (1) Hyperemia, chemosis, and papillary hypertrophy may be noted in the upper and lower conjunctiva.
      (2) Ulceration of superior cornea or small subepithelial infiltrates (Trantas dots) may be noted.
   f. Etiology. Seasonal inflammation of the conjunctiva associated with hay fever or other atopic disease.

      g. Diagnostic evaluation. Differential diagnosis includes mild allergic conjunctivitis, trachoma, and giant papillary conjunctivitis.

      h. Treatment

        (1) "Pulse dose" of 1% prednisolone 3–4 ×/day for 1 week followed by .12% prednisolone 3–4 ×/day—often for months.

        (2) As vernal conjunctivitis is brought under control, milder steroids, such as fluorometholone, may be useful.

        (3) Mast cell stabilizers may be safely used on an ongoing basis.

      i. Follow-up. Every few weeks.

6. Herpes simplex conjunctivitis

      a. Follicular conjunctivitis due to HSV 1.

      b. Symptoms. Foreign body sensation and tearing.

      c. Clinical signs

        (1) Hyperemia and lid vesicles if the lid is involved.

        (2) If the cornea is involved, a dendritic ulcer may be noted.

      d. Etiology

        (1) Conjunctival infection due to herpes simplex virus (HSV 1).

        (2) May be associated with injury or other ocular disease.

      e. Diagnostic evaluation

        (1) Careful slit lamp examination with attention to the cornea.

        (2) Sodium fluorescein staining may be useful to identify associated dendritic ulcer.

        (3) Differential diagnosis includes bacterial and chlamydial infection.

      f. Treatment

        (1) Trifluorothymidine 1% (Viroptic) 4–5 ×/day may be useful until the conjunctivitis has cleared.

        (2) If a dendritic ulcer is present, antiviral must be used more frequently (every 1–3 hours).

      g. Follow-up. 2–3 days to monitor cornea.

7. Pharyngoconjunctival fever (PCF)

      a. Syndrome of viral infection of eyes, nose, and throat.

      b. Symptoms. Sore throat and ocular foreign body sensation.

      c. Clinical signs

        (1) Hyperemia and teary, watery discharge.

        (2) Diffuse conjunctival redness may also be observed.

      d. Etiology. Adenovirus that typically affects nose, throat, and upper respiratory system.

      e. Diagnostic evaluation. Differential diagnosis includes bacterial, allergic, and herpes simplex conjunctivitis.

      f. Treatment

        (1) Management is essentially supportive.

        (2) A broad-spectrum antibiotic used 3–4 ×/day may be used for prophylactic cover but this has little value in treatment of the primary infection.

        (3) Disease is self-limiting, typically lasting 2–3 weeks.

      g. Follow-up. Recheck weekly.

8. Epidemic keratoconjunctivitis (EKC)

      a. Highly contagious form of conjunctivitis and keratitis.

      b. Symptoms. Foreign body sensation and decreased vision.

      c. Clinical signs

        (1) Chemosis, petechial hemorrhages, and subepithelial infiltrates may be noted.

        (2) May be associated with preauricular adenopathy.

      d. Etiology. Adenovirus types 8 and 17.

      e. Diagnostic evaluation

        (1) Careful slit lamp evaluation to rule out corneal involvement (subepithelial infiltrates).

       (2) Palpate the preauricular node to identify swelling.

       (3) Differential diagnosis of other red eye types.

  f. Treatment

       (1) Supportive therapy with artificial tears.

       (2) Coverage with broad-spectrum antibiotic may have some value if corneal epithelium is affected.

       (3) If subepithelial infiltrates reduce vision or are uncomfortable, steroids (0.12% or 1% prednisolone tid or qid) may provide some improvement.

       (4) Steroids must be tapered if they are used.

       (5) Cycloplegics such as 5% homatropine bid will help reduce photophobia.

  g. Follow-up

       (1) 1–2 weeks if cornea involved.

       (2) May have to taper steroids over several weeks.

       (3) In monitoring IOP, be sure to disinfect tonometer tips.

9. Inclusion (chlamydial) conjunctivitis

  a. Symptoms. Foreign body sensation, photophobia, and discharge.

  b. Clinical signs

       (1) Mucopurulent discharge, follicular and papillary hypertrophy.

       (2) Preauricular adenopathy may be found.

       (3) Frequently chlamydial conjunctivitis has been misdiagnosed as bacterial conjunctivitis and does not respond to topical antibiotics.

  c. Etiology

       (1) Conjunctival inflammation secondary to chlamydial infection.

       (2) Sexually transmitted disease.

  d. Diagnostic evaluation

       (1) Slit lamp examination to rule out other anterior segment disease.

       (2) Palpation of preauricular area of adenopathy.

       (3) Conjunctival smears show intracellular inclusion bodies.

  e. Treatment

       (1) Oral tetracycline 250 mg qid for 10 days (erythromycin 250 mg may be substituted in pregnant or lactating women, or children).

       (2) Topical antibiotics used 3–4 ×/day may provide useful coverage for secondary infection.

       (3) Disease is highly contagious and is sexually transmitted.

  f. Follow-up. 1–2 weeks until clear.

10. Toxic follicular conjunctivitis

  a. An acute inflammatory reaction secondary to irritation by injurious agent or drug.

  b. Symptoms

       (1) Mild irritation and some tearing.

       (2) Nonresponse to medicines previously or currently being used.

  c. Clinical signs

       (1) Follicular hypertrophy noted along with diffuse redness.

       (2) Toxic agent may be seen within the cul-de-sac.

  d. Etiology

       (1) Chemical injury.

       (2) Topical medication use.

       (3) Ocular foreign body.

  e. Diagnostic evaluation. Careful slit lamp examination to rule out other red eye types.

  f. Treatment

       (1) Removal of toxic agent.

       (2) Symptomatic treatment of red eye may include ocular lubricants, topical antibiotics, or, in some cases, topical anti-inflammatories.

  g. Follow-up. Varies with severity and etiology.

11. Oculodermatologic conjunctivitis
   a. A variety of conjunctivitis associated with dermatologic conditions (for a more complete discussion, see Chapter 6).
   b. Common dermatologic problems that manifest in the conjunctiva are:
      (1) Acne rosacea.
      (2) Psoriasis.
      (3) Atopic dermatitis.
12. Mucous membrane disorders and the conjunctiva
   a. A variety of conjunctival complications are associated with mucous membrane disorders.
   b. Benign mucous membrane pemphigoid (BMMP) results in tissue destruction of the conjunctiva.
   c. Erythema multiforme (Stevens-Johnson syndrome) causes dryness and inflammation of the conjunctiva as well (see Chapter 6).
13. Pinguecula
   a. Hyperplasia of elastic tissue of the conjunctiva.
   b. Most pingueculae are found nasally.
   c. Symptoms. Subjectively patients complain of burning and often a cosmetic problem.
   d. Clinical signs. An elevated vascular lesion may be noted nasally.
   e. Etiology
      (1) The hyperplasia of the elastic tissue of the conjunctiva may be stimulated by irritation from dust, wind, and sunlight (UV).
      (2) Pingueculae are found primarily in individuals who spend a great deal of time outdoors.
   f. Diagnostic evaluation
      (1) Careful slit lamp examination to rule out other causes of irritation in this area of the conjunctiva is indicated.
      (2) Differential diagnosis includes pterygium and malignant conjunctival lesion.
   g. Treatment
      (1) Supportive therapy such as copious use of ocular lubricants or vasoconstrictors as indicated.
      (2) Particularly inflamed pinguecula (pingueculitis) will respond to the use of mild topical steroids (0.12% prednisolone or fluorometholone) used several times a day on a short-term basis.
      (3) Sunglasses may reduce UV radiation.
      (4) Surgical removal is indicated if the cosmetic problem is severe, lid function is impaired, or contact lens fitting is affected.
   h. Follow-up
      (1) Monitor IOP if patient is using steroids.
      (2) Semiannual or annual follow-up in other cases.
14. Superior limbic keratoconjunctivitis (SLK)
   a. Inflammation and vascularization of the superior bulbar conjunctiva.
   b. Symptoms. Subjectively patients complain of foreign body sensation, pain, and occasional photophobia.
   c. Clinical signs. The superior bulbar conjunctiva is hyperemic and there may be superior punctate keratitis.
   d. Etiology
      (1) Frequently associated with contact lens wear.
      (2) May be associated with hyperthyroid disease.
   e. Diagnostic evaluation
      (1) Differential diagnosis includes other types of conjunctivitides.
      (2) Slit lamp examination should be completed with lid eversion to rule out foreign body of the upper tarsus.

       f. Treatment
         (1) Supportive therapy through the use of artificial tears.
         (2) Proper diagnosis is essential in ruling out thyroid dysfunction.
         (3) Bandage lens may give some relief.
         (4) 0.5–1% silver nitrate may be applied to superior conjunctiva.
         (5) Cautery or superior conjunctival resection may be necessary.
         (6) Once primary cause is determined, SLK may resolve.
       g. Follow-up. A few weeks to several months depending upon etiology.

15. Subconjunctival hemorrhage
       a. Rupture of fragile conjunctival vessels.
       b. Symptoms
         (1) Sudden onset of redness in the eye.
         (2) There is no pain and vision is unaffected.
       c. Clinical signs. Objectively a bright, reddish lesion is noted.
       d. Etiology. Rupture of fragile conjunctival vessels following trauma, coughing, or straining.
       e. Diagnostic evaluation. Careful slit lamp examination to rule out other red eye types.
       f. Treatment
         (1) Management essentially supportive.
         (2) Initially cool compresses may cause localized vasoconstriction to reduce bleeding.
         (3) Later warm compresses hasten reabsorption of blood.
         (4) There is no indication for antibiotic or steroid therapy in subconjunctival hemorrhage.
       g. Follow-up. The red eye will clear in 7–21 days.

III. Episclera and Sclera

A. *General assessment of episclera and sclera*
1. Note color of the sclera—dark or blue indicates thinning, redness suggests inflammation, yellow suggests jaundice or fatty deposition within the stroma.
2. Note presence and distribution of redness.
3. Note presence of nodule formation.

B. *Pathophysiology of symptoms—episclera and sclera*
1. Inflammation of the episclera is fairly common and may be associated with systemic disease. Inflammation of the sclera is rather uncommon and signals serious collagen disease of the body.
2. Redness may be localized or diffuse.
3. Pain—stimulation of the extensive network of long and short posterior ciliary nerves from inflammation will result in pain.
4. Edema—the episclera is particularly susceptible to fluid accumulation.
5. Lymphocytic infiltration—nodular formation in episcleritis is the result of lymphocytic infiltration.

C. *Inflammatory disease of the episclera and sclera*
1. Episcleritis
       a. Nonspecific inflammation of the episcleral vessels.
       b. Symptoms
         (1) Acute unilateral redness.
         (2) Patients may complain of mild discomfort and pain on convergence due to pulling at the insertion of the muscle of the inflamed area of the sclera.
       c. Clinical signs
         (1) Diffuse episcleritis manifests as a large area or quadrant of episcleral inflammation.

(2) Nodular episcleritis presents as a localized area of hyperemia and inflammation usually resulting in an elevated purplish nodule.

d. Etiology
  (1) Often associated with rheumatoid arthritis.
  (2) May be associated with stress, poor nutrition, or fatigue.

e. Diagnostic evaluation
  (1) Careful slit lamp evaluation to rule out other types of red eye such as conjunctivitis or iritis.
  (2) Cells and flare may be noted in episcleritis or scleritis due to the common vascular supply shared with the iris and limbus.
  (3) Episcleritis may be differentiated from conjunctivitis by the application of 0.12% phenylephrine to the cul-de-sac. In conjunctivitis the vessels will blanch, whereas in episcleritis the vessels will remain red.

f. Treatment
  (1) Careful evaluation for systemic disease is indicated, as episcleritis may be associated with autoimmune collagen disorders such as rheumatoid arthritis.
  (2) Systemic evaluation is particularly indicated when episcleritis is recurrent.
  (3) Episcleritis is frequently self-limiting.
  (4) Clinical course may be hastened by the use of topical decongestants as well as mild topical steroids 4–5 ×/day.
  (5) Topical steroids should be tapered to lessen the likelihood of rebound.

g. Follow-up. 2–4 weeks if steroids are used. Monitor IOP.

2. Scleritis
  a. A serious autoimmune response that results in destruction of scleral tissue.
  b. Symptoms. Patients complain of pain, decreased vision, and tenderness to touch.
  c. Clinical signs. Diffuse inflammation and thinning of the sclera resulting in a bluish-red appearance may be noted.
  d. Etiology. The underlying causes of scleritis are frequently rheumatoid arthritis, systemic lupus erythematosus, or polyarteritis nodosa, as well as herpetic disease.
  e. Diagnostic evaluation
    (1) It is important to accurately diagnose scleritis, as this represents a sight-threatening red eye.
    (2) Identify underlying systemic etiology.
  f. Treatment
    (1) Referral is always indicated, as scleritis is best handled on a secondary or tertiary level with coordination of medical care.
    (2) Aggressive systemic treatment with antibiotics, antivirals, or antimetabolites is usually indicated.
    (3) Scleral grafts may be required when a scleral perforation occurs.

IV. Cornea

A. *Features of the cornea*
  1. The cornea is the chief refractive surface of the eye, accounting for approximately two-thirds of its refractive power.
  2. The normal cornea is transparent.
  3. The average corneal diameter measures 11.7 mm in the horizontal and 10.8 mm in the vertical.
  4. Histologically, the cornea is composed of the epithelium, stroma, and endothelium.
  5. The basement membrane of the epithelium lies on Bowman's membrane, which is located in the anterior stroma.

6. Descemet's membrane serves as the posterior limit of the stroma and is secreted by the endothelium.
7. Physiologically, the high metabolic rate of the epithelium is sustained by oxygen from the atmosphere, limbal circulation, and tear film.
8. Water is removed from the collagenous stroma by the active transport pumping of the endothelium.

B. *General assessment of the cornea*
   1. Note corneal luster on external examination.
   2. Look for corneal opacification in the form of edema, infiltration, ulceration, scarring, or vascularization.
   3. Note any associated lid or conjunctival disease.

C. *Pathophysiology of symptoms*
   1. Staining—staining with sodium fluorescein or rose bengal indicates epithelial disease. Pattern of staining may give clue to etiology (see Figure 5-4).
   2. Infiltrates—lymphocytic infiltration in response to a cornea challenged by infection, toxicity, or hypoxia.
   3. Edema—accumulation of fluid within the cornea. May be limited to the stroma or epithelium.
   4. Ulceration—a complete loss of epithelium as a result of an infectious process—usually with lymphocytic infiltration or marked edema.
   5. Vascularization—any abnormal ingrowth of blood vessels in response to chronic hypoxia, infectious disease, or chronic allergy.

D. *Infection and inflammation*
   1. Superficial punctate keratitis (SPK)
      a. Fine, pinpoint epithelial defects of the cornea.
      b. Symptoms. Foreign body sensation, redness, photophobia, and occasionally pain.
      c. Clinical signs
         (1) Localized or diffuse epithelial staining.
         (2) May be unilateral or bilateral.
         (3) May be associated redness, foreign body sensation, or pain.
         (4) May be associated with conjunctival or lid disease.
      d. Etiology
         (1) May have various causes.
         (2) Infective—blepharitis, conjunctivitis, rosacea.
         (3) Degenerative—dry eye syndrome, exposure keratopathy, trichiasis.
         (4) Toxic—drug toxicity (neomycin, gentamicin, and many others), contact lens solutions.
         (5) Allergic.
         (6) Traumatic—eye rubbing, contact lenses, foreign body under the upper eyelid.
      e. Diagnostic evaluation
         (1) Differential diagnosis includes corneal abrasion, subepithelial infiltrates, herpes simplex keratitis.
         (2) Careful history will help delineate possible etiologies.
         (3) Clinical appearance of staining will give clue to etiology (see Figure 5-2).
      f. Treatment
         (1) Non-contact lens wearers with mild SPK may be managed with copious use of artificial tears in the daytime and lubricating ointment at night.
         (2) Non-contact lens wearers with significant SPK should be treated the same as for a corneal abrasion with antibiotics, cycloplegics, and pressure patch.

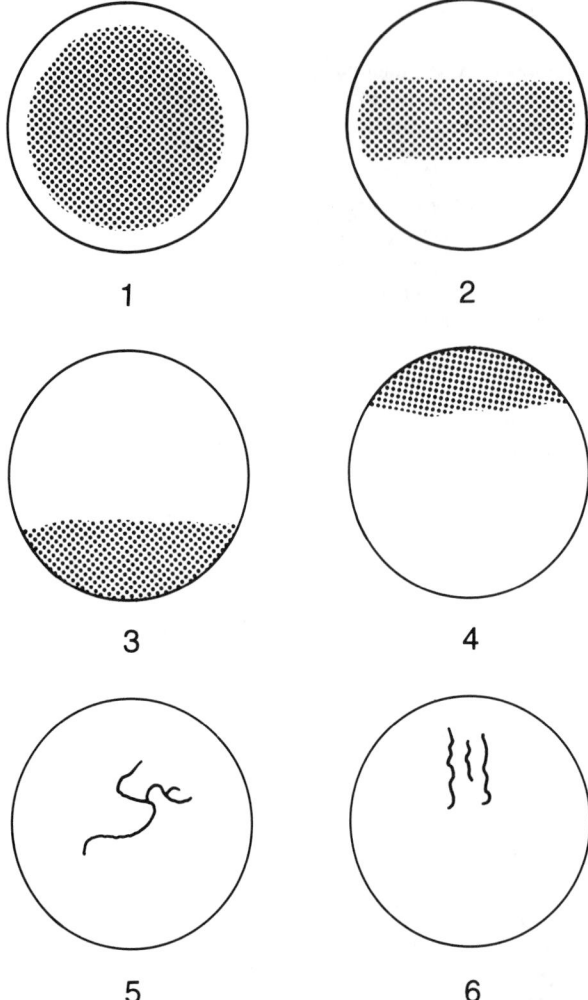

Figure 5-2. Corneal staining and associated etiologies. (1) Diffuse: bacterial and viral keratoconjunctivitis, drug toxicity. (2) Middle one-third: exposure, dry eye, lagophthalmos. (3) Lower one-third: blepharoconjunctivitis, acne rosacea, trichiasis. (4) Upper one-third: vernal conjunctivitis, trachoma, giant papillary conjunctivitis, superior limbic keratoconjunctivitis. (5) Dendritic: herpes simplex keratoconjunctivitis. (6) Linear: abrasion, foreign body under upper lid.

        (3) Contact lens wearers should discontinue contact lens wear and be treated as above.

    g. Follow-up

        (1) SPK frequently is a long-term problem.

        (2) Contact lens wearers may not resume contact lens wear until the SPK has totally resolved.

        (3) Patients should be seen at least weekly until SPK has resolved.

  2. Infectious infiltrate or ulcer

    a. Symptoms

        (1) Decreased visual acuity.

        (2) Pain or photophobia.

        (3) Red eye.

        (4) Discharge—may have associated conjunctivitis.

b. Clinical signs
    (1) Stromal opacity which consists of white blood cell infiltration and edema.
    (2) By definition, an ulcer exists in deepithelialized cornea *with substance loss.*
    (3) May be associated conjunctival disease or lid disease.
    (4) May have significant anterior chamber reaction including hypopyon.
    (5) May have associated generalized corneal edema.

c. Etiology
    (1) Bacterial—particularly when associated with mucopurulent conjunctivitis.
    (2) Herpes simplex virus—may have associated herpes simplex conjunctivitis or herpes simplex keratitis.
    (3) Fungal—often associated with "tree branch" injury.
    (4) *Acanthamoeba*—associated with poor contact lens hygiene and homemade saline, public swimming pools.

d. Diagnostic evaluation
    (1) Careful history required to determine presence of associated disease, history of contact lens wear, trauma, or systemic disease.
    (2) Careful slit lamp examination to determine extent of corneal disease, presence of associated conjunctival lid disease, presence of anterior chamber reaction.
    (3) Conjunctival culture may be helpful in ascertaining etiology.
    (4) Corneal scrapings for smears and cultures are mandatory when infiltrate has ulcerated (see Clinical Procedure).
    (5) Differential diagnosis includes subepithelial infiltrates associated with viral conjunctivitis, marginal infiltrates associated with staphylococcus hypersensitivity, stromal inflammation associated with foreign body.

e. Treatment (assuming bacterial)
    (1) Topical antibiotics
        (a) Small infiltrates may be treated with broad-spectrum antibiotics such as tobramycin q 2–4 hours or ciloxan q ¹/₂–1 hour.
        (b) Large infiltrates or frank ulcers should be covered with topical antibiotics q ¹/₂–1 hour in the case of tobramycin, and q 15–30 minutes with ciloxan. Fortified tobramycin is also useful for severe ulcers (see Clinical Procedure for fortified Tobramycin) every q 1 hour.
    (2) Pain may be mediated by cycloplegic (atropine 1% bid or homatropine 5% tid–bid); may also use oral analgesics such as acetaminophen.
    (3) No patch.

f. Follow-up
    (1) Daily observation with careful notation of the size of the lesion.
    (2) Modify antibiotic therapy if culture indicates an organism that is not susceptible to the antibiotic that you have started.
    (3) As ulcer improves, may taper drug therapy.
    (4) If ulcer is central, or if severe corneal thinning is observed, may refer to corneal specialist.

Clinical Alert

An eye with a corneal ulcer or infection is *never* pressure patched.

---

3. Fungal keratitis
    a. Symptoms
        (1) Decreased visual acuity.

    (2) Pain and photophobia.
    (3) Red eye and/or discharge.
    (4) Previous history of trauma (contact with vegetable matter).
    (5) May have history of topical steroid use.
- b. Clinical signs
    (1) Stromal opacity with feathery borders.
    (2) Opacity may appear several days or even weeks after trauma to the cornea.
    (3) May have satellite lesions, anterior chamber reaction, or hypopyon.
- c. Etiology. Several fungal species—*Candida, Fusarium,* and *Aspergillus.*
- d. Diagnostic evaluation
    (1) History to determine associated trauma.
    (2) Slit lamp examination to determine extent of disease.
    (3) Corneal scrapings may be useful in identifying fungi.
- e. Treatment
    (1) Natamycin 5% q 1–2 hours while awake and q 2 hours at night.
    (2) Cycloplegic homatropine 5% TID
    (3) Note: Topical steroids are *not* used.
    (4) The eye is not patched.
- f. Follow-up
    (1) Daily observation carefully noting the size of the lesion.
    (2) If after several days the cornea does not improve or stroma becomes involved, refer patient to cornea specialist.
    (3) As epithelium and ulcer improves, drug may be tapered.
    (4) Severe corneal thinning should be evaluated by a cornea specialist for possible keratoplasty.

Clinical Procedure—Corneal Scraping

Description/Purpose: To obtain material from corneal ulcers for culture or smear.

Materials/Equipment: Topical anesthetic. Kimura spatula or sterile knife blade. Culture media (blood agar, chocolate agar, Sabouraud's agar) and thioglycolate broth (transport tube). Microscope slides for Gram's and Giemsa stain.

Procedure: Scraping and Culture
Anesthetize the cornea.
Have patient fixate point across room.
Using the back side of sterile knife blade or spatula sterilized over flame, scrape the ulcer starting on the bed moving toward edge. Try to obtain as much material for culture without using excessive force.
Plate material on each of the respective agar plates and thioglycolate broth. Sterilize spatula or blade after each sample is plated.
Label each sample and send to laboratory.
Scraping and Smears
Anesthetize cornea and obtain scrapings as above.
Spread material across slide, fix, and send to laboratory for Gram's or Giemsa stain.

```
┌─────────────────────────────────────────────────────────────────┐
│              Clinical Procedure—Making Fortified Tobramycin        │
│                                                                     │
│ Description/    To provide fortified antibiotics for treatment of   │
│ Purpose         corneal ulcers.                                     │
│ Materials/      Ampule 40 mg/ml tobramycin                          │
│ Equipment       5-ml bottle of tobramycin 0.3% ophthalmic solution. │
│ Procedure       Withdraw 2 ml of the 40 mg/ml tobramycin and        │
│                 deposit in the 5-ml bottle of 0.3% tobramycin.      │
│                 This mixture results in 7 ml of 15 mg/ml tobramycin.│
│                 Preparation should be refrigerated.                 │
│                                                                     │
│ From Cullom RD, Chang B. The Wills Eye Manual. Philadelphia: JB     │
│ Lippincott, 1994 p 459.                                             │
└─────────────────────────────────────────────────────────────────┘
```

4. Viral keratitis
  a. Herpes simplex virus (HSV)
    (1) Symptoms
       (a) Usually painful, unilateral red eye.
       (b) May be previous history of cold sores.
       (c) May be associated with history of HSV lid disease or conjunctivitis.
       (d) May have history of previous episodes.
    (2) Clinical signs
       (a) Corneal epithelial disease usually represented by a dendritic lesion.
       (b) Epithelial disease may manifest as superficial punctate keratitis or even geographic ulcer.
       (c) May have decreased corneal sensitivity.
       (d) May be areas of previous scarring.
       (e) Corneal stromal disease is identified by a disc-shaped grayish patch which may be central or peripheral.
       (f) Stromal disease usually has associated keratic precipitates.
       (g) Stromal disease may be associated with elevated intraocular pressure.
    (3) Etiology. Herpes simplex virus type 1.
    (4) Diagnostic evaluation
       (a) Careful slit lamp evaluation with staining to identify dendrite or other epithelial defects.
       (b) With cotton wisp, compare corneal sensitivity between two eyes.
       (c) Differential diagnosis includes linear corneal abrasion resembling dendrite, recurrent corneal erosion, herpes zoster keratitis (the latter is associated with painful skin vesicles that do not cross the midline).
    (5) Treatment
       (a) Trifluridine 1% drops (Viroptic) q 1–2 hours, up to 9 ×/day.
       (b) Vidarabine 3% ointment (Vira-A) 5 ×/day may be used as an alternative.
       (c) Cycloplegic agent if patient photophobic.
       (d) Steroids not used in presence of epithelial disease.
       (e) Debridement is effective in conjunction with topical therapy.
       (f) If stromal disease is present and epithelial disease absent, 1% prednisolone qid may be added in conjunction with antiviral therapy.
    (6) Follow-up
       (a) Patients with epithelial disease should be examined within the first 2–4 days and weekly thereafter.
       (b) Antivirals should not be used longer than 2–3 weeks.

        (c) If treating stromal disease, steroids should be tapered once cornea is clear.
- b. Adenovirus keratitis
  - (1) Symptoms. Decreased vision, pain, redness, tearing.
  - (2) Clinical signs
    - (a) Conjunctival hyperemia.
    - (b) Subepithelial infiltrates with minimal staining.
    - (c) Anterior chamber usually quiet.
  - (3) Etiology
    - (a) Adenovirus types 8 and 19 (epidemic keratoconjunctivitis).
    - (b) Other adenoviral types 3, 4, and 7.
  - (4) Diagnostic evaluation
    - (a) Careful slit lamp examination with fluorescein staining.
    - (b) Differential diagnosis includes superficial punctate keratitis, herpes simplex keratitis, toxicity due to previous use of medicine, subepithelial infiltrates associated with contact lens wear hypoxia, chlamydial infection.
  - (5) Treatment
    - (a) If symptoms mild, artificial tears are usually satisfactory.
    - (b) If patient exhibits reduced visual acuity or is very symptomatic, topical steroids (0.12%–1% prednisolone bid–qid) may be used.
    - (c) Photophobic patients may be treated with cycloplegic.
  - (6) Follow-up
    - (a) 7–10 days, then every 14 days thereafter.
    - (b) As cornea clears, steroids may be tapered.
    - (c) Clinical course may last weeks or even months.

Clinic Alert

If the possibility of herpes simplex keratitis exists, steroids should not be used. The long-term use of topical steroids may result in steroid-induced glaucoma or suprainfection.

---

5. Drug-induced keratitis
   - a. Punctate keratitis seen following long-term use of topical medicine.
   - b. Symptoms. Chronic red eye, associated with scratchiness and burning.
   - c. Clinical signs
     - (1) Punctate staining of the cornea.
     - (2) Conjunctival hyperemia.
     - (3) Filamentary keratitis.
   - d. Etiology. Long-term exposure to topical medicines, including aminoglycosides, antivirals, atropine, and virtually any other topical medicine.
   - e. Diagnostic evaluation
     - (1) Careful slit lamp evaluation to rule out other causes.
     - (2) Differential diagnosis includes superficial punctate keratitis associated with conjunctivitis and other anterior segment problems.
   - f. Treatment
     - (1) Discontinuation of topical medicine.
     - (2) May use nonpreserved artificial tears for symptomatic relief.
   - g. Follow-up. Patients are generally asymptomatic within 5–7 days.
6. Marginal infiltrates and ulcers
   - a. Symptoms
     - (1) Redness and irritation usually unilateral.
     - (2) Visual acuity usually unaffected.

b. Clinical signs
   (1) A grayish oval lesion near limbus.
   (2) There is usually a clear space between the lesion and the limbus.
   (3) There may be some staining with fluorescein.
c. Etiology
   (1) Occur secondary to acute or chronic bacterial conjunctivitis.
   (2) Associated with staphylococcal blepharitis.
   (3) Lymphocytic infiltration due to staphylococcal toxins.
   (4) Area is not a primary bacterial infection.
d. Diagnostic evaluation
   (1) Careful slit lamp examination with fluorescein staining.
   (2) Differential diagnosis includes phlyctenular conjunctivitis, scarring from corneal foreign body, and herpes keratitis.
e. Treatment
   (1) Treat primary cause such as conjunctivitis or blepharitis.
   (2) Broad-spectrum topical antibiotic drops several times a day for the first few days.
   (3) If area does not resolve, may add steroid in form of antibiotic–steroid combination drug tid or qid.
f. Follow-up
   (1) Initial return visit 4–5 days after commencing treatment.
   (2) Examine weekly thereafter.

Clinical Alert

If marginal infiltrate is associated with contact lens wear, contact lens wear may not resume until area has completely resolved (small grayish stromal scar may remain).

---

7. Phlyctenular keratoconjunctivitis
   a. Symptoms
      (1) Tearing, pain, redness, photophobia.
      (2) May have history of previous episodes.
   b. Clinical signs
      (1) Corneal phlyctenule appears as a small, grayish-white, raised lesion at or near the limbus.
      (2) There are usually dilated conjunctival blood vessels.
      (3) May be associated corneal neovascularization.
      (4) Usually bilateral.
   c. Etiology
      (1) Staphylococcal blepharitis.
      (2) Possibly tuberculosis.
   d. Diagnostic evaluation
      (1) Careful slit lamp examination of all ocular structures including cornea, conjunctiva, and lid margins.
      (2) Differential diagnosis includes marginal corneal ulcer, early pterygium, herpes simplex keratitis.
      (3) Refer to internist to rule out systemic cause such as tuberculosis.
   e. Treatment
      (1) For very symptomatic patients, 1% prednisolone used several times a day is helpful.
      (2) For patients with minimal symptoms, artificial tears may be helpful.
      (3) Antibiotic drops or ointments may be used in conjunction with topical steroids.

f. Follow-up
    (1) 4–5 days after initial visit.
    (2) Should see every 10 days to 2 weeks after that.
8. Neurotrophic corneal ulcers
    a. Symptoms. Redness, tearing, foreign body sensation.
    b. Clinical signs
        (1) Marked conjunctival hyperemia.
        (2) Eyelids may be swollen from excessive tearing.
        (3) Epithelial staining ranging from fine punctate to severe ulceration.
    c. Etiology
        (1) Damaged trigeminal nerve (by trauma, surgery, tumor, or inflammation).
        (2) Seen often after stroke.
        (3) May be seen with infection following fifth cranial nerve such as herpes zoster or herpes simplex.
    d. Diagnostic evaluation
        (1) Careful slit lamp evaluation to determine extent of corneal disease.
        (2) In-depth history to ascertain primary cause.
        (3) Differential diagnosis includes other causes of punctate keratitis and corneal ulcer.
    e. Treatment
        (1) Mild forms may be treated with artificial tears and ointment used several times a day.
        (2) If epithelial defect only, should be treated with antibiotic ointment and pressure patched.
        (3) Corneal ulcers should be treated aggressively as outlined previously.
    f. Follow-up
        (1) Mild forms may be seen every 1–2 weeks.
        (2) More severe forms should be followed daily until clear.
9. Exposure keratitis
    a. Symptoms. Scratchiness, foreign body sensation, redness.
    b. Clinical signs
        (1) Conjunctival redness.
        (2) Punctate staining, especially in the lower one-third of the cornea.
        (3) May have associated marginal infiltrate.
    c. Etiology
        (1) Incomplete lid closure (lagophthalmos).
        (2) Nocturnal lagophthalmos (incomplete closure while sleeping).
        (3) Exophthalmos associated with thyroid disease.
        (4) Bell's palsy.
        (5) Postsurgical.
    d. Diagnostic evaluation
        (1) General observation.
        (2) Identify incomplete lid closure (see clinical procedure identifying incomplete lid closure).
        (3) Careful slit lamp evaluation to determine corneal involvement.
        (4) Differential diagnosis includes other types of corneal epithelial problems.
    e. Treatment
        (1) Mild forms may be treated with artificial tears and lubricants.
        (2) Corneal epithelial loss or ulceration should be treated appropriately.
        (3) Severe forms may be treated with tarsorrhaphy (partially suturing lids together at the outer canthus).

E. *Degenerative conditions*
    1. Keratoconus
        a. Symptoms
            (1) Blurred vision in early stages.

      (2)   Advanced keratoconus may be associated with pain, tearing, and marked decrease in vision.

  b. Clinical signs

      (1)   Visual acuity not corrected with spectacles.

      (2)   Large, rapid change in refraction (particularly cylinder).

      (3)   Corneal thinning.

      (4)   Irregular mires on keratometry.

      (5)   Poor retinoscopic reflex.

      (6)   May be unilateral or bilateral.

      (7)   On down gaze, cornea pushes lower eyelid out (Munson's sign).

      (8)   Iron deposits in epithelium at the base of the cone (Fleischer's ring).

  c. Etiology

      (1)   Etiology unknown.

      (2)   May be associated with eye rubbing.

  d. Diagnostic evaluation

      (1)   Careful slit lamp evaluation to determine presence of cone.

      (2)   Refractive procedures to identify cornea as cause of reduced vision.

      (3)   May improve vision by refracting over diagnostic rigid contact lens.

  e. Treatment

      (1)   Best corrected vision obtained with spectacles in early stages.

      (2)   Advancing keratoconus may be best corrected with rigid contact lenses.

      (3)   Corneal graft may be indicated when glasses or contact lenses no longer correct vision or cornea thins excessively.

  f. Follow-up

      (1)   Mild forms of keratoconus may be followed every 6–12 months.

      (2)   Advanced keratoconus, where corneal thinning and perforation is a concern, should be followed more frequently.

2. Band keratopathy

  a. Symptoms

      (1)   Decreased visual acuity.

      (2)   Patient may complain of white area on cornea.

  b. Clinical signs

      (1)   White deposition of calcium in anterior cornea.

      (2)   Area of deposition is usually within the palpebral aperture and extends from 3:00 to 9:00.

  c. Etiology

      (1)   Chronic inflammatory disease such as pars planitis or chronic iritis.

      (2)   May be associated with long-standing glaucoma.

      (3)   May be associated with phthisis bulbi.

  d. Diagnostic evaluation

      (1)   Careful slit lamp evaluation to determine extent of band keratopathy.

      (2)   Complete history to ascertain previous inflammatory disease or systemic illness.

      (3)   Differential diagnosis includes corneal scarring and other types of corneal dystrophy.

  e. Treatment

      (1)   Primary disease needs to be identified and treated.

      (2)   Mild forms of band keratopathy may be treated with lubricants such as artificial tears and ointments.

      (3)   Severe band keratopathy may be referred for surgical removal with the chelating agent ethylenediaminetetraacetate. (EDTA).

  f. Follow-up. Mild forms may be followed at approximately 6- to 12-month intervals.

3. Corneal dystrophies

  a. Features

      (1)   Corneal dystrophies are usually bilateral and are considered hereditary.

      (2)   Corneal dystrophies may be classified as anterior, stromal, or posterior.

  b. Anterior membrane corneal dystrophies
   (1) Meesman's dystrophy—microcystic changes in the epithelium. Slowly progressive with onset in early childhood.
   (2) Cogan's dystrophy—characterized by comma-shaped, grayish epithelial opacities, usually central. Maplike opacities may be seen at the level of the basement membrane. These patients are predisposed to develop recurrent corneal erosion.
   (3) Fingerprint dystrophy—fine, wavy lines (mare's tails) located anterior to Bowman's membrane. Patients are usually asymptomatic but are predisposed to develop recurrent corneal erosion.
  c. Stromal corneal dystrophies
   (1) Granular dystrophy—whitish granular changes noted within the stroma. Visual acuity may be slightly reduced. Dystrophy may appear in early childhood.
   (2) Macular dystrophy—characterized by dense, gray, central opacity at level of Bowman's membrane. Visual acuity is usually markedly affected.
   (3) Lattice dystrophy—fine linear opacities in Bowman's membrane in the central cornea emanating to the periphery. Recurrent corneal erosion may occur. Visual acuity rarely affected.
  d. Posterior corneal dystrophies
   (1) Fuchs' dystrophy—endothelial dystrophy beginning in third or fourth decade. Disease characterized by guttata and defects in endothelium. Decompensation of endothelium leads to stromal and epithelial edema. Glaucoma is sometimes associated with this disease. Bullous keratopathy is found in the extreme variations of Fuchs' endothelial dystrophy.
   (2) Posterior polymorphous dystrophy—calcium crystals found in deep stromal layers along with edema. Patients usually asymptomatic.
  e. Treatment
   (1) Anterior membrane dystrophies
    (a) Frequently require no treatment.
    (b) Sometimes respond to artificial tears.
    (c) If recurrent corneal erosion results from anterior membrane dystrophy, patient should be treated with pressure patching (see IV.E.4).
   (2) Stromal corneal dystrophies
    (a) Rarely require treatment.
    (b) If visual acuity is severely compromised, consider corneal graft.
   (3) Posterior corneal dystrophies
    (a) No treatment required for early Fuchs' dystrophy.
    (b) As Fuchs' dystrophy proceeds, stromal and epithelial edema may be treated with 2% or 5% sodium chloride drops several times a day. This may be supplemented with 5% sodium chloride ointment at bedtime.
    (c) Pain and discomfort from bullous keratopathy may be treated with soft contact lens.
    (d) Associated glaucoma should be treated aggressively.
 4. Recurrent corneal erosion
  a. Chronic loss of corneal epithelium.
  b. Symptoms. Sudden onset of foreign body sensation, scratchiness, red eye, decreased visual acuity.
  c. Clinical signs
   (1) Fluorescein stain shows epithelial disruption.
   (2) Conjunctival hyperemia.
   (3) Excessive tearing.

d. Etiology
   (1) Acquired forms are associated with previous history of corneal injury.
   (2) Familial is usually bilateral and occurs more frequently in women.
   (3) Erosion associated with corneal dystrophy is seen most often with Cogan's and fingerprint dystrophy.
e. Diagnostic evaluation
   (1) Careful slit lamp examination to identify epithelial defect.
   (2) Must rule out primary corneal abrasion.
   (3) Must rule out corneal ulcer.
f. Treatment
   (1) Cycloplegia, antibiotic ointment, and pressure patch.
   (2) Once epithelium has closed, prophylactic use of bland ointments is helpful.
   (3) Severe forms of recurrent corneal erosion respond to use of hypertonic saline (5% sodium chloride) ointment at bedtime.
   (4) Debridement sometimes of value.
5. Corneal pigmentation
   a. Krukenberg's spindle
      (1) Deposition of pigment on endothelium.
      (2) Associated with pigment dispersion syndrome and pigmentary glaucoma.
   b. Blood staining. Deposition of hemosiderin in corneal stroma associated with hyphema.
   c. Hudson-Stahli line
      (1) Horizontal brown line in the inferior one-third of the cornea.
      (2) Probably represents iron deposits at the level of Bowman's membrane.
      (3) Very common.
   d. Fleischer's ring
      (1) Brownish ring seen at base of cone in keratoconus.
      (2) Probably represents hemosiderin at level of Bowman's membrane.
      (3) Best seen with cobalt filter.
6. Keratoplasty
   a. Corneal transplant surgery.
   b. Penetrating keratoplasty—full thickness cornea replacement.
   c. Lamellar keratoplasty—partial thickness replacement.
   d. Indications—corneal scarring, thinning, irregularity, persistent edema.

F. *Corneal trauma*
   1. Abrasion
      a. Symptoms. Pain, foreign body sensation, tearing, reduced vision.
      b. Clinical signs
         (1) Area of epithelial loss observed with fluorescein stain.
         (2) Marked limbal injection.
         (3) Anterior chamber reaction possible.
      c. Diagnostic evaluation
         (1) Careful slit lamp evaluation with fluorescein staining.
         (2) Rule out corneal ulcer.
      d. Treatment
         (1) Cycloplegia for photophobia and pain.
         (2) Antibiotic ointment.
         (3) Pressure patch.
      e. Follow-up
         (1) Patient should be seen in 24 hours.
         (2) Repatch if epithelial defect is significant.
         (3) If cornea has reepithelialized, artificial tears may be useful for an additional day or two.

Clinical Procedure—Pressure Patching

Description/Purpose	Purpose of pressure patching is to tightly close the lids to promote corneal healing. The lack of blinking keeps the epithelium from lifting and speeds healing.
Equipment	Sterile gauze eye pads. Adhesive tape (author prefers a 1-inch paper hypoallergenic tape). Cycloplegic (5% homatropine or 0.25% scopolamine). Antibiotic ointment (bacitracin or tobramycin).
Procedure	Anesthetize cornea to minimize irritation and facilitate handling. Instill drop of cycloplegic. Instill ½-inch antibiotic ointment and close eyelids. Place one or two eye pads over closed lids. Place large strip of adhesive tape diagonally across eye pad starting with tape adherent to the cheek. Holding eye pad in place, pull on the cheek to create tension and affix the other end to a clean forehead. Affix tape over entire eye pad. Ask patient to attempt to open the eye—if able, eye pad has not been properly placed. NOTE: Never keep eye patched longer than 24 hours.

---

2. Burns
   a. Chemical
      (1) Contact with acid or alkaline chemicals results in loss of epithelium.
      (2) Symptoms. Burning, decreased vision, photophobia, redness.
      (3) Clinical signs
          (a) Minimal—superficial punctate keratitis.
          (b) Advanced—large area of denuded epithelium.
          (c) Alkaline burns tend to cause more damage to epithelium.
      (4) Etiology. Chemical injury to cornea.
      (5) Diagnostic evaluation
          (a) Careful slit lamp evaluation to determine extent of epithelial loss.
          (b) Differential diagnosis includes corneal ulcer.
      (6) Treatment
          (a) Immediate copious irrigation (20–30 minutes with saline solution; if saline not available, water may be used).
          (b) Once eye has been flushed, cycloplegic instilled.
          (c) Antibiotic ointment and pressure patching is indicated.
          (d) Oral analgesics are helpful.
      (7) Follow-up. Patient should be seen in 24 hours.
   b. Thermal
      (1) Symptoms. Decreased vision, pain, and photophobia following thermal burn.
      (2) Clinical signs. Coagulated epithelium.
      (3) Etiology. Thermal burn usually due to curling iron or steam.
      (4) Diagnostic evaluation
          (a) Differential diagnosis includes corneal ulcer.
          (b) History usually indicates cause.
      (5) Treatment
          (a) Cycloplegic for pain and photophobia.
          (b) Topical antibiotic ointment.
          (c) Pressure patching.

          (d) Epithelial debridement is not essential.

          (e) Oral analgesics may be helpful.

    (6) Follow-up. Patient should be seen in 24 hours.

  c. Ultraviolet burn

    (1) Symptoms. Pain, decreased vision, photophobia following exposure to UV light source.

    (2) Clinical signs. Superficial punctate keratitis.

    (3) Etiology

          (a) UV exposure to sunlight or sun lamps.

          (b) Electric arc welding.

    (4) Diagnostic evaluation

          (a) Careful slit lamp examination to reveal extent of epithelial loss.

          (b) Differential diagnosis includes other types of superficial punctate keratitis.

    (5) Treatment

          (a) Mild forms treated with artificial tears and lubricating ointments.

          (b) Oral analgesics may be of some use.

          (c) Severe UV burns may be pressure patched.

    (6) Follow-up. Patient should be seen in 24 hours.

3. Corneal foreign body

  a. Symptoms. Pain, decreased vision, photophobia, redness.

  b. Clinical signs

    (1) Corneal foreign body may be seen on slit lamp examination.

    (2) Foreign object may be metallic or nonmetallic.

  c. Etiology

    (1) Metallic foreign bodies result from grinding, welding, or striking metal with hammer.

    (2) Nonmetallic foreign bodies frequently seen in children.

  d. Diagnostic evaluation

    (1) Careful slit lamp examination to rule out other possible causes for red eye.

    (2) Differential diagnosis includes corneal ulcers.

    (3) Rule out penetrating intraocular injury.

  e. Treatment

    (1) Removal of corneal foreign body (see Clinical Procedures).

    (2) Cycloplegia for photophobia.

    (3) Treatment with topical antibiotics (such as tobramycin drops q.i.d. ×48 hours).

    (4) If epithelial defect severe, pressure patching is indicated.

  f. Follow-up

    (1) Patient should be seen in 24 hours if epithelial defect is severe.

    (2) If defect is minimal, no follow-up required.

Clinical Procedure—Corneal Foreign Body Removal

Description/Purpose: Purpose is to remove corneal foreign body with minimum of trauma to surrounding tissue.

Equipment: Various instruments are useful in the removal of corneal foreign bodies. Among them are:
Large gauge (18 to 25) hypodermic needle.
Foreign body spud.
No. 3 or No. 5 jeweler's forceps.
Nylon loop.

(continued)

Clinical Procedure (*continued*)

Procedure	Anesthetize the cornea with proparacaine or Fluress.
	Place patient at the slit lamp with forehead firmly against the head rest.
	Ask patient to fixate distant point.
	Bring instrument in from the side, out of patient's line of sight. Superficial foreign bodies may be removed easily with little effort.
	Embedded corneal foreign bodies may require lifting the foreign body with upper edge of the needle or forceps and then lifting the material away from the eye.
	NOTE: Author's choice is jeweler's forceps, as they afford a fairly sharp point to lift an embedded corneal foreign body without the likelihood of corneal penetration. The forceps offer the additional advantage of immediate pickup of the foreign material.
	Most corneal foreign bodies without rust ring leave only a small epithelial defect and, therefore, do not require patching.
	Large epithelial defect may be treated with topical antibiotic drops 3–4 ×/day for 48 hours.

Clinical Procedure—Corneal Rust Ring Removal

Description/ Purpose	To remove rust ring left by metallic corneal foreign body.
Equipment	Alger brush or dental burr with $\frac{1}{2}$- or 1-mm burr.
Procedure	After corneal foreign body has been removed, alger brush is lightly applied to area of rust.
	Rust and necrotic epithelium are removed until area is clear. Some staining of Bowman's membrane may remain.
	If epithelial defect is large (greater than 3 mm across) or patient is in extreme pain, pressure patching with cycloplegic and antibiotic is appropriate.
	If defect is small, treatment with topical antibiotic drops 4 ×/day for 48 hours is satisfactory.

V. **Uvea**

A. *Uveal tract*

1. Uveal tract is composed of three parts: iris, ciliary body, and choroid.
2. Iris sphincter and dilator muscles are found in the anterior stroma of the iris and effect changes in pupil size.
3. Ciliary body has large surface area and is highly vascularized. Two inner layers of ciliary epithelium are external pigmented and internal nonpigmented. The nonpigmented epithelium is important in the secretion of aqueous.
4. Ciliary muscles (longitudinal, radial, and circular) are responsible for ciliary body contraction. Contraction of the ciliary body results in accommodative changes of the lens.
5. The pars plana is a thin layer of ciliary muscle and vessels covered by ciliary epithelium and represents transition to retina.
6. Choroid is bounded internally by Bruch's membrane and externally by the suprachoroid. The pigment epithelium of the retina rests on Bruch's membrane.

7. Choroid is highly vascularized and vessels are fenestrated (sodium fluorescein leaks, resulting in "choroidal flush" during fluorescein angiogram).
8. Rich vascular network of choroid supplies nourishment to outer portions of the retina.

B. *General assessment of the uveal tract*
1. Note circumcorneal redness suggestive of anterior uveitis.
2. Note anterior chamber for presence of white cells, red cells, or flare.
3. Look at surface of the iris for neovascularization (rubeosis).
4. Note retrolental space for presence of white cells suggestive of inflammation of the ciliary body or pars plana.
5. Examination of choroid is done during ophthalmoscopy. Note should be made of subretinal blood, vascularization, pigmentation, or raised lesions.

C. *Pathophysiology of symptoms—uveal tract*
1. Keratic precipitates and cells and flare in the anterior chamber may account for reduced vision.
2. Vitreous cells and flare may account for glare or blurred vision.
3. Inflammation of the iris or ciliary body may result in pain owing to abundant pain receptors in the anterior uvea (this may be manifested by photophobia or pain on accommodation or on pupil constriction in response to light).
4. Choroidal disease itself seldom results in pain or blurred vision unless the macula is affected.

D. *Uveitis—inflammation of the uveal tract*
1. Anterior uveitis
   a. The most common inflammation of the uveal tract.
   b. Symptoms
      (1) Usually acute onset of pain.
      (2) Photophobia.
      (3) Blurring of vision.
      (4) Red eye (circumcorneal flush).
      (5) Small pupil.
      (6) Usually no discharge.
      (7) Usually unilateral.
   c. Clinical signs
      (1) Circumcorneal injection.
      (2) Cells and flare in the anterior chamber (graded 1+ through 4+).
      (3) Keratic precipitates may be small and fine (acute, nongranulomatous) or large and hyalinized (chronic, granulomatous).
      (4) Pupil is usually miotic.
      (5) IOP is usually low but may be elevated.
      (6) Posterior synechiae may be present.
   d. Etiology
      (1) Nongranulomatous
         (a) Trauma.
         (b) Postoperative following intraocular surgery.
         (c) UGH syndrome (uveitis-glaucoma-hyphema)—inflammation caused by anterior chamber intraocular lens irritating the iris.
         (d) Juvenile rheumatoid arthritis—seen frequently in young girls.
         (e) Reiter's syndrome.
         (f) Ankylosing spondylitis—seen most frequently in young adult males, associated with low back pain.
         (g) Inflammatory bowel disease.
         (h) Behçet's disease (seen most frequently in young adults).

(i) Glaucomatocyclitic crisis (Posner-Schlossman syndrome)—recurrent episodes of elevated intraocular pressure and mild, subclinical iritis.

(j) Fuchs' heterochromic iridocyclitis.

(2) Chronic, granulomatous

(a) Sarcoidosis (usually blacks).

(b) Syphilis.

(c) Tuberculosis.

e. Diagnostic evaluation

(1) Careful slit lamp examination to determine extent of iritis, looking carefully for cells and flare in the anterior chamber and keratic precipitates on endothelium.

(2) *All* patients with anterior uveitis require a dilated fundus examination looking for evidence of posterior disease.

(3) Systemic workup is indicated for bilateral, recurrent, or granulomatous anterior uveitis and may include the following:

(a) ESR—erythrocyte sedimentation rate.

(b) CBC—complete blood count.

(c) ANA—anterior nuclear antibody test.

(d) Veneral Disease Research Laboratory (VDRL) test.

(e) Fluorescent treponemal antibody absorption (FTA-ABS).

(f) Purified protein derivative (PPD) and anergy panel.

(g) Chest x-ray.

NOTE: If above testing, history, or other symptoms are positive for systemic disease, then patient should be referred for complete workup to rule out associated systemic disease.

f. Treatment

(1) Cycloplegic drops—cyclopentolate 1% used 3–4 ×/day for mild iritis, homatropine 5% bid-qid for moderate inflammation, atropine 1% tid-qid for severe inflammation.

(2) Topical steroid drops—1% prednisolone q 1–6 hours depending upon severity.

(3) Associated elevated IOP should be treated with β-blockers if possible (steroid responder may be managed by discontinuing or reducing the steroids).

(4) Chronic, long-term iritis may be managed with cycloplegic alone once severe inflammation is brought under control.

g. Follow-up

(1) Patient should be seen every 1–5 days in the acute phase.

(2) Once iritis is brought under control, steroids should be tapered gradually over 1–3 weeks depending upon the severity and the duration of therapy.

(3) Once iritis is quiet, patient should be seen every 4–6 months.

(4) Chronic low-dose steroids or nonsteroidal anti-inflammatory drugs may be needed to control chronic iritis.

2. Posterior uveitis

a. Symptoms

(1) Blurred vision.

(2) Floaters.

(3) Photophobia.

(4) (Occasional) pain.

(5) (Occasional) redness.

b. Clinical signs

(1) Vitritis (white cells in vitreous matrix).

(2) Retinal infiltrates or exudate.

(3) Retinal vasculitis.

(4) Retinal edema.

(5) May have associated anterior uveitis.

Clinical Alert

Patients with anterior uveitis should *always* have a dilated fundus examination with scleral depression to rule out posterior involvement.

---

   c. Etiology
     (1) Toxoplasmosis—retinochoroiditis resulting in usually a single retinal inflammatory lesion.
     (2) Ocular histoplasmosis—a chorioretinitis usually associated with yellow-white choroidal spots that may affect the peripapillary area, macula, and far periphery. This disease is endemic in the Ohio and Mississippi River valley in the USA.
     (3) Syphilis.
     (4) Sarcoidosis.
     (5) Pars planitis.
   d. Diagnostic evaluation
     (1) Dilated fundus examination looking for evidence of posterior inflammation.
     (2) Binocular indirect ophthalmoscopy with scleral depression useful in detecting peripheral snow banking associated with pars planitis.
     (3) Slit lamp examination to rule out anterior segment disease.
     (4) Differential diagnosis includes optic neuritis, vascular occlusive disease, hypertensive retinopathy.
   e. Treatment. Specific treatment depends on etiology. Posterior uveitis should be referred to a retina specialist for evaluation and treatment, and coordination with the appropriate medical specialist. Associated anterior uveitis should be treated as outlined in V.D.1.
3. Pars planitis
   a. Symptoms
     (1) Decreased visual acuity.
     (2) Floaters.
   b. Clinical signs
     (1) Decreased visual acuity.
     (2) Cells in the vitreous.
     (3) Snow banking in peripheral retina (white exudative material seen in peripheral retina with binocular indirect ophthalmoscopy and scleral depression).
     (4) Other possible signs include retinal inflammation, cystoid macular edema, posterior subcapsular cataract, band keratopathy.
     (5) Signs of anterior uveitis are usually absent.
   c. Etiology
     (1) Unknown inflammatory etiology.
     (2) Usually seen in patients aged 15–40 years.
   d. Diagnostic evaluation
     (1) Binocular indirect ophthalmoscopy with scleral depression.
     (2) Slit lamp examination to evaluate anterior segment.
   e. Treatment
     (1) In asymptomatic patients treatment is not necessary.
     (2) If visual acuity is decreased, then treatment with topical steroid (1% prednisolone) q 3–6 hours may be initiated.
     (3) If cystoid macular edema (CME) is present, steroids must be used more frequently—q 1–2 hours. May require retrobulbar steroids or oral anti-inflammatories.
   f. Follow-up
     (1) This is a chronic disease and needs to be followed carefully.

      (2) In acute phase, patient should be seen every 1–4 weeks with steroids adjusted according to response.

      (3) Low-dose steroids may be required for the long term to control inflammation.

  E. *Uveal tumors*

    1. Malignant melanoma of the iris

      a. Symptoms. Generally asymptomatic.

      b. Clinical signs

        (1) Unilateral mass lesion of the iris (usually dark).

        (2) Usually slow-growing.

        (3) Lesion may be vascularized.

        (4) Anterior chamber may exhibit cells and flare.

        (5) May have associated elevated IOP.

        (6) Tumor may be localized or diffuse.

      c. Etiology. Primary and malignant melanoma.

      d. Diagnostic evaluation

        (1) Careful slit lamp examination.

        (2) Intraocular pressure measurement.

        (3) Differential diagnosis includes iris nevi, iris cyst, iris heterochromia, pigment dispersion.

        (4) Dilated fundus examination to rule out posterior lesion.

        (5) Photograph lesion and record dimensions.

      e. Treatment

        (1) Observe and watch for change (patient should be seen every 3–12 months).

        (2) If change is noted or other suspicious signs appear, patient should be referred for workup and possible treatment.

    2. Malignant melanoma of the choroid

      a. Symptoms

        (1) Patients may be asymptomatic.

        (2) Reduced visual acuity.

        (3) Visual field defect may be present.

        (4) Signs and symptoms of retinal detachment may be present.

      b. Clinical signs

        (1) Grayish mass lesion in posterior pole or periphery.

        (2) Malignant melanoma may be amelanotic or whitish.

        (3) Lesion may be vascularized.

        (4) May have associated retinal detachment.

      c. Etiology. Primary or metastatic lesion.

      d. Diagnostic evaluation

        (1) Dilated fundus examination with careful attention to posterior pole and periphery.

        (2) Slit lamp examination to rule out anterior segment disease.

        (3) Differential diagnosis includes other pigmented lesions of the retina and choroid, including nevi, retinal pigment epithelial hypertrophy.

        (4) Additional workup: diagnostic B scan ultrasound, fluorescein angiography.

      e. Treatment. Treatment of malignant melanoma of the choroid is controversial and includes observation, enucleation, radiation, or a resection of the lesion.

      f. Follow-up. Depends on the severity of the lesion and/or treatment.

VI. The Lens

  A. *Features of the lens*

    1. The lens is a multicellular structure consisting of long epithelial cells growing circumferentially, meeting to form the Y sutures.

    2. The anterior Y suture is upright; the posterior Y suture is upside down.

3. Isoindicial layers are identified anatomically: nucleus (embryonic, fetal, adult), cortex, the capsule.
4. Lens maintains clarity by complex biochemical processes. Disturbance of these biochemical processes affects clarity.
5. Ability of lens to change shape accounts for changing focus from distance to near (ocular accommodation).
6. Contraction of the ciliary muscle releases tension on the zonules, allowing the center of the lens to thicken due to normal elasticity of the capsule.
7. With aging, elasticity of the capsule is lost and accommodative ability decreases.

B. *General assessment of the lens*
   1. Note lens clarity.
   2. If opacity is noted, identify depth of opacity relative to anatomic features of the lens.
   3. Observe lens with pupil dilated in both direct illumination and retroillumination for best views.

C. *Pathophysiology of symptoms—lens*
   1. Loss of transparency (cataract) is the most common lens problem observed by optometrists.
   2. Loss of transparency results in decreased visual acuity.
   3. Light scatter or glare—may cause reduced visual acuity in bright light.
   4. Some types of cataracts may cause decreased accommodative ability in young people.

D. *Cataract*
   1. Defined as loss of transparency of the lens.
   2. Symptoms
      a. Blur—distance vision may decrease while near vision improves (second sight).
      b. Glare—one of the earliest signs of cataract. Particularly bothersome in patients when driving at night due to oncoming headlights.
      c. Double vision—irregular refractive changes within the lens may result in monocular diplopia.
      d. Changes in color perception—increasing sclerosis of the lens causes lens nucleus to yellow, resulting in loss of color perception, particularly in blue end of spectrum.
   3. Etiology
      a. Loss of transparency of the lens may be congenital or acquired, or due to trauma, disease processes, medications, or radiation.
      b. Congenital
         (1) Metabolic disorders such as galactosemia, hypoglycemia, and galactakinase deficiency may result in cataracts.
         (2) Dislocated lenses are associated with Marfan's syndrome or Marchesani's syndrome.
         (3) Rubella cataracts are the result of fetal infection before the ninth week of gestation. This tends to affect the central nucleus. Prominent sutures are sometimes observed.
      c. Acquired. Senile types are due to a progression of sclerosis of the nucleus, cortex, or capsule.
      d. Traumatic. Blunt trauma to the lens may result in lens opacity frequently of the anterior capsule or posterior subcapsular area.
      e. Disease processes. Cataracts may be seen in undiagnosed or poorly managed diabetes. Diabetic cataracts frequently appear as "snowflake" opacities observed in the cortex. Opacities may disappear once treatment is initiated. Early diabetic changes in refractive power (usually myopic) of the lens may be due to fluctuating blood glucose levels, resulting in an unstable refraction.
      f. Pharmacologically induced cataracts
         (1) Corticosteroids (both systemic and topical) may cause lens opacifi-

cation. Generally such cataracts appear after long-term use. Steroid-induced cataracts tend to be limited to the posterior subcapsular area.

(2) The anticholesterol agent mevacor has been associated with cortical opacities of the lens.

(3) Indirect acting parasympathomimetics (miotics such as echothiophate, DFP, and demecarium bromide) are associated with anterior subcapsular cataracts in children.

(4) Patients taking medications on a long-term basis should be monitored annually or semiannually for the development of cataracts.

g. Radiation

(1) Cataracts may form following electrocution.

(2) UV radiation may be related to the development of senile cataracts. UV-absorbing tints may be of some value as protection.

(3) X-rays produce posterior subcapsular cataracts. Patients frequently exposed to x-ray radiation should be monitored carefully.

(4) Microwaves (in everyday dosage levels) have not been found to be associated with cataract formation.

4. Diagnostic evaluation

a. History—careful history regarding onset and severity of vision loss is helpful. Questions regarding systemic disease, medications, and/or trauma should be included in the general medical history.

b. Best corrected visual acuity—visual acuity with best refraction is useful in quantifying vision loss. Frequently a shift towards myopia will be found.

c. Glare acuity—visual acuity under glare conditions is helpful in ascertaining functional vision. Light scattering due to cataract formation will reduce visual acuity due to a loss of contrast sensitivity. Two methods to measure glare acuity are outlined in Clinical Procedures.

d. Potential Acuity Measurement (PAM)—the Guyton-Minkowski PAM, a slit lamp-mounted PAM unit, utilizes a Maxwellian viewing system to project a visual acuity chart on the retina. Such a system bypasses small lenticular opacities, giving the examiner an idea of postoperative visual acuity (see Clinical Procedures).

e. Biomicroscopy—direct visualization of the lens with the biomicroscope permits detailed evaluation of the cataract. Both direct illumination and retro-illumination are helpful in ascertaining the density of opacification.

f. Cataracts may be named by their location within the lens or by specific etiology.

g. Density of cataracts may be quantified using scale of 1+ to 4+ (densest).

h. Ophthalmoscopy—both direct and indirect can be used to evaluate cataracts by viewing the dark cataract against the red reflex.

i. Retinoscopy—cataracts may be viewed against the red reflex in a manner similar to ophthalmoscopy.

j. Ultrasonography—both A and B scan ultrasonography may be used to detect cataracts owing to the increased acoustic reflectivity of the dense lens. A scan ultrasonography may be used to determine the axial length of the eye, which is useful in calculating the power of the intraocular lens. B scan ultrasonography is useful in determining the presence of a retinal detachment in a patient with an extremely opaque lens.

Clinical Alert

Accurate description of the cataract, including type and severity (based on acuity), is important for medical/legal documentation prior to surgery.

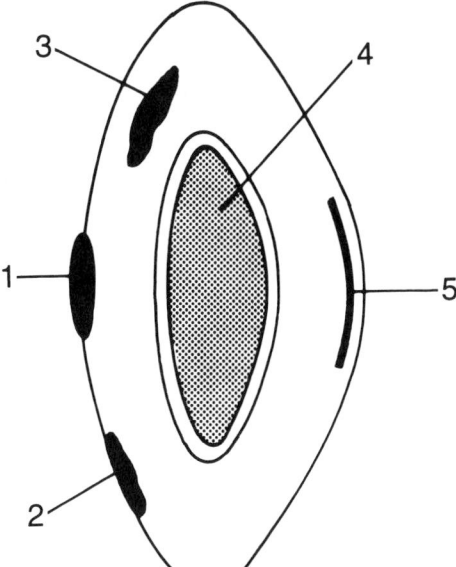

Figure 5-3. Naming cataracts based on location. (1) Anterior polar cataract, (2) anterior subcapsular cataract, (3) cortical cataract, (4) nuclear cataract, (5) posterior subcapsular cataract.

5. Treatment
   a. If visual acuity is not severely compromised, or patient complaints are minimal, patients may be followed at 3-, 6-, or 12-month intervals until such time as symptoms warrant referral for cataract surgery.
   b. Visual acuities worse than 20/40 to 20/60 often interfere with patient's activities (such as reading or driving).
   c. Such patients are candidates for cataract surgery and should be offered the opportunity for surgical consult.
   d. Preoperative evaluation of cataract patients may take place in the optometrist's office (see Clinical Procedures).

Clinical Procedure—Brightness Acuity Testing	
Description/ Purpose	Brightness acuity testing is helpful in ascertaining the functional loss of vision. It is useful as a guide to help decide when to remove cataracts.
Equipment	Brightness acuity tester (Mentor) or slit lamp biomicroscope.
Procedure	One eye is occluded and the brightness acuity tester is brought before the eye to be tested.
	Visual acuity is obtained without illumination.
	Visual acuity is then obtained utilizing the low, medium, and high illuminations, recording each acuity with the respective illumination.
	The fellow eye is then tested in the same manner.
	An alternative method uses the slit lamp biomicroscope light source.
	Using a 1-mm slit just inside the pupillary margin to simulate glare conditions, the patient is asked to read the acuity chart. Patients with clinically significant cataracts usually experience marked reduction in visual acuity under these conditions.

Clinical Procedure—Potential Acuity Measurement (PAM)

Description/ Purpose	Purpose of PAM is to obtain preoperative indication of the potential visual function of an eye following cataract surgery.
Equipment	Potential acuity meter (Mentor PAM). The PAM utilizes a Maxwellian viewing system to project a visual acuity chart on the retina past the lenticular opacities. Dilated pupil is recommended.
Procedure	Pupils are dilated with mydriatic. Set relative level of ametropia on the diopteric power scale, located on the side of the instrument. With the slit lamp locate relatively clear areas of the lens. Focus the PAM beam at a pinpoint through the clear areas. Once clear areas are found, patient should be able to read the chart. Ask patient to read smallest line possible. Record potential acuity. NOTE: "False-positive results" may be obtained in spite of disease processes such as macular degeneration, macular holes, or vascular occlusive disease; therefore, the PAM is only a guide and does not represent a guaranteed postoperative visual acuity.

---

6. Follow-up
   a. Postoperative care of the cataract patient may be comanaged by the surgeon and the optometrist.
   b. It is recommended that the surgeon see the patient initially at the first postoperative visit (many surgeons prefer to see the patient for the first and second postoperative visits).
   c. Suggested postoperative visits in an uncomplicated recovery may occur at 1 day (surgeon), 1 week, 1 month, 2 months, and 3 months.
   d. With small-incision cataract surgery, final postoperative prescription may be obtained as early as 3 weeks.

VII. Vitreous

   A. *Features of the vitreous*
      1. Vitreous comprises two-thirds of the volume of the globe.
      2. Vitreous composition is 99% water with the remainder collagen and hyaluronic acid.
      3. Outer surface of the vitreous is called the hyaloid membrane.
      4. Vitreous is firmly attached to pars plana epithelium and retina near ora serrata.
      5. Vitreous is loosely attached to optic nerve head and posterior lens capsule.
      6. Cloquet's canal traverses the center of the vitreous from the nerve head to the posterior lens capsule. Before birth this canal contains the hyaloid artery. Remnants of the artery may remain and be visible ophthalmoscopically. Attachment of hyaloid artery at the posterior lens is occasionally visible (Mittendorf's dot).

   B. *General assessment*
      1. Normally vitreous is not visible with the direct or indirect ophthalmoscope.
      2. Vitreous structure or pathology is best viewed with the slit lamp biomicroscope utilizing the direct beam.
      3. Retroillumination will afford an excellent view of opacities within the vitreous such as a ringlike opacity seen in posterior vitreous detachment.
      4. Advent of the Volk 90 or 78 diopter lens extends the capacity of the biomicroscope to evaluate the vitreous.

5. B scan ultrasonography may be used to evaluate vitreous cavity in cases of vitreous hemorrhage.

C. *Pathophysiology of symptoms*
   1. Pathology related to vitreous frequently affects its gel-like nature, causing the vitreous to become fluid. Particulate or cellular material within the vitreous will appear to move around following liquefaction, resulting in the complaint of floating spots.
   2. Vitreous liquefaction or detachment will allow the vitreous to mechanically stimulate the retina, resulting in flashing lights (photopsia).

D. *Disease entities*
   1. Vitreous syneresis
      a. Liquefaction, shrinkage and collapse of the normal gel-like vitreous.
      b. Symptoms
         (1) Photopsia.
         (2) Occasionally floaters.
      c. Clinical signs
         (1) Floaters and vitreous fibrils may be seen against red reflex or with direct illumination with the slit lamp biomicroscope.
         (2) There is an absence of anterior or posterior vitreous detachment.
         (3) There is an absence of retinal pathology.
      d. Etiology
         (1) Normal aging process (65% of persons over 60 years of age exhibit vitreous syneresis).
         (2) Myopia.
      e. Diagnostic evaluation
         (1) Careful biomicroscopy to identify vitreous syneresis.
         (2) Rule out vitreous detachment.
         (3) Careful binocular indirect ophthalmoscopy with scleral depression to rule out retinal tear or detachment.
         (4) Goldmann three-mirror evaluation to rule out other vitreoretinal pathology.
      f. Treatment. Essentially none.
      g. Follow-up. Patients should be monitored carefully for the development of retinal tear (suggest 6- to 12-month follow-up visit).
   2. Vitreous detachment
      a. Separation of the anterior or posterior hyaloid membrane from its attachment.
      b. Symptoms
         (1) Sudden onset of floating spots.
         (2) Photopsia.
         (3) Occasionally decreased visual acuity (if large vitreous opacity is located centrally).
      c. Clinical signs
         (1) Anterior vitreous detachment is identified by the anterior hyaloid membrane detaching and falling backward (as seen with dilated pupil and biomicroscope).
         (2) Posterior vitreous detachment is identified by the presence of a circular or incomplete circular midvitreal ring (Vogt's ring).
      d. Etiology
         (1) Anterior vitreous detachment results when the vitreous detaches from its insertion near the ora serrata and occasionally from its attachment to the posterior lens surface.
         (2) Posterior vitreous detachment results when the vitreous detaches from its attachment near the optic nerve head.

(3) Both types of detachments are a normal course of aging or associated with myopia.

(4) Occasionally vitreous detachment is seen following trauma.

e. Diagnostic evaluation

(1) Careful slit lamp examination to rule out anterior segment pathology and observe the anterior vitreous.

(2) Binocular indirect ophthalmoscopy with scleral depression to rule out peripheral retinal disease or retinal break.

(3) Goldmann three-mirror evaluation to rule out peripheral retinal disease or retinal break.

f. Treatment

(1) In the absence of retinal pathology, there is no specific treatment for vitreous detachment.

(2) Reassurance is necessary as patient will be quite apprehensive.

g. Follow-up

(1) Patients with anterior or posterior vitreous detachment should be seen in approximately 3–4 months and then annually thereafter to rule out retinal disease.

(2) Patient should be advised of the signs and symptoms of retinal detachment and such advice documented in the patient's record.

Clinical Alert

Patients with recent onset of symptoms of flashes and floaters who exhibit blood in the vitreous should be assumed to have a retinal tear until proven otherwise.

---

3. Asteroid hyalosis

a. Calcium soaps located within the matrix of the vitreous.

b. Symptoms

(1) Usually none.

(2) Occasionally decreased visual acuity or complaint of floaters.

c. Clinical signs

(1) On indirect ophthalmoscopy numerous yellowish particles will be seen entrapped in the vitreous matrix. These particles tend to move when the eyes are moved but generally return to their original position.

(2) Usually unilateral but may be bilateral.

d. Etiology

(1) Associated with aging.

(2) Associated with diabetes.

e. Diagnostic evaluation. Careful peripheral retinal examination to rule out pathology.

f. Treatment

(1) Essentially no treatment required.

(2) In extreme cases of asteroid hyalosis where visual acuity is markedly reduced (20/100 or worse), vitrectomy is possible.

g. Follow-up. Only routine examination is required.

4. Vitreous hemorrhage

a. Symptoms

(1) Sudden onset of decreased visual acuity.

(2) Sudden onset of floaters.

b. Clinical signs

(1) Blood may be identified by slit lamp examination.

(2) Retinal details are obscure on ophthalmoscopy.

c. Etiology
   (1) Numerous causes.
   (2) Vascular conditions of the retina most common—diabetes, hypertension, branch vein occlusion, sickle cell disease.
   (3) Vitreous hemorrhage frequently associated with retinal tear or detachment.
   (4) Trauma.
d. Diagnostic evaluation
   (1) Careful funduscopic examination to ascertain source of bleeding.
   (2) If vitreous is filled with blood, B scan ultrasound may be required to rule out retinal disease.
e. Treatment
   (1) Treatment of primary cause such as photocoagulation in diabetes.
   (2) If unable to ascertain cause of bleeding, referral to retinal specialist is mandatory.
f. Follow-up. Depends on cause.
5. Vitrectomy. Vitrectomy is a surgical procedure used to remove opacified vitreous, or vitreous which is causing traction on the retina which may lead to retinal detachment.

VIII. Retina

A. *Features of the retina*
   1. Retina is derived from neuroectoderm and consists of 10 distinct layers.
   2. Retina extends from optic nerve to ora serrata.
   3. Macula contains the fovea and represents the area of the sharpest vision having the highest concentration of cones.
   4. Thickness of the retina varies from 300 μm near the macula to 150 μm or less near the ora serrata.
   5. Retina receives blood supply from two sources. Choriocapillaris in contact with Bruch's membrane supplies outer one-third of the retina. Inner two-thirds of the retina are nourished by branches of the central retinal artery.
   6. Fovea centralis supplied by choriocapillaris only.

B. *General assessment*
   1. Note red reflex in all 360°.
   2. Optic nerve should appear pink with minimal cupping. Border of optic nerve head should be distinct. Optic nerve should not be raised.
   3. Note course and caliber of vessels.
   4. Note arteriolar light reflex relative to vessel width (should be less than 1:2).
   5. Observe avascular zone. Macular pigmentation should be regular, and foveal light reflex should be bright.
   6. Peripheral retina is best observed with the indirect ophthalmoscope.

C. *Retinal examination procedures*
   1. Ophthalmoscopy
      a. Direct ophthalmoscopy affords an excellent view of the retina, especially at the disc and macula.
      b. Indirect ophthalmoscopy provides a good view of the periphery as well as stereopsis to aid in the detection of elevated lesions such as tumors, detachments, or serous elevation of the retina. The view is inverted and reversed.
      c. Contact lens/biomicroscope evaluation of the retina with the Goldmann three mirror lens gives a clear, detailed view of the peripheral retina as well as the macula.
      d. Indirect biomicroscopy
         (1) Volk lens (78 or 90 diopters) is useful in examining the posterior pole and some peripheral retinal lesions. The view, however, is inverted and reversed.

    (2) Hruby lens yields a direct, upright view. It is particularly useful in evaluating the disc and macula problems. The peripheral fundus is difficult to observe with this lens.

  2. Retinal function assessment

    a. Snellen visual acuity gives the clinician an indication of macular function.

    b. Contrast sensitivity is a measure of the resolving ability of the retina as well.

    c. A potential acuity measurement/interferometer is particularly useful in assessing retinal function when media opacities exist.

    d. Color vision is a good indicator of macular function because of the high concentration of cones. Poor color vision can be indicative of macular dysfunction.

    e. Amsler grid testing is particularly useful in ruling out macular disease. Subtle macular changes will result in metamorphopsia or disturbance of the grid.

    f. Visual field. Both the sensitivity of the retina and the extent of the visual field may be determined by a threshold visual field test.

    g. Measurement of dark adaptation times is useful in assessing rod function, particularly in conditions such as retinitis pigmentosa. Similar information may be obtained with a photo stress test. In this test the patient's visual acuity is measured prior to a 30-second exposure to the ophthalmoscope light. The time it takes for the patient's visual acuity to return to within one level of pretest acuity is an indicator of the ability to dark adapt. Increased time, especially when comparing one eye to the other, is indicative of disease.

  3. Fluorescein angiography. Intravenous fluorescein angiography is useful in evaluating retinal circulation. Detection of retinal damage in diabetes, macular edema, and subretinal neovascularization is greatly enhanced with this technique.

  4. Electrophysiology

    a. Electroretinogram. Electroretinogram (ERG) is useful in detecting diffuse retinal damage. ERG is usually performed under both photopic (light-adapted and scotopic dark-adapted conditions). Macular disease is not usually detected by ERG testing.

    b. Visually evoked response (VER) is a measurement of the visually evoked cortical potential. Patient is shown a light stimulus and the nerve impulses are registered in the occipital cortex by a computer. VER is useful in the detection of subclinical lesions along the visual pathway, in nonresponsive patients or infants, and in the evaluation of amblyopia.

D. *Pathophysiology of symptoms*

  1. Retinal diseases affecting the macula generally result in reduced central visual acuity.

  2. Peripheral retinal disease may affect side vision, patient mobility, and night vision.

  3. There are no pain receptors in the retina, so pain is absent in retinal disease.

E. *Disease entities: Vascular diseases*

  1. Central retinal artery occlusion (CRAO)

    a. Symptoms

      (1) Acute, unilateral loss of vision.

      (2) No pain.

    b. Clinical signs

      (1) White, edematous retina.

      (2) May have cherry red spot.

      (3) May have evidence of arteriolar occlusive disease such as Hollenhorst plaque.

      (4) May have afferent pupillary defect.

          (5)   May involve entire central retinal artery or a branch of the central retinal artery.

    c. Etiology
        (1)   Usually embolic phenomenon related to the carotid artery or heart.
        (2)   Thromboembolic phenomenon possible.
        (3)   Giant cell arteritis.

    d. Diagnostic evaluation
        (1)   Careful evaluation of the fundus to ascertain retinal details.
        (2)   Careful history to uncover related medical history such as carotid artery disease or valvular heart disease.
        (3)   Differential diagnosis includes ischemic optic neuropathy and central retinal vein occlusion.

    e. Treatment (acute)
        (1)   Digital massage of the eye (forces embolus to a smaller branch).
        (2)   Increase partial pressure of CO_2 by breathing into a paper bag.
        (3)   Immediate referral to ophthalmologist for anterior chamber paracentesis (lowering of IOP by removing small amounts of aqueous to allow embolus to move to smaller branch).
        (4)   Acetazolamide (250 mg tablets ×2) in conjunction with topical β-blocker in an effort to lower IOP.
        (5)   Patient will need a complete medical workup to rule out carotid artery disease, valvular heart disease, and giant cell arteritis.

    f. Follow-up. Patient should be seen several weeks after the event to be certain that no sequelae such as rubeosis or neovascular glaucoma have developed.

Clinical Alert

Central retinal artery occlusion is a true ocular emergency. (If the blockage can be caused to move to a smaller branch, patient's vision may improve.)

---

  2. Central retinal vein occlusion (CRVO) and branch retinal vein occlusion (BRVO)
    a. Symptoms
        (1)   Acute, unilateral loss of vision.
        (2)   No pain.

    b. Clinical signs
        (1)   Marked retinal hemorrhages in all quadrants in the case of the CRVO.
        (2)   Retinal hemorrhages in one quadrant in the case of a BRVO.
        (3)   Additionally cotton-wool spots, edema, or shunt vessels on the disc may be observed.
        (4)   Examiner should look carefully for neovascularization of the disc or iris.

    c. Etiology
        (1)   Sclerosis of adjacent retinal arterioles causing compression on the vein.
        (2)   Associated with hypertension.
        (3)   Often associated with glaucoma or elevated IOP.

    d. Diagnostic evaluation
        (1)   Dilated fundus examination to determine all of the retinal findings.
        (2)   Slit lamp examination to rule out neovascularization of the iris.
        (3)   Differential diagnosis includes relative retinal ischemia due to carotid occlusive disease, diabetic retinopathy, papilledema, or papillitis.

    e. Treatment
        (1)   Treat associated systemic disorders such as hypertension.
        (2)   Lower IOP if elevated.

      (3) Consider panretinal photocoagulation if neovascularization of the iris or optic nerve is present, or if retinal ischemia is observed on fluorescein angiogram.

      (4) Consider focal or grid laser if macular edema is marked in branch retinal vein occlusion.

      (5) Advise internist of condition as it may be prudent to discontinue medications that may contribute to vascular occlusion, such as oral contraceptives or inappropriate hypertensive medications.

      (6) Anticoagulative therapy may be of some value (aspirin).

3. Diabetic retinopathy

  a. Retinal changes associated with both insulin-dependent and non-insulin-dependent diabetes. Diabetic retinopathy may be divided into background, preproliferative, and proliferative diabetic retinopathy.

  b. Symptoms

    (1) Background diabetic retinopathy: Bilateral appearance of microaneurysms, dot and blot hemorrhages, lipoidal (hard) exudates), and macular edema.

    (2) Preproliferative diabetic retinopathy: all of the findings in background diabetic retinopathy. Additionally intraretinal microvascular abnormalities (IRMAs), cotton-wool spots, and marked capillary nonperfusion (seen on fluorescein angiogram).

    (3) Proliferative diabetic retinopathy: bilateral findings. Usually the changes noted in nonproliferative and preproliferative diabetic retinopathy are present. Additionally neovascularization of the disc (NVD) or neovascularization elsewhere (NVE) is present. In severe forms of proliferative diabetic retinopathy, retinal detachment, vitreous hemorrhage, and proliferation of fibrovascular tissue are evident. Marked macular edema may be noted as well.

  c. Etiology

    (1) Vascular changes occur due to the affect of diabetes on the small blood vessels.

    (2) Neovascular and proliferative changes result from ischemia.

    (3) Very poor correlation between the presence of retinal disease and the relative control of the diabetes.

  d. Diagnostic evaluation

    (1) Careful evaluation of the fundus with the direct and indirect ophthalmoscope to identify diabetic findings.

    (2) Biomicroscopy with a Volk lens or contact lens is useful in detecting macular edema and neovascular changes. Biomicroscopy is indicated to rule out iris neovascularization.

    (3) Fluorescein angiogram should be obtained to determine extent of diabetic changes as well as presence of capillary nonperfusion (capillary nonperfusion leads to proliferative changes).

    (4) Differential diagnosis includes central retinal vein or branch retinal occlusion, hypertensive retinopathy, and sickle cell retinopathy.

  e. Treatment

    (1) Mild forms of nonproliferative diabetic retinopathy may be simply monitored (retinal photography useful).

    (2) Consider referral to retina specialist (see Clinical Alert—Guidelines for Referral).

  f. Follow-up

    (1) All diabetics should receive at least an annual examination.

    (2) Patients with moderate background diabetic retinopathy should be seen every 6 months.

    (3) Patients with preproliferative or proliferative changes should be seen every 2–4 months depending on severity.

Clinical Alert—Guidelines for Referral of Diabetic Retinopathy

Best corrected visual acuity 20/40 or less, regardless of clinical appearance.
Observable diabetic retinopathy within 500 μm of the center of the macula.
Lipoidal exudates within 500 μm of the center of the macula.
Macular edema.
Disc neovascularization.
Iris neovascularization.
Any other proliferative change.
Vitreous hemorrhage.

---

    g. Treatment
      (1) Panretinal photoablation is an effort to reduce areas of hypoxic retina. Large areas of retina are burned with the argon or krypton laser up to the disc on the nasal side and to the temporal border of the macula. Occasionally 2,000 to 3,000 burns may be required.
      (2) Focal treatment. Individual leaking microaneurysms may be treated, especially close to the macula where they may contribute to macular edema.
      (3) Vitrectomy. Removal of vitreous blood which has been present for longer than 6 months is accomplished by pars plana vitrectomy. Pars plana vitrectomy is usually followed up with panretinal photocoagulation.
4. Hypertensive retinopathy
    a. Symptoms
      (1) Usually patients are asymptomatic.
      (2) Severe forms of hypertensive retinopathy may cause reduced visual acuity.
    b. Clinical signs
      (1) Bilateral A/V crossing phenomenon.
      (2) Narrowing of retinal arterioles.
      (3) Widening of arteriolar reflex (greater than 1:2).
      (4) Flame hemorrhages and occasional microaneurysms.
      (5) Cotton-wool spots (localized areas of ischemia.
      (6) Hard exudates (in "macular star" formation).
      (7) Occasionally will be associated with central retinal vein occlusion.
    c. Etiology
      (1) Hypertension.
      (2) May be associated with other systemic disease such as kidney disease.
    d. Diagnostic evaluation
      (1) Careful funduscopic evaluation to determine extent of changes.
      (2) Complete medical history
      (3) Determine state of control of blood pressure.
      (4) If high blood pressure has been previously undiagnosed, referral to internist is indicated.
    e. Treatment
      (1) Proper control of hypertension.
      (2) If papilledema is present, should be referred to internist or family practitioner immediately.
    f. Follow-up
      (1) Every 2–4 months depending on the severity.
      (2) Once hypertensive retinopathy has cleared, then annual examination is indicated.
      (3) At each visit should communicate findings to managing internist or family practitioner.

F. *Disease of the macula*
1. Central serous choroidopathy
    a. Localized detachment of sensory retina.
    b. Symptoms
        (1) Usually occurs in middle-aged males.
        (2) Patient complains of blurred or decreased vision.
        (3) Patient may complain of blind spot in central field.
        (4) May experience differences in color perception between the two eyes.
    c. Clinical signs
        (1) Localized serous elevation of the retina; no blood or evidence of subretinal neovascularization is usually present.
        (2) Visual acuity may be only slightly affected in the 20/25 range or may be reduced to the 20/80 to 20/100 level.
        (3) May have Amsler grid distortions or central scotoma.
    d. Etiology
        (1) Defect in pigment epithelium allows fluid to accumulate in the subretinal space.
        (2) Etiology unknown but may be related to stress.
    e. Diagnostic evaluation
        (1) Differential diagnosis includes subretinal neovascular membrane, pigment epithelial detachment, retinal detachment.
        (2) Careful macular evaluation required using contact lens or Volk 78 or 90 diopter lens.
        (3) Fluorescein angiography is helpful in definitive diagnosis, ruling out a subretinal membrane, or identifying area of pigment disruption for laser treatment.
        (4) Classic fluorescein angiographic finding is "smoke stack" hyperfluorescence.
    f. Treatment
        (1) Most cases are followed every 1–2 months until resolution.
        (2) If visual acuity does not improve after 4–6 months, patient may be candidate for laser photocoagulation.
        (3) Recurrent cases may also be indication for laser treatment
2. Pigment epithelial detachment
    a. Focal detachment of pigment epithelium resulting in blisterlike elevation of the retina.
    b. Symptoms
        (1) Patient may be asymptomatic if lesion is away from the fovea.
        (2) Decreased visual acuity is commonly reported.
    c. Clinical signs
        (1) Well-defined area of elevation of pigment epithelium which may mask choroidal details.
        (2) Patient may have Amsler grid distortion.
    d. Etiology
        (1) May be idiopathic.
        (2) Often associated with subretinal neovascular membrane.
    e. Diagnostic evaluation
        (1) Careful evaluation of the retina with the indirect ophthalmoscope to rule out retinal detachment.
        (2) Evaluation of the macula with the contact lens or the Volk 78 or 90 diopter lens to rule out subretinal neovascularization.
        (3) Fluorescein angiogram shows early fluorescence which persists throughout the study. If subretinal neovascularization is present will be seen in early views.

    f. Treatment
      (1) Idiopathic pigment epithelial detachments may resolve spontaneously.
      (2) May be treated with photocoagulation if persistent or associated with subretinal neovascular membrane.
3. Age-related macular degeneration
    a. Two forms: nonexudative or dry, and exudative or wet.
    b. Nonexudative (dry form)
      (1) Symptoms
          (a) Usually occurs in patients over the age of 50.
          (b) Patients complain of gradual reduction in visual acuity.
      (2) Clinical signs
          (a) Drusen may be small, or large and coalesced.
          (b) Pigment epithelial hypertrophy or pigment epithelial atrophy.
          (c) Amsler grid defects.
      (3) Etiology
          (a) Irregular thickening of Bruch's membrane resulting in drusen.
          (b) Cause of disruption of Bruch's membrane is unknown.
      (4) Diagnostic evaluation
          (a) Careful evaluation of the macula with contact lens or Volk lens to rule out other macular disease.
          (b) Differential diagnosis may include old inflammatory scarring.
          (c) Fluorescein angiography to differentiate between dry and wet forms of age-related macular degeneration.
      (5) Treatment
          (a) Essentially none.
          (b) Patient should be monitored to be alert to formation of subretinal neovascular membrane.
          (c) Patient should monitor vision at home with Amsler grid.
          (d) When visual acuity is markedly reduced, low-vision aids may be helpful.
          (e) Use of vitamin supplements is controversial.
      (6) Follow-up
          (a) Every 6 to 12 months depending on severity
    c. Exudative (wet form)
      (1) Symptoms
          (a) Usually an acute, sudden loss of visual acuity or distortion of vision.
          (b) Patient may complain of central scotoma.
      (2) Clinical signs
          (a) Associated drusen, usually large and coalesced.
          (b) May have hemorrhage, exudate, or fluid.
          (c) Subretinal neovascular membrane.
      (3) Etiology. Defects in pigment epithelium and Bruch's membrane allow choroidal vessels to develop beneath the retina.
      (4) Diagnostic evaluation
          (a) Differential diagnosis includes high myopia, inflammatory disease, pigment epithelial detachment, choroidal rupture.
          (b) Examination should include careful evaluation with contact lens or Volk 78 or 90 diopter lens.
          (c) Amsler grid to demonstrate central loss.
          (d) Fluorescein angiography will identify subretinal neovascular membrane early in the study and continue to leak throughout.
      (5) Treatment
          (a) Referral to retinal specialist.

    (b) Treatment of extrafoveal, juxtafoveal, and even subfoveal subretinal neovascular membranes has been shown to be effective.

   (6) Follow-up

    (a) Reccurrence is common in patients with subretinal neovascular membranes.

    (b) Amsler grid should be used daily.

    (c) Patients should be followed every 3–6 months

4. Presumed ocular histoplasmosis syndrome

 a. Inflammatory disease of the retina characterized by macular lesion, peripapillary lesion, and peripheral punched-out lesions.

 b. Symptoms

  (1) May be asymptomatic.

  (2) Patients may report decreased visual acuity or distortion of central vision.

 c. Clinical signs

  (1) Yellow, white, or "punched-out" peripheral lesions.

  (2) Macular subretinal neovascular membrane or pigment epithelial atrophy.

  (3) Peripapillary atrophy.

  (4) Usually minimal vitreous haze

 d. Etiology

  (1) Usually occurs between age 20 and 50.

  (2) Appears to be endemic to the Ohio-Mississippi River valley in the USA.

  (3) History of exposure to histoplasma capsulatum fungi which is carried by droppings from pigeons, chickens, or other birds.

 e. Diagnostic evaluation

  (1) Differential diagnosis includes age-related macular degeneration, high myopia, angioid streaks, toxoplasmosis.

  (2) Careful evaluation with contact lens or Volk lens to rule out other macular pathology.

  (3) Fluorescein angiography may identify active subretinal neovascular membrane.

  (4) Amsler grid test to demonstrate central defect.

 f. Treatment

  (1) If lesions are not active, treatment is not indicated.

  (2) Laser treatment is appropriate if subretinal neovascular membrane is identified.

 g. Follow-up

  (1) Patients with quiet lesions should be followed every 6–12 months.

  (2) Patients who have had subretinal neovascular membrane should be followed every 3–6 months and monitor their vision at home with an Amsler grid.

5. Macular hole

 a. Loss of retinal tissue in macula.

 b. Symptoms. Markedly decreased vision—20/200 or worse.

 c. Clinical signs

  (1) Round, reddish lesion in the avascular zone not associated with hemorrhage.

  (2) May also have grayish halo or yellow spots within the center.

 d. Etiology

  (1) Usually associated with vitreo-retinal traction.

  (2) May be associated with persistent macular edema.

 e. Diagnostic evaluation

  (1) Differential diagnosis includes macular pucker (surface wrinkling retinopathy) with pseudohole formation, hereditary macular dystrophies, solar burns of the macula.

        (2) Examination should include evaluation with contact lens or Volk lens.

        (3) Occasionally fluorescein angiography is helpful to make definitive diagnosis.

    f. Treatment. Vitrectomy surgery may be helpful in selected cases.

    g. Follow-up. Examination every 6–12 months.

6. Angioid streaks

    a. Brown, irregular bands radiating from the disc.

    b. Symptoms

        (1) Usually asymptomatic.

        (2) If associated with subretinal neovascular membrane, may have markedly reduced vision.

    c. Clinical signs

        (1) Brownish or gray irregular bands radiating from the disc.

        (2) May have associated pigment epithelial disruption.

        (3) May have associated hemorrhage in conjunction with subretinal neovascular membrane.

    d. Etiology

        (1) Breaks in Bruch's membrane.

        (2) May be associated with Paget's disease, sickle cell disease, and pseudoxanthoma elasticum.

    e. Diagnostic evaluation

        (1) Differential diagnosis includes myopic degeneration (due to lacquer cracks in Bruch's membrane).

        (2) Examination includes contact lens or Volk evaluation.

        (3) Fluorescein angiography is helpful to determine presence of subretinal neovascular membrane.

    f. Treatment

        (1) If no subretinal neovascular membrane, treatment is not required.

        (2) Management of associated systemic disease—referral to internist or family physician is indicated.

    g. Follow-up

        (1) Fundus examination every 6–12 months.

        (2) Monitor at home with Amsler grid.

G. *Disease of the peripheral retina*

1. Retinal holes

    a. May represent retinal tear with operculum or atrophic retinal hole.

    b. Retinal tear

        (1) Symptoms

            (a) Acute onset of flashes and floaters.

            (b) May have reduced vision if associated with retinal detachment involving macula.

        (2) Clinical signs

            (a) Full thickness retinal tear with operculum (overlying retina which has detached in an area of hole).

            (b) Vitreous floaters—may represent red blood cells or liberated pigment cells.

        (3) Etiology

            (a) Vitreous traction.

            (b) Vitreous syneresis found in myopia and aging eyes.

            (c) Retinal thinning found in myopia and in peripheral retinal degenerations such as lattice degeneration.

        (4) Diagnostic evaluation

            (a) Differential diagnosis includes lattice degeneration, cobblestone degeneration.

          (b) Workup includes fundus examination with binocular indirect ophthalmoscope and scleral depression.

          (c) Evaluation with Goldmann three-mirror lens is useful.

          (d) Most retinal tears are found in the superior temporal quadrant.

    (5) Treatment

          (a) Most flap tears in symptomatic patients are treated.

          (b) Treatment is recommended if there has been a detachment in either eye.

          (c) Patients who are highly myopic or aphakic should be treated.

    (6) Follow-up

          (a) Untreated patients should be followed at 3- to 6-month intervals.

          (b) Once stable, treated patients should be seen annually.

          (c) Patients should be advised of the signs and symptoms of retinal detachment, and instructed to seek attention at once should they become symptomatic.

  c. Atrophic retinal holes

    (1) Symptoms. Patients are generally asymptomatic.

    (2) Clinical signs. Generally a reddish, full-thickness hole without operculum.

    (3) Etiology. Progressive retinal thinning due to high myopia or retinal degeneration.

    (4) Diagnostic evaluation

          (a) Differential diagnosis includes lattice degeneration, cobblestone degeneration, and retinoschisis.

          (b) Evaluation should include careful binocular indirect evaluation with scleral depression.

          (c) Goldmann three-mirror evaluation is useful to rule out localized subretinal fluid.

    (5) Treatment

          (a) Most atrophic retinal holes are untreated

          (b) Treatment is recommended if there has been a retinal detachment in either eye or if patient is symptomatic.

    (6) Follow-up

          (a) Patients with atrophic retinal holes should be followed at 6- to 12-month intervals.

          (b) Patient should be advised of the signs and symptoms of retinal detachment.

2. Retinal detachment

  a. Separation of the retina from the pigment epithelium.

  b. Symptoms

    (1) Flashes and floaters.

    (2) May have reduced visual acuity if macula is involved.

    (3) May complain of a "curtain" coming across the vision.

  c. Etiology

    (1) Most retinal detachments are tear-induced (rhegmatogenous).

    (2) Retinal detachments may be caused by a serous elevation of the retina associated with other retinal disease such as an optic pit or choroidal effusion, or by vitreous traction, or choroidal tumor.

  d. Diagnostic evaluation

    (1) Differential diagnosis includes retinoschisis and choroidal detachment.

    (2) Examination includes binocular indirect ophthalmoscopy with scleral depression.

    (3) Goldmann three-mirror evaluation is useful in locating retinal hole.

    (4) B-scan ultrasound is helpful in detecting retinal detachment beneath vitreous hemorrhage or dense cataract.

    e. Treatment
- (1) Patients with retinal detachment with the macula on should be treated expediently, usually within 1–2 days.
- (2) Treatment usually consists of cryopexy with scleral buckle.
- (3) Macula off retinal detachments are usually treated within several days and do not represent an emergency.

    f. Follow-up
- (1) Patients who have had surgical repair of retinal detachment should be examined every 6–12 months.
- (2) Examiner should note that the buckle is well anterior and that there are no new retinal breaks.
- (3) There is usually increased myopia following a scleral buckle procedure.

3. Senile retinoschisis
- a. Splitting of retina into two layers between inner and outer plexiform layers.
- b. Symptoms. Generally asymptomatic.
- c. Clinical signs. Transparent, smooth "blister" of tissue extending forward into vitreous.
- d. Etiology
  - (1) May have associated peripheral cystoid degeneration.
  - (2) Juvenile retinoschisis is congenital and thought to be genetically X-linked.
- e. Diagnostic evaluation
  - (1) Differential diagnosis includes retinal detachment and choroidal detachment.
  - (2) Examination includes binocular indirect ophthalmoscopy with scleral depression.
  - (3) Goldmann three mirror evaluation is helpful in locating inner or outer layer holes.
- f. Treatment
  - (1) Generally retinoschisis is not treated.
  - (2) If outer layer hole forms, treatment may be indicated.
  - (3) If macula is threatened, treatment, such as photocoagulation or cryopexy or scleral buckling, may be indicated.
- g. Follow-up. Asymptomatic, untreated patients should be seen at 6- to 12-month intervals.

4. Peripheral cystoid degeneration
- a. Accumulation of clear material between layers of the retina.
- b. Symptoms. Generally asymptomatic.
- c. Clinical signs. Small areas of cystlike spaces in far periphery.
- d. Etiology. Present in patients of all ages; increases with age.
- e. Diagnostic evaluation
  - (1) Differential diagnosis includes lattice degeneration or paving stone degeneration.
  - (2) Careful evaluation with the indirect ophthalmoscope and scleral depression is indicated.
- f. Treatment. No treatment is required.
- g. Follow-up. Annual examination with indirect ophthalmoscope is adequate.

5. Paving stone degeneration
- a. Absence of pigment epithelium in outer retinal layers.
- b. Symptoms. Generally asymptomatic.
- c. Clinical signs. Large areas of pigment epithelial atrophy in far periphery.
- d. Etiology. Loss of pigment epithelium with age.
- e. Diagnostic evaluation
  - (1) Differential diagnosis includes lattice degeneration and inflammatory retinal disease.

(2) Examination should include binocular indirect ophthalmoscopy with scleral depression.

    f. Treatment. Generally not treated.

    g. Follow-up. Annual examination indicated.

6. Lattice degeneration

    a. Localized area of retinal atrophy associated with hyalinized retinal vessels.

    b. Symptoms. Generally asymptomatic; however, may have symptoms if associated with retinal break.

    c. Clinical signs

      (1) Elongated, excavated areas of peripheral retina.

      (2) May have overlying hyalinized white blood vessels (lattice).

      (3) Overlying vitreous may be liquefied.

    d. Etiology. Lattice degeneration is associated commonly with high myopia.

    e. Diagnostic evaluation

      (1) Differential diagnosis includes other types of retinal degenerations, flap tears, atrophic retinal holes.

      (2) Examination should include binocular indirect ophthalmoscopy with scleral depression and Goldmann three-mirror evaluation.

      (3) Examination should include careful evaluation for retinal breaks (retinal breaks associated with lattice degeneration are a major cause of rhegmatogenous retinal detachment).

    f. Treatment

      (1) Most cases of lattice degeneration are untreated.

      (2) Treatment is recommended if there is an associated retinal break or history of retinal detachment in either eye.

    g. Follow-up. Untreated patients with lattice degeneration should be seen every 6–12 months.

IX. Glaucoma

A. *Features of glaucoma*

1. Complex of eye diseases generally characterized by elevated IOP, optic disc damage, and visual field loss.

2. The incidence of glaucoma in the US population is between 1% and 2% in people over the age of 40.

B. *Anatomy and physiology*

1. Aqueous humor is produced by nonpigmented epithelium of the ciliary body.

2. Aqueous drains from the eye via the trabecular meshwork and into Schlemm's canal.

3. IOP is determined by rate of aqueous production and outflow.

C. *General assessment*

1. IOP by Goldmann applanation tonometry should be obtained on all patients whenever possible. Although damage can occur at any pressure level, IOPs greater than 21 mm Hg are suspicious.

2. Optic nerve evaluation is optimized by pupillary dilation and binocular examination techniques. A cup-to-disc ratio greater than 0.5 or asymmetry of 0.2 or more is suspicious.

3. Threshold visual fields provide a sensitive assessment of the extent of the field. Paracentral or nasal loss may represent early signs of glaucoma. Field loss close to fixation is usually associated with extensive optic disc damage and should be treated aggressively.

4. Gonioscopy reveals whether angle is open or closed. Additional abnormalities such as pigmentation, rubeosis, or peripheral anterior synechia may be observed. See Figure 5-4 for normal angle features.

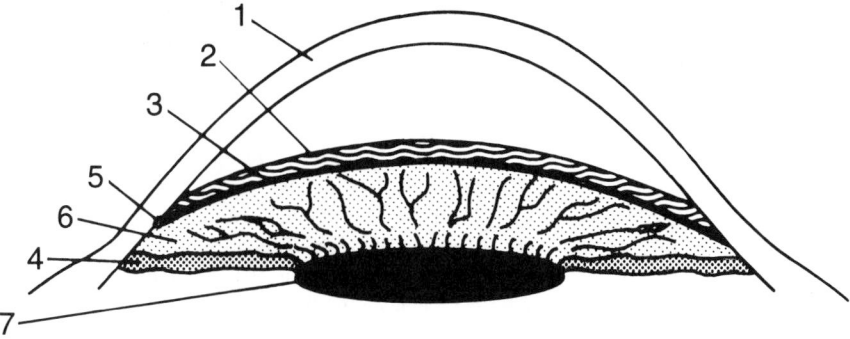

Figure 5-4. Angle anatomy. (1) Cornea, (2) Schwalbe's line, (3) trabeculum, (4) sclera, (5) scleral spur, (6) iris, (7) pupil.

D. *Pathophysiology of symptoms*
1. Generally patients with glaucoma are asymptomatic due to the insidious nature of the disease.
2. Blurred vision or halos around lights may be caused by corneal edema associated with acute rises in IOP.
3. Ocular pain and headache are associated with acute rise in IOP.

E. *Primary open angle glaucoma (POAG)*
1. 90% of cases of primary glaucoma are open angle.
2. Symptoms. Generally patients are symptomatic.
3. Clinical signs
    a. Enlarged cup-to-disc ratio (greater than 0.5), or asymmetry between the two discs.
    b. Elevated IOP—generally greater than 21 mm Hg.
    c. Visual field defects (nasal, paracentral, or arcuate loss found early in the disease).
    d. Anterior chamber generally deep and angle open.
4. Etiology
    a. Probably familial or genetically determined disorder.
    b. Elevated IOP, generally thought to be caused by poor outflow due to degenerative changes in the trabeculum or Schlemm's canal.
    c. Optic nerve damage may be due to vascular insufficiency.
    d. Risk factors include previous personal or family history of glaucoma, systemic vascular disease such as hypertension, arteriosclerotic disease or diabetes, myopia, and increased incidence in blacks.
5. Diagnostic evaluation
    a. Complete workup for glaucoma includes dilated fundus examination with binocular observation of optic nerve, IOP measurement, threshold visual fields, and gonioscopy.
    b. Differential diagnosis includes other glaucoma types such as secondary or angle closure glaucoma as well as low tension glaucoma. The differential diagnosis should also include other types of optic atrophy.
6. Treatment
    a. Patients with mildly elevated IOP (21–28 mm Hg), normal optic nerve, and no visual field loss may be followed without treatment as glaucoma suspects.
    b. Patients with normal IOP but suspicious optic nerves or visual fields should be followed. Stereo disc photographs are helpful in determining baseline appearance of the optic nerve. Suspicious or unreliable visual fields should be repeated at a later date, usually within 1–3 months.

    c. Patients with elevated IOP pressure, obvious optic nerve damage, or visual field loss should be treated. If intraocular pressure is mildly elevated, a single drug is used initially. β-Blockers or adrenergic drugs bid usually represent the first line of treatment. A uniocular trial is helpful. Usual target pressure is approximately 30% lower than baseline IOP. Patients should be rechecked in 3–5 weeks.

    d. Patients with marked elevation in IOP, severe optic nerve damage, and/or extensive visual field loss should be treated aggressively. Multiple medications may be started to lower pressure as quickly as possible. If the visual field loss is extensive or optic nerve damage profound, referral for surgical consult may be appropriate even at initial diagnosis. If the IOP is brought under control with the multiple medications, the drugs may be removed from the regimen one at a time to determine the efficacy of fewer medications.

    e. Once IOP has been lowered, patients should be followed at 3- to 6-month intervals. Threshold visual fields should be performed every 6–12 months to determine if the disease is progressing. If there is progressive visual field loss, then medication should be added to lower IOP further. Dilated optic nerve examinations and gonioscopy should be performed annually.

    f. Patients exhibiting extensive optic nerve damage or field loss within 1–10 degrees of fixation may be candidates for trabeculectomy and should be referred for surgical consult.

F. *Low tension glaucoma (LTG)*

    1. Glaucoma associated with various etiologies in which the intraocular pressure is less than 21 mm Hg and the patient exhibits optic nerve damage and/or visual field loss.

    2. Symptoms
      a. Generally asymptomatic.
      b. Advanced low tension glaucoma patients may complain of difficulties with peripheral vision.

    3. Clinical signs
      a. IOP less than 21 mm Hg.
      b. Enlarged cup-to-disc ratio in one or both eyes.
      c. Asymmetry in cup-to-disc ratio between the two eyes.
      d. Visual field loss.
      e. Splinter hemorrhages at the optic nerve.

    4. Etiology
      a. Previous history of primary open angle glaucoma.
      b. Wide diurnal variation.
      c. History of anemia or blood loss resulting in poor perfusion of the optic nerve.
      d. Previous episode of secondary glaucoma resulting in poor outflow.

    5. Diagnostic evaluation
      a. Differential diagnosis of other glaucomas.
      b. Careful evaluation of IOP, optic nerve, and visual fields.
      c. Detailed medical history.
      d. CT scan of head is sometimes indicated to rule out other causes of disc change.

    6. Treatment
      a. Target pressures for low tension glaucoma are 10–12 mm Hg.
      b. If IOP is already in the 10–12 mm Hg range, then patient should be followed with frequent visual fields (usually 3- to 6-month intervals).
      c. Treatment protocols are the same as for primary open angle glaucoma

    7. Follow-up
      a. In "stabilized" low tension glaucoma, patients should be followed at 3- to 4-month intervals
      b. Visual fields should be completed every 6–12 months.

G. *Acute angle closure glaucoma*

1. Glaucoma associated with a sudden increase in IOP pressure due to blockage of outflow at the anterior chamber angle by the root of the iris.

2. Acute angle closure glaucoma causes severe pain and sudden vision loss and thus represents a true ocular emergency.

3. Symptoms. Pain, hazy vision, or halos around lights, headache, nausea.

4. Clinical signs
   a. Severely elevated IOP.
   b. Corneal edema.
   c. Closed angle as viewed with gonioprism.
   d. Usually mid-dilated, fixed pupil.

5. Etiology
   a. Physiologically shallow anterior chamber. Shallow anterior chambers may be identified with the shadow test or Van Herrick test.
   b. Physiologic pupillary block. Pupillary block is common in hyperopic eyes and eyes with posterior synechiae from previous inflammation.
   c. Plateau iris. Plateau iris exists when the central anterior chamber is of moderate depth but the peripheral iris bulges into the chamber angle causing blockage.
   d. Closure of the angle due to anterior displacement of the lens caused by the following factors:
      (1) Increased size of the lens.
      (2) Choroidal detachment or swelling.
      (3) Posterior segment tumor.
      (4) Accommodation.

6. Diagnostic evaluation
   a. IOP measurement.
   b. Biomicroscopy carefully assessing presence of corneal edema and anterior chamber depth. Frequently corneal edema precludes careful evaluation of the anterior chamber for depth and/or cells and flare. If unable to see anterior chamber structures, anterior chamber depth may be assessed in the fellow eye.
   c. Pupillary responses.
   d. Differential diagnosis includes secondary inflammatory glaucoma, pigmentary glaucoma, glaucomatocyclitic crisis (Posner-Schlossman syndrome), phacolytic glaucoma.

7. Treatment
   a. Topical β-blocker (Timoptic 0.5% BID).
   b. Carbonic anhydrase inhibitor (acetazolamide 250 mg tablets ×2).
   c. Osmotic agents (osmoglyn or isosorbide).
   d. Pilocarpine 2% q 15 minutes for 2–3 applications (contraindicated in pseudophakic pupillary block).
   e. Apraclonidine 0.1% for one instillation.
   f. If IOP does not drop within 1 hour, laser or surgical peripheral iridectomy is required. If IOP drops, patient should be continued on pilocarpine 1%–2% qid until a laser peripheral iridectomy can be performed.
   g. If angle of fellow eye is narrow, may consider prophylactic treatment with $1/2$%–1% pilocarpine qid.

8. Follow-up. Once IOP has been stabilized, visual fields and optic nerves need to be evaluated.

H. *Angle recession glaucoma*

1. Trauma-induced unilateral secondary glaucoma.

2. Symptoms
   a. Usually asymptomatic.
   b. History of previous contusion injury.

3. Clinical signs
   a. Elevated IOP.
   b. Enlarged cup-to-disc ratio or disc asymmetry between the two eyes.
   c. Visual field loss.
   d. Deep anterior chamber.
   e. Wide ciliary band noted on gonioscopy especially compared to the fellow eye.
4. Etiology. Contusion to the eye causes the iris to tear at the root resulting in damage to the trabecular meshwork.
5. Diagnostic evaluation
   a. Differential diagnosis includes primary open angle glaucoma.
   b. IOP measurement, disc evaluation, and visual fields helpful.
   c. Definitive diagnosis is made by gonioscopy/comparing the two eyes.
6. Treatment
   a. Protocols similar to primary open angle glaucoma usually successful.
   b. Argon laser trabeculoplasty is less effective than with other types of glaucoma and, therefore, patient may proceed to trabeculectomy sooner.
7. Follow-up
   a. Patients with glaucomatous damage should be followed every 3–6 months.
   b. Patients without glaucomatous damage should be monitored annually.

I. *Inflammatory glaucoma*
   1. Secondary glaucoma due to uveitis.
   2. Symptoms. Blurred vision, pain, photophobia.
   3. Clinical signs
      a. Acute rise in IOP.
      b. Hazy or cloudy cornea.
      c. Cells and flare in the anterior chamber.
      d. May have other signs of iritis such as keratic precipitates, miotic pupil, ciliary flush.
   4. Etiology
      a. Iritis.
      b. Trauma.
   5. Diagnostic evaluation
      a. Differential diagnosis includes angle closure glaucoma, glaucomatocyclitic crisis (Posner-Schlossman syndrome), and pigmentary glaucoma.
      b. Careful slit lamp evaluation is required to identify signs of anterior segment inflammation.
      c. IOP measurement.
      d. Gonioscopy to rule out angle closure.
      e. Previous history of anterior segment inflammatory disease.
   6. Treatment
      a. Topical β-blocker (timolol ¼% or ½% bid).
      b. Topical steroid (prednisolone acetate 1% q 1–6 hours depending on the severity of the iritis).
      c. Cycloplegic (homatropine 5% or atropine 1% bid-qid depending upon severity).
      d. If IOP is extremely high, as in angle closure glaucoma, carbonic anhydrase inhibitor or hyperosmotic agents may be employed (under no circumstances should pilocarpine be used, as it will aggravate the inflammation).
   7. Follow-up
      a. Patients are seen every few days following the initial episode.
      b. Steroids and antiglaucoma medicines may be tapered as inflammation and IOP return to normal.

c. Patients on therapy for several weeks may exhibit persistent elevated IOP. One should consider steroid-induced glaucoma in these cases.

J. *Pigmentary glaucoma*

1. Glaucoma caused by the deposition of pigment in the trabecular meshwork impeding outflow.
2. Symptoms
    a. Generally asymptomatic.
    b. Typically occurs in males.
3. Clinical signs
    a. Elevated IOP.
    b. Deposition of pigment band on corneal endothelium (Krukenberg's spindle).
    c. "Slitlike" defects in the iris as seen by retroillumination.
    d. Optic nerve cupping and/or visual field loss.
    e. Dense pigment band noted in trabeculum on gonioscopy.
    f. Large fluctuation in IOP possible during the day.
4. Etiology
    a. Pigmentary glaucoma appears to have a hereditary basis.
    b. Many patients exhibit pigmentary changes without elevated IOP and should be regarded as "glaucoma suspects."
    c. May be structural abnormality in myopes.
5. Diagnostic evaluation
    a. Measurement of IOP.
    b. Evaluation of disc and visual field.
    c. Biomicroscopy identifying Krukenberg's spindle and iris defects.
    d. Gonioscopy identifying pigment deposition in the trabeculum.
    e. Differential diagnosis includes inflammatory open angle glaucoma and pseudoexfoliation syndrome.
6. Treatment
    a. Protocols for primary open angle glaucoma are usually effective.
    b. As pigmentary glaucoma patients are generally younger, patient may be reluctant to use pilocarpine.
    c. Argon laser trabeculoplasty is effective.
    d. Trabeculectomy if other measures are not successful.
7. Follow-up
    a. Pigmentary glaucoma patients should be seen every 3 months or more often if the glaucoma is severe.
    b. Visual fields should be accomplished every 6–12 months.

K. *Steroid-induced glaucoma*

1. Elevated IOP following long-term use of topical or systemic steroids.
2. Symptoms
    a. Generally asymptomatic.
    b. Steroid-induced glaucoma unchecked will result in a loss of central vision.
3. Etiology. Long-term use of topical or systemic steroids.
4. Diagnostic evaluation
    a. Careful history to identify use of topical or systemic steroids.
    b. Measurement of IOP.
    c. Evaluation of optic nerve and visual fields.
    d. Differential diagnosis includes primary open angle glaucoma, inflammatory glaucoma.
5. Treatment
    a. Discontinue steroid or reduce frequency or concentration of steroid.
    b. Use less potent steroid (fluorometholone vs dexamethasone).

         c. Antiglaucoma therapy as in primary open angle glaucoma.

         d. As IOP is reduced, antiglaucoma medications may be discontinued.

L. *Neovascular glaucoma*

  1. Elevated IOP and glaucoma secondary to neovascularization of the iris and angle structures.

  2. Symptoms. Usually asymptomatic; however, may have pain and decreased vision associated with acute rise in IOP.

  3. Clinical signs. Elevated IOP associated with vascularization of iris and angle structures (rubeosis).

  4. Etiology

      a. Diabetic retinopathy.

      b. Vascular occlusive disease (particularly ischemic central retinal vein occlusion).

      c. Branch retinal vein occlusion.

      d. Carotid occlusive disease.

      e. Intraocular tumors.

      f. Other vascular disorders.

  5. Diagnostic evaluation

      a. Differential diagnosis includes primary open angle glaucoma and inflammatory glaucoma.

      b. Careful history to determine possible systemic etiology.

      c. IOP measurement.

      d. Gonioscopy to identify vessels in the anterior chamber angle.

      e. Evaluation of optic nerve and visual fields.

      f. Fluorescein angiogram to evaluate retinal condition if present.

  6. Treatment

      a. IOP is controlled with topical β-blockers, carbonic anhydrase inhibitors, hyperosmotic agents.

      b. Miotics and epinephrine compounds are generally avoided as they may exacerbate iris inflammation.

      c. Retinal condition should be fully evaluated and treated (e.g., panretinal photocoagulation and diabetes).

      d. Laser photocoagulation of vessels in the angle may be helpful.

      e. Trabeculectomy or valve implants if other medical and laser procedures fail.

      f. Anterior segment inflammation should be treated with steroids and cycloplegics.

  7. Follow-up

      a. Neovascular glaucoma is difficult to manage and should be followed carefully.

      b. Patients under control should be followed at 3-month intervals.

M. *Glaucoma procedures*

  1. Argon laser trabeculoplasty (ALT)

      a. The mechanism by which ALT lowers IOP is poorly understood. ALT results in an increase in aqueous outflow.

      b. 80–100 applications of laser energy are directed to the anterior half of the pigmented trabecular meshwork.

      c. Patients are generally placed on topical steroids qid for several days following the procedure and are checked within 2–4 weeks.

      d. The procedure is effective in 70% to 80% of the patients.

      e. Complications are rare.

  2. Peripheral iridectomy/iridotomy

      a. Surgical or laser procedure creating opening in peripheral iris for direct communication from posterior chamber to anterior chamber (generally done with laser).

      b. Most useful in pupillary block angle closure glaucoma.

c. Argon laser or YAG laser energy is directed to the peripheral iris until opening is observed.

d. Patients may be placed on topical steroids for several days to 1 week following the procedure.

e. IOP is checked within a few hours following the procedure. If pressure is decreasing, the patient continues on antiglaucoma medicines and steroids until seen in a few days.

f. If IOP is under control, patient is seen again in 1–2 months.

g. Anterior chamber angle should be evaluated postoperatively. Angle structures should be observed.

3. Glaucoma filtering surgery (trabeculectomy)

a. Filtering surgery creates an opening from the anterior chamber to the subconjunctival space.

b. Glaucoma filtering surgery generally reserved for cases where medical or laser therapy has failed, although the trend is to proceed to trabeculectomy sooner.

c. There are three types of filtering operations:
   (1) full thickness procedures;
   (2) partial thickness procedures;
   (3) tube or valve implantations.

d. 5-Fluorouracil (5-FU) or mitomycin are antimetabolites used postoperatively in patients who are at risk of scarring. Such patients are those who have had previous filtering operations which have failed or other intraocular surgery.

e. Filter surgery is most successful in primary open angle glaucoma.

f. Patients should be followed carefully for several weeks.

g. Patients exhibiting conjunctivitis or external disease following filtering surgery should be treated aggressively and promptly, as endophthalmitis may result.

X. Neuro-Ophthalmology

A. *Features of neuro-ophthalmic problems*

1. Problems with cranial nerves II, III, IV, V, VI, and VII may result in ocular complaints.

2. Neuro-ophthalmic problems are unique in that they do not lend themselves to single tissue examination as do other eye problems.

3. Neuro-ophthalmic problems are frequently identified by patient complaints or symptoms (often multiple symptoms).

4. Careful history including onset, frequency, and duration of symptoms can be helpful in deciding which symptoms require further investigation.

5. Optometrist must develop "framework of clinical reference" to recognize patients requiring consultation with neurologist, neurosurgeon, neuro-ophthalmologist, internist, or other practitioner.

B. *Neuro-ophthalmic examination*

1. Expanded ophthalmic exam, special attention to visual function, muscle function, and visual fields.

2. Visual function

a. Want best corrected visual acuity or pinhole acuity.

b. Differences in monocular color vision may indicate optic nerve disease.

c. Red cap test (compare appearance of red bottle cap in each eye) may result in desaturation of red color in eye with optic nerve disease.

d. Brightness comparison test. Patient looks at flashlight monocularly. Brightness seen with good eye is assigned "100 units." Examiner asks how bright light seems with affected eye. Optic nerve disease frequently results in decreased brightness perception.

3. Visual fields
   a. Confrontation fields are useful as quick screen or in difficult or uncooperative patients.
   b. Amsler grid useful in identifying central scotoma.
   c. Tangent screen will identify most neurologic field problems, as most affect central 30° of field.
   d. Automated bowl perimeter utilizing threshold strategies for central 30° (Humphrey 30-2) or suprathreshold strategies for full field (Humphrey 120 point).
4. Ocular motility
   a. Observe patient's ability to fixate.
   b. Conduct versional testing in six cardinal positions of gaze.
   c. Present target to elicit convergence.
   d. Perform cover test to determine nature of muscle imbalance if history of diplopia.
5. Pupillary examination
   a. Examine in semidarkened room (semidilated).
   b. Examine prior to instillation of dilating drops.
   c. Note pupil size and any anisocoria (20% of "normals" exhibit some anisocoria).
   d. Note presence of direct and consensual light reflex.
   e. Observe pupillary constriction on convergence/accommodation.
   f. Test for afferent pupillary defect utilizing swinging flashlight test.

Clinical Procedure—Swinging Flashlight Test

Description/ Purpose	To determine the presence of afferent pupillary defect (APD or Marcus-Gunn pupil). Will find positive APD in optic nerve disease.
Equipment	Flashlight or illuminator.
Procedure	Conduct examination in semidarkened room. Shine light into good eye and note pupillary constriction (direct and consensual in fellow eye). "Swing" light to affected eye and look for relative pupillary dilation. Positive APD suggests optic nerve disease or other problem along prechiasmal afferent pathway.

---

6. Eyelids
   a. Note position of both eyelids, looking for evidence of ptosis or narrowed palpebral aperture. Ptosis of sudden onset may indicate third nerve problem. Bilateral ptosis worse in day suggests myasthenia gravis.
   b. Note levator function. Poor levator function may be associated with third nerve problem.

C. *Neuro-ophthalmic considerations*
   1. Optic nerve disease
      a. Papilledema
         (1) Swelling of optic nerve head associated with increased intracranial pressure.
         (2) Symptoms
             (a) Headache, nausea, vomiting.
             (b) Usually visual acuity is good.

   (3) Clinical signs
    (a) Bilateral swelling of optic nerve.
    (b) Absence of venous pulse.
    (c) Visual acuity normal.
    (d) Normal color vision.
    (e) Normal pupillary responses.
    (f) May exhibit peripapillary hemorrhages.
   (4) Etiology
    (a) Increased intracranial pressure of any cause.
    (b) Intracranial space occupying lesion.
    (c) Inflammatory disease of brain.
    (d) Intracranial hemorrhage.
   (5) Diagnostic evaluation
    (a) Complete ophthalmic exam.
    (b) In-depth medical/ophthalmic history.
    (c) Blood pressure
    (d) Order computed tomography (CT) or magnetic resonance imaging (MRI) to rule out intracranial lesion.
   (6) Treatment
    (a) Management of underlying cause.
    (b) Referral to neurologist or neurosurgeon.
  b. Pseudotumor cerebri
   (1) Papilledema associated with obesity, headache, and no other findings.
   (2) Symptoms
    (a) Headache.
    (b) Usually female.
    (c) Transient visual complaints.
   (3) Clinical signs
    (a) Bilateral papilledema.
    (b) Normal CT or MRI.
    (c) No other signs of intracranial disease.
   (4) Etiology
    (a) Obesity.
    (b) Medications: steroids, tetracycline, vitamin A, oral contraceptives.
   (5) Diagnostic evaluation
    (a) Complete ophthalmic workup.
    (b) CT or MRI normal.
    (c) Visual field (should be normal).
    (d) High cerebrospinal fluid pressure on lumbar puncture.
    (e) Diagnosis made by exclusion.
   (6) Treatment
    (a) Referral to neurologist.
    (b) Usually self-limiting.
 (c) Swollen disc associated with sudden vision loss
  (1) Symptoms. Reduced vision (usually unilateral, sudden).
  (2) Clinical signs
   (a) Reduced visual acuity—often to hand motion.
   (b) Monocular color defects.
   (c) Swollen disc with edema and flame hemorrhage.
   (d) Afferent pupillary defect (Marcus-Gunn pupil).
   (e) Central scotoma or other field loss.
   (f) Jaw pain or head pain (associated with temporal arteritis).
   (g) Disc appearance may be normal in retrobulbar neuritis.

      (h) If gradual vision loss, must consider possible optic nerve or intracranial tumor.

(3) Etiology

    (a) Etiology of optic nerve swelling associated with vision loss generally varies with age of patient.

    (b) Young (<55 years of age)

        i. Optic neuritis most likely cause of disc swelling in middle-aged patients.

        ii. Causes Viral causes in children.
Associated with demyelinating disease in middle-aged patients.
Granulomatous infection.
Idiopathic.
Optic nerve tumor (if vision loss gradual).

    (c) Older (age 55 and older)

        i. Anterior ischemic optic neuropathy (AION) most common in older patients.

        ii. Two general categories of AION
Arteritic AION—associated with giant cell arteritis.
Nonarteritic AION—associated with hypertension, arteriolar sclerosis, diabetes, tumor.

(4) Diagnostic evaluation

    (a) Complete ophthalmic exam.

    (b) Swinging flashlight test for afferent pupillary defect.

    (c) Visual field testing.

    (d) Monocular color vision.

    (e) Blood tests (CBC, sedimentation rate, FTA-ABS, ANA).

    (f) CT or MRI if blood work normal.

    (g) Temporal artery biopsy if suspect giant cell arteritis.

(5) Management/follow-up

    (a) Optic neuritis

        i. Observation—treatment with oral steroids is controversial.

        ii. Consider referral to neurologist for evaluation for demyelinating disease.

        iii. Follow-up in 1 month.

    (b) Arteritic AION

        i. Temporal artery biopsy.

        ii. STAT ESR rate.

        iii. Oral or iv steroids (oral steroids should be used in consultation with patient's internist).

        iv. Steroids may be tapered after ESR normalizes.

        v. Treatment may last several months.

        vi. Follow-up and ESR rate monthly.

    (c) Nonarteritic AION

        i. If ESR normal and no other symptoms of arteritic AION (jaw claudication, then no treatment is indicated).

        ii. Follow-up 1 month.

Clinical Alert

Gradual, progressive vision loss associated with optic nerve swelling may be indicative of a compressive optic nerve tumor at any age.

d. Optic atrophy
  (1) Disc pallor following loss of ganglion cells.
  (2) Symptoms. Loss of visual acuity (may be congenital, often progressive).
  (3) Clinical signs
     (a) Primary optic atrophy—sharp disc margins, enlarged physiologic cup, lamina cribosa visible, pale white color.
     (b) Secondary optic atrophy—blurred disc margins, filling in of physiologic cup, poor visibility of lamina crirbosa, gray-white glial veil overlying disc.
     (c) Reduced visual acuity.
     (d) Afferent pupillary defect.
  (4) Etiology
     (a) Consecutive optic atrophy following retinal disease such as retinitis pigmentosa.
     (b) Secondary optic atrophy often follows papilledema or papillitis.
     (c) Optic atrophy of glaucoma may be differentiated from other primary forms by nasal displacement of the blood vessels and prominent lamina.
     (d) Retrobulbar neuritis.
     (e) Compressive lesions such as optic nerve glioma or meningioma.
     (f) Toxic—alcohol and drugs such as chloroquine, digitalis, and lead.
  (5) Diagnostic evaluation
     (a) Differential diagnosis includes all possible causes of disc pallor—congenital, acquired, glaucoma.
     (b) Complete ophthalmic examination with attention to visual acuity, pupillary responses, visual fields.
  (6) Treatment
     (a) Patients with progressive or previously undiagnosed optic atrophy should receive complete workup by neurologist or neuro-ophthalmologist.
     (b) Documented, nonprogressive optic atrophy is not treated.
     (c) Low vision evaluation if appropriate.
  (7) Follow-up. Every 6–12 months.

Clinical Alert

Reduced visual acuity may herald the presence of optic nerve disease, carotid-occlusive disease, or intracranial disease.
Patients with progressive visual acuity loss without obvious ocular basis should receive a complete neuro-ophthalmic evaluation.

---

2. Neuro-ophthalmic conditions resulting in diplopia
  a. History
     (1) Is diplopia monocular or binocular?
     (2) Onset, duration, frequency.
     (3) Any other associated symptoms (decreased visual acuity, pain, pupil disturbances)?
     (4) General medical health.
  b. Systemic etiologies
     (1) Stroke.
     (2) Thyroid disease.
     (3) Diabetes.
     (4) Myasthenia gravis.

   c. Third nerve (oculomotor) palsy

     (1) Third nerve innervates inferior rectus, inferior oblique, medial rectus, superior rectus, and levator and parasympathetic fibers to iris sphincter and ciliary muscles.

     (2) Internal ophthalmoplegia is loss of autonomic innervation to iris and ciliary body with sparing of innervation to extraocular muscles.

     (3) External ophthalmoplegia is loss of extraocular muscle innervation with sparing of autonomics.

     (4) Symptoms. Isolated third nerve palsy usually results in diplopia and ptosis.

     (5) Clinical signs

       (a) Inability to look in all fields except temporal.

       (b) Ptosis.

       (c) Dilated, unreactive pupil.

     (6) Etiology

       (a) If pupil involved, consider aneurysm or tumor.

       (b) If pupil spared, consider diabetes or hypertension.

     (7) Diagnostic evaluation

       (a) Examine extraocular muscle movements in all cardinal positions of gaze.

       (b) Evaluate pupil size and response.

       (c) Look for ptosis.

       (d) Differential diagnosis includes thyroid disease, myasthenia gravis, orbital disease, midbrain lesion (symptoms usually bilateral).

     (8) Treatment

       (a) Complete ophthalmic examination.

       (b) Referral to neurologist if no specific ocular basis for diplopia.

       (c) CT or MRI.

       (d) If acute third nerve palsy is associated with dilated pupil, must refer emergently—possible aneurysm.

       (e) Tensilon test to rule out myasthenia gravis.

       (f) Treat systemic disease if related.

       (g) Patch to eliminate diplopia.

       (h) Observation if no underlying problem.

     (9) Follow-up. If third nerve palsy has no obvious cause, recheck every 6–8 weeks. Third nerve function should be improved in 2 to 3 months from onset. If no improvement, refer to neurologist.

   d. Fourth nerve (trochlear) palsy

     (1) Fourth nerve innervates superior oblique muscle.

     (2) Symptoms. Vertical (and torsional) diplopia.

     (3) Clinical signs

       (a) Inability of eye to look downward and nasally.

       (b) Three-step test indicates superior oblique problem.

     (4) Etiology. Most common is trauma.

     (5) Diagnostic evaluation

       (a) Complete ophthalmic examination.

       (b) Three-step test (see Clinical Procedures).

       (c) Maddox rod testing and cover test to identify hyperdeviation.

       (d) Look for head tilt.

     (6) Treatment

       (a) Treatment of injury.

       (b) Observation if no underlying cause.

     (7) Follow-up. Every 3–4 months while resolving, annual exam thereafter.

Clinical Procedure—Three-Step Test

Description/ Purpose — To identify faulty muscle in patient presenting with vertical diplopia.

Procedure — STEP 1—Determine right or left hypertropia, thus isolating four muscles.

Example: Left hypertropia isolates weak left depressors: left inferior rectus and left superior oblique or weak right elevators: right superior rectus and right inferior oblique.

STEP 2—Determine if deviation is greater in right or left gaze. This eliminates two of the four possible muscles. (Note: remaining two muscles will both be either intortors or extortors with respect to cyclo movement. To help remember which are intortors or extortors, use mnemonic SIN: superior—intortors).

Example: Left hypertropia increases in right gaze isolates: right superior rectus and left superior oblique.

STEP 3—Determine if deviation is worse with head tilt to left or right. This utilizes cyclorotational tendencies of the eye to isolate intortor or extortor function.

Example: Left hypertropia increases with right gaze and head tilt right. Isolated muscles right superior rectus and left superior oblique are intortors. If hyper deviation increases with head tilt right, right intortor is defective; therefore, right superior rectus is identified as faulty muscle.

---

    e. Sixth nerve (abducens) palsy
      (1) Sixth nerve innervates the lateral rectus muscle.
      (2) Symptoms. Binocular horizontal diplopia (maximal when turning eye to affected muscle, minimal when turning eye away).
      (3) Clinical signs
        (a) Noncommitant esotropia, inability to turn eye outward.
        (b) Head turn toward paretic muscle.
      (4) Etiology. Vascular lesions, trauma, demyelinating disease, infectious disease, aneurysm, stroke, increased intracranial pressure.
      (5) Diagnostic evaluation
        (a) Complete ophthalmic examination.
        (b) Differential diagnosis includes thyroid disease, myasthenia gravis, Duane's syndrome.
      (6) Treatment
        (a) Refer to neurologist.
        (b) CT or MRI.
        (c) If no underlying disease, observation.
      (7) Follow-up. Examine every 6 to 8 weeks until resolved.
  3. Pupil disturbance
    a. Adie's tonic pupil
      (1) Unilateral, dilated pupil with minimal reaction to light.
      (2) Symptoms
        (a) Generally asymptomatic.
        (b) May complain of blurred vision.
      (3) Clinical signs
        (a) Unilateral, slightly dilated pupil.
        (b) Sluggish response to direct and consensual stimulation.
        (c) 80% occur in women.

      (4) Etiology

         (a) Idiopathic.

         (b) May be associated with loss of deep tendon reflexes.

      (5) Diagnostic evaluation

         (a) Observe pupil for sluggish constriction on direct stimulation.

         (b) Adie's pupil is hypersensitive to 0.12% pilocarpine and constricts more than normal, fellow eye.

         (c) Anisocoria may be observed in old photographs.

      (6) Treatment. None.

      (7) Follow-up. Routine examinations.

b. Marcus-Gunn pupil

      (1) Afferent pupil defect discussed in optic nerve section.

      (2) Detected with swinging flashlight test.

c. Argyll-Robertson pupil

      (1) Anisocoria associated with tertiary syphilis

      (2) Symptoms. Usually none.

      (3) Clinical signs

         (a) Miotic pupils (usually bilateral).

         (b) Does not react to light.

         (c) Constricts with accommodation.

      (4) Etiology

         (a) Usually associated with tertiary syphilis.

         (b) May be associated with other central nervous system disorders.

      (5) Diagnostic evaluation

         (a) Complete ophthalmic examination

         (b) Dilated fundus examination looking for chorioretinitis.

         (c) VDRL or FTA-ABS to rule out syphilis.

      (6) Treatment

         (a) Treat underlying disease—refer to internist.

         (b) Observation if no underlying disease.

      (7) Follow-up. Routine exams if stable.

d. Horner's pupil

      (1) Miosis associated with Horner's syndrome.

      (2) Symptoms

         (a) May be asymptomatic.

         (b) Anisocoria.

         (c) Ptosis, miosis, anhydrosis (loss of ability to sweat) on affected side of face.

         (d) Pupil responses are normal.

      (3) Etiology

         (a) Disruption of efferent sympathetic pupillary pathway.

         (b) Preganglionic (first or second order)—stroke, tumor, aneurysm.

         (c) Postganglionic (third order)—vascular headache syndromes, herpes zoster.

      (4) Diagnostic evaluation

         (a) Complete ophthalmic exam.

         (b) Testing with hydroxyamphetamine (1% paredrine).

         (c) Failure of pupil to dilate with hydroxyamphetamine indicates postganglionic lesion.

         (d) CT or MRI.

         (e) Chest and cervical spine x-rays.

         (f) Blood work/CBC.

      (5) Treatment. Treat underlying disorder—refer to internist.

      (6) Follow-up. Once stabilized—regular examinations.

Clinical Alert

Horner's syndrome of sudden onset may be life-threatening and should be immediately referred to internist or neurologist.

Clinical Alert—Malingering

Clinicians should be alert to special motivations of patients who may be feigning visual loss (legal, financial, disability, etc.)
When attempting to "discover" a malingerer, use objective tests (pupil functions, optokinetic nystagmus, electrodiagnostics).

Clinical Alert—Visual Fields and Neuro-Ophthalmology

Certain visual field results should bias clinician toward neuro-ophthalmic diagnoses.
Unilateral central scotoma is common with optic (or retrobulbar) neuritis.
Bitemporal hemianopia is associated with pituitary tumors.
Homonymous hemianopia is common with intracranial disease such as tumor, aneurysm, or stroke.

---

4. Migraine headache
    a. Classic migraine is a syndrome consisting of an aura of neurologic disturbance (usually visual) followed by headache.
    b. Symptoms
        (1) Prodromal symptoms usually last 15–20 minutes.
        (2) Visual symptoms include blurred vision, scintillations, scotomata.
        (3) May have dizziness, paresthesia.
        (4) Above symptoms followed by headache, nausea, and vomiting.
    c. Clinical signs
        (1) Few.
        (2) Visual field loss observed if testing done during prodromal phase.
    d. Etiology
        (1) Prodromal symptoms are associated with vasoconstriction of external carotid artery and its branches.
        (2) Headache associated with vasodilation of external carotid artery and its branches.
    e. Diagnostic evaluation
        (1) Complete ophthalmic examination.
        (2) Full field visual field testing to help rule out other neurologic problems affecting visual pathway.
        (3) Neurologic consult if uncertain as to diagnosis.
    f. Treatment
        (1) Referral to neurologist, internist, or family practitioner.
        (2) Avoid triggering agents which initiate attack (foods, drink, medication, or emotional causes).
        (3) Analgesics for pain.
        (4) Ergotamine tartrate in severe forms.
    g. Follow-up. Routine examinations.

Clinical Alert—Ocular Migraine

Vasoconstriction of external carotid artery and its branches without vasodilation can occur and will result in visual disturbances without headache (ocular migraine).

Such disturbances usually last 15–20 minutes.

Suggested Readings

Alexander LJ. *Primary Care of the Posterior Segment.* East Norwalk, CT: Appleton and Lange, 1994.

Bartlett JD, Jaanus SD. *Clinical Ocular Pharmacology.* Boston: Butterworth, 1989.

Fingeret M, Casser L, Woodcome HT. *Atlas of Primary Eye Care Procedures.* East Norwalk, CT: Appleton and Lange, 1990.

Cullom RD, Chang B. *The Wills Eye Manual.* Philadelphia: J.B. Lippincott, 1994.

Lewis TL, Fingeret M. *Primary Care of the Glaucomas.* East Norwalk, CT: Appleton and Lange, 1993.

Spalton DJ, Hitchings RA, Hunter PA. *Atlas of Clinical Ophthalmology.* 2nd ed. St. Louis: Mosby, 1994.

Tasman W, Jaeger E. *Duane's Clinical Ophthalmology.* Philadelphia: J.B. Lippincott, 1994.

Vaughan D, *General Ophthalmology.* 13th ed. East Norwalk, CT: Appleton and Lange, 1992.

Kevin L. Alexander. *The Lippincott Manual of Primary Eye Care*. Copyright © 1995 by J.B. Lippincott Company.

CHAPTER **6**

The Eye in Systemic Disease

J. James Thimons

I. **Infectious Diseases**

A. *The broadest category of diseases that produce ocular manifestations are the infectious diseases. Ranging from bacterial infection to protozoan disease, this group of clinical entities is a continuing challenge for clinicians.*

B. *Bacterial infections*
   1. Brucellosis
      a. A worldwide disease, uncommon in the United States, brucellosis is associated with infected domestic animals (dairy cattle, etc.) and exposure to contaminated products.
      b. Ocular/systemic signs. Ocular involvement is related to neuro-ophthalmic disease associated with meningitis (retrobulbar neuritis, papilledema, cranial nerve palsy).
      c. Etiology. Chronic disease can demonstrate ocular inflammation (uveitis, scleritis/episcleritis).
      d. Diagnostic evaluation.
         (1) Blood cultures to identify organism.
         (2) Serum agglutination testing.
         (3) General optometric examination.
      e. Treatment
         (1) Identification of underlying disease and treatment with doxycycline for 7–10 weeks in acute disease.
         (2) Chronic disease—may require therapy for up to 6 months.

Clinical Alert

Although the disease is rare, certain occupations demonstrate increased risk of infection. Individuals exposed to animals (veterinarians, farmers, etc.) or their by-products are at risk.

---

   2. Metastatic bacterial infections
      a. Infection of globe secondary to systemic bacterial infection. Reduced incidence currently due to early treatment of physical disease.
      b. Symptoms. Pain, decreased vision, redness.
      c. Ocular/systemic signs. Ocular involvement is primarily inflammatory (iritis, vitritis, keratitis).

    d.   Etiology. History of intravenous drug abuse common.

    e.   Diagnostic evaluation. Laboratory testing to identify causative organism (blood cultures).

    f.   Treatment. Antibiotic therapy is based on causative organism.

Clinical Alert

In any patient with advanced idiopathic inflammation, endophthalmitis should be considered.

---

3.   Mycobacterial disease (leprosy)

    a.   Worldwide disease characterized by tissue destruction and infiltration with subsequent damage to neural and cutaneous tissue which produces contractures and deformities.

    b.   Symptoms. Irritation, redness, discomfort, vision reduction.

    c.   Ocular/systemic signs

        (1)   Ocular involvement is generally noted to be inflammatory (iritis or iridiocyclitis).

        (2)   Late stage can show adnexal scarring.

    d.   Etiology

        (1)   The disease is due to *Mycobacterium leprae*.

        (2)   Route of transmission is still not well defined.

    e.   Diagnostic evaluation. Blood titers for *M. leprae* are the best mechanism of identification.

    f.   Treatment

        (1)   Oral therapy with both sulfones and rifampin must be continued for the life of the patient.

        (2)   Topical therapy for inflammation is cycloplegics and steroids. Dosage is based on severity.

Clinical Alert

Regular optometric examination is critical to long-term management of anterior segment complications. Patient compliance must be stressed due to chronicity of disease.

---

4.   Tuberculosis

    a.   A common communicable disease that is seen in areas of poor sanitation and hygiene. Secondary to exposure to *Mycobacterium tuberculosis* it can present as either a chronic or an acute multisystem disease.

    b.   Symptoms. Fatigue, chronic chest infections, ocular discomfort, decreased acuity.

    c.   Ocular/systemic signs

        (1)   Anterior segment involvement is mixed presentation with a follicular, purulent conjunctivitis.

        (2)   Inflammation is common with uveitis (granulomatous), choroiditis, optic neuritis.

        (3)   Phylctenulosis can be an early eye sign.

    d.   Etiology

        (1)   Causative agent is *M. tuberculosis*.

        (2)   Mode of transmission is through contact with infected individual.

    e.   Diagnostic evaluation

        (1)   Most common testing is purified protein derivative (PPD).

      (2)   Chest x-ray.

      (3)   Refer to internist.

   f. Treatment

      (1)   Oral therapy with izoniazid and rifampin for up to 1 year.

      (2)   Ethambutol can be substituted in cases resistant to rifampin.

Clinical Alert

Tuberculosis is increasing rapidly in urban areas in the United States, and ocular complications, once uncommon, are now more frequently seen, particularly in patients with AIDS and intravenous drug abusers.

---

5. Trachoma and inclusion conjunctivitis (TRIC) infection

   a. Obligate intracellular organism that bears similarities to both bacteria and virus. It is classically divided into *Chlamydia trachomatis* and *Chlamydia psittaci* and is the causative agent in both trachoma and inclusion conjunctivitis.

   b. Symptoms. Ocular infection which occasionally is accompanied by concurrent systemic symptoms of genitourinary disease, pneumonitis, etc.

   c. Ocular/systemic signs

      (1)   Acute infection with purulent discharge.

      (2)   Corneal involvement with sub-epithelial infiltrates typical in chlamydia. Vascularization and scarring common with trachoma.

      (3)   Lid scarring seen in advanced trachoma.

   d. Etiology

      (1)   *Chlamydia trachomatis* is causative agent.

      (2)   Nature of disease is related to serotype (A–C trachoma; D–K chlamydia).

      (3)   Trachoma is associated with poverty, poor sanitation, etc.

      (4)   Chlamydia is commonly transferred through sexual contact.

   e. Diagnostic evaluation

      (1)   In-office testing utilizes immunofluorescent antibody testing.

      (2)   More definitive testing is done with McCoy cell culture.

   f. Treatment

      (1)   Systemic—usually tetracycline or erythromycin 500 mg po bid ×7–10 days.

      (2)   Ocular—tetracycline or erythromycin ointment bid-qid for 4–6 weeks. Oral tetracycline or erythromycin may be helpful.

Clinical Alert

Chlamydia is rapidly becoming one of the most common causes of conjunctivitis in the 20- to 40-year-old age group. Diagnosis of eye findings can be crucial because of silent nature of disease and lack of systemic symptoms.

C. *Spirochetal disease*

   1. The family of diseases associated with the spirochete is diverse and produces significant ocular findings that encompass all tissues. Systemic complications involve both chronic and acute multisystem disease.

   2. Lyme disease

     a. An endemic disease in the Northeast United States that affects the entire globe. Secondary to exposure to ticks infected by *Borrelia burgdorferi*.

b. Symptoms. Flulike malaise, joint pain, eye discomfort, blurred vision, redness, swelling. Usually begins as a rash.

c. Ocular/systemic signs

(1) Ocular involvement can encompass entire globe—most common is conjunctivitis, corneal infiltrate, uveitis, optic neuritis.

(2) Systemic disease is diffuse multisystem. Can involve heart, cortex, joints, skin, etc.

d. Etiology

(1) Secondary to the spirochete *Borrelia burgdorferi*.

(2) Most common transmission is via infected ticks from deer, and disease is endemic in northeastern United States.

e. Diagnostic evaluation

(1) Enzyme-linked immunosorbent assay (ELISA) is most definitive test. (NOTE: There may be variability in the quality of this test)

(2) Erythrocyte sedimentation rate (ESR) can be used to assess inflammation levels.

f. Treatment

(1) Adult therapy is best accomplished with tetracycline 250 mg qid ×21 days (or doxycycline 50 mg bid).

(2) Pencillin can be used for children below age 8. (50 mg/kg divided into 4 doses).

(3) Erythromycin 250 mg qid can be substituted for tetracycline-sensitive patients.

Clinical Alert

Like some spirochete diseases (syphilis), Lyme disease can mimic a wide variety of ocular and systemic disease and must be considered in any patient with appropriate history and clinical findings.

---

3. Syphilis

a. Spirochetal infection which is commonly transmitted through sexual contact. Is classified as either first degree, second degree, or third degree in its effect on the human organism.

b. Symptoms. Dependent on stage of disease.

c. Ocular/systemic signs

(1) Primary disease—chancre, regional lymphadenopathy, maculopapular rash, uveitis, vitritis.

(2) Secondary disease—mucous membrane eruptions with diffuse lymphadenopathy perivasculitis, and interstitial keratitis.

(3) Tertiary disease—neurologic involvement (cranial nerve palsy, cognitive dysfunction, etc.) concurrent sexually transmitted diseases, optic atrophy.

d. Etiology. Infection by *Treponema pallidum* via sexual contact.

e. Diagnostic evaluation

(1) Laboratory testing with Venereal Disease Research Laboratory (VDRL) test, fluorescent treponemal antibody absorption, or microhemagglutination assay for antibodies to treponema pallidum is most common.

(2) Cerebrospinal fluid examination is generally considered definitive.

f. Treatment

(1) Based on level of disease benzathine penicillin G in 2.4 million units/week x3 weeks is most common.

(2) Ocular treatment involves inflammation management with cycloplegics,

steroids, and ocular antihypertensives for intraocular pressure (IOP) control.

Clinical Alert

Inadequate treatment can permit continued existence of the organism and persistence of disease. Patients should be followed regularly after treatment to substantiate decline of symptoms and signs of infection.

---

   4. Leptospirosis
      a. Spirochetal infection is endemic in areas where exposure to domestic animals is frequent. Commonly noted in farmers, cattle veterinarians, and fishermen. Infection is secondary to direct penetration through compromised cutaneous tissue. Dissemination throughout the body initiates as in onset of symptoms.
      b. Symptoms. Most common are headaches, skin rashes, nausea, vomiting, muscle ache, flulike presentation.
      c. Ocular/systemic signs
         (1) Atypical—conjunctival engorgement is most common. Iritis, uveitis are typical in late stage disease.
         (2) Severe disease can produce optic nerve and retinal inflammation.
      d. Etiology.
         (1) Caused by *Leptospira interrogans* (170 serotypes) harbored by domestic animals.
         (2) Contact with urine or feces of infected animals.
      e. Diagnostic evaluation. Agglutination testing is done to isolate the serotype.
      f. Treatment
         (1) No specific therapy, but the use of penicillin G iv 2.4 million units qd is recommended.
         (2) Ocular treatment with cycloplegics and steroids is indicated concurrently if inflammation is present.

Clinical Alert

Late onset disease is challenging due to lack of historical data and nonspecific ocular findings.

   D. *Viral disease*
      1. Viral disease associated with the eye has classically been related to herpetic infection. Although this disease is still prevalent, other significant viral entities have been identified and are now a part of the optometric practitioner's differential diagnosis when considering viral disease.
      2. Human immune deficiency virus (HIV) infection
         a. The newest of the viral diseases, acquired immunodeficiency syndrome (AIDS), is a complex, diffuse system disease that has risen to epidemic proportion. Routes of transmission are sexual contact, blood transfusion from contaminated products, infected needles, and via the birth canal.
         b. Symptoms. Patients present with nonspecific diffuse disease which can include weight loss, secondary infection, and relapsing illness.
         c. Ocular/systemic signs
            (1) Ocular involvement is not common in the early phases of the disease.

(2) Primary manifestations include cytomegalovirus (CMV) retinitis, HIV retinitis, neuro-ophthalmic involvement, and rarely conjunctival Kaposi's sarcoma.

(3) Systemic disease is related to opportunistic infections (herpes simplex virus, herpes zoster virus, toxoplasmosis, *Pneumocystis carinii,* fungal disease, etc).

d. Etiology

(1) Infection occurs following exposure to the HIV organism via sexual contact, IV drug abuse, transfusions.

(2) Other routes of exposure are not well documented.

e. Diagnostic evaluation

(1) Blood titers to demonstrate presence of the disease.

(2) Complete optometric examination

(3) Comanagement with patient's physician to monitor ocular complications.

f. Treatment

(1) Current therapy is designed to minimize impact of opportunistic infections.

(2) Azidothymidine (AZT) is most common anti-HIV agent.

(3) Ganciclovir and Foscarnet are the only agents currently used in the treatment of CMV retinitis.

Clinical Alert

HIV infection has become epidemic worldwide. Practitioners should adopt appropriate protocols for in-office prevention of disease transmission.

---

3. Cytomegalovirus (CMV)

a. Common viral entity (80% penetration) among normal population. Acquisition is through multiple sources, and once infected, host sheds virus for extended period.

b. Symptoms. Muscle fatigue, gastrointestinal involvement, blurred vision, floaters.

c. Ocular/systemic signs

(1) The hallmark sign is a necrotizing retinitis with large areas of infiltration and hemorrhage.

(2) Patients frequently present with initial vitritis which can present with floaters.

d. Etiology. Common viral organism; exposure in general population is near universal.

e. Diagnostic evaluation. Primary diagnosis is frequently based on the presence of opportunistic disease in an otherwise nonsymptomatic patient.

f. Treatment

(1) Ganciclovir and Foscarnet are used to treat active CMV retinitis.

(2) Infectious disease specialist manages systemic treatment.

Clinical Alert

CMV retinitis is rarely noted in nonimmunosuppresed individuals. If diagnosed, HIV infection must be suspected.

---

4. Epstein-Barr virus (EBV)

a. Virus with strong association with infectious mononucleosis.

b. Symptoms
   (1) Chronic fatigue which can last months to years.
   (2) Occasional visual complaints including discomfort, pain, and vision reduction.
c. Ocular/systemic signs
   (1) Inflammation (iritis, iriocyclitis, uveitis, choroiditis) is sometimes noted.
   (2) Occasional conjunctivitis of a follicular variety.
d. Etiology
   (1) EBV is a commonly observed virus and is endemic in the community. Routes of transmission are not well defined.
   (2) The disease is frequently associated with mononucleosis.
e. Diagnostic evaluation. The laboratory diagnosis can be based on either VCA (viral capsid antigen) levels or EBNA (Epstein-Barr nuclear antigen).
f. Treatment. Although no therapy is definitive, acyclovir is currently considered the best treatment option.

5. Herpes simplex virus (HSV)
   a. DNA complex virus which commonly produces infection of the mucous membranes and, in the immunocompromised host, diffuse systemic involvement.
   b. Symptoms. Febrile illness, oral and genital sores, recurrent pattern to disease state.
   c. Ocular/systemic signs
      (1) Primary disease usually involves mucous membranes (mouth, genitalia, ocular).
      (2) Initial episode is usually minor.
      (3) Secondary disease involves cornea (epithelium or stroma). Recurrence is 25%.
   d. Etiology
      (1) HSV is endemic in population, with up to 90% of patients greater than 15 years old having positive titer.
      (2) Route of inoculation is related to contact with infected host and direct transfer.
   e. Diagnostic evaluation. Immunoassay is possible in office; McCoy cell culture is most accurate.
   f. Treatment
      (1) Epithelial disease is best managed by topical antiviral therapy. (Trifluridine q 3 hours is recommended.)
      (2) Cycloplegia is useful if discomfort (homatropine 5% bid) is present.
      (3) Stromal disease is managed with both steroids and antivirals, initially in matching doses, then tapering.

Clinical Alert

Treatment of corneal epithelial disease is limited to topical antivirals. Steroids are only used in treatment of stromal disease to decrease inflammation.

---

6. Herpes zoster virus (HZV)
   a. Varicella zoster is the agent responsible for chickenpox and adult onset vesicular disease. The human organism is the only host for this organism, and its distribution is via airborne droplets.
   b. Symptoms. Malaise, fever, and pain along dermatome.
   c. Ocular/systemic signs
      (1) Ocular involvement is diffuse with multitissue disease.

(2) Conjunctivitis, keratitis, episcleritis, uveitis in acute phase. Occasional rare involvement of optic nerve, glaucoma.

(3) Systemic disease can be severe, with vesicular rash and visceral involvement.

d. Etiology. HZV is the adult manifestation of the varicella virus. Distribution is by airborne transfer via droplets.

e. Diagnostic evaluation

(1) Physical exam is most common method for diagnosis due to typical presentation.

(2) Occasionally physical signs will not be present at initial complaint of pain. Cautious observation can be productive.

f. Treatment

(1) Immediate initiation of oral acyclovir (800 mg q 5x/day) reduces postherpetic neuralgia.

(2) Oral steroids are still mainstay of treatment.

(3) Topical therapy is oriented toward inflammation and pain management (steroids, cycloplegics).

(4) Monitoring IOP is crucial.

Clinical Alert

Early intervention with acyclovir has been shown to decrease postherpetic neuralgia.

---

7. Molluscum contagiosum

a. Pox-virus-related skin disease that produces lesions which are raised, circumscribed, and umbilicated and has been shown to be self-limiting.

b. Symptoms. Itching, occasional infected lesion, injection, recurrent red eye.

c. Ocular/systemic signs

(1) Follicular conjunctivitis, sub-epithelial infiltrates (SEIs), subconjunctival hemorrhage, lymphadenopathy are commonly noted together.

(2) Recurrent nature of disease with treatment failure is common due to misdiagnosis.

d. Etiology. Pox-virus disease with contact as source of infection.

e. Diagnostic evaluation

(1) Physical examination of head and neck is usually sufficient to identify lesions.

(2) Biopsy confirmation is diagnostic if uncertain.

f. Treatment

(1) Most effective method of treatment is removal.

(2) Chemical cautery, cryopexy, surgical excision are most common.

Clinical Alert

Chronic conjunctivitis must be investigated as possibly related to molluscum. Examination of lids and adnexa for disease is necessary in identification.

E. *Protozoan disease*

1. Infestation with protozoan organisms, although not common, can have significant ocular complications. Involvement is somewhat tissue-specific relative to individual organism. The following are the most common protozoan infections.

2. Toxoplasmosis
   a. *Toxoplasma gondii* is the causative organism in this common disease. Transmission is via direct contact with contaminated soil. The cat is the host most frequently associated with the disease.
   b. Symptoms. Blurred vision, ocular discomfort, and redness.
   c. Ocular/systemic signs
      (1) Ocular manifestations include uveitis, vitritis, retinochoroiditis (macular and peripheral lesions).
      (2) Systemic disease is multisystem with visceral involvement common.
      (3) Rare to have systemic and ocular disease simultaneously.
   d. Diagnostic evaluation
      (1) Physical exam frequently gives classic "headlight in fog" appearance in active lesions.
      (2) ELISA testing is most accurate and should accompany toxotiters for definitive diagnosis.
   e. Treatment
      (1) Therapy is complex and requires use of pyrimethamine and sulfonamides administered orally.
      (2) Oral steroids are essential to control sequelae of disease when treating central lesion.
      (3) Topical therapy with cycloplegics or steroids is based on level of disease.

Clinical Alert

Toxoplasmosis scars are able to develop new vessel activity. Careful examination is indicated to rule out neovascular changes.

---

3. Amebiasis
   a. A broad group of protozoan agents can affect the human species. Most common is the Entamoebidae family and the free-living *Acanthomoeba*. Both have been implicated in serious eye infections but are not common entities.
   b. Symptoms. Patients present with general constitutional malaise which includes headache, weight loss, nausea, vomiting, and fever.
   c. Ocular/systemic signs
      (1) Identification of disease in patients with systemic symptoms is difficult due to vague nature of disease.
      (2) Ocular involvement is diffuse and includes HSV-like keratitis, conjunctivitis, SEIs, scleritis, and iritis.
   d. Etiology of eye-related disease
      (1) Poor contact lens hygiene.
      (2) Homemade contact lens saline.
   e. Diagnostic evaluation
      (1) Blood studies are essential to identify the organism.
      (2) Antibody titers can be useful in evaluating exposure and current level of involvement.
   f. Treatment
      (1) Broad-spectrum treatment is required to manage disease.
      (2) This entails use of bacitracin, gentamicin, vidarabine, and amphotericin B.
      (3) Topical anti-inflammatory therapy is warranted if anterior chamber reaction is present.

Clinical Alert

Acanthamoeba is particularly difficult to diagnosis due to its similarities to other disease states and its low incidence; clinicians should be alert to diagnosis when corneal lesion is recalcitrant to topical therapy.

---

    4. Malaria

        a. Worldwide disease with significant implications for both ocular and systemic disease. Endemic areas are well described but the disease persists in large numbers. Route of transmission is the *Anopheles* mosquito.

        b. Symptoms. Diffuse disease is hallmark of malaria. Malaise syndrome including fever, chills, sweating, and headaches is typical of disease.

        c. Ocular/systemic signs

            (1) Ocular involvement is unpredictable, with minimal anterior chamber activity.

            (2) Retinal hemorrhages and exudates with papilledema are most notable.

            (3) Severe cases can cause extraocular muscle palsies and nystagmus.

        d. Etiology

            (1) Occurs secondary to bite of an infected mosquito (*Anopheles*), blood transfusion, or IV drug abuse.

            (2) Can have localized epidemics related to population movements (armies, etc.).

        e. Diagnostic evaluation

            (1) Antibody identification is the most common form of analysis.

            (2) Blood smears can show active organism.

        f. Treatment

            (1) Chloroquine administered orally is the drug of choice with therapy of acute disease lasting up to 2 weeks.

            (2) Ocular therapy is aimed at treating associated disease (HSV keratitis).

Clinical Alert

Malarial ocular complications are infrequent except in the severe falciparum form of the disease.

   F. *Mycotic infection*

      1. Fungal infection is a common component of ocular and systemic disease. Histoplasma is frequently suspected in fungal eye disease and is endemic throughout many parts of the United States (Mississippi River Valley).

      2. Histoplasmosis

        a. A fungal disease which has multisystem effects on the human body. Infection is related to inhalation of the *Histoplasma capsulatum* organism. Soil contaminated by infected avians is the most common cause.

        b. Symptoms. The disease has few or no symptoms unless macular vision is involved, when visual loss can be dramatic.

        c. Ocular/systemic signs

            (1) Primary sign is choriodopathy which produces peripapillary, peripheral, and occasionally macular lesions.

            (2) Although systemic involvement is possible, it is uncommon. The most typical change is noted as hilar adenopathy on routine x-ray.

        d. Etiology. *Histoplasma capsulatum* is the causative organism, but active organisms are not found in lesions. Exposure to soil, avian droppings, etc. has been implicated in spreading of disease.

e. Diagnostic evaluation. ELISA testing is also useful in those instances in which diagnosis is equivocal.

f. Treatment. Retinal complications (macular) require angiography and laser if possible to treat subretinal neovascular membrane (SRNVM).

Clinical Alert

No clear indication for treatment exists beyond laser for SRNVM. Regular follow-up should be instituted to ascertain status of lesions and provide intervention. Home Amsler grid testing is indicated for all patients with posterior pole involvement.

II. **Endocrine Disorders**

A. *Endocrine function is a vital component of normal metabolism throughout the body. Abnormalities produce multisystem involvement which is both complex and potentially life-threatening. Ocular manifestations are frequently the first sign of disease.*

B. *Thyroid dysfunction*
1. The thyroid gland secretes T_3 and T_4 hormones which are mediated by thyroid-stimulating hormone (TSH). This mechanism has cortical control via the hypothalamus and thyrotropin-releasing hormone (TRH). The imbalance of this complex system accounts for the two basic presentations of this disease.
2. Hyperthyroidism
   a. Autoimmune or idiopathic disease characterized by an oversecretion of thyroid hormones which results in classic ocular and systemic manifestations. Excessive secretion can be attributed to numerous causes, including Graves' disease, toxic goiter, and subacute thyroiditis.
   b. Symptoms
      (1) Patients frequently report irritability, nervousness, weight loss, and fatigue.
      (2) Palpitations and sweating are also common.
   c. Ocular/systemic signs
      (1) Ocular involvement can be pronounced, with a multitude of presentations. These include lid retraction, lagophthalmos, proptosis, and conjunctival edema.
      (2) More advanced disease involves optic nerve and extraocular muscle dysfunction secondary to edema of orbit and muscle fibrosis.
      (3) Associated disease includes superior limbic keratoconjunctivitis and exposure keratitis.
   d. Etiology. Imbalance of thyroid production which causes excessive thyroid hormone.
   e. Diagnostic evaluation
      (1) Standard workup uses T_3, T_4 levels.
      (2) Up to 20% of patients have normal T_3, T_4 (euthyroid in presence of disease). Orbital computed tomography (CT) or magnetic resonance imaging (MRI) is definitive in symptomatic patients.
      (3) TSH serum levels can be evaluated in equivocal cases.
   f. Treatment
      (1) Palliative therapy is usually sufficient early in disease. Lubricants, taping lids shut at night, patching, etc. all limit exposure of cornea and desiccation.
      (2) Surgical intervention is sometimes required for acute decompression of orbit in severe cases.

Clinical Alert

As orbital changes progress in thyroid disease, potential sight-threatening involvement of the optic nerve can take place. Frequent optometric examination is indicated along with comanagement with endocrinologist or internist.

---

3. Hypothyroidism
   a. Condition in which a decrease in thyroid secretions produces a diminution of basal metabolic function with subsequent multisystem effects.
   b. Symptoms
      (1) Fatigue, lethargy, dryness of skin, and coarse hair are all typical of the disease.
      (2) Onset is usually insidious and diagnosis can be elusive initially.
   c. Ocular/systemic signs
      (1) Most common of the clinical signs are disturbances of function, e.g., weight loss, menstrual difficulties, appetite reduction, etc.
      (2) Ocular involvement is usually subtle and involves corneal edema, lash loss, blepharoptosis, conjunctival edema.
      (3) Severe cases can develop papilledema and optic atrophy.
   d. Etiology. Insufficient supply of thyroid hormone due to generalized dysfunction of gland.
   e. Diagnostic evaluation. The standard laboratory evaluation includes T_3, T_4, TSH serum levels.
   f. Treatment
      (1) Supplemental therapy with thyroid replacement is the most common means of successful treatment.
      (2) Lifelong treatment is usually required to manage disease.
      (3) Ocular signs and symptoms diminish with successful systemic treatment.

Clinical Alert

Conjunctival and periorbital edema are common in this disease and should be monitored when patient is on treatment to ensure compliance.

C. *Diabetes mellitus*
   1. A deficiency of insulin (either secretion or metabolic ineffectiveness) which produces hyperglycemia. Two classes of the disease exist: juvenile and adult onset.
   2. Symptoms
      a. Polydypsia, polyphagia, and polyuria are the classic triad of complaints. These are frequently seen in the early phase of the disease. Fatigue and weight fluctuation are also common.
      b. Vision reduction is most commonly noted as early ocular symptom due either to cataract or to refractive error.
   3. Ocular/systemic signs
      a. Refractive fluctuation is one of the most common signs and frequently is the first presentation in the optometric examination.
      b. Other metabolic problems, such as cataracts, healing delays, etc., are typical of the underlying disease.
      c. Advanced involvement includes retinopathy (background diabetic retinopathy [BDR], proliferative diabetic retinopathy [PDR], macular edema) all of which can compromise vision.

       d. Neuro-ophthalmic disease involves diplopia and is most typically seen as sixth cranial nerve palsy.

4. Etiology
   a. Secondary to a deficiency in insulin (secretion or metabolic ineffectiveness) which produces hyperglycemia.
   b. There is a strong genetic relationship between parents and offspring.
   c. Differentiation of disease is between juvenile and adult onset (insulin-dependent vs non-insulin-dependent disease.) Juvenile diabetes mellitus is due to massive loss of beta cells with little if any production.

5. Diagnostic evaluation
   a. Traditional testing included urine evaluation, postprandial assessment, and testing blood sugar.
   b. Current testing includes OGTT (oral glucose tolerance testing) and glycosolated hemoglobin (A1H) which measures glucose levels over time.

6. Treatment
   a. Therapy is directed at early diagnosis with thorough optometric examination.
   b. Comanagement of systemic disease with dietary restriction, oral hypoglycemic agents, and insulin.
   c. Cataracts are removed surgically.
   d. Retinal complications are evaluated with fluorescein angiography and treated with panretinal photocoagulation (PRP), focal laser, and macular grid laser for edema, if indicated.

Clinical Alert

Diabetes is a life-long disease once diagnosed. Frequent examination is indicated for early detection of retinopathy and successful management. Hypertension can accelerate diabetic disease. Blood pressure measurements should be a part of all eye examinations of diabetics with referral to the patient's physician when not well controlled.

III. Collagen Disorders

A. *This category of systemic disease manifests itself in a variety of presentations which are related to inflammatory disease of a multisystem nature. Although it encompasses a wide range of conditions, the primary diseases associated with this entity are:*

B. *Polyarteritis nodosa*
   1. Vasculitis of medium and small arteries of unknown etiology. Usual onset in 4th–5th decades with multisystem presentation of necrotizing arteritis, predominantly male 3:1.
   2. Symptoms.
      a. A general decrease in well-being is frequently the earliest sign of this disease.
      b. Weight loss, appetite decrease, fever, muscle pain, joint discomfort, are typical in early phases.
   3. Ocular/systemic signs
      a. Ocular involvement can be significant. Anterior segment changes include conjunctival edema and injection, keratitis sicca, and ulcerative keratitis.
      b. Retinal changes include nerve fiber layer infarction (NFLI), exudates, hemorrhages, and vasculitis.
      c. Inflammation is typical (uveitis).
      d. Optic nerve involvement in late stages can be severe (papilledema/optic atrophy).
   4. Etiology. The disease is secondary to vasculitis of small to medium arteries. The etiology is unknown but males predominate.

5. Diagnostic evaluation. Serum IgM, IgE levels are helpful in isolating disease.
6. Treatment
   a. Therapy is directed at systemic manifestations. Corticosteroids are primary modality of therapy along with cyclophosphamide for severe necrotizing vasculitis.
   b. Topical ocular therapy includes steroids and cycloplegics and ocular lubricants for surface disease.

Clinical Alert

Cytotoxic agents used for treatment have significant complications and require regular monitoring.

C. *Polymyositis*
   1. A nonsuppurative inflammatory disease characterized by diffuse involvement of skeletal muscles and frequently associated with other collagen diseases.
   2. Symptoms
      a. Skin changes commonly noted by patient include "butterfly" mask, facial rash, etc.
      b. Ocular symptoms include extraocular muscle disturbances which are transient initially.
   3. Ocular/systemic signs
      a. Diplopia is one of the more common complaints related to the disease and is frequently associated with progressive muscle weakness systemically.
      b. Occasionally patients will complain of respiratory distress in conjunction with the disease.
   4. Etiology. Results from diffuse inflammation of muscle fibers and subsequent decrease in function.
   5. Diagnostic evaluation
      a. Typically creatinine and kinase levels are reviewed for elevation.
      b. Definitive testing is accompanied by electromyography (EMG) and muscle biopsy testing.
   6. Treatment
      a. Therapy is directed at controlling systemic inflammation with oral steroids and immunosuppressive agents.
      b. Recent work with plasmapheresis has shown some success.

D. *Systemic lupus erythematosus (SLE)*
   1. Autoimmune disease characterized by antibody production against cellular-nuclear antigens with diffuse inflammation and immunologic abnormalities.
   2. Symptoms
      a. Cutaneous changes of the upper back, neck, and arms are a common complaint. This is frequently accompanied by a "butterfly" facial rash.
      b. Complaints of muscle weakness and pain can sometimes be an early manifestation.
   3. Ocular/systemic signs
      a. Chronic conjunctivitis associated with drying of the mucous membranes is not uncommon.
      b. Retinal changes include NFLI, hemorrhage, arteritis, and branch retinal artery occlusion.
      c. Neuro-ophthalmic disease involves edema, optic nerve head atrophy, optic neuritis, as well as extraocular muscle palsies.
   4. Etiology. Autoimmune disease with development of specific antibodies against cellular nuclear antigens which produces significant inflammation.

5. Diagnostic evaluation. Specific lab tests include antinuclear antibody (ANA) and DNA double-strand test. ANA is nonspecific but indicative of the disease.
6. Treatment
   a. Therapy is similar to that of other collagen disorders in that systemic steroids, cyclosporine, and chloroquine have all been used to treat the disease.
   b. Essential management is still oral steroids.
   c. Topical therapy is directed at ocular surface disease with lubricants, punctal plugs, etc.

Clinical Alert

Systemic drug therapy can produce significant ocular complications. Frequent optometric examination is necessary during active therapy of FLE.

E. *Scleroderma (systemic sclerosis)*
   1. Connective tissue disorder of unknown etiology that produces small vessel damage with secondary fibrous scarring of associated tissue and organs.
   2. Symptoms
      a. Typical early symptoms include dry eye problems associated with skin changes (thickening and then tightening).
      b. Occasionally myopathy and myalgia are noted.
      c. Late in disease patient complains of lid abnormalities.
   3. Ocular/systemic signs
      a. Ocular complications are most commonly seen as dry eye and early conjunctival edema with some scarring.
      b. Common systemic changes with little ocular impact (vasculitis, pericarditis).
      c. Retinal disease involves NFLI hemorrhage, edema, with occasional papilledema.
   4. Etiology. This disease has no known etiology, but damage takes place secondary to fibrous scarring of associated tissue organs.
   5. Diagnostic evaluation. ANA and thorough optometric examination. Rarity of disease makes diagnosis difficult and clinically challenging.
   6. Treatment
      a. No specific treatment known at this time but dry eye treatment is crucial. Palliative treatment for symptoms is best initial therapy.
      b. Management of secondary infection (with topical antibiotics) is important to long-term success.

Clinical Alert

Ocular surface disorders must be managed aggressively to minimize long-term complications. Retinal findings are identical to malignant hypertension and must be managed accordingly.

F. *Juvenile rheumatoid arthritis (JRA)*
   1. Name used to describe a variety of childhood-based arthritic diseases which manifest themselves with specific presentations related to the "subgroup" classification.
   2. Symptoms
      a. Common symptoms include fever, flulike malaise, blurred vision.
      b. In advanced disease the patient notices fatigue and abnormal growth.

3. Ocular/systemic signs
   a. The primary ocular involvement is "white" iritis and associated findings. These include cataract, band keratopathy, synechia, glaucoma, and macular edema—all secondary to uveitis.
   b. Systemic disease is noted to produce organomegaly, growth retardation, anemia, and leukocytosis.
4. Etiology
   a. The disease is a grouping of a variety of disorders under a single heading. Each entity has a different clinical expression.
   b. Pauciarticular is the subgroup most likely to produce uveitis.
   c. Girls are most likely to present with the disease (9:1).
5. Diagnostic evaluation
   a. The key to diagnosis is thorough physical exam because of the typical changes noted.
   b. Laboratory tests specific for the disease are HLA-B27, HLA DRW5, and ANA.
6. Treatment
   a. Therapy is aimed at minimizing sequelae and maintaining patient comfort.
   b. Topical treatment utilizes steroids and cycloplegics in the acute phase and mydriatics between exacerbations to prevent synechiae.
   c. In chronic disease, IOP and cataract management (surgical) can be complex.

Clinical Alert

The chronicity of this disease necessitates long-term steroid treatment. Patients must be monitored for development of IOP elevation and cataracts. Hydroxychloroquine has been implicated in retinal pigmentary disturbance.

G. *Adult rheumatoid arthritis*
1. Common condition which affects multiple joints with inflammatory disease. More commonly found in females (2–3 times) and usually first noted in the 4th–5th decades.
2. Symptoms
   a. Joint pain and stiffness is the most typical early complaint of the patient.
   b. Occasionally vision is blurred and ocular discomfort is present in acute disease.
3. Ocular/systemic signs
   a. Systemic disease is represented by rheumatoid nodules, vasculitis, muscle atrophy, and pulmonary fibrosis.
   b. Most commonly seen ocular component is dry eye disorders. Frequently the patient will present with a unilateral uveitis, episcleritis, or scleritis.
   c. Severe disease can demonstrate scleromalacia and optic nerve involvement.
4. Etiology. Adult onset immune-mediated disease that is more common in females than males.
5. Diagnostic evaluation
   a. Thorough physical examination.
   b. Laboratory tests including erythrocyte sedimentation rate (ESR) and
   c. rheumatoid factors.
   d. Synovial fluid exam.
   e. x-ray studies of joints.
6. Treatment
   a. Symptomatic, rest, proper nutrition.
   b. Drug therapy including nonsteroidal anti-inflammatory drugs (NSAIDs), oral gold, hydroxychloroquine, corticosteroids.

Clinical Alert

Early diagnosis of ankylosing spondylitis is critical to effective management of disease complications. Practitioners should always consider this process when presented with recurrent uveitis in a young male.

H. *Ankylosing spondylitis*

1. An inflammatory disease which selectively affects the sacroiliac area. It is most commonly seen in young males.
2. Symptoms. Stiffness of the lower back, blurred vision, redness, pain.
3. Ocular/systemic signs
   a. Low back pain in conjunction with iritis is the classic presentation of this disease. In severe cases it can demonstrate ulcerative colitis and pulmonary fibrosis.
   b. The iritis is acute and can be dramatic. 30% of patients have recurrences.
4. Etiology. One of the family of autoimmune-mediated diseases. Specific expression is in young males and initiates in the sacroiliac area.
5. Diagnostic evaluation
   a. Physical examination and appropriate lab tests are the best mechanism for accurate diagnosis.
   b. HLA-B27 has a high association with the disease.
6. Treatment. Therapy is aimed at systemic inflammation and may involve use of NSAIDs or steroids. Primary concern is management of pain and limitation of scarring. Ocular treatment is similar to other uveitis presentations, with steroids and cycloplegics being used primarily.

I. *Phakomatoses*

1. The phakomatoses represent a category of diseases that commonly present with hamartomas of the central nervous system (CNS), ocular tissue, cutaneous system, and internal organs.
2. Sturge-Weber syndrome
   a. Nongenetic congenital vascular condition characterized by triad of cutaneous, CNS, and eye abnormalities.
   b. Symptoms. Primary complaint usually involves skin disorders (nevus flammeus, etc.) minimal ocular involvement.
   c. Ocular/systemic signs
      (1) Classic skin involvement (nevus flammeus) can be associated with cerebral angioma and epilepsy.
      (2) There is possibility of calcification of intracranial structures.
      (3) Hemangiomas of the ciliary body, iris, and episclera are common.
      (4) Port wine stains, hemangioma of the choroid, glaucoma in late stage disease.
   d. Etiology. Abnormal development of hamartomas of the CNS. No specific genetic predispostion.
   e. Diagnostic evaluation. CT of cortex is indicated to rule out cranial involvement, IOP monitoring throughout life, and complete physical examination.
   f. Treatment
      (1) Therapy is directed at managing complications of disease.
      (2) IOP monitoring to rule out glaucoma, and dermatology consultation to manage port wine stain.
3. Neurofibromatosis
   a. Common inherited disorder of neural tissue cell production. Classified into three main groups.
   b. Symptoms. Common symptoms include skin disease (café-au-lait spots) and neurofibromas.

    c. Ocular/systemic signs

       (1) Systemic involvement is significant with neural crest tumors, severe disorders, and retardation common. Ocular changes include iris hamartomas, ptosis secondary to lid neurofibroma, optic nerve glioma, and retinal hamartoma.

       (2) Late onset glaucoma is common and occasionally pulsating exophthalmos is noted.

    d. Etiology

       (1) Inherited disorder related to development of neural tissue.

       (2) Primary expression is neurofibromas and hamartomas which produce complications.

    e. Diagnostic evaluation

       (1) CT scan is indicated regularly to assess cortical involvement.

       (2) Audiometry can demonstrate presence of eighth cranial nerve lesion.

    f. Treatment. The most important element is early diagnosis and appropriate genetic counseling. Surgical intervention can be undertaken to relieve severe disease or complications.

Clinical Alert

Significant risk of malignancy development throughout the patient's lifetime warrants continued observation.

---

   4. Tuberous sclerosis (Bourneville's disease)

    a. A genetic disorder characterized by hamartoma in the majority of body systems.

    b. Symptoms. Major patient symptoms involve skin disorders.

    c. Ocular/systemic signs

       (1) Cutaneous signs include hypomelanotic lesions, facial angiofibromas, and shagreen patches.

       (2) CNS findings include seizures, mental retardation, giant cell astrocytoma, hydrocephalus.

       (3) Cardiac signs include rhabdomyomas.

    d. Etiology. Genetic disorder which involves the development of hamartomas.

    e. Diagnostic evaluation

       (1) CT/MRI for cerebral lesions.

       (2) Echocardiogram for heart disorders.

       (3) Neuro-ultrasound/physical ultrasound.

       (4) Serial visual fields.

    f. Treatment

       (1) Genetic counseling is critical in preventing recurrence.

       (2) Surgical treatment of complications is recommended.

Clinical Alert

Onset of symptoms is not consistent with severity of disease. Clinician should examine patient regularly even when asymptomatic.

---

   5. Von Hippel-Lindau disease

    a. A genetic disease of neuroectoderm/mesoderm development with characteristic angiomatosis of retina, CNS hemangioblastomas, and thoracic angiomas.

  b. Symptoms
   (1) Minimal symptomatology in early disease.
   (2) Occasionally blurred vision is present if macular involvement.
  c. Ocular/systemic signs
   (1) Systemic complications include cerebellar hemangioblastoma (35%), renal carcinoma (30%), polycythemia (10%–25%), chromocytoma.
   (2) Ocular signs include classic presentation of angiomatosis retinae (vascular tumor associated with artery and vein).
   (3) Exudation common and can progress to exudative detachment.
  d. Etiology. Congenital disease that produces capillary angiomatous hamartomas that involve the retina and optic nerve.
  e. Diagnostic evaluation. Symptoms are nonspecific and therefore a full medical/neurologic evaluation is warranted if retinal findings are present.
  f. Treatment
   (1) Laser therapy of retinal lesions is possible, although not always successful.
   (2) Cryotherapy and diathermy have also been used to treat retinal lesions.

Clinical Alert

Large tumor treatment is complex and can lead to significant complications, including retinal detachment. Post-treatment patients should be monitored closely for development of retinal breaks, hemorrhage, detachment.

IV. Hematologic Diseases

 A. *The blood system is responsible for a wide variety of body functions, and abnormalities of this system can produce significant alterations of physical health. Although the number of conditions associated with hematologic abnormalities is myriad, those commonly associated with ocular disorders are represented by the following.*

 B. *Anemia*
  1. A group of disorders related to a decrease in red blood cell (RBC) volume. Hematocrit value decrease is noted in this condition in conjunction with RBC volume or as an independent findings.
  2. Symptoms
   a. Fatigue, weakness, and brittle nails (iron deficiency) are hallmark symptoms of this disease.
   b. Ocular complaints are minimal but may involve fluctuating vision or transient vision loss.
  3. Ocular/systemic signs
   a. Retinal hemorrhages of all types are common. NFLI and hard exudates are also noted.
   b. The classic finding is a "Roth spot" which is seen secondary to ischemia and hemorrhage.
   c. Unless posterior pole is involved, visual acuity is usually not disturbed.
  4. Etiology. Anemia is a decrease in hemoglobin secondary to either a decrease in RBC production or an abnormal shape of the cell.
  5. Diagnostic evaluation. The standard evaluation includes a CBC (complete blood count), fasting blood sugar, platelet levels, and physical exam. This profile permits differential diagnosis of the disease state and appropriate treatment.

6. Treatment
    a. Treatment of underlying disease is the key to successful management, in that ocular findings diminish when systemic treatment is undertaken.
    b. Routine ocular follow-up is recommended.

Clinical Alert

Retinopathy secondary to anemia is rare with hemoglobin titers greater than 8 g/100 ml. If above this level, consider other etiology for retinopathy.

C. *Leukemia*
    1. Abnormal white cell levels (elevated) associated with dysfunction of bone marrow production. Classification is related to age of onset, type of cell involved, and chronicity.
    2. Symptoms
        a. General decline in physical health is typical of disease. Patients experience weight loss, fatigue, and frequent infections.
        b. Ocular involvement in late phase can significantly affect vision, and patient may experience spontaneous subconjunctival hemorrhage.
    3. Ocular/systemic signs
        a. Systemic disease exhibits lymph node involvement, visceral infiltration, infection, and hemorrhage.
        b. Ocular complications are diverse and include iritis, spontaneous hyphema, and limbal degeneration.
        c. Retinal findings show infiltration and thickening of the choroid, hemorrhages, and tortuosity.
        d. Optic nerve compression is possible in late phase of disease.
    4. Etiology. Leukemia is most typically a disease of bone marrow dysfunction that causes a decrease in white cell production.
    5. Diagnostic evaluation
        a. Standard testing involves CBC with differential and physical examination.
        b. Suspicious findings should be investigated with bone marrow aspiration or lymph node biopsy.
    6. Treatment
        a. Typically treatment is aimed at stabilizing bone marrow production with transfusions, bone marrow transplants, etc.
        b. Irradiation and chemotherapeutic agents are also used in managing the disease.

Clinical Alert

Infiltration can occur in any tissue and should be suspected as a possible cause of any orbital abnormalities in children.

D. *Platelet disease*
    1. Abnormality of platelet function secondary to either functional disturbance (thrombocytopenia) or impaired platelet generation.
    2. Symptoms
        a. Patients may complain of abnormal bleeding or being easily bruised with only minor trauma.

   b. Minimal ocular complaints are noted unless central vision is affected.

  3. Ocular/systemic signs

   a. Typically patients show ocular hemorrhages which can involve any or all structures.

   b. In more severe cases, epilepsy and papilledema have been noted.

  4. Etiology. Abnormality of platelets secondary to decreased production or abnormal function.

  5. Diagnostic evaluation

   a. Analysis of platelet function can be done by assessing prothrombin time (PTT). Occasionally bone marrow studies can be done to assess diagnosis. Management of underlying disease will resolve ocular complications.

   b. Regular follow-up examinations to assess for exacerbation should be done.

E. *Sickle cell disorder*

  1. Disease characterized by predominance of hemoglobins. Classification is based on structure of the gene.

  2. Symptoms. Pain in extremities, loss of vision (sudden), and fatigue are most common signs of disease.

  3. Ocular/systemic signs

   a. "Sea fan" neovascularization is pathognomonic of the disease.

   b. Associated with the neovascularization is vitreal hemorrhage, spontaneous hyphema, and tractional detachment.

   c. "Comma" signs are frequently noted in patients with advanced disease.

  4. Etiology. Abnormal hemoglobin production and metabolism.

  5. Diagnostic evaluation. Laboratory blood work should include CBC and sickle cell preparation to identify the disease.

  6. Treatment

   a. Common treatment involves analgesics for pain, and management of secondary infections.

   b. Blood transfusions are helpful but do not provide permanent resolution.

   c. Laser therapy of "sea fan" lesions may be indicated to prevent vitreous bleeding. Cryotherapy can also be used to treat more peripheral lesions.

Clinical Alert

Elevated IOP due to hyphema produces more significant damage to ONH even at lower pressures due to poor perfusion of microvascular anatomy of the optic nerve. Treatment of pressure should be aggressive to minimize damage. Do not give Diamox to manage pressure due to hyphema as it will likely cause more sickling.

F. *Polycythemia*

  1. Hyperviscosity syndromes caused by increased RBCs, increased white cells, and abnormal plasma proteins result in increased blood volume and decreased blood flow.

  2. Symptoms

   a. Headaches, dizziness, weight loss, and weakness are typical complaints associated with the disease.

   b. Specific ocular complaints relate to visual loss, such as transient changes, scotomas.

  3. Ocular/systemic signs

   a. Ocular involvement shows stasis of veins, scattered hemorrhages, retinal edema, and central retinal vein occlusion.

   b. Advanced disease shows optic nerve edema.

       c.   Systemic complications are spontaneous epistaxis and ecchymosis. Occasionally, visceral bleeding is present with tenderness of the abdomen.

4. Etiology. Increased viscosity of RBCs, WBCs, and plasma blood elements. Can be related to general disease or specific stimulus.
5. Diagnostic evaluation. As with other blood dyscrasias, CBC and platelet studies are useful in identifying the process. Ocular findings are specific enough that the clinical exam can be helpful in diagnosis.
6. Treatment. Medical management of underlying disease is required to relieve ocular complications.

Clinical Alert

Visual abnormalities are frequently the first presenting sign of disease. Recognition of color variation and vascular abnormality is instrumental in early recognition.

V. Gastrointestinal Diseases

A. *The relationship between gastrointestinal disease and ocular manifestations is well accepted, but the specific etiology is still not established. Ocular manifestations involve an inflammation of the uveal tract with specific clinical features.*

B. *Crohn's disease/ulcerative colitis*
1. Inflammatory bowel disease is not an uncommon problem in the United States and has both chronic and acute ocular complications.
2. Symptoms
   a. Patients frequently present for diagnosis of red, painful eye and have history of gastrointestinal disease.
   b. Ocular complaints involve inflammatory disease (e.g., episcleritis scleritis, iritis, uveitis, papillitis).
   c. Can have symptoms of fever, malaise, weight loss due to diarrhea.
3. Ocular/systemic signs
   a. Intestinal distress is common with rectal bleeding, diarrhea, malaise.
   b. Ocular manifestations include diffuse inflammatory disease. Can also demonstrate orbital inflammation.
   c. Patient can have induced ocular complications from chronic treatment.
4. Etiology. Cause of this disease is unclear. The apparent etiology is an immune-mediated process.
5. Diagnostic evaluation. Laboratory testing is indicated to confirm findings from physical exam. HLA-B27 is common in this group but not specific.
6. Treatment
   a. Medical/surgical treatment of bowel disease is indicated to reduce symptoms and exacerbations.
   b. Topical management with cycloplegics and steroids during acute episodes is indicated.
   c. Careful monitoring of potential side effects of chronic treatment (cataracts, IOP, etc.) should be undertaken.

Clinical Alert

Diagnosis of etiology of anterior uveitis is crucial to appropriate therapy of systemic disease. Ocular manifestations may be first sign of significant bowel disease.

VI. Inflammatory Diseases

A. *Inflammatory disease is a common component of ophthalmic practice. Although the majority of conditions are well established regarding their etiology and mechanisms, some inflammatory disorders still are unresolved. This section discusses those conditions which have no specific cause.*

B. *Sarcoidosis*
  1. A granulomatous disease of unknown etiology that is most commonly noted in young adults. The effect of the disease is multisystemic in nature and related to activated T-helper cells and their effect on cell differentiation.
  2. Symptoms. Most common symptoms of early disease are related to ocular problems. Decreased vision with pain or discomfort may be the most typical presentation.
  3. Ocular/systemic signs
     a. Granulomatous uveitis is a hallmark sign. It frequently involves both anterior and posterior structures.
     b. Retinopathy is composed of granulomas, hemorrhage (secondary to neovascularization), and phlebitis.
     c. Systemic manifestations include pulmonary lymphadenopathy, hemoptysis, arthritis (late phase), and visceral involvement.
  4. Etiology. This granulomatous disease is of unknown etiology but is related to changes in activated T-helper cells.
  5. Diagnostic evaluation
     a. The most useful battery of tests for this condition is the ACE (angiotensin-converting enzyme) and chest x-ray.
     b. Further confirmation can be achieved by using the gallium scan and biopsy of suspected lesions.
  6. Treatment
     a. Topical and oral steroids (depending on disease state) are employed to treat the inflammation that accompanies the disease.
     b. Cycloplegics are necessary to limit sequelae associated with anterior segment inflammation.

Clinical Alert

The decision to treat systemically is related to the ocular findings. Most experts agree ocular involvement warrants initiation of therapy; therefore early diagnosis of eye findings is essential to proper management.

C. *Behçet's syndrome*
  1. An idiopathic inflammatory disease which is commonly seen in Asia, the Mediterranean, and parts of the European continent. It is multisystem in presentation and is normally noted in the 3rd and 4th decades.
  2. Symptoms. Symptoms are generally related to inflammatory disease: blurred vision, discomfort, and redness. Patients also complain of oral and genital ulcerations.
  3. Ocular/systemic signs
     a. Anterior chamber reaction can be severe, with hypopyon common. Episcleritis, scleritis, vitritis, and choroiditis can all be present.
     b. Severe disease can show optic nerve involvement with eventual atrophy.
     c. Systemic disease involves skin (acne erythema nodosum), joint (arthritis), and vascular (cardiac, thrombophlebitis).

4. Etiology
   a. The disease is idiopathic and is primarily seen in Asians and Mediterranean individuals.
   b. It appears to be an immune-mediated condition.
5. Diagnostic evaluation
   a. Specific lab testing for this condition involves HLA-B51.
   b. The physical examination is crucial and diagnostic criteria have been developed to assist in identification.
6. Treatment
   a. Immunosuppressive therapy is the primary treatment with agents such as cyclophosphamide, cyclosporine, and steroids being used concurrently.
   b. Topical therapy includes steroids and cyclophosphamide as well as ocular antihypertensives for IOP control.

Clinical Alert

Practitioner must be alert to serious side effects of immunosuppressive agents and follow patient frequently during and after treatment.

D. *Vogt-Koyanagi-Harada (VKH) syndrome*
1. A broad-based disease process of unknown etiology. Characteristically it presents with inflammation and cutaneous changes and is observed more frequently in individuals of Asian descent.
2. Symptoms
   a. Fever, headache, tinnitis, as well as hair loss and hearing impairment are the most typical symptoms.
   b. Visual involvement is related to complications from the inflammatory process, e.g., blurred vision, pain, redness, etc.
3. Ocular/systemic signs
   a. The hallmark sign is the exudative choroiditis. This is frequently accompanied by neovascularization and exudative detachment.
   b. Anterior segment involvement includes uveitis and marked poliosis.
   c. Systemic presentations include vertigo, alopecia, auditory loss, and cervical rigidity.
4. Etiology. VKH syndrome is an idiopathic disease that has a predilection for the choroid and hair of the head and neck. It is much more frequent in individuals of Asian descent.
5. Diagnostic evaluation
   a. Physical exam is critical in diagnosis because of unique presenting signs.
   b. Electroretinography (ERG) or Electro-oculogram (EOG) can be helpful in defining the disease.
   c. Fluorescein angiography has also been demonstrated to be useful in difficult cases.
6. Treatment
   a. Oral and topical steroids for inflammation management.
   b. Periocular injections have been successful when topical therapy is not sufficient.

Clinical Alert

Disease has potential for severe complications and treatment must be individually adjusted to minimize secondary effects of drugs and limit sequelae of disease.

VII. Dermatologic Disorders

    A. *The eye may exhibit numerous conditions that relate to cutaneous disease. These vary from infectious disease to autoimmune syndromes and affect primarily external tissue.*

    B. *Cicatricial pemphigoid*

       1. A chronic, idiopathic disease which produces bullous lesions of the mucosal surface and scarring. The mechanism is thought to be related to the type II hypersensitivity response.

       2. Symptoms

          a. Initial complaints of dry eye are common.

          b. Foreign body sensation and irritation are typical.

       3. Ocular/systemic signs

          a. Systemic disease is manifested by bullous eruptions, erythematous plaques, and scarring.

          b. Inflammation initially, followed by keratization and cicatrization of the globe is typical as disease progresses.

          c. Corneal involvement includes pannus, keratitis, stromal necrosis, and eventually ulcerative lesions.

          d. Late stage developments include lacrimal duct obstruction and cataract.

       4. Etiology. This disease is idiopathic and constitutes an essentially immune-mediated condition. The response is typical of type II hypersensitivity and the clinical presentation is consistent with this process.

       5. Diagnostic evaluation

          a. HLA-B27 and serum IgA levels are the most appropriate lab tests to assist in diagnosis.

          b. The retinal presentation can be very minimal, and most of these patients are treated for some time for the presentation of dry eye before diagnosis is completed.

       6. Treatment

          a. Treatment initially is palliative and oriented toward dry eye management and tissue conservation.

          b. As the disease progresses, surgical intervention for trichiasis, entropion, exposure, etc. is required.

          c. In significant disease, oral immunosuppressive agents are required.

Clinical Alert

Ocular damage occurs most frequently due to the chronic nature of the disease. Clinicians must take an active role in prevention of sequelae and treatment of secondary infection to prevent visual loss.

    C. *Erythema multiforme*

       1. Idiopathic inflammatory disease characterized by cutaneous lesions of varying severity. The extreme form of the disease is Stevens-Johnson syndrome, a systemic process that affects the entire body.

       2. Symptoms

          a. Primary ocular symptoms involve the conjunctiva (redness, swelling, hemorrhage, etc.).

          b. As disease progresses, corneal involvement ensues with decreased vision and discomfort.

       3. Ocular/systemic signs

          a. Ocular signs include conjunctival disease (conjunctivitis, chemosis, hemorrhage) as well as corneal disease (neovascularization, cicatrization, and infiltration).

          b. In advanced disease, inflammation is dramatic with uveitis which can progress to endophthalmitis, and panophthalmitis.

      c.   Flulike symptoms are typical of systemic manifestations: malaise, fever, arthralgia, and skin lesions are typical.

    4. Etiology. Idiopathic immune-mediated disease. The primary expression in this entity is cutaneous.

    5. Diagnostic evaluation. The clinical examination findings are the most important component in the diagnosis, since laboratory testing is not particularly productive.

    6. Treatment

      a.   Because of the possibility of an idiosyncratic reaction to certain pharmaceuticals, identification of the causative agent is crucial.

      b.   Palliative therapy is used for managing anterior segment complications. Bandage contact lenses are helpful.

      c.   Oral antibiotics and steroids are used in extreme cases as surgery for cicatricial changes in the adnexa.

Clinical Alert

Practitioners must monitor ocular status frequently to ensure control of secondary infections and ocular surface disturbances. Aggressive intervention is indicated to limit sequelae.

  D. *Acne rosacea*

    1. Dermatologic condition which primarily involves the facial area and is related to acneform lesions associated with telangectasia and erythema. Ocular involvement occurs in more than half the patients with the disease.

    2. Symptoms

      a.   Dry eye, recurrent red eye, irritation, and, in late stages, decreased visual acuity, and photophobia.

      b.   Occasionally the patient will complain of skin lesions in association with the disease.

    3. Ocular/systemic signs

      a.   Acneform lesions, telangectasias, and comedones are the cutaneous involvement most commonly noted.

      b.   Ocular involvement includes blepharitis, conjunctivitis, infiltration, neovascularization, and opacification.

    4. Etiology. Adult onset skin disease which is related to *Staphylococcus aureus* colonization and metabolism of sebaceous glands.

    5. Diagnostic evaluation

      a.   The physical examination is critical in the diagnosis because of the classic presentation of the disease.

      b.   Vital dyes and culture and sensitivity technique are useful but not definitive.

    6. Treatment

      a.   Oral tetracycline or erythromycin 250 mg qid for a minimum of 2 weeks is the treatment most commonly used in the acute phase. It can be continued on a daily basis for several weeks.

      b.   Topical therapy involves lid hygiene, steroids, antibiotics, metronidazole (Metrogel), and dry eye management.

      c.   A dermatologic consult is indicated if long-term therapy is anticipated.

Clinical Alert

Although severe corneal involvement is not common, practitioners should carefully monitor ocular status with regular eye health examinations.

VIII. **Vascular Diseases**

    A. Disease characterized by increasing rigidity and thickening of the arterial wall of vessels of variable size. It is classified into three distinct groups.

    B. Hypertension

       1. An elevation of blood pressure which is initiated by the process of peripheral vascular resistance and progresses to target organ damage if left untreated.

       2. Symptoms. Symptoms are dependent on level of disease. Early changes include breathlessness, tinnitus, dizziness, lightheadedness, and headache.

       3. Ocular/systemic signs

          a. Arteriolar attenuation, hemorrhages, NFLI, exudative maculopathy, and optic nerve head edema.

          b. Branch retinal vein occlusion and central retinal vein occlusion are both seen in significant hypertensive disease.

       4. Etiology. The primary mechanism is peripheral vascular resistance which increases central pressure and damage to heart and vascular organs. There is a reasonable genetic factor involved in acquisition.

       5. Diagnostic evaluation. Blood pressure measurement accomplished serially is the most effective means to identify hypertension. Since readings can be influenced by a variety of exogenous factors, multiple readings are helpful.

       6. Treatment

          a. Primary treatment involves dietary restrictions (salt, alcohol, etc.) as well as weight loss and exercise.

          b. Secondary and tertiary level care utilizes pharmaceuticals (diuretics, β-blockers, calcium channel blockers, ACE inhibitors) to control pressure.

          c. Comanagement should be instituted and dilated fundus evaluation should be accomplished regularly to maintain retinal status.

Clinical Alert

Minimal relationship between retinal findings and blood pressure in essential hypertension. Malignant hypertension is likely if significant retinal findings are observed. Optometric exam of the hypertensive patient should include blood pressure measurement and communication with the primary care physician regarding findings.

    C. Carotid artery disease

       1. Alteration of blood flow, either by embolization or reduction in diameter, to produce symptomatic effect on end organ function. Commonly seen as ocular or cerebral symptomatology that involves neural function.

       2. Symptoms. Patients have symptoms associated with cerebral hypoperfusion. These include transient vision loss, strokelike signs (tingling, numbness, paralysis, cognitive dysfunction, etc.) and can be transient (transient ischemic attack [TIA]) or completed (cerebrovascular accident [CVA]).

       3. Ocular/systemic signs

          a. The classic ocular manifestation of the disease is the Hollenhorst plaque.

          b. Retinal emboli can be fibroplatelet, cholesterol, or calcific, and produce branch retinal artery occlusion, central retinal artery occlusion, or no apparent obstruction of flow.

          c. Can see emboli in patients with heart valve disease.

       4. Etiology. Deposition of blood elements (cholesterol) in vessel produces turbulence of flow and allows formation of thrombi. Breakup of this material with movement to smaller arterial system can produce typical signs and symptoms.

       5. Diagnostic evaluation

a. Complex vascular analysis is required to diagnose and manage the condition. Carotid analysis with Doppler scanning, ausculation, digital subtraction angiography (DSA), and ocular pneumoplethysmography is required.

b. Visual field testing can be useful in identifying cerebral involvement and can be a useful indicator for the use of CT or MRI.

c. Traditional arterial angiography has been associated with morbidity and mortality and should be used only when indicated.

6. Treatment
   a. Symptomatic patients should be referred to a vascular surgeon.
   b. Surgical correction is accomplished by endarterectomy.

APPENDIX 1

Ocular Involvement in Selected Systemic Diseases

	Conjunctiva	Cornea	Sclera	Anterior Chamber	Lens	Intraocular Pressure	Vitreous	Retina	Choroid	Optic Nerve Head
Brucellosis	+	+	+	+	+ late	+ late	−	+	−	+
Metastatic bacterial inection	+	+	+	+	−	+/−	+	+	+	+
Leprosy	−	+	−	+	−	+/−	−	−	−	−
Tuberculosis	+	+	+	+	−	+/−	+	+	+	+
TRIC infection	+	+	+	+/−	−	−	−	−	−	−
Lyme disease	+	+	+	+	−	−	+	+	+	+
Syphilis	+	+	+	+	−	+/−	+	+	+	+
Leptospirosis	+	+	+	+	−	−	+	+	+	+
HIV infection	+	−	−	+	−	+/−	+	+	+	+
Cytomegalovirus	−	−	−	+	−	+/−	+	+	+	+
Epstein-Barr virus	+	+	+	+	−	−	−	+	+	+
Herpes simplex	+	+	+	+	−	+/−	−	−	−	−
Herpes zoster	+	+	+	+	−	+	−	−	−	+

(continued)

Appendix 1 (*Continued*)

	Conjunctiva	Cornea	Sclera	Anterior Chamber	Lens	Intraocular Pressure	Vitreous	Retina	Choroid	Optic Nerve Head
Molluscum	+	+	−	−	−	−	−	−	−	−
EKC/PCF	+	+	+	−	−	−	−	−	−	−
Toxoplasmosis	−	−	+	+	−	+/−	+	+	+	+
Amebiasis	+	+	+	+	−	−	−	+	−	−
Malaria	+	−	−	−	−	−	−	+	+	+
Histoplasmosis	+	+	−	−	−	−	−	+	+	+
Hyperthyroid	+	+	−	−	+	−	−	−	−	+
Hypothyroid	+	+	−	−	−	−	−	−	−	+
Diabetes	−	+	−	−	+	−	−	+	+	+
Polyarteritis	+	+	+	+	+	−	−	+	+	+
Polymyositis	+	−	−	−	−	−	−	+	−	−
Systemic lupus erythematosus	+	−	−	−	−	−	−	+	+	+
Scleroderma	+	+	−	−	−	−	−	+	−	+
Juvenile rheumatoid arthritis	+	+	+	+	+	+/−	−	+	−	+
Rheumatoid arthritis	+	+	+	+	+	+	−	−	−	−
Ankylosing spondylitis	+	+	+	+	−	−	−	−	−	−
Sturge-Weber syndrome	−	−	+	+	−	−	−	−	+	−
Neurofibromatosis	+	−	−	−	−	−	−	+	+	+
Tuberous sclerosis	−	−	−	−	−	−	−	+	+	+
Von Hippel-Lindau disease	−	−	−	−	−	−	−	+	+	+
Anemia	+	−	−	−	−	−	−	+	+	+
Leukemia	+	+	+	+	−	−	+	+	+	+
Platelet disorder	+	−	−	+	−	−	+	+	+	+
Sickle cell	+	−	−	−	−	−	+	+	+	+
Polycythemia	+	−	−	−	−	−	+	+	+	+
Crohn's disease	−	+	+	+	−	−	+	−	−	+
Sarcoidosis	+	+	+	+	−	+/−	+	+	+	+
Behçet's disease	−	−	+	+	−	+	+	+	+	+
Vogt-Koyanagi-Harada syndrome	+	−	+	+	−	−	+	+	+	+
Pemphigoid	+	+	+	−	+/−	+/−	−	−	−	−
Erythema multiforme	+	+	+	+	+	−	−	−	−	−
Rosacea	+	+	+	+/−	−	−	−	−	−	−
Arteriosclerosis	−	−	−	−	−	−	−	+	−	+
Hypertension	−	−	−	−	−	−	−	+	−	+
Carotid disease	−	−	−	−	−	−	−	+	−	+

Kevin L. Alexander. *The Lippincott Manual of Primary Eye Care*. Copyright © 1995 by J.B. Lippincott Company.

CHAPTER **7**

Clinical Refraction

Michael Polasky

I. **Examination**

A. *Incidence of ametropia*
1. Myopia: 10% to 15% of adults $\geq$ -1.00 D. Majority are less than -1.50 D. Incidence of -0.25 D or more of myopia in children age 6 very low (1%–2%) but climbs to 25%–35% by age 14.
2. Hyperopia: 10% to 20% of young adults $\geq$ $+1.00$. Majority are less than $+1.50$ but incidence of hyperopia increases steadily and significantly above age 40. Incidence of $+0.50$ D or more of hyperopia in children age 6 very high, 70%–90%.
3. In addition to age, variables affecting the incidence of refractive error include, but are not limited to, heredity, culture, race, and environment.

B. *Principles of optical correction*
1. Refractive error: Refractive error is expressed in terms of the characteristics of the lens required to correct the optics of the eye such that an image at infinity will be in focus on the retina with the accommodation of the eye in a relaxed state.
    a. Emmetropia: The convex surfaces of the optical elements of the eye focus light from a distant object on the retina.
    b. Myopia: Distant objects form a focus in front of the retina, and a correcting lens with minus power is required to diverge incoming light and push the focus back to the retina.
    c. Hyperopia: Distant objects form a focus behind the retina, and a correcting lens with plus power is required to converge incoming light and pull the focus up to the retina.
    d. Astigmatism: The amount of correction required varies with different meridians, and requires a lens with different powers in different meridians.
    e. The powers of the lenses used to correct myopia, hyperopia, and astigmatism may be expressed using an optical cross (power diagram) or in a prescription using sphero-cylinder form. The sphero-cylinder prescription may be written in plus or minus cylinder form as discussed in Chapter 8.
2. Lens characteristics
    a. Effectivity
        (1) The closer a correcting lens is placed to the eye, the more plus (less minus) power will be required to correct the eye.
        (2) Refracting the eye with lenses at a specific distance requires the final correcting lenses to be placed at the same distance.
        (3) Differences between refracting distance and fitting distance become significant with refractive errors over 4.00 D, and critical with errors over 10.00 D.

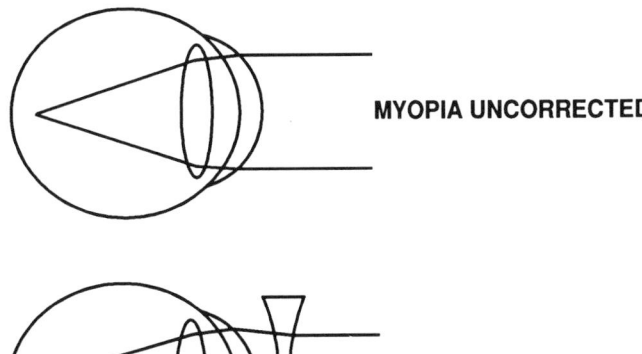

MYOPIA UNCORRECTED

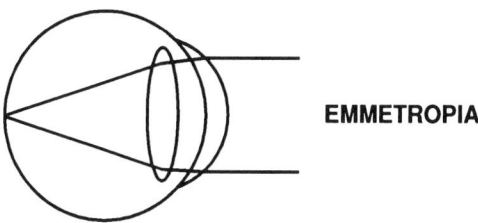

EMMETROPIA

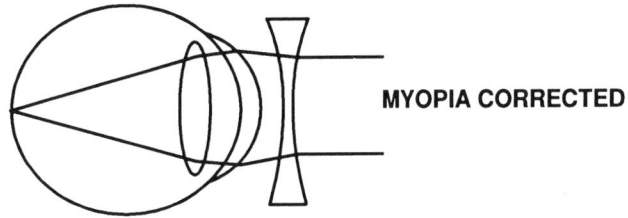

MYOPIA CORRECTED

Figure 7-1.   Emmetropia: No correction required when viewing a distant object.

Figure 7-2.   Myopia: Image forms in front of retina. Correction diverges light to form focus of distant object on retina.

     (4)   A common clinical error is to refract a patient at a distance which is longer than the distance at which the spectacle lenses will be fit. This will result in insufficient plus power being prescribed for the hyperope and too much minus power being prescribed for the myope.

     (5)   Because of effectivity, the clinician may find it necessary to confirm prescriptions of significant power using trial lenses placed in the proper spectacle plane.

  b. Prism

     (1)   Prism will be used as part of refractive testing and, on occasion, as part of the optical correction.

     (2)   Although light is refracted towards the base of a prism, it is more useful to remember that the image of an object viewed through a prism is displaced in the direction of the apex of the prism.

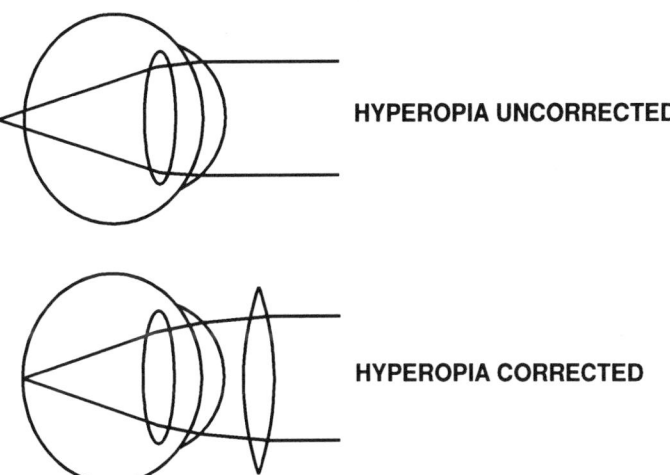

HYPEROPIA UNCORRECTED

HYPEROPIA CORRECTED

Figure 7-3.   Hyperopia: With accommodation at rest, image forms behind retina. Correction converges light to form focus of distant object on retina.

          (3)   Prism moves the image seen by the eye, not the eye. The eye may or may not move in the direction of the image.

          (4)   Prism is generated when viewing off the optical center of an ophthalmic lens. This may be used effectively when prescribing corrective lenses, but it may also affect certain aspects of refractive testing and must be carefully controlled.

      c.   Tilt-cylinder

          (1)   If an observer views an object through the optical center of a lens, but the lens is tilted such that the observer's eye is not on the optic axis of the lens, unwanted cylinder will be produced.

          (2)   The amount of unwanted cylinder caused by tilting an ophthalmic lens increases with the power of the lens and the amount of the tilt.

          (3)   Unwanted cylinder caused by lens tilt may cause errors in refraction, and if spectacle lenses are improperly fit, unwanted cylinder may contaminate an otherwise accurate prescription.

      d.   Combining cylinders

          (1)   When a cylinder lens is used to correct a cylinder error, the two cylinders must have the same axis.

          (2)   If the correcting cylinder is of the correct power but does not have the correct axis, a resultant cylinder will be created which has an axis approximately 45° away from the axis of the correcting cylinder.

          (3)   This optical effect will be applied to both objective and subjective techniques used to determine the refractive error.

      e.   Image size

          (1)   Correcting a refractive error, especially astigmatism, will produce differences in retinal image size which can cause serious adaptation problems with an optical correction.

          (2)   Unequal refractive errors produced by refractive surgery, especially cataract extraction with intraocular lens implantation, can cause serious image size differences when the correction is made with spectacle lenses.

          (3)   Problems with image size differences due to astigmatism and surgery are virtually eliminated when corrected with contact lenses.

   3.   Pupil size

      a.   Pupil size controls the amount of retinal blur produced by a given amount of uncorrected refractive error. A small amount of refractive error may produce significant blur if it is associated with a large pupil. Likewise, large refractive errors may produce only small amounts of blur when associated with small pupils.

      b.   During the course of the examination, the clinician may generate different refractive errors as part of testing and may alter pupil size as well. The resulting optical affects must be anticipated.

  C.   *History and symptoms of ametropia*

   1.   Myopia

      a.   The age of onset of simple, benign myopia is usually during the peak growth years, ages 7 to 14 years.

      b.   Subjective complaints almost always include problems seeing distant objects. Complaints are often associated with specific tasks such as difficulty seeing the chalkboard at school, the screen in a movie theater, or TV screen at home, or seeing the ball while playing baseball or tennis.

      c.   The onset of myopia is usually slow, which may leave the patient unaware that his or her vision is worse than that of other people.

      d.   A sign of myopia often observed by teachers, parents, or friends of the patient is "squinting" of the eyelids when attempting to view distant objects. These observations often lead to a referral or recommendations for an eye examination whether or not the patient has observed a reduction in distance vision.

  e. Occasionally the repeated effort of trying to narrow the palpebral aperture (squint) will lead to headache or other symptoms of asthenopia.

  f. Avoid diagnosing the amount of myopia from the subjective complaint of the amount of blur. Some patients will report only a slight level of blur and have a significant uncorrected refractive error, while others will report huge amounts of blur and require only a small correction.

  g. Patients who are already myopic will usually tolerate less blur than they did before their first pair of glasses. Once the effect of wearing glasses has been experienced by the patient, they will often return with symptoms of distance blur which require only a -0.25 or -0.50 D sphere to correct.

  h. The onset of myopia at an early age (birth through age 6) or the continuation of increases in myopia after age 25 may indicate the presence of a degenerative or pathological myopia.

2. Hyperopia

  a. Hyperopia of less than 2.00 D is commonly found in young children and tends to decrease in amount through the growth years.

  b. Hyperopia above 5.00 D will probably not decrease through the growth years and may show some increase with age.

  c. Since simple hyperopia can be overcome using accommodation, a large percentage of hyperopic patients will not complain of blurred vision.

  d. Symptoms of hyperopia usually include some form of asthenopia or headache, often associated with near work. The symptoms may be driven by excessive use of accommodation, an accommodative eso deviation, or a combination of both.

  e. More subtle symptoms may include a lack of interest in reading or performing near work. In young patients, this may lead to poor performance in school and weak study habits.

  f. Without symptoms of blurred vision, the acceptance of a correction for hyperopia is often poor.

  g. Since the hyperopic patient often uses accommodation to correct the refractive error, symptoms increase in frequency and severity as presbyopia approaches.

  h. If symptoms suggest the possibility of uncorrected hyperopia but none is found using a manifest refraction, a cycloplegic refraction may be useful in revealing any "latent" hyperopia. Special care is often necessary to effectively prescribe for latent hyperopia.

3. Astigmatism

  a. Since astigmatism is associated with either myopia or hyperopia, the symptoms associated with this refractive condition often add to the symptoms associated with the other refractive error.

  b. Symptoms of uncorrected astigmatism may include blur, headache, and asthenopia. Headaches and asthenopia may be due to efforts on the part of the accommodative system to achieve an accurate focus.

  c. Since uncorrected astigmatism tends to blur an image in only one meridian, patients can often perform quite well with significant amounts of uncorrected astigmatism.

  d. Symptoms of blur are more common when the axis of the uncorrected astigmatism is oblique.

  e. If the uncorrected astigmatism is with-the-rule (axis 180), the patient may narrow the palpebral aperture (squint) to improve vision.

4. Presbyopia

  a. The loss of accommodation results in a variety of symptoms depending on whether there is any other uncorrected refractive error present at the same time. The onset of symptoms commonly occurs around the age of 40.

  b. Inability to see objects clearly at near is the most common symptom of presbyopia. Patients may complain they must hold reading material too far away to see clearly.

      c.   Less obvious symptoms include the need for high levels of illumination in order to be able to read. Fatigue while reading and feeling sleepy while reading may also be symptoms of presbyopia.

      d.   If there is any uncorrected hyperopia present, it will often bring on symptoms several years earlier.

      e.   Because of effectivity, myopia corrected with spectacles will delay the onset of presbyopia. Symptoms may be delayed to age 44 to 45 years.

      f.   A patient who has uncorrected myopia in one eye only may never complain of symptoms of presbyopia, since one eye is used to see clearly at distance and the myopic eye is used to see clearly at near.

5. Anisometropia

      a.   Uncorrected anisometropia rarely results in symptoms of blur, but complaints of headache, asthenopia, and lack of depth perception are fairly common.

      b.   Small amounts of uncorrected anisometropia often produce more symptoms than do large amounts. When the uncorrected anisometropia is greater than 1.00 D, the patient is more likely to choose one eye to view with and suppress the other eye.

      c.   Since suppression often accompanies uncorrected anisometropia, amblyopia is a distinct possibility.

      d.   Amblyopia is more likely with uncorrected anisometropic hyperopia than with anisometropic myopia. In the case of uncorrected anisometropic hyperopia, one eye always requires more accommodation than the other eye to see clearly. The eye requiring less accommodation to see clearly will be the preferred eye, while the other eye may be suppressed, leading to functional amblyopia.

      e.   In certain cases, the correction of anisometropia will lead to symptoms of headache, asthenopia, and visual distortions. This is commonly due to unwanted induced prism generated when patients view objects through the peripheral portion of their spectacle lenses. In certain cases, aniseikonia may be produced by the correction of anisometropia. This is most common when the anisometropia is corrected with spectacle lenses and there is an unequal amount of astigmatism present in each eye, or equal amounts of astigmatism at unequal, oblique axes.

D. *Visual acuity*

1. Visual acuities are part of almost every vision examination. They are typically taken early in the examination, often immediately after the case history.

2. Typical visual acuity testing is done using targets with high contrast and very fine detail. Less commonly, visual acuity may be tested under conditions of reduced contrast.

3. Many types of targets are used to measure visual acuity. Many times the patient is asked to identify a familiar shape (recognition acuity). The shape may be a number, letter, or drawing of a familiar object. Other targets require the patient to identify the position of a gap or other characteristic of the target. Since the patient does not need to identify the object, this type of acuity may be considered resolution acuity.

4. Many types of charts are available for testing visual acuity.

      a.   Projected visual acuity charts are often used to test distance acuity. Slides are available which test recognition acuity using letters, numbers, and simple drawings of common objects. Slides are available to test resolution acuity using tumbling "E" and Landolt "C" characters.

      b.   For calibration purposes, it is useful to remember that a 20/200 character is approximately 88 mm high (top to bottom) when projected at 20 feet. Adjustments in image size follow a linear relationship. If the chart is to be viewed at 10 feet, the projected image must be adjusted such that the image of a 20/200 character is only 44 mm high.

      c.   Wall charts are also available for testing visual acuity. They do not have the

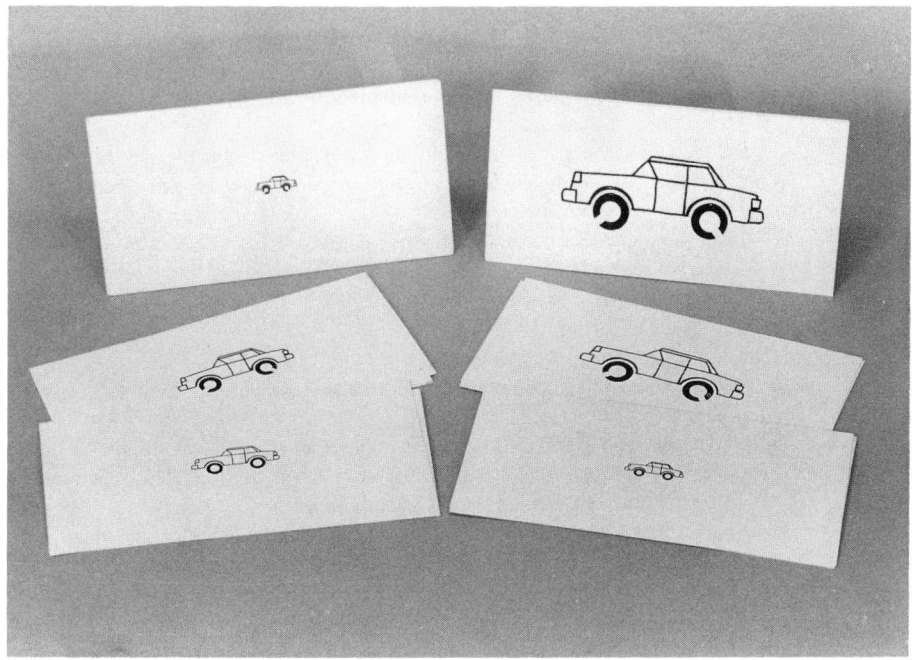

Figure 7-4.   "Broken Wheel" cards for testing visual acuity.

flexibility of the projection systems for testing distance visual acuity. They are, however, much less expensive.

    d.   Near point acuity is commonly tested with a printed card. Cards are available with the same types of characters (optotypes) that are used for testing distance acuity. In addition, some unique cards such as the "broken wheel" cards are available for testing acuity in young children.

5. Testing

    a.   Typical visual acuity testing begins by testing under monocular conditions at distance. An occluder is held over one eye, either by the patient or by the clinician.

    b.   Have the patient begin with larger characters and work towards the smaller ones.

    c.   If acuity is to be measured without correction, measure the unaided acuity before measuring acuity with correction.

    d.   Record as the visual acuity the row in which the patient reads half or more of the characters. (NOTE: Some standards require the patient to read more than half of the characters before receiving credit for the row.)

    e.   Encourage the patient to guess.

    f.   The most clinically significant visual acuity is often the corrected acuity at distance. If no correction is available and the clinician suspects a nonrefractive cause for reduced visual acuity, measuring the acuity through a pinhole may provide useful information, as an improvement in visual acuity suggests an uncorrected refractive error.

    g.   Avoid conditions that would reduce contrast or provide distracting glare.

    h.   Variations in testing are common. If the patient cannot read the largest letters on the distance chart, move the patient closer to the chart. Record the test distance over the smallest letter the patient can read. For example, 10/400 would indicate the patient could read the 400 acuity letter at 10 feet. Some clinicians prefer to convert the 10/400 fraction to an equivalent 20-foot distance or 20/800.

    i. Isolating a line of letters or other test characters may help to simplify the test and minimize confusion. Isolating letters, however, may provide acuities which are better than expected with patients who are amblyopic. For this reason, full line acuities should be taken whenever amblyopia is a possibility.

    j. Recording: Visual acuity is often recorded as a Snellen fraction where the numerator is the test distance and the denominator is the distance at which the smallest letter read subtends an overall angle of 5′ of arc or the detail within the character subtends 1′ of arc. An acuity of 20/200 indicates the patient was 20 feet from the chart and the smallest character the patient was able to read subtends an angle of 5′ when viewed at a distance of 200 feet. Obviously when the character is viewed at 20 feet it subtends an much larger angle, specifically 50′ of arc.

6. Consider all aspects of the patient when testing acuity.

    a. Acuities should always be taken prior to installation of drops or manipulation of the eye.

    b. Young patients fear punishment if they make an error and are often unwilling to guess. Acuities taken at the end of the exam when the child is more comfortable with the clinician and the setting often produce better results.

    c. Large pupils, natural or drug induced, result in more blur and thus poorer acuities with the same amount of uncorrected refractive error.

    d. Patients who oppose having one eye covered are likely to have very poor acuity in the other eye.

    e. Patients who need good acuity for acceptance into specific programs or licensure to perform certain activities may attempt to "cheat" on the test. Watch for narrowing of the palpebral aperture ("squinting"), looking past the edge of the occluder, and any indication the chart has been memorized.

    f. Patient may malinger during visual acuity testing, resulting in much worse acuity than expected. Usually a goal of financial reward is being sought, often from an insurance company or other third party.

    g. Visual acuity improves through infancy to about age 5 or 6 where it remains fairly constant until the mid to late 40s when a slight reduction in best corrected acuity may begin. It should be noted that many patients maintain good visual acuity well into their 60s and beyond.

7. Variables and expected values

    a. If testing conditions are kept similar, visual acuity varies little from day to day.

    b. Poor quality charts and distracting test conditions such as glare may reduce acuity by a line or two.

    c. Uncorrected myopia of −1.00 D should reduce distance visual acuity to approximately 20/50, −2.00 should result in 20/150, and −3.50 should give 20/300.

    d. Uncorrected hyperopia in patients with adequate accommodation often produces little reduction in acuity through 3 D of uncorrected refractive error, since the patient can correct the hyperopia with his or her accommodation.

    e. Uncorrected astigmatism tends to produce about half the reduction in acuity when compared to an equal amount of uncorrected simple myopia. This is a very general rule, since the acuity will vary with the type and axis of the astigmatism.

E. *Retinoscopy (static)*

1. The purpose of retinoscopy is to provide the clinician with an objective measure of the refractive error. In addition, retinoscopy provides information on the clarity of the media and the uniformity of the optical elements of the eye.

2. Instrumentation is fairly similar from manufacturer to manufacturer. Today's instruments are typically streak retinoscopes which incorporate controls for focus and rotation of the streak as well as illumination control of a halogen light source. Additional features may include polarizing filters and attachments to aid in performing near point retinoscopy.

3. The focus system of the retinoscope has a wide range of adjustment, permitting the

clinician to image the lamp of the retinoscope in front of the clinician (real image) or behind the clinician (virtual image). When this convergent or divergent light beam from the retinoscope is directed into a patient's eye, the image of the lamp becomes the object for the image formed on the patient's retina. For the following discussion, it is assumed the light coming from the retinoscope is made of parallel or slightly divergent rays.

4. When the light from the retinoscope is moved across the patient's pupil, the clinician is moving the location of the source of the light, and therefore the light coming out of the pupil appears to change its position. Interpretation of this movement of the light or "reflex" from the patient's eye allows the clinician to determine the patient's refractive error.

5. The movement of the retinoscopy "reflex" observed by the clinician is based on the location of the patient's far point relative to the position or "working distance" of the clinician.

6. To minimize errors due to changes in distance, the clinician should work as far away from the patient as practical. Limitations include the apparent size of the pupil and access by the clinician to various lenses or lens systems. Working distances of 66 or 50 cm are common.

7. If the clinician moves the light across the patient's pupil and the reflex moves in a direction opposite to the light from the retinoscope (against motion), the far point of the patient is located between the clinician and the patient. This would indicate myopia of a value greater than the working distance. If the clinician is working at 66 cm, the myopia present would be greater than 1.50 D.

8. If the clinician moves the light across the patient's pupil and the reflex moves in the same direction as the light from the retinoscope ("with motion"), the far point of the patient may be located behind the clinician. This would indicate myopia of a value less than the working distance. If the working distance is 66 cm, the myopia would be less than 1.50 D. With motion is also produced if the patient's far point is at infinity (emmetropia), or if the patient's far point is behind the patient. In this case, the light is diverging as it comes from the patient's eye, which defines the condition of hyperopia.

9. If the far point of the patient falls exactly at the clinician's eye, no motion or neutrality is observed. The reflex is bright and appears to flash on and off as the streak is moved across the pupil. With a working distance of 66 cm, the patient's refractive error would be exactly 1.50 D.

10. When the amount of uncorrected refractive error is great, the reflex will appear narrow and dim and will move only slightly with the movement of the streak from the retinoscope. As the refractive error is reduced, the retinoscopy reflex becomes brighter and wider and moves more quickly.

11. The clinical procedure for performing static retinoscopy uses lenses to move the patient's far point from its initial uncorrected position to a position which is exactly at the clinician's eye (neutrality). Since the position of the clinician is known, it is then possible to change the power of the lens in front of the patient's eye to move the patient's far point from the clinician's position out to infinity. This lens power should provide the patient with the proper optical correction for distance vision.

12. Spherical refractive errors
    a. If "against motion" is observed at the start of retinoscopy, use minus lenses to achieve neutrality. Once neutrality is achieved, add additional minus power to move the far point from the position of the examiner out to infinity. If a 66-cm working distance was used, an additional -1.50 D of power must be added to the power that produced neutrality. For example, if -2.25 D was required to achieve neutrality, the final prescription is -1.50 D more or -3.75 D.
    b. If with motion is observed at the start of retinoscopy, use plus lenses to achieve neutrality. Once neutrality is achieved, again add minus power to move the far point from the position of the examiner out to infinity. For example, if $+2.25$ D was required to achieve neutrality, the final prescription adds -1.50 for a 66-cm working distance for a final prescription of $+0.75$ D.

13. Spherocylinder corrections; minus cylinder refractor
   a. Assume all patients have a spherocylinder refractive error. Begin by moving the streak through different meridians and look for a difference in the reflex. When significant cylinder is present, the reflex will rotate away from the streak of the retinoscope towards a principal meridian. Rotate the streak from the retinoscope to match the position of the reflex. (If no difference in the reflex is seen, move the streak through the horizontal meridian and use spherical lenses to neutralize the reflex. Now add an additional −1.00 D of minus sphere and proceed as describe in I.C.13.c below.)
   b. Rotate the streak 90° and observe the reflex in the other principal meridian. If against motion is observed in both meridians, choose the meridian with the brighter, wider, faster reflex. Add sphere power to neutralize this meridian and then add an additional −1.00 D of minus power to produce an easy-to-see with motion. If with motion is observed in both meridians, choose the meridian with the narrower, slower, dimmer reflex and proceed as before. If the reflex in one meridian shows with motion and the other against motion, choose the with motion meridian to neutralize first. Remember to add an additional −1.00 D of minus power to refine the position for the cylinder correction. This additional power will be removed later.
   c. With the additional −1.00 in place, rotate the axis of the streak back and forth to identify the position where the reflex and the streak are perfectly matched and the reflex is as narrow as possible while showing with motion. The axis for the correcting minus cylinder is now placed 90° away from this position. Before adding any minus cylinder power, reduce the minus sphere power such that the meridian that was showing with motion now shows neutrality. The other principal meridian should now show against motion. Move the streak through the meridian showing against motion and add minus cylinder power until the against motion is neutralized.
   d. Rotate the streak once more to see that all meridians show neutrality.
   e. Add sufficient minus sphere power to compensate for the working distance (i.e., remove the working lens) and record the final combination of sphere and cylinder as the optical correction.
   f. To improve the sharpness of the reflex, try changing the focus of the streak. This is known as enhancing. Enhancing improves the appearance of the reflex by making the difference between the bright and dark areas of the reflex more obvious. If with motion is present, try adjusting the focus from a fully divergent beam to a slightly convergent beam. Do not focus the streak at the patient's eye, since this will eliminate the motion of the reflex. If against motion is observed adjust the focus to a convergent beam which focuses at a point between the patient and the clinician. This will produce a more clearly defined reflex and convert the against motion into a pseudo with motion.

F. *Subjective methods of refraction (dry)*
   1. General concepts
      a. Use questions and answers to adjust sphere and cylinder values.
      b. Test using distance targets with accommodation at rest.
      c. Adjust prescription for each eye so that both eyes will be in focus at the same time on any target at any distance.
      d. The distance sphere correction, whether monocular or binocular, should be the most plus (least minus) lens which grants the patient the best visual acuity.
      e. Begin with the monocular subjective.
   2. Sphere correction: monocular
      a. Begin with estimate of refractive correction such as the retinoscopy finding, the previous Rx, lensometer results, or automated refractor results.
      b. Patient views a letter chart with letters close to the patient's visual acuity threshold.

    c.   Add sphere in a plus direction to "fog" patient and place accommodation at rest.

    d.   Reduce plus sphere until there is no improvement in performance.

    e.   Do not make additional changes of lenses in a minus direction if the letter chart "looks the same" or the letters just look "darker."

3.   Cylinder correction: Jackson cross cylinder test—monocular procedures for minus cylinder refractor

    a.   Place Jackson cross cylinder device in place to check cylinder axis and power.

    b.   If axis tested first, test cylinder power second, then retest cylinder axis. If cylinder power is tested first, test axis second, then retest cylinder power.

    c.   Use a letter chart with letters two to three lines larger than the patient's best acuity. 20/25, 20/30, and 20/40 are common letter sizes.

    d.   To test cylinder axis, set cross cylinder device with the dots marking the principal meridians of the cross cylinder device straddling cylinder axis in refractor.

    e.   Flip the cross cylinder device and ask the patient which of the two choices appears clearer; which choice allows the patient to read more letters.

    f.   Leave the cross cylinder device in the preferred position and turn the cylinder axis in the refractor towards the meridian marked by the red dots on the cross cylinder device. Turn the axis in the refractor only a small amount, no more than 10° or 15°.

    g.   Continue to present paired choices to the patient making smaller changes, 2° or 3°, as the axis is refined, especially when the cylinder power is high.

    h.   Leave the correcting cylinder axis in the position where the patient reports the two choices to be equally clear (equally blurred).

    i.   To test cylinder power, align the axis markings of the cross cylinder lens with the axis of the correcting cylinder in the refractor.

    j.   Flip the cross cylinder lens in the same manner as with axis.

    k.   In the case of a minus cylinder refractor, increase the power of the refractor cylinder if the patient prefers the cross cylinder with red dots aligned with refractor axis. Decrease power if white dots are preferred.

    l.   Stop when patient reports both choices equally blurred.

    m.   If in between two cylinder powers, one too weak, one too strong, use weaker cylinder power as correction.

4.   Repeat test for sphere using small letters. Measure and record visual acuity along with monocular subjective results.

5.   Additional cylinder testing: clock dial—monocular

    a.   Project clock dial pattern.

    b.   Begin with retinoscopy finding (or other approximate Rx) and remove cylinder correction.

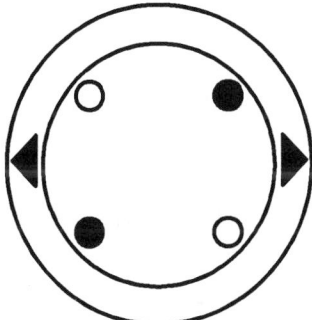

Figure 7-5. Cross cylinder device positioned to test cylinder axis.

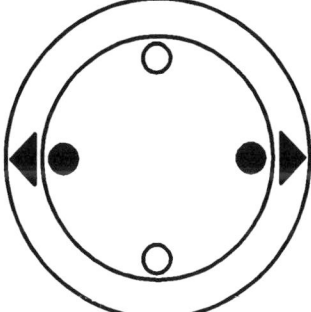

Figure 7-6. Cross cylinder device positioned to test cylinder power.

    c.   Add plus sphere fog until all lines are blurred. OK if some lines are better than others, but best lines must be blurred. Alternate method for determining plus blur: blur until 20/40 letters just readable.

    d.   Reduce plus sphere until one set of lines is clear. If all lines are clear at the same time, no cylinder needed.

    e.   If one set of lines begins to clear first, but as plus power is reduced another set of lines becomes clearer, may have reduced plus sphere too much. Confirm that clearest set of lines is slightly blurred.

    f.   Identify clearest and next clearest set of lines by clock face numbers. Example: 1:00 to 7:00 o'clock.

    g.   Correcting cylinder axis = smallest number on clearest line × 30°. Example: 1:00 to 7:00 o'clock clearest. Set axis at 30°. If 1:00 to 7:00 o'clock and 2:00 to 8:00 o'clock are equally clear, set axis at 45°. If 1:00 to 7:00 o'clock is clearest and 2:00 to 8:00 o'clock is *next* clearest, set axis at 37°.

    h.   Set cylinder axis in refractor and add cylinder power. Patient to watch *only* lines which started as clearest and lines 90° away which are the most blurred.

    i.   Stop adding power when blurred lines are as clear as original clear set. Example: 1:00 to 7:00 o'clock is clearest at start. Patient instructed to watch blurred lines at 4:00 to 10:00 o'clock as clinician adds cylinder power axis 30°. Stop adding cylinder power when lines at 4:00 to 10:00 o'clock are as clear as lines at 1:00 to 7:00 o'clock. *If patient now reports a new set of lines as clearest, axis will need to be adjusted slightly.* See next step.

    j.   Refine cylinder axis by asking patient to compare clarity of lines either side of original clearest set. To help patient make judgment, blur chart slightly with plus sphere, and reduce plus sphere while patient watches to see which lines clear first.

    k.   Turn correcting cylinder axis *slightly* toward axis indicated by clearer lines. Example: Lines at 1:00 to 7:00 o'clock were clearest at start. After adding cylinder power axis 30°, the patient is instructed to look at the 11:00 and 12:00 o'clock lines and compare them with the 2:00 and 3:00 o'clock lines, and to pick the clearest. The patient reports the 12:00 to 6:00 o'clock lines to be the clearest. The clinician should turn the correcting cylinder axis *slightly* toward the 60° axis, about 5° or 10°. With the new correcting cylinder axis of 35°, once again ask the patient to compare the lines either side of the original clearest set. When the lines either side appear equally clear, the axis is correct.

    l.   Recheck cylinder power by having patient compare original clearest set of lines with lines 90° away. If original set is clearest, add additional cylinder power. If lines 90° away are clearer, reduce cylinder power until the two sets are equally clear. If an exact match is impossible, go with lesser amount of cylinder power.

    m.   Repeat test for sphere using small letters. Measure and record visual acuity along with monocular subjective results.

6.   Additional sphere test: bichrome (may be done monocularly but more stable when done binocularly)

    a.   To refine final sphere value using bichrome technique, add a small amount of plus sphere fog, about +0.50.

    b.   Select chart, split chart if available, with some letters near patient's visual acuity threshold and add red/green filter overlay.

    c.   Turn out all room lights and darken room as much as possible.

    d.   Ask patient on which side of the chart are the letters clearer and blacker: red or green.

    e.   Red side should be clearer to start. If not, add plus until red is clearer.

    f.   Reduce plus until red = green or first green (clinician's discretion).

    g.   Record and compare with other sphere test data.

7.   Balancing: dissociated blur; works well when best visual acuity for each eye is the same

    a.   Set dissociating prism, 3 base up for one eye, 3 base down for the other (occlude one eye during the process).

    b.   Chart = group of lines (20/30, 20/25, 20/20) or one line, either 20/30 or 20/40.

    c. With both eyes open, add plus sphere blur to both eyes. Letters should be blurred but readable.

    d. Ask patient which chart is clearer, upper or lower.

    e. Add plus blur to better eye until charts are equally blurred. If no match is possible, leave with closest match.

    f. Reduce plus blur and have patient compare upper and lower charts with minimal blur using small letters (20/25, 20/30). Add additional plus sphere to better eye if necessary to equalize clarity. No more than 0.25 D change in balance is anticipated at this level.

    g. If dissociated blur balance is attempted with patient with unequal best corrected visual acuities, use letters 2 lines larger than best visual acuity for weaker eye and use more plus sphere blur. Do not reduce the plus blur to confirm the balance as described in I.F.7.f.

    h. Proceed to final binocular sphere check.

8. Balancing: Vectograph—good balance, fast, accurate; patient must be binocular with little or no suppression; best visual acuity may be reduced one line due to filters and reduced contrast of chart.

    a. Polarizing filters in front of patient's eyes; patient has both eyes open.

    b. Project Vectograph chart on "silver" screen.

    c. Top part of chart (slide) seen by right eye only; left eye sees empty boxes.

    d. Perform sphere and cross cylinder tests on right eye, directing patient to watch appropriate rows of letters on upper part of chart.

    e. Repeat sphere and cylinder tests for left eye using second portion of chart (slide). Left eye sees letters, right eye sees empty boxes.

    f. Confirm final sphere finding for each eye by adding (+) 0.25 DS to each eye, one eye at a time. Acuity should reduce. If not, sphere is over minused. Add additional (+) sphere until chart appears worse. Reduce (+) sphere 0.25 D and sphere should be correct. (Reduced contrast of chart through polarizing filters tends to cause clinician to over minus patient.)

    g. Demonstrate differences in right and left eye performance using split chart. Do *not* blur better eye to match weaker eye.

9. Balancing: alternate occlusion

    a. Begin with monocular subjective findings.

    b. Have patient view acuity chart with both eyes open.

    c. Alternately occlude right and left eyes while asking the patient which eye has the clearer image.

    d. Add plus to better eye to equalize the clarity of the two eyes.

    e. Repeat sphere check under binocular conditions.

10. After completing balance, perform final binocular sphere check.

    a. If visual acuities are good, add plus sphere to both eyes simultaneously until 20/20 letters are not readable binocularly.

    b. Reduce plus sphere until 20/20 just readable. Letters should not be clear.

    c. Continue reducing plus sphere until there is no further improvement in clarity of the acuity chart. Make no more than -0.75 DS change in power to accomplish this effect (-0.50 D change is common).

    d. If visual acuity less than 20/20 best corrected, add plus sphere to reduce acuity slightly. Add minus sphere until no further improvement in performance. Avoid adding minus lenses when patient says chart looks better but there is no change in visual acuity performance.

    e. This binocular sphere endpoint may be checked using the bichrome test.

G. *Drugs in refraction*

1. Mydriatics/cycloplegics: since mydriatic/cycloplegic agents are used on almost all patients, consider the following:

    a. If refraction is done under effect of drug, compare to nondrug results.

    b. Large pupil causes shallow depth of focus, possible shift in spherical refraction, possible shift in cylinder power (and possibly axis), possible reduced "best visual acuity" due to spherical aberrations, and photophobia.

    c. Loss of accommodation provides information on latent hyperopia and pseudomyopia but eliminates immediate near testing and may have subtle affects on near performance for more than 24 hours.

    d. Partial cycloplegia tends to increase the measured accommodation to convergence ratio (AC/A): increased effort required to see clearly results in excessive convergence.

2. If mydriatic/cycloplegic exam is planned, complete all tests related to accommodation and/or convergence first, or schedule additional visit for these tests.

3. Side effects of drug may affect patient behavior during exam. Atropine and cyclopentolate systemic effects may include restless and irritable behavior as well as other central nervous system (CNS) effects which may affect ability to subjectively test refraction, accommodation, muscle balance, etc.

4. Consider all side effects, ocular and systemic, before using drug. Consider impact on testing and patient's life style for duration of action of drug. Use minimum concentration to produce effect and use drug with minimum side effects; especially important with cycloplegia in children.

5. Counsel patient/parent on expected drug effects and their time course.

6. For most patients, 1 or 2 drops of 1% cyclopentolate 30 min prior to refraction yields satisfactory results.

7. For young or uncooperative children, or when suspecting latent hyperopia, 1% atropine solution is prescribed 2 or 3 times a day for 1 or 2 days prior to examination. NOTE: Atropine may cause fever in children and should be discontinued should the parent report symptoms.

H. *Ancillary refractive techniques: Pinhole/stenopaic slit*

1. Pinhole is universal sphere, stenopaic slit is universal cylinder.

2. Use for screening; is reduced acuity due to optical problem or a possible disease process?

3. If acuity will not improve with pinhole, it will not improve with a lens.

4. Acuity which improves with a pinhole may still not improve with a lens if the optics of the eye are irregular or distorted, such as with a distorted cornea or cataract.

5. 2 mm is effective; wider reduces effect; smaller reduces light level and generates diffraction from edge of aperture, which reduces effectiveness.

6. Use when other techniques are unsuccessful at improving visual acuity.

7. Use when monocular diplopia is present to confirm optical origin.

I. *Refracting difficult eyes*

1. High Rx, (+) and (−)

    a. Measure and control vertex distance during refraction. Common to refract at distance longer than fitting distance. Will refract too much minus or not enough plus if refraction is done at longer distance than fitting distance. Unless cylinder is very high, error will only be with sphere. Tell patient to keep face in contact with refractor.

    b. Rx must be fit well or power will be in error. If Rx correctly matches fitting distance but Rx slides down nose slightly (due to weight), myopic patient will be undercorrected and hyperopic patient (aphakia) will be overcorrected due to changes in lens effectivity.

    c. No pantoscopic tilt on phoropter, tilt generates unwanted cylinder. If final spectacle Rx is to have pantoscopic tilt, lower optical centers of spectacle Rx such that optical center line of lens passes through center of rotation of eye. Should have no unwanted cylinder.

    d. Use trial frame or patient's old Rx to confirm final sphere values. Most powerful lens should be in back lens cell of trial frame. Be sure all lens power labels are visible from front of frame.

 e. Problems of diplopia during binocular testing are usually due to induced prism. Be sure patient is centered behind lenses. Be sure PD is accurate.

2. Reduced visual acuity: distorted or cloudy media, retinal damage, amblyopia

 a. Use letters patient can see. Make large changes in sphere, cylinder power, and cylinder axis; large enough that patient can detect change in spite of reduced visual acuity.

 b. Room illumination may affect testing. Determine effects of bright room, dark room, stray light.

 c. Contrast sensitivity test may reveal correlation between patient's symptoms of poor performance in low contrast settings.

 d. If available, use flip cross cylinder lens of higher power, ± 0.50 D.

 e. Traditional refraction techniques may enhance ghost images (monocular diplopia) in cases of distorted media (cataract). Consider trial modification of both sphere and cylinder for best performance and patient acceptance.

 f. Isolation of acuity letters may be useful, but do not use when amblyopia is suspected. Will produce a false visual acuity relative to expected performance when reading or performing other "crowded" visual acuity tasks. Isolated line visual acuity is acceptable.

 g. In amblyopia, expect patient to read acuity letters out of sequence, read only the first and last letters of a row, report "Letters are clear but I cannot read them."

3. Geriatric examinations

 a. Special attention should be given to communication. Tests may seem confusing, annoying.

 b. Small pupils often reduce the blur associated with lens changes. Make larger changes in lens power; small lens changes may produce no effect.

 c. Sudden changes in refraction may indicate incipient cataract or systemic diseases such as diabetes. Large changes in Rx may prove to be unwearable, especially if change is monocular. Consider compromise Rx. Demonstrate using trial lenses.

J. *Measurement of accommodation*
Normal = 18.5 D. −0.3(age).
Minimum = 15 D. −0.25(age).

1. Donder's push up

 a. Present patient with a near point chart with small letters.

 b. Initial position should be within range of accommodation, and any refractive error, especially astigmatism, should be corrected.

 c. Use letters as small as patient can read. Chart will be brought toward the patient and letters will increase in angular size. 20/20 letter at 40 cm becomes 20/80 at 10 cm.

 d. Bring chart toward patient until patient reports blur. Measure distance of chart from patient's spectacle plane. Convert distance to diopters. Repeat test 3 times for each eye independently. If amplitude of accommodation decreases with repetition, there is fatigue of accommodation and vision therapy or a near add may be indicated.

 e. Repeat amplitude measurement under binocular condition. Problems with fusion may reduce the measured amplitude under binocular conditions.

 f. Test facility of accommodation by having patient switch focus from a distance target to a near target and back to distance. Each switch should take no more than a second. Reduced facility is best managed with vision therapy, although near adds are sometimes effective. To test facility, the distance refraction must be accurate and in place, and the near target must be within the range of accommodation. Facility of accommodation is not performed with a presbyopic patient.

    g.   To measure amplitude of accommodation with early presbyopia, place +2.00 sphere over distance refraction and have patient view near point letter chart at 40 cm. Bring near point chart toward patient until letters blur. Measure distance from spectacle plane and convert to diopters, subtract 2.00 D and record as amplitude. May be done monocularly or binocularly.

    h.   Rule for tentative add: allow patient to use half of accommodative ability, supply additional power necessary to clear near target in form of add. Example: Patient has amplitude of accommodation of 2.00 D and reading distance is 40 cm. Let patient use 1.00 D of accommodation; tentative add is +1.50 to achieve total of 2.50 D necessary for 40 cm near task.

2. Minus lens to blur

    a.   With letter chart at 40 cm and refractive error fully corrected, add minus lenses until chart blurs. To obtain amplitude of accommodation, add 2.50 D to power of minus add. Test is commonly done through refractor, but a lens bar will provide a rough estimate.

    b.   Unless amplitude of accommodation is reduced, the (−) add should not be used binocularly, since the amplitude of accommodation will usually not be reached due to limit of negative fusional vergence.

    c.   Binocular amplitude of accommodation may be measured using minus lens to blur when the amplitude of accommodation is reduced (especially presbyopia). With near point letter chart at 40 cm, add (+) sphere if necessary to clear near chart. Then, reduce (+) or add (−) until chart blurs. If value is more (+) than distance refraction, subtract this add from 2.50 D and record as amplitude of accommodation. If value is more (−) than distance refraction (nonpresbyope), add the value to 2.50 D. as in I.J.2.a above.

    d.   If patient is becoming presbyopic and first blur occurred as the initial (+) add was being reduced, a tentative add for presbyopia may be determined by adding +0.50 D sphere to value noted when first blur occurred. Record this value as an add relative to the distance refraction. Example: When presbyopic patient first views near point card at 40 cm with distance refraction, chart is blurred and clinician must add plus sphere to both eyes to clear chart. The clinician reduces the plus sphere add until the card blurs. The clinician notes there is still +1.00 D in the refractor over the distance refraction values. The tentative add for presbyopia is +1.00 (+) +0.50 or +1.50 add. Maximum add for 40 cm = +2.50. NOTE: with advancing presbyopia, there may be only one or two lenses that produce clear vision at near and the formula need not be used.

3. Accommodative response/lag of accommodation

    a.   Binocular near cross cylinder test

        (1)   Near cross cylinder target at 40 cm, patient has both eyes open with cross cylinder lenses placed minus cylinder axis 90° in front of both eyes. Illumination is moderate to dim.

        (2)   Begin with distance refraction (or monocular cross cylinder finding) and add plus sphere lenses equally to both eyes until vertical lines are darker than horizontal.

        (3)   Reduce plus sphere equally to both eyes. Stop when vertical and horizontal lines are equally clear or when horizontal lines are first clearer than vertical. Average add over distance refraction = +0.50 D.

        (4)   In nonpresbyopic patients, values over +0.50 may indicate the need for an add, especially with esophoria. Binocular cross cylinder finding is the power of the add to prescribe.

        (5)   In presbyopic patients, target will be blurred to start. Add plus sphere as above, and as target clears, patient will identify which set of lines is clearest.

        (6)   As before, reduce plus sphere until lines are equal or select the first lens which makes horizontal clearer than vertical. If more than one lens causes

horizontal and vertical to appear equal, use least plus lens. The amount of the binocular cross cylinder add is the tentative add for presbyopia.

    b. Dynamic retinoscopy (Nott technique): a measure of accommodative "posture" under normal reading conditions. While patient reads near point chart, clinician locates where the patient's eyes are actually focusing (neutrality) using a retinoscope and compares its location with location of target. Focus behind card = positive lag. Focus in front of card = negative lag. Normal lag is slightly behind the target or +0.50 D lag. Excessive lag may result in near symptoms and may be managed with vision therapy or lenses.

       (1) May be done through refractor or outside in normal space.

       (2) Illumination: as bright as practical. Clinician must be able to see retinoscopy reflex.

       (3) Nearpoint card at normal reading distance, often 40 cm. Distance refractive error corrected, with or without near adds.

       (4) Patient has both eyes open.

       (5) While patient reads near point card, clinician locates patient's far point by performing retinoscopy and moving closer and farther from the patient to locate neutrality. Commonly, neutrality point is slightly behind near point card.

       (6) Take difference between location of near point card and neutrality point in diopters, and record.
Example: Near point card is at 40 cm, clinician locates neutrality at 67 cm. 40 cm = 2.50 D and 67 cm = 1.50 D.
Difference = 1.00 D. Since neutrality point was behind card, difference is recorded as a positive lag or +1.00 D lag.

    c. Dynamic retinoscopy (monocular estimation method or MEM technique) While patient reads near point card, clinician measures difference in accommodative response from accommodative stimulus using trial lenses.

       (1) Done outside refractor in free space with distance refraction corrected, with or without adds.

       (2) Setup same as Nott dynamic.

       (3) Clinician keeps retinoscope in plane of near point card and does not move while patient reads near point card.

       (4) Trial lens placed in front of patient's eye, one eye at a time, while performing retinoscopy. Lens that produces neutrality is amount of lag. Lens must not be in front of patient's eyes for more than 2 or 3 seconds. Remove lens and replace for another 2 or 3 seconds if needed.

K. *Measurement of heterophorias, vergences (see Chapter 10, Binocular Vision Problems)*

    1. Cover test: identifies phoria (latent) or tropia (manifest) ocular deviations, and provides information on amount, direction, and type of deviation.

      a. Patient fixates small target at distance or near with both eyes open and good illumination on patient's eyes.

      b. Each eye must be capable of independent, steady fixation or test may not be possible.

      c. Clinician covers left eye while watching right. If right eye does not move when left eye is covered, right eye is fixating target.

      d. Clinician covers right eye while watching left. If left eye does not move when right eye is covered, left eye is fixating target and no strabismus (squint) is present. If one eye moves when the other is covered, the eye which moved is deviating and a strabismus is present. Clinician should cover and uncover same eye at least three times to be sure fusion is not easily broken down by cover—uncover exercise.

      e. Clinician should watch eyes carefully when testing of right eye is complete and testing of left eye is about to begin to be sure patient does not alternate fixation. If patient can alternate fixation, movement of one eye will be seen when the other eye is covered, but not when it is uncovered. Example: Right eye moves out when left eye is covered, but remains stationary when left eye is uncovered = alternating strabismus.

   f. Determine direction of deviation using alternate cover test. Watch one eye as the cover is alternated from right to left and back to right again. Watch one eye as it is uncovered for any motion. If it moved out to take up fixation, the deviation was eso. Movement in = exo, up = hypo, down = hyper. Top turns in = excyclo, top turns out = encyclo.

   g. To measure, place prism (loose prism or prism bar) in front of one eye and perform alternate cover test again. Base of prism in proper direction to move image in the direction of the deviation. Example: Base in prism measures exo deviation. Add enough prism to produce no motion. Gradually add too much prism to produce a reversal of motion. If more than one prism power produced no motion before reversal occurred, record the larger amount of prism as the correct amount and identify the deviation as latent.

   h. Record amount, direction (eso or exo), and type of deviation (tropia or phoria). If no deviation, record as orthophoria.

2. Von Graefe phoria test: designed to measure direction and amount of deviation but does not differentiate phoria from tropia. Suppression prevents test from being performed.

   a. Commonly done through refractor. May be done distance or near. Use a small fixation target. Small detail in target important for near testing. Occlude one eye or have patient close eyes during setup.

   b. 6 PD vertical "dissociating" prism in front of one eye. Risley prism in front of other eye, set to produce lateral prism.

   c. Remove occluder or have patient open eyes. Should report diplopia.

   d. Have patient watch target seen by eye with vertical prism. Example: If BU prism used, patient watches lower target.

   e. Patient asked to report if upper target is to the right or left of lower target. Use lateral prism (Risley) to move upper image directly over lower image. Bracket by bringing upper image from both left and right side. May flash upper target using cover paddle, covering and uncovering one eye to minimize residual fusion clues.

   f. Record amount and direction of lateral deviation. Base in (BI) prism = exo; base out (BO) = eso.

   g. Measure vertical using 10–15 PD BI dissociating prism. Risley prism in front of other eye, set to produce vertical prism.

   h. Patient watches image seen by eye with BI prism.

   i. If images not same height, level with each other, adjust vertical Risley prism to level images. Increase and decrease vertical prism power to bracket end point.

   j. If distance refraction over 1.00 D in vertical meridian, perform distance test through pinholes to minimize induced prism. Cannot use pinholes during near test, will loose accommodation and convergence.

   k. Record amount and direction of vertical deviation. BD = hyper, BU = hypo.

3. Maddox rod phoria test: Similar to Von Graefe. Gives information on direction and amount of ocular deviation.

   a. May be done through refractor using Maddox rod and Risley prism. May be done outside refractor using Maddox rod and loose or bar prism. It is recommended the refractive error be corrected.

   b. Test requires small point source of light; penlight works well.

   c. Lighting should be uniform; no other point sources of light in the field of view.

   d. To measure lateral deviation, ribs of Maddox rod should run back and forth. Ribs up and down to measure vertical.

   e. With the refractive error corrected and both eyes open, place Maddox rod device in front of one eye and turn on point source of light. Direct patient to keep both eyes open and look at the light.

f. Patient should report seeing light and line. Line will be vertical if measuring lateral deviation and horizontal if measuring vertical deviation.

g. If line appears to pass through light, no deviation is present (ortho). If light is off line, add prism to place light on line. BI prism = exo, BO = eso, BD = hyper, BU = hypo.

h. Example: With Maddox rod before patient's right eye to measure a lateral deviation, ribs back and forth, the patient reports seeing a vertical line and a light, with the light to the right of the line. 8 PD BI prism is placed over the Maddox rod to place the line on the light. 8 PD exo is recorded.

i. If test is done outside refractor, through refractive correction, the effect of induced lateral or vertical prism may be measured. This is especially valuable in solving down-gaze reading problems caused by induced vertical phoria with anisometropia.

4. Thorington: Near test for lateral or vertical phoria using Maddox rod and Thorington near point card.

a. Test in refractor with refraction corrected and refractor set for near point testing, with both eyes open.

b. Maddox rod in front of one eye.

c. Thorington near point card mounted on near point rod at 40 cm. Card has small hole in center with a row of numbers or letters proceeding laterally (or vertically) away from the hole. Numbers and letters are 1 PD apart.

d. With penlight held behind hole in card, patient sees card with one eye and line from Maddox rod with other eye.

e. Patient is asked through which number or letter the line passes. Direction and amount of deviation may be recorded immediately without the use of prism.

f. Modified Thorington card has letters and numbers proceeding outward from the center hole at a 45° angle, allowing easy measurement of either a lateral or a vertical deviation.

g. Distance Thorington test possible with special chart with "muscle light" in center.

5. Stereoscope: Tests for lateral and vertical phoria commonly part of screening series but may be used at any time.

a. Similar to Thorington test, but no Maddox rod or penlight is required. Refraction should be corrected for best results.

b. Phoria test card for stereoscope has dissimilar pictures for right and left eye to prevent fusion. Commonly a line for one eye and a row of numbers and letters for the other eye.

c. Patient indicates number or letter on which the line is superimposed. Numbers and letters are 1 prism diopter apart to allow immediate interpretation of amount and direction of deviation.

d. Separate cards are used for distance and near as well as horizontal and vertical deviations.

6. Risley vergences: Measure range of fusion using refractor and Risley prism.

a. If possible, test with refractive error corrected.

b. For lateral vergences, position Risley prism in front of each eye, set to produce lateral prism. Test BI before BO to minimize aftereffects of convergence generated by BO vergences.

c. Patient must be binocular, have both eyes open, and have no significant level of suppression.

d. For distance, isolate a vertical row of 20/20 or 20/25 letters for typical patient.

e. Add BI prism gradually before both eyes until patient reports the letters either blurring or splitting into two charts. If blur occurs, note prism diopter value and continue adding prism until diplopia occurs and note prism diopter value.

f. After chart doubles, reduce the prism power gradually before both eyes until chart becomes single again and note the prism diopter value.

g. Record the prism diopter values in sequence: blur/break/recovery. Example: 8/14/6.

h. If no blur occurs, only diplopia, record an X for the blur finding. Example: X/10/7.

i. If no break occurs, patient can fuse maximum amount of prism, indicate maximum prism used followed by a (+), and indicate no recovery finding. Example: 18/40±. Be sure patient is binocular; suppression or the presence of an occluder before one eye may give the impression of very high vergence ability. If during testing the target appears to be moving steadily to the right or left, the patient is monocular, and the test should be stopped until the problem is corrected.

j. For near testing, use a well-illuminated small target with some vertical contour and sufficient detail to detect blur. A near point card with a vertical row of 20/20 or 20/25 Snellen letters would be ideal, but many charts are possible.

k. Expected (Morgan): distance, BI = X/7/4, BO = 9/19/10. Near, BI = 13/21/13, BO = 17/21/11.

7. Bar vergences: Similar to Risley vergences but done outside refractor in free space.

a. Test with refraction corrected, good light, both eyes open with no suppression.

b. Distance target: vertical row of 20/20 or 20/25 letters. Near target: any small chart or target with some vertical contour and sufficient detail to detect blur.

c. Test BI before BO. Testing BO first results in a residual tonicity in the convergence muscle system leading to an artificially reduced BI finding. The divergence system has much less of the residual affect.

d. Use prism bar before one eye only. Increase prism power by moving prism bar from section to section, allowing patient a chance to fuse each increase in prism power. A very brief period of diplopia with each increase in prism power is not uncommon. Be careful not to position the prism bar so the patient is viewing through a junction or seam between two prism sections.

e. Measure and record, in sequence, the prism power necessary to produce first blur, diplopia (break), and then reduce prism until recovery (see Risley vergences, I.K.6 above).

8. Lateral phoria and vergence analysis. Treat to eliminate symptoms or improve performance (reduced stereo acuity, suppression, amblyopia).

a. If patient has exophoria, the measured compensating vergence, base out, should be at least twice the phoria (Sheard). Example: Phoria = 8 exo. Base out vergences should measure 16 or greater (use blur finding or break if no blur occurs).

b. If BO vergences are less than twice the phoria, consider vision therapy to increase vergence ability or prism to decrease the phoria and increase the relative vergence value. Example: Phoria = 8 exo, BO vergences = 7/16/10. Phoria = 8, increase BO blur finding from 7 to at least 16 through vision therapy. Prism solution gives patient 3 BI. Phoria now measures 5 exo instead of 8 exo, and BO now measures 10 instead of 7.

c. If patient has esophoria, evaluate both BI and BO vergence values (Percival). BO vergence value (blur) should not be greater than twice the base in value. If treatment is indicated due to symptoms or performance problems, use vision therapy, lenses, or prisms to reduce difference between BI and BO blur findings. Example: BI = 5/12/3, BO = 16/25/16. Use vision therapy to improve BI vergences (blur) to at least 8. Use BO prism. Prescribing 2 BO will increase the measured BI blur value to 7 and decrease the measured BO blur value to 14, exactly twice the BI value.

d. If an eso deviation is present at near, an add may be used instead of prism. The power of the add required is a function of the patient's accommodation to convergence ratio (AC/A). The higher the AC/A, the more effective an add becomes.

9. Fixation disparity: commonly fixation disparity measurements are actually the amount of prism required to eliminate the disparity. This value is the "associated

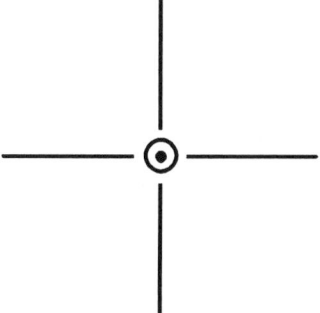

Figure 7-7. Test pattern used to detect fixation disparity.

phoria." Usually lateral deviations require actual measurement of the fixation disparity under various levels of fusion load (prism) to be of value. The "associated
phoria" may be useful, however, in the diagnosis and management of vertical
deviations.

   a. May be done distance or near if appropriate charts are available.

   b. Chart separates images for right and left eye, usually using polarizing filters or
red-green filters.

   c. A common chart is a "plus" sign with the upper half of the vertical line seen by
the right eye and the lower half by the left eye. The horizontal line is split in a
like manner, with the right side seen by the right eye and the left side seen by the
left eye.

   d. The horizontal line is used to measure the vertical associated phoria. While
viewing through the appropriate filters, the patient is asked if the right half of the
horizontal line is higher or lower than the left.

   e. If the lines are even, no disparity is present and 0 is recorded. If the two halves
are misaligned, prism is added to determine the minimum amount of prism to
place the lines in alignment. This value is recorded as the associated vertical
phoria and may be considered as a good starting value when prescribing for
vertical deviations.

  L. *Automated refraction*

    1. Auto refractors provide a quick (1–5 seconds) objective measure of refractive error
which can be easily performed by a trained assistant.

    2. Most accurate on refractive errors under 4 D.

    3. Less accurate when media are disrupted and/or refractive error is high.

    4. Placing accommodation at rest can be a problem. If distance fixation target is not at
infinity but imaged at infinity, proximal awareness may trigger accommodation and
result in overcorrection in minus direction.

    5. Newest models are available with auto keratometer results as well.

    6. Operation very simple. Most units use a video display for focus and alignment.
Follow manufacturer's instructions.

II. Diagnosis and Management

  A. *Myopia*

    1. Symptoms: distance blur (may be unaware with gradual onset). Headaches and
asthenopia possible but rare.

    2. Signs: "squinting" of eyelids, staring, rubbing eyes, moving close to object of
regard (TV, chalk board, etc.).

    3. Onset at any age but common between ages 7 and 20.

    4. Uncorrected distance visual acuity reduced, near visual acuity good.

    5. Retinoscopy, monocular and binocular subjective usually match. Overcorrection
possible if accommodation unstable, especially with history of excessive near

work. Final refraction should be no more than -0.50 D more minus than first readable 20/20 finding. Cycloplegic refraction should be used if accommodation is unstable and pseudomyopia a possibility.

6. Corrected visual acuity may be slightly reduced while wearing full correction, but will often improve to normal levels with full-time wear of correction for 2 to 3 weeks.

7. With high levels of myopia, vertex distance is important. If refraction is done with a long vertex distance and patient is fit with shorter vertex distance, correction will be too strong.

8. Tests of accommodative ability may show reduction in performance. Patient is used to "add" of uncorrected myopia. Accommodative performance usually improves with wear of distance correction. Vision therapy is indicated if accommodative insufficiency persists after wear of distance Rx.

9. Acceptance of spectacle Rx is usually good due to dramatic improvement in distance vision which masks most adaptation problems.

10. Possible spectacle adaptation problems include: Walls, doors appear bowed outward (barrel distortion). Floor appears raised due to base down prism effect. Objects straight ahead appear farther away due to minification. Reading is more difficult since accommodation not used to working as much at near. Objects may appear to move when patient moves head while wearing Rx (swimming sensation); effect caused by variable amounts of induced prism. Cosmetic appearance of "glasses." Correction with contact lenses eliminates all but accommodation problems listed.

11. Myopia control is incomplete science. Bifocals may be effective in some cases where patient is eso at near with correction. Vision therapy may be effective when accommodative spasm creates pseudomyopia. Contact lens correction may be effective in some but not all cases due to unknown factors. Many theories exist, but none "airtight." Success of control should be based on objective measurements, not visual acuity.

12. If subjective exam calls for a reduction in minus power, consider that patient may have adapted to over-minus Rx similar to hyperopic patient. Reduction of power may produce symptoms of loss of contrast and sharpness, even though acuity remains the same. If a significant reduction in correction is indicated, consider leaving the patient with a -0.25 Diopter overcorrection. Demonstrate any planned change using trial lenses.

B. *Hyperopia*

1. Symptoms: many young patients asymptomatic. Symptoms include headaches and asthenopia, especially while reading. Reports of transient blur, especially when tired.

2. Signs: rubbing eyes, intermittent or constant esotropia.

3. Low hyperopia common in young children, often decreasing in amount towards emmetropia.

4. Any child with esotropia should be carefully examined for hyperopia using a cycloplegic exam.

5. Retinoscopy, monocular subjective and binocular sphere check often produce different results. The most plus power measured is probably the most correct. The patient will often accept more plus under binocular conditions than monocular.

6. Perform binocular sphere check carefully to determine wearable Rx. During binocular sphere check, add plus sphere to fog 20/20 visual acuity letters. Wait 10 to 15 seconds to see if patient will relax accommodation and allow letters to clear. If letters clear, add additional plus sphere to both eyes until the patient reports the letters remain slightly blurred, but a few of the 20/20 letters are readable. From this point, reduce plus sphere to both eyes by 1.00 D. This Rx will most likely be wearable by the patient. In cases of significant esophoria or esotropia, a reduction of 0.50 D of plus sphere may be the best choice.

7. Measuring monocular visual acuity with full plus correction may be difficult. Consider the following options:

    a. Do not occlude the eye not being tested but rather fog this eye by $+1.00$ to $+1.75$ D of additional plus sphere.

    b. If the patient can be trusted not to "cheat" on the test, leave both eyes open but add vertical prism to dissociate the visual acuity chart and have the patient read the upper and lower chart to measure right and left eye visual acuity. This procedure should be used with caution on patients who might have reduced vision and are trying to achieve a goal such a driver's license, pilot's license, or other occupational requirement. Realize, however, that most patients will not be aware that the right eye is seeing only one of the images and the left eye, the other image.

    c. With final Rx in place, have patient view the acuity chart with both eyes open. While patient watches smallest row readable, cover one eye and see if letters are still readable using uncovered eye. Letters may remain clear for only a few seconds, but this is adequate to confirm good acuity. If letters appear instantly blurred, look for possible error in balance or amblyopia.

8. Acceptance of plus correction is often poor. Hyperopic patients usually see more clearly without their glasses than with. Biggest benefit is usually comfort. If glasses slip down patient's nose, effective strength of prescription increases, which may result in overcorrection and blur. Hyperopic patients often notice distortions, swimming sensations, and image displacement more with their spectacle corrections since they do not have the dramatic improvement in visual acuity to psychologically mask these effects. Demonstrate final Rx in trial frame before prescribing and emphasize benefits of correction. Partial correction of hyperopia is common. A gradual increase in correction strength over several years is an option.

C. *Astigmatism*

1. Symptoms: headache, blurred vision, asthenopia.
2. Signs: squinting of eyelids, tilting of spectacle correction.
3. If acuity is reduced, it will usually be reduced at both distance and near.
4. Usually in combination with myopia or hyperopia and therefore adds to the problems already present.
5. Power and axis of correction often remains stable over many years.
6. Retinoscopy, keratometry, and subjective testing should have good correlation. If patient rejects cylinder power using Jackson cross cylinder test, retest cylinder power using a line astigmatic chart such as the clock dial or sun burst.
7. As with myopia, initial corrected acuity may not be as good as expected but will often improve with full-time wear of the correction.
8. Patients vary dramatically as to their acceptance of astigmatic corrections. Correction of astigmatism is best done with contact lenses, since correction with spectacle lenses results in a change in the retinal image size and shape. If the two eyes do not have identical optical corrections, significant problems of aniseikonia often result.
9. Common complaints with the spectacle correction of astigmatism include spatial distortions, dizziness, headache, asthenopia and a general feeling that something is wrong with the glasses.
10. Options include fitting the patient with contact lenses, reducing cylinder power while modifying the sphere power to partially compensate (equivalent sphere), rotating cylinder axis toward the 90° or 180° axis or designing special iconic lenses (rare).
11. Since many patients adapt to these optical effects, demonstrate the correction before prescribing or modifying a prescription. If the patient is advised that many

of these initial sensations are normal and may disappear with constant wear, patient acceptance of the correction is often significantly improved.

12. Wearability is often improved if the prescription is fabricated in a small eye size frame and fit close to the face. Consider increasing pantoscopic tilt and wrap or "face form" of the frame.

13. If the patient has more than one pair of glasses, change all corrections since significant problems often occur if the patient is allowed to switch back to a previous prescription (sunglasses).

D. *Anisometropia*

1. Uncorrected anisometropia symptoms: asthenopia, headache, a sense that the two eyes are not working together. Symptoms may be absent if suppression is present.

2. Uncorrected anisometropia may cause reduced stereo acuity, even with good monocular visual acuity. If anisometropia has been uncorrected for some time, and suppression is active, amblyopia is possible.

3. Anisohyperopia (one eye more hyperopic than the other) is a high risk for the development of amblyopia and should be corrected immediately. Set balance using standard balance procedures, retinoscopy, and binocular refraction techniques if available. Do *not* modify the balance between right and left eye based on monocular visual acuities. It is common for accommodation to be unstable under monocular, noncycloplegic conditions, resulting in poor monocular acuities—consider cycloplegic refraction. If the balance has been confirmed using several techniques and the binocular visual acuity is good, prescribe the full difference in refractive error, especially with children.

4. Anisomyopia (one eye more myopic than the other) may often produce no symptoms and, in low amounts of anisometropia, may have some beneficial effects. In the case of presbyopic contact lens wearers, the intentional creation of an uncorrected myopic anisometropia is used as a technique for managing the presbyopia (monovision). One eye is corrected for distance and the other eye is corrected for near, resulting in clear vision at both distances for some patients, along with slightly compromised binocularity. Higher amounts of anisomyopia may result in suppression similar to hyperopic case. Important clinical considerations with anisomyopia include:

   a. Refraction is usually stable with objective tests closely matching subjective data.

   b. Adaptation to spectacles is not as good as with equal amounts of myopia in both eyes, but is better than hyperopic anisometropia.

5. Anisoastigmatism: unequal cylinder power and/or different axes

   a. Symptoms: headache and asthenopia are common. NOTE: If one eye is significantly worse than the other, suppression may be triggered and symptoms may be reduced. Visual distortions are usually found only in the corrected state.

   b. Since astigmatism is usually longstanding, ask about previous attempts at treatment. If patient reports previous Rx had to be remade several times before it was correct, proceed with changes carefully. Rx was probably "correct" the first time, but unwearable.

   c. Cylinder is always refractive and usually corneal. Retinoscopy, keratometry, and subjective should match closely.

   d. Caution: long-standing uncorrected cylinder is often rejected during the Jackson cross cylinder test. Note the reduced amount and retest with a line astigmatic chart such as the clock dial or sun burst.

   e. Contact lenses provide the best correction with the fewest symptoms. A complex contact lens fit may be required.

   f. Spectacle correction of unequal astigmatism may produce symptoms of asthenopia, headache, and distortion. The cause is aniseikonia and induced prism. Both are eliminated with contact lenses.

    g. Before prescribing, demonstrate the cylinder correction in a trial frame. Tell the patient the Rx is correct optically, but it may require a period of adaptation. If the patient is not advised, and there is a problem with adaptation, the patient will assume the clinician made a mistake.

    h. If Rx is not wearable, options include: (1) a reduction in cylinder power with a compensating change in sphere. Example: If cylinder is reduced from -3.00 DC to -2.00 DC, add -0.50 DS to the sphere correction. (2) Rotate the cylinder axis in small amounts toward the 90° or 180° meridian while checking acuity to be sure there is no major reduction. (3) Perform a combination of the two previous steps. (4) Design special isokonic lenses (bitoric design).

6. Anisometropia and multifocals

    a. An add forces patient to look away from the optical centers of lenses, and induced vertical prism results.

    b. "Slab off" prism is often helpful but is cosmetically noticeable and produces significant "jump" at junction line. Minimum amount = 1.5 PD.

    c. Optically, slab off is the same as holding a loose prism over the multifocal portion of a spectacle lens.

    d. On glass lenses, slab off is typically ground on the front of the lens.

    e. On plastic lenses, slab off may be ground base up on the back of the lens by the local surfacing laboratory or ready-made, molded base down on the front surface in combination with a flat top bifocal (D-28 Younger). If molded on the front surface, the local laboratory need only surface the back of the lens as they would any other bifocal. No special grinding operations are involved. This reduces the chance for error and speeds delivery time (if the blanks are available). Remember, with the ready-made variety, the prism is always base down. When slab off is ground on the back surface of a lens, it is always base up prism.

    f. Measure need for prism with Maddox rod test at near. Prism required may be less than amount predicted optically.

    g. The slab off prism value may also be determined using a vectograph slide from an acuity projector. Hold the slide over a white card at the near working distance with head, eyes, and target in normal reading positions. The patient views fixation disparity portion of the slide through polarizing filters.

    h. Add enough vertical prism to level horizontal line of fixation disparity target. Prescribe this amount for slab off.

    i. To avoid using slab off prism, lower distance optical center slightly, fit multifocal high, and instruct patient on using upper portion of multifocal (easier when seg is "no jump" style).

7. General considerations: Most adaptation problems are related to induced prism when looking away from the optical centers. Lateral induced prism is often more of a problem than vertical.

8. Correct anisometropia with contact lenses whenever possible. NOTE: Aniseikonia is usually present when axial anisometropia is corrected with contact lenses or refractive anisometropia is corrected with spectacles. If aniseikonia is predicted with contact lenses, attempt a contact lens correction anyway. Aniseikonia problem may not be as great as induced prism, weight, and cosmetic problems associated with glasses.

9. If spectacle lenses must be used, fit Rx close to the face to reduce vertex distance. Use a frame with adjustable pads and small eye size. Instruct the patient to use the center of lenses whenever possible; learn to turn head instead of eyes.

10. Use slab off prism in down gaze with multifocal lenses only. Slab off prism usually causes more problems than it eliminates in single vision design.

11. Demonstrate the final Rx in a trial frame but realize the final spectacle Rx will be in a larger frame and may cause problems not found with trial lenses.

E. *High prescription power/aphakia*

1. Measure and control vertex distance. Fit Rx at the same distance as the refraction distance. Use a frame with adjustable pads to allow for adjustment at dispensing. If Rx fits closer than refraction, effective power will be too much minus or not enough plus. Reverse is true if Rx is too far away from the eyes (Rx slides down patient's nose). As a rule: *Refract and fit the Rx with as short a vertex distance as possible.* This results in better optics, less magnification or minification, and better cosmetic appearance.

2. Drop optical centers to match pantoscopic tilt. If lenses are tilted without dropping optical centers, a large amount of unwanted cylinder will be generated. Test at dispensing by having patient fixate a penlight while the clinician sights directly over penlight with one eye. The clinician moves up, down, left, or right until the reflections from the front and back of the spectacle lens are stacked, one on top of the other. The clinician is now looking down the optic axis of the lens. With the patient looking at the penlight, the stacked reflections from the lens should appear approximately in the center of the patient's pupil and should align with the reflection from the patient's cornea. If this does not occur, adjust the pantoscopic tilt, level of the Rx, and face form of the Rx until this alignment occurs.

3. Use aspheric design to improve peripheral optics. Consider benefits of high index optical materials, tints, and coatings.

4. Be aware of prismatic effects of high Rx. Aphakia is large change in Rx resulting in significant image displacement which may lead to serious mobility problems. If phoria is different, consider decentering lenses to provide partial prism correction. Bifocal segments may be ordered with a wider or narrower separation to partially offset the induced lateral prism at near.

5. Advise the patient that spectacle adjustment is critical to optimal performance, and regular visits to readjust the Rx are common.

6. Contact lenses usually produce *significantly* better optical performance than spectacle lenses in this power range.

F. *Amblyopia*

1. The following characteristics of amblyopic vision may be discovered during the typical vision examination:

   a. The presence of an uncorrected anisometropia (especially anisohyperopia) or strabismus or both.

   b. Reduced visual acuity in one eye, where: acuity improves with isolation of letters (or other characters); letters in an acuity row are read out of order, or an extra letter is added, or a letter is omitted; the first and last letters of an acuity row are read but the others are missed; the letters of the chart appear to change as the patient observes the chart; the chart appears gray and dim like a poor-quality photocopy; the patient reports there appears to be a shadow or hazy spot between the patient and the chart.

   c. Reduced amplitude of accommodation in the amblyopic eye.

   d. Unsteady fixation with the amblyopic eye, possible eccentric fixation.

   e. Suppression of the amblyopic eye during binocular testing.

   f. Poor ability to make a position judgment during lateral phoria tests (if suppression can be broken down).

   g. During subjective refraction patient reports chart becoming clearer but cannot read any more letters. "The chart is clear, I just can't read it."

2. The proper balance is important. Remember, if a dissociated blur balance is attempted with a patient with unequal best corrected visual acuities, use letters 2 lines larger than best visual acuity for the weaker eye and use more plus sphere blur. Do not reduce the plus blur to confirm the balance. When there is a signifi-

cant reduction in visual acuity (20/100 and worse) associated with amblyopia, objective tests like static and dynamic retinoscopy or autorefraction may provide better information about the balance than a subjective balance.

3. If testing involving diplopia (balance, phorias) cannot be performed due to suppression, try:
   a. Reduce room illumination to a minimum (*dark* room).
   b. Increase the separation of the two images.
   c. Increase the size of each image.
   d. Perform a brief period of alternate occlusion to demonstrate to the patient the location of the two images.
4. Treatment involves treating the cause for the suppression which resulted in the amblyopia.
   a. If anisometropia is the cause, correct the full amount of the anisometropia. Trust the data from retinoscopy and the balance. Do not reduce plus power before the amblyopic eye based on *monocular* visual acuity findings.
   b. If strabismus is the cause, consider all options, including vision therapy, prism, and surgery. Consider alternate fixation if correction of the strabismus is unsuccessful.
   c. Antisuppression and antiamblyopia therapy should be initiated as soon as possible. In the case of amblyopia due to uncorrected anisometropia, the visual acuity in the amblyopic eye will often improve dramatically over the first 6 to 8 weeks of wear of corrective spectacle lenses without any special therapy techniques. After this time period, however, therapy should be pursued aggressively.

Suggested Readings

Amos, JF. *Diagnosis and Management in Vision Care*. Stoneham, MA: Butterworth, 1987.

Borish IM. *Clinical Refraction*. Chicago: Professional Press, 1975.

Eskridge JB, Amos JF, Bartlett JD. *Clinical Procedures in Optometry*. Philadelphia: Lippincott, 1991.

Grosvenor TP. *Primary Care Optometry*. New York: Professional Press, 1989.

Von Noorden GK. *Binocular Vision and Ocular Motility*. St. Louis: CV Mosby, 1980.

CHAPTER **8**

Ophthalmic Optics

William L. Brown

I. **Prescription Writing. Spherocylinder Form**

A. *The optical cross is a very convenient and powerful way of describing the powers and directions of the principal meridians of an ophthalmic lens.*

1. A cross is drawn with its limbs parallel to the principal meridians of the lens (left side of Figure 8-1).

2. At one end of each limb is written the meridian being represented, 070 and 160 in Figure 8-1.

3. At the other end of each limb is written the power of the lens in that principal meridian, −0.75D in 160 and +1.50D in 070 in Figure 8-1.

B. *Powers are communicated more commonly in written form using spherocylinder notation.*

1. When the powers are written in spherocylinder form, the lens is considered to be composed of a spherical lens power (equal power in all meridians) combined with a simple cylinder (zero power in one principal meridian and maximum power in the other).

   a. Principal meridians are the directions in the lens having the two extreme powers, the maximum and the minimum.

   b. The spherocylinder form of a lens prescription consists of three numbers—the sphere power, the cylinder power, and the cylinder axis.

   c. The lens denoted in the optical cross (Figure 8-1) can be divided into a spherical component having +1.50D in all meridians and a simple cylinder component having its axis (with zero power) in meridian 070 and its maximum power (−2.25D) in meridian 160.

      (1) The powers from the sphere and cylinder components in meridian 070 (+1.50D and 0.00D) total +1.50D, as shown on the cross.

      (2) The powers from the two components in meridian 160 (+1.50D and −2.25D) total −0.75D.

      (3) Since the power of the simple cylinder in this combination is minus, this is the minus cylinder representation of the lens, written +1.50 −2.25 × 070.

         (a) Sphere power is followed by cylinder power and then by cylinder axis.

         (b) "Axis" is abbreviated "X."

      (4) The axis is always written as a number greater than zero and less than or equal to 180.

      (5) The use of three digits for all axes (including leading zeros for one and two-digit axes such as "005" instead of "5") can reduce the potential for misinterpretation.

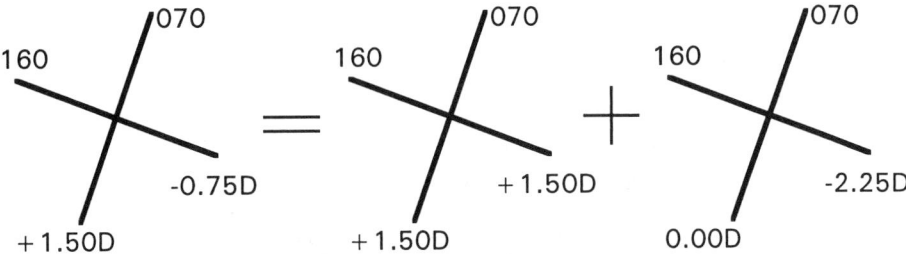

Sphero-cylinder   =   Sphere   +   Cylinder

=   +1.50DS   +   -2.25DC X 070

Figure 8-1.   The optical cross shows the powers in the principal meridians of a spherocylinder lens: +1.50D in meridian 070 and −0.75D in 160. The spherocylinder can be represented as the combination of a sphere (+1.50D) and simple cylinder (−2.25D × 070).

d.   The lens can be represented in the plus cylinder form by considering the power in the other principal meridian (−0.75D) to be the sphere.
  (1)   The axis of the simple cylinder component, with zero power, is meridian 160.
  (2)   The powers in the axis meridian 160 total −0.75D.
  (3)   The maximum power of the simple cylinder, +2.25D, is in meridian 070, 90° away from the axis.
  (4)   The total power in meridian 070 is the required +1.50D.
  (5)   The plus cylinder form of the Rx is −0.75 +2.25 × 160.

2.   In summary, the following steps are used to write the lens prescription in spherocylinder form from the optical cross.
  a.   The sphere power is chosen from the powers in the principal meridians.
    (1)   For minus cylinder form, the power of greater plus or lesser minus (depending on whether the powers are plus or minus) is chosen to be the sphere: +1.50D in the example.
    (2)   For plus cylinder form, the power of lesser plus or greater minus is chosen: −0.75D in the example.
  b.   The cylinder power is determined by calculating the difference between the powers of the two principal meridians, subtracting the sphere power from the power in the other principal meridian.
    (1)   In the example for minus cylinder form, −0.75 −(+1.50) = −2.25D.
    (2)   For plus cylinder form, +1.50 −(−0.75) = +2.25D.
    (3)   The cylinder power has the same magnitude in both forms but opposite signs.
  c.   The axis meridian for the cylinder power is the meridian of the sphere power.
    (1)   In the example, the cylinder axis for minus cylinder form is meridian 070, the sphere meridian.
    (2)   For plus cylinder form, the axis is meridian 160.
  d.   Figure 8-2 shows the same prescription written in both plus cylinder and minus cylinder forms.
    (1)   The right eye shows the Rx in minus cylinder form: +1.50 −2.25 × 070.
    (2)   The left eye shows the same Rx in plus cylinder form: −0.75 +2.25 × 160.

R͓		SPHERICAL	CYLINDRICAL	AXIS	PRISM	BASE
D.V.	O.D.	+1.50	-2.25	070		
	O.S.	-0.75	+2.25	160		
N.V.	O.D.					
	O.S.					

FOR_____ DATE_____

ADDRESS_____

REMARKS_____

_____ , O.D.

Figure 8-2.   The same lens prescription is written in minus cylinder form (right eye) and in plus cylinder form (left eye).

3. The choice of which cylinder form to use is generally determined by the type of cylinder in the photopter used.
   a. Optometrists most commonly use minus cylinder phoropters and therefore typically write prescriptions directly in minus cylinder form.
   b. Ophthalmologists commonly use plus cylinder phoropters and typically write prescriptions in plus cylinder form.
   c. Regardless of the form of the written prescription, the cylinder will be placed on the rear surface of the spectacle lens, with rare exceptions.
4. A lens prescription can be placed on an optical cross as follows:
   a. The sphere power from the Rx is placed in the cylinder axis meridian. (In the minus cylinder example above, +1.50D is placed in meridian 070.)
   b. The cylinder power is added to the sphere power to find the power in the other principal meridian [+1.50 +(−2.25) = −0.75D in meridian 160].

C. *An Rx in one spherocylinder form (either plus or minus) can be transposed to the other cylinder form as follows:*
   1. The new sphere power is found by adding the sphere and cylinder power algebraically [+1.50 +(−2.25) = −0.75D].
   2. The new cylinder power retains the same magnitude but the sign is changed (−2.25D becomes +2.25D).
   3. The new axis is found by changing the original axis by 90°, keeping it a positive angle less than or equal to 180 (70 + 90 = 160).
   4. The plus cylinder form of +1.50 −2.25 × 070 is −0.75 +2.25 × 160.

II.   Frames

A. *Parts*
   1. The frame, which is used to mount spectacle lenses in front of the eyes, consists of two major components, the front and the temples.
   2. The front is the part of the frame which holds the lenses at the proper distance from the eyes with the proper separation between the lenses.
      a. The front has two eyewires which hold the lenses (Figure 8-3a); the beveled edges of the lenses are inserted into grooves around the inside of the eyewires (Figure 8-3b).

(a)

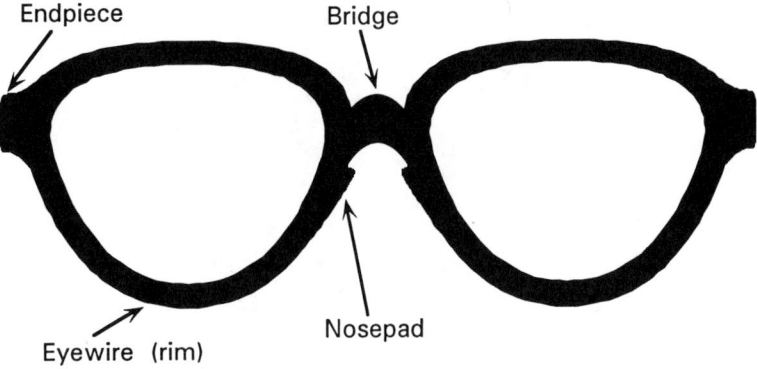

Endpiece   Bridge

Eyewire (rim)

Nosepad

(b)

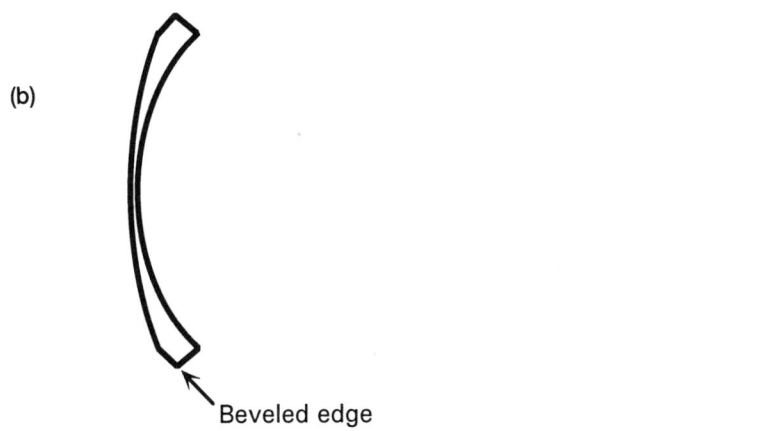

Beveled edge

Figure 8-3.   (a) The parts of a frame front are diagrammed. (b) Ophthalmic lenses have beveled edges to fit into the groove inside the eyewire.

b. The bridge is the part of the front which holds the eyewires together and helps support the front on the patient's nose.
(1) The saddle bridge is rounded to fit the patient's nose, with the weight of the front supported by the top as well as the sides of the bridge of the patient's nose (Figure 8-4a).
(2) The keyhole bridge is narrower at the top of the bridge than the saddle bridge (Figure 8-4b).
(a) The top of the bridge does not rest on the patient's nose.
(b) The front is held higher in front of the eyes than with a saddle bridge.
(3) The adjustable bridge has plastic nose pads which are attached to the nasal eyewires by thin strands of metal (Figure 8-4c).
(a) The pads rest against the sides of the nose to support the frame.
(b) Because the separation between the pads and the angle of the pads can be changed to improve the fit on the patient's nose, adjustable pads are helpful for a patient whose bridge is difficult to fit with fixed pads.
(c) Compared to older adjustable pads, most current adjustable pads have a very limited range of adjustment for changing the vertical position of the frame and the vertex distance of the lenses.

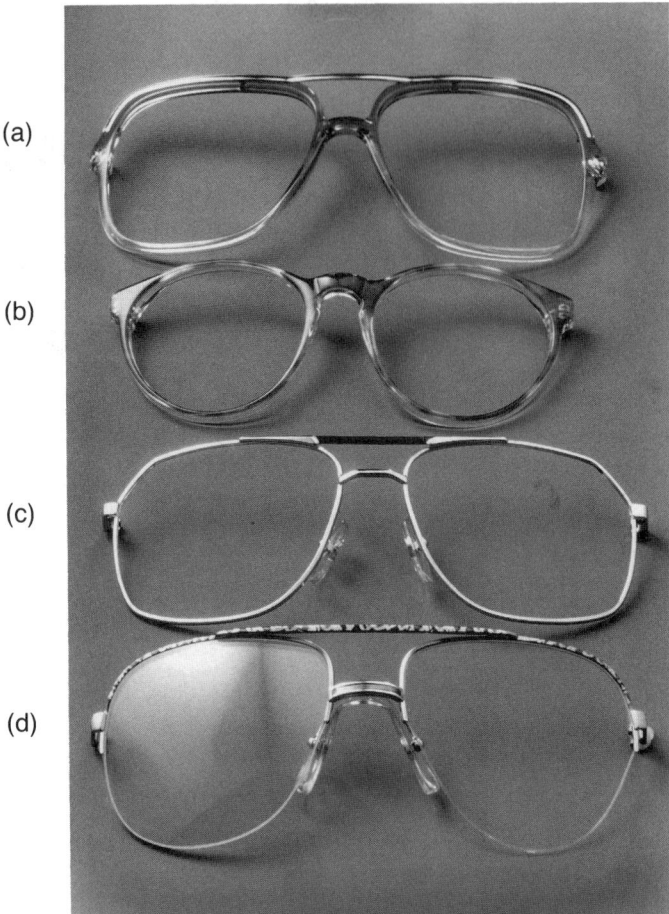

Figure 8-4. Each of the four frames has a different type of bridge: (a) saddle bridge, (b) keyhole bridge, (c) adjustable pads, (d) form fit bridge.

       (d) Frames without adjustable pads have fixed nose pads, which are a broadening of the nasal eyewires where they rest on the nose to increase the surface area supporting the weight of the frame.

       (e) Adjustable pads can be added to some frames having fixed bridges.

    (4) The form fit bridge is a soft plastic bridge (Figure 8-4d).

       (a) It fits inside the nasal parts of each eyewire and under the cross piece between the eyewires.

       (b) The weight of the frame is equally distributed on the top and both sides of the nose.

  3. The temples attach to the front and support the frame by resting on or hooking around the ears.

    a. The most commonly used temple, the skull temple, extends back from the frame front to the top of the ear, at which point the temple bends approximately 45° to fit behind the upper portion of the ear (Figure 8-5a).

    b. The comfort cable temple extends from the temple front back to the ear, where the temple becomes flexible, following snugly around the entire back of the ear (Figure 8-5b).

      (1) The comfort cable is much less likely to slide down a patient's nose or come off a patient's face than a skull temple.

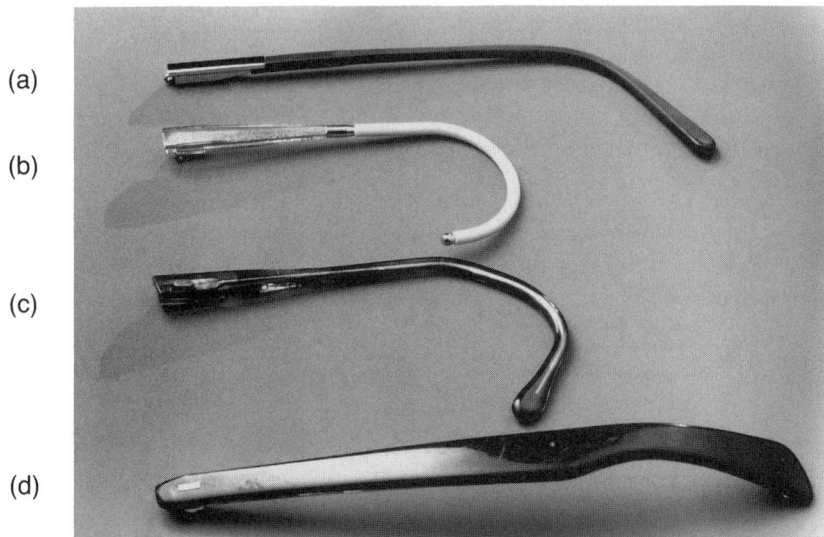

Figure 8-5. Four types of temples are illustrated: (a) skull, (b) comfort cable, (c) riding bow, (d) library.

           (2)   Comfort cable temples are useful for active patients, including small children, and for patients for whom the bridge is difficult to fit.

      c.   The riding bow temple is similar to the comfort cable, except that the curved portion which fits behind the ear is solid rather than flexible material (Figure 8-5c).

      d.   The library (paddle) temple extends straight back from the front and rests on the top of the ear (Figure 8-5d).

           (1)   A portion of the bottom of the temple may be cut out at the top of the ear.

           (2)   These temples are designed for ease of removal from the ears, and are designed for glasses which are removed quite often (such as a reading-only Rx).

  B.   *Measurements*

     1.   Frame measurements in the United States are based on the boxing system.

      a.   Each lens is "boxed" with two horizontal lines, one tangent to the highest point on the lens and one tangent to the lowest point on the lens, and with two vertical lines, one tangent to the most nasal point and one through the most temporal point (Figure 8-6).

      b.   The lines pass through the outermost points on the lenses, which for a beveled lens are on the outer edge of the bevel.

           (1)   The bevel extends approximately 0.5 mm into the groove of the frame.

           (2)   Approximately 1 mm of the total horizontal width of the lens (0.5 mm on each side) and 1 mm of the vertical height of the lens are hidden from view when the lens is mounted in the eyewire.

      c.   The "A" dimension is the horizontal width of the box.

      d.   The "B" dimension is the vertical height of the box.

      e.   When the A and B dimensions are measured using the edges of visible lens, 1 mm is added to each to account for the bevel hidden in the eyewire groove.

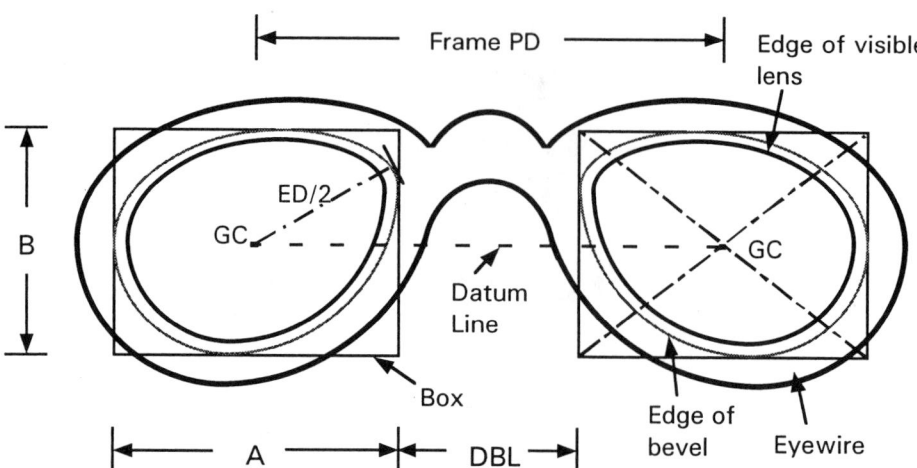

Figure 8-6.   Dimensions of a frame front and lenses as defined by the boxing system. The lens is boxed with lines tangent to the innermost, outermost, uppermost, and lowermost edges of the lens bevel (hatched line), which are hidden in the groove of the eyewire. A is the horizontal lens size, B is the vertical lens size, GC is the geometrical center of the lens, frame PD is the distance between the two GCs, ED is the effective diameter of the lens, and DBL is the distance between the innermost edges of the two lenses.

f. The DBL (distance between lenses) is the distance between the closest points on the two lenses.
    (1) It is the distance between the nasal vertical lines of the boxes for the two lenses.
    (2) Subtract 1 mm from the distance between the closest points in the lenses visible in the frame to compensate for the hidden bevels.
g. The geometrical center (GC) of a lens is equidistant from the two sides of the box and from the top and bottom of the box; it is the intersection of the two diagonals of the box.
h. The frame PD (also called DBC, or distance between centers) is the distance between the geometrical centers of the two eyewires: Frame PD = A + DBL.
i. The effective diameter (ED) of the lens is twice the distance from the geometrical center of the lens to the most distant point on the lens.
    (1) It is sometimes estimated clinically by measuring the longest dimension of the lens.
    (2) The longest dimension is usually from the inferior temporal to the superior nasal corner.
j. The datum line is the line connecting the geometrical centers of the two lenses.
k. Two numbers are usually found stamped on a frame, the eyesize and the bridge size, e.g., 52-17.
    (1) These two numbers are used as stock numbers or reference numbers for cataloging the frame and are not necessarily true dimensions of the frame.
        (a) The eyesize is not necessarily the A dimension.
        (b) The bridge is not necessarily the DBL.
    (2) If the numbers are separated by a box (e.g., 52[]17), then presumably the eyesize is the A dimension and the bridge size is the DBL.
        (a) Quality control may keep the true dimensions of the frame from equaling the numbers stamped on the frame, so it is wise to

measure the dimensions of the individual frame when there is any question.

(b) Discrepancies between the markings and the frame dimensions are most apparent in some imported frames for which the boxing system is not used.

1. The overall temple length (OAL) is the distance from the hinge end of the temple to the posterior tip.

(1) If the temple is bent, as in a skull temple, the length is measured around the bend by adding the distance from the anterior end to the bend to the distance from the bend to the posterior end (Figure 8-5a).

(2) The temple length may be designated in either millimeters or, less commonly, in inches.

(a) Lengths in millimeters usually are in 5-mm increments, such as 130, 135, 140 mm.

(b) Lengths in inches are usually in $1/4''$ increments, such as $5 1/2$, $5 3/4$, 6 inches.

(3) Temple length is usually stamped on the inside of the temples.

C. *Materials*

1. Frames are made from a variety of materials, principally categorized as plastic and metal.

2. Common materials and their characteristics are listed in Tables 8-1 and 8-2.

Table 8-1. Common Plastic Frame Materials and Their Characteristics

Name	Material	Heat Level for Adjusting	Size Variability	Other Characteristics
Zyl	Cellulose acetate	Medium to high	Can be stretched or shrunk	Most common material
Propionate	Cellulose propionate	Low	No size/shape memory after stretching	Hypoallergenic Lightweight No alcohol/acetone Cold snap lens
Polyamide	Nylon base	Low	Shrinks when overheated	Hypoallergenic Lightweight No acetone Cold snap lens
Carbon	Carbon front Metal temples	No heat	Cannot be stretched	Lightweight Exact lens size Holds adjustment
Carbon 22	Carbon and nylon	Low	Eyewire not split like carbon frame	Hypoallergenic Lightweight
Optyl	Epoxy resin	High—do not water cool	Shape and size memory when heated	Hypoallergenic Lightweight
Nylon	Nylon	Hot water; hold adjustment until cool	Does not shrink or stretch	Strong Flexible Hypoallergenic Soak periodically to avoid drying out

Modified from *Common Plastic Frame Materials* by Walman Optical Company, 801 12th Avenue, North, Minneapolis, MN 55411, 1992.

Table 8-2.   Common Metal Frame Materials and Their Characteristics

Name	Material	Characteristics	Corrosion Resistance	Finishes	Frame Parts
Monel	68% nickel 30% copper 2% iron	Easy to shape	Good	Can be coated for many color treatments	Used in temples, endpieces and front; not a material of choice for eyewire
Nickel	Nickel	Easy to shape	Good		Good overall frame material
Nickel silver	62% copper 20% zinc 18% nickel	Rigid and lustrous Not easy to shape Metal of choice for gold-filled frames	Very poor	Cannot be plated	Used for bridges, endpieces
Phosphor-bronze	75% copper	Variation is bronze beryllium Returns to shape when bent	Poor	Easily electro-plated	Used for temples
Stainless steel	67% iron 18% chrome	Durable, flexible, strong	Excellent		Good overall frame material
Titanium	Rare earth material	Lightweight Easy to adjust Expensive	Excellent	Coloration limited	
Aluminum	Aluminum	Cannot be welded or soldered	Good	Can be chemically anodized and treated with broad range of colors	Limited to designs which use screws, rivets to attach frame sections
Beryllium	Blend of metals	Light, strong			Used for frames
Cobalt	Primarily cobalt	Durable, flexible, lightweight Resilient	Good	Takes all colors	Frames can be thin

Modified from *Common Frame Materials* by Walman Optical Company.

    D.   *Adjustments*
        Appendix 2 summarizes the most common problems regarding adjustment of glasses and possible solutions.

III. Lens Materials

    A.   *Lens characteristics and materials*
        1.   A variety of materials are currently available for ophthalmic lenses, having different indices of refraction, specific gravities, and Abbe values.
            a.   If two lenses of the same power are made of different materials, the lens made of the higher-index material will have flatter surfaces (see Index of Refraction in Appendix 1.E).
               (1)   The edge thickness of a minus lens and the center thickness of a plus lens are reduced in a high-index lens, both primary reasons for the popularity of "high-index" materials.

        (2)   The volume of material in the lens is reduced accordingly in the higher-index lens.

   b.   Specific gravity (density) is the weight per cubic centimeter.

        (1)   The weight of a lens depends upon the volume of the lens and the specific gravity.

        (2)   Although a high-index lens has less volume, it may not be lighter in weight than a lower-index lens if the density of the high-index lens is significantly larger than the density of the lower-index lens.

   c.   Abbe value is a measure of the amount of chromatic aberration which is evident in a lens (see discussion of Abbe value in "Light within an optical material" and chromatic aberration in "Aberrations" in Appendix 1, I.E.5).

        (1)   Current materials for ophthalmic lenses have Abbe values ranging from about 30 to 60.

        (2)   A high Abbe value, in the 50s, indicates that the lens will have little chromatic aberration.

        (3)   A low Abbe value, in the 30s, indicates that the lens will have relatively large chromatic aberration.

   d.   Table 8-3 lists the values for index of refraction, Abbe value, and specific gravity of several of the lens materials which are currently available.

Table 8-3. Optical Characteristics of Commonly Available Ophthalmic Lens Materials

Lens Material/ Trade Name	Index Refraction (see note 1)	Abbe Value (see note 2)	Specific Gravity/Weight (see note 3)	Approx. Transmission at 380 nm (see note 4)
CR-39 plastic	1.498	57.8	1.32	43%
Crown glass	1.523	58.5	2.54	87%
Spectralite	1.537	47.0	1.21	15%
HI—RI plastic	1.556	37.7	1.22	59%
High X plastic	1.565	36.0	1.17	1%
Polycarbonate	1.586	30.0	1.20	1%
1.6 index plastic	1.596	36.0	1.34	1%
1.66 BI-concave	1.660	32.0	1.35	1%
1.7 index glass	1.701	30.8	2.99	57%
1.8 index glass	1.805	25.4	3.39	72%

NOTE 1—The HIGHER the number, the THINNER the lens for equal power. (Polycarbonate may be surfaced to 1.5 center thickness and both polycarbonate and high-index 1.6 plastic are available in finished at 1.5 C.T.; this reduced C.T. further reduces edge thickness on minus powered lenses.)

NOTE 2—The LOWER the number, the GREATER the image distortion away from the center of the lens (chromatic aberration). Put another way, because ALL powered lenses have this property, the lower the number, the closer to the center of the lens noticeable distortion will occur. Further, the higher the power, the more noticeable this becomes.

NOTE 3—Weight compared to an equal volume of water (with a value of 1.00). The HIGHER the number, the HEAVIER the material. (NOTE: Because higher index materials use flatter base curves to achieve equal powers, they will be thinner and therefore contain less material. Even if the specific gravity of two lenses were equal, for equal powers, the lens with the higher index of refraction will weigh less.)

NOTE 4— UV radiation is recognized by ANSI to be radiation up to 380 nm. This figure shows the relative effect of various lenses on blocking UV. The LOWER the number, the more effective the lens material.

Used by permission of Walman Optical Company.

2. Glass was the first material used for ophthalmic lenses and is still used for a substantial number of lenses because of its scratch resistance.
   (1) Ophthalmic crown glass is used for most glass single-vision lenses.
      (a) It is also used for most glass progressive addition lenses and for the distance lens portion of most glass bifocals and trifocals.
      (b) The major ingredients of ophthalmic crown glass are silica, sodium oxide, and calcium oxide.
      (c) Its index of refraction, 1.523, is the standard for comparing other materials.
      (d) The Abbe value is high.
   (2) Barium crown glass is used for segments in some fused bifocals.
      (a) The name is derived from the significant amount of barium oxide in the glass.
      (b) The Abbe value is high.
   (3) Flint glass is also used for segments in fused bifocals.
      (a) Lead oxide is a principal component of flint glass.
      (b) Abbe value is low, so chromatic aberration is greater.
   (4) High-index glass of 1.60, 1.70, and 1.80 is available for high-power lenses.
      (a) Titanium oxide is a principal component in these glasses.
      (b) The density is generally very high, so for lower powers the lens is heavier in these materials than in an ophthalmic crown lens, even though the higher-index lenses are thinner.
      (c) In powers above approximately 6-8D, the high-index glass lenses are lighter than ophthalmic crown lenses. (see Section IV.G.5)
      (d) Abbe values are generally low.
b. In the 1970s plastic lenses (hard resin) gained in popularity because of their light weight.
   (1) CR-39®, chemically known as allyl diglycol carbonate, is the trade name of Pittsburgh Plate Glass Industries.
      (a) Hard resin is a term used to refer to this material; it is sometimes used to refer to plastics in general.
      (b) The index of refraction is slightly less than ophthalmic crown, so hard resin lenses are thicker than glass lenses.
      (c) The density is approximately half that of ophthalmic crown, so hard resin lenses are lighter for all powers.
      (d) Abbe value is high.
   (2) Polycarbonate is a high-index plastic which has excellent impact resistance.
      (a) The density is very low, lower than that of hard resin, so polycarbonate lenses of all powers are not only thinner but also lighter than hard resin lenses.
      (b) Abbe value is very low, so chromatic aberration is great.
   (3) Other high-index plastics are available.
      (a) The specific gravities are generally slightly higher than for hard resin.
      (b) Abbe values are generally low.

B. *Impact resistance*
1. The Food and Drug Administration requires that dress ophthalmic lenses be sufficiently impact resistant to pass a drop ball test as specified by ANSI Z80.1-1987.
  a. ANSI Z80.1 is a Federal standard for ophthalmic lenses used for dress wear, most recently revised in 1987; Z87.1-1989 applies to safety lenses used for occupational safety.
  b. The drop ball test consists of dropping a ⅝-inch diameter steel ball weighing 16g (0.56 ounces) onto the convex surface of the lens from a height of 50 inches.

2. In order to pass the drop ball test, glass lenses must be treated.
   a. Heat treatment (thermal tempering) is one way to increase the impact resistance of a glass lens.
      (1) The lens is heated to close to softening (about 650°C), which causes the surface to expand.
      (2) The lens is rapidly cooled with a sudden blast of air, which solidifies the surface.
      (3) As the interior of the lens cools more slowly, it shrinks, placing the surface under tension and creating a layer of surface compression approximately 600 μm thick.
      (4) Heat-tempered glass is approximately 2–3× more impact resistant than untempered glass.
      (5) A few lenses are treated at a time; the process takes approximately 5–10 minutes depending on lens power and thickness.
      (6) Heat tempering was the first method for tempering lens, but now it has been largely replaced in large-scale laboratories by chemical tempering.
   b. Chemical tempering involves placing the lens in a molten chemical bath.
      (1) For ophthalmic crown glass, the bath is potassium nitrate heated to about 450°C.
         (a) This is much cooler than heat tempering and warpage is much less likely.
         (b) For other types of glass, other ionic baths may be used, such as sodium nitrate and potassium nitrate for photochromic glass.
      (2) Sodium ions in the surface of the lens are replaced by larger potassium ions in the bath.
      (3) The forcing of larger ions into the surface forms a layer of compression at the surface about 75 mm thick.
      (4) Chemically tempered glass is 7–10× more impact resistant than untempered glass.
         (a) Minimum thickness of lenses can be made smaller.
         (b) Typical minimum thickness is 1.8 mm compared to 2.0 mm for a thermally hardened lens.
      (5) The process takes several hours, much longer than heat tempering, but several hundred lenses can be done at one time in the larger units.
   c. Anything which pierces the compression layer of a tempered glass lens, whether heat or chemical, will significantly reduce the impact resistance.
      (1) Scratches affect both, but chemically hardened lenses are affected more.
      (2) Edging a tempered lens destroys the compression layer.
         (a) A heat-tempered lens may shatter; it should be heated to remove the compression before reedging and then retempered after edging.
         (b) A chemically treated lens can be edged but must be retempered afterwards.
3. Hard resin lenses (with no additional impact resistance treatment) have approximately the same impact resistance as chemically hardened glass lenses.
   a. Chemically tempered lenses tend to be more resistant to large-mass, low-velocity missiles.
   b. Hard resin tends to be more resistant to small-mass, high-velocity, sharply pointed objects.
4. Polycarbonate (PC) has approximately 10–20× more impact resistance than untreated glass, making it the material of choice when the greatest impact resistance is desired.
   a. PC should be considered for active children, for protection of the good eye for a monocular patient for athletics, and for industrial safety glasses.

b. Patients in occupations in which scratching is likely, such as auto mechanics and farmers, often reject polycarbonate lenses after trying them once because of the low scratch resistance compared to glass.

5. Glass lenses have superior scratch resistance, followed by hard resin; polycarbonate has the poorest scratch resistance of the more commonly used materials.

IV. Single-Vision Lenses

A. *Uses*

1. A single-vision lens has only one power, either spherical or sphero-cylindrical, in contrast to a multifocal lens, which has more than one power.
2. The power of the lens is dependent on its use.
   a. The lens power may correct the patient for distance vision.
      (1) If the patient has sufficient accommodation, near tasks can be seen clearly while wearing the glasses.
      (2) If the patient does not have sufficient accommodation for near work, the glasses are essentially for distance only.
   b. The lens power may be the algebraic sum of the distance Rx and the required add to provide a single-vision, reading-only Rx or an occupational/avocational lens for an intermediate distance.

B. *Decentration*

1. The major reference point (MRP) is the point in the lens which has the proper refractive power and proper amount of prism as specified in the prescription (Figure 8-7).

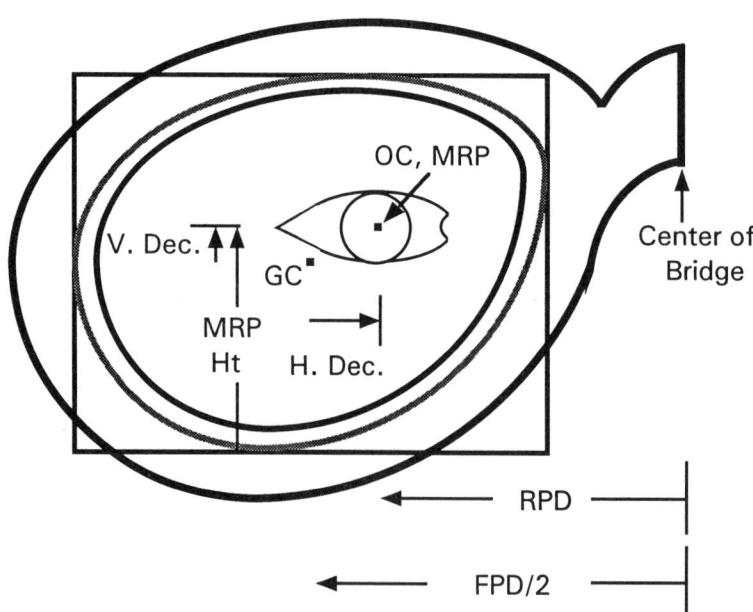

Figure 8-7. Elements of decentration are shown for a right lens for which the MRP (major reference point) is at the OC (optical center), both of which are at the eye. The rectangle is the box tangent to the extreme points on the lens bevel (hatched line). The MRP is located at the RPD (right monocular PD); MRP Ht is the distance from the lowest edge of the lens to the MRP. FPD/2, half the frame PD, is the distance from the center of the bridge to the GC. The vertical decentration (V.Dec) is the vertical distance from the GC to the OC; horizontal decentration (H.Dec) is the horizontal distance from the GC to the OC.

2. Most prescriptions specify zero prism, which occurs when the lens is positioned so the line of sight passes through the optical center (OC) of the lens.
   a. The OC is the MRP in this case.
   b. If the patient's PD equals the frame PD (PPD = FPD), zero prism results when the OC of the lens is at the GC of the frame.
   c. The eyesizes of most frames are large enough, however, that the frame PD is larger than the patient's PD.
      (1) The OC must be moved from the GC of the frame to the patient's line of sight for zero prism.
      (2) The distance from the GC to the OC is termed decentration.
         (a) The decentration required to place the OC of the lens at the patient's line of sight is: Decentration = (FPD − PPD)/2.
         (b) This expression for decentration assumes the eyes are symmetrically placed about the center of the bridge of the nose (equal monocular PDs).
         (c) If the monocular PDs are unequal, decentration must be calculated separately for each eye: Decentration = (FPD/2) − Monocular PD.
         (d) For example if the frame has A = 50, DBL = 20, and the patient's left and right monocular PDs are 33 and 31, respectively, the decentrations are calculated separately.
            i. The frame PD is 50 + 20 = 70 mm.
            ii. Decentration for the right lens is (70/2) − 33 = 2 mm in.
            iii. Decentration for the left lens is (70/2) − 31 = 4 mm in.
            iv. If the total PD is used, the decentration for each lens is (FPD − PPD)/2 = (70 − 64)/2 = 3 mm in.
            v. The use of total PD instead of monocular PD's may have significant effects in higher lens powers.
      (3) Maximum decentration (Max Dec) depends upon the size of the lens blank (blank diameter, BD) from which the lens is to be cut and the effective diameter (ED) of the lens.
         (a) Max Dec = (BD − ED)/2.
         (b) The minimum blank diameter (MBD) required for a particular decentration is given by: MBD = ED + 2(Dec).
         (c) Blank diameters available vary with the type of lens and manufacturer, with the more commonly used lens powers and materials available in greater numbers of blank diameters.
   d. The vertical position of the OC (or more generally the MRP) can also be specified.
      (1) The distance from the lowest point on the bevel of the lens (bottom side of the "box") to the OC (or MRP) can be specified as the "MRP level" or MRP height.
      (2) Alternatively the distance from the GC (at the vertical midpoint of the frame) to the OC (or MRP) can be used to specify a vertical decentration: Vert Dec = MRP level − B/2, where B is the vertical dimension of the frame.
      (3) If the OC is placed at the level of the line of sight, zero vertical prism results, but this is not the position for best off-axis lens performance.
      (4) If no vertical position is specified, the laboratory will place the OC at the vertical level of the GC, the vertical midpoint of the lens (B/2).
3. If prism is specified in the prescription, the OC is not the MRP and will not be located at the line of sight (Appendix 1.V).

C. *Lens thickness*
   1. Lens thickness is important in the design of any lens.
      a. It is usually preferable to have the lens as thin as possible in order to reduce the bulk of the lens, reduce its weight, and improve its cosmetic appearance.

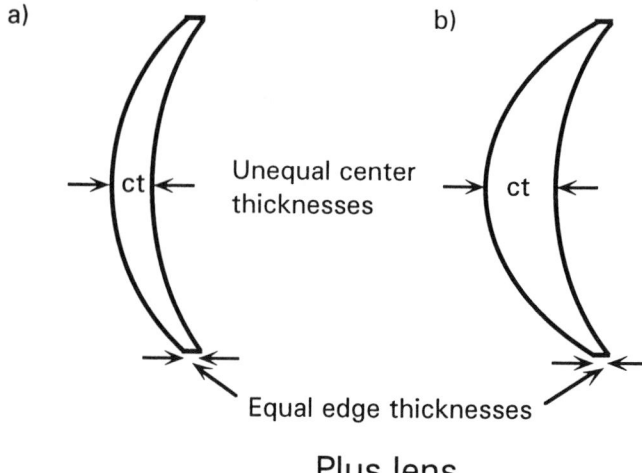

Plus lens

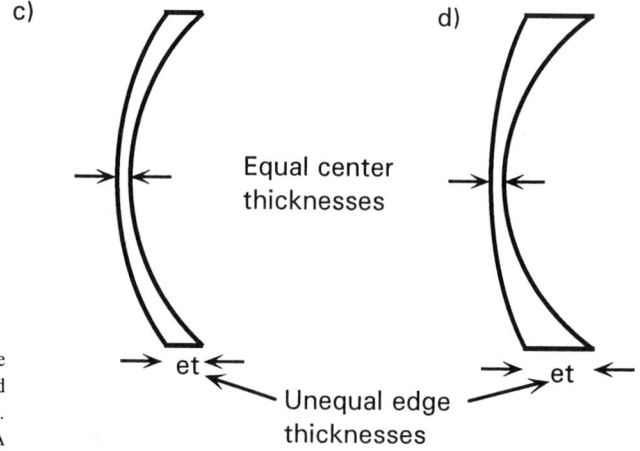

Figure 8-8. (a) A plus lens has a larger center thickness than edge thickness. (b) A stronger plus lens having the same edge thickness and diameter as the first has a larger center thickness than the weaker lens. (c) A minus lens has a larger edge thickness than center thickness. (d) A stronger minus lens having the same center thickness and diameter as the first minus lens has a larger edge thickness than the first.

Minus Lens

    b.   In addition to these considerations, the center thickness of a lens affects the power of the lens and its magnification.

2.   For a plus lens the thickness is greatest at the center (OC) and smallest at the edge (Figure 8-8a and 8-8b).

    a.   The edge of a plus lens, its weakest part, must be kept thick enough to permit the lens to pass the drop ball test.

       (1)   For low plus lenses the minimum edge thickness might be 1.8 mm, while for high plus lenses it might be reduced to 1.0 mm to shave as much thickness as possible off the lens.

       (2)   In general, however, this change in the minimum thickness at the edge of a plus lens is fairly small compared to the changes in center thickness which occur from lens to lens.

          (a)   For a given lens power and diameter, the center thickness will vary considerably according to the lens material.

          (b)   An advantage of a high-index lens is that the surface curvatures are flatter and the center thickness is reduced.

    b. When the OC of a plus lens is decentered from the GC, the thinnest part of the
        edge is farthest from the OC.
        (1) In the usual case of the OC decentered in, the temporal edge of the lens is
             thinnest, and the nasal edge is thickest.
        (2) If too much decentration is required, a larger blank size is necessary,
             resulting in a larger center thickness and a heavier lens.
3. For a minus lens the thickness is greatest at the edge and thinnest at the center (OC)
    (Figures 8-8c and 8-8d).
    a. The center thickness is generally kept constant for various minus lens powers
        and diameters, thick enough to pass the drop ball test.
        (1) For most lenses, the minimum center thickness is 2.0 mm.
        (2) Some PC lenses are made with center thicknesses of 1.5 mm ("polythin")
             and 1.0 mm to reduce edge thickness.
    b. The thickest part of the edge is farthest from the OC; when a minus lens is
        decentered in, the temporal edge is thicker than the nasal edge.
4. The relationships between center thickness CT (at the OC) and edge thickness ET of a
    lens which were just discussed are summarized in the following first-order equation:
    $ET = CT + (Fh^2)/2(n - 1)$ where F is the approximate power in the meridian of
    interest, h is the distance from the optical center to the edge, and n is the index of
    refraction of the lens.
5. For a spherocylinder, the edge thickness changes around the perimeter of the lens not
    only due to the varying distance from the OC of the lens but also because of the
    changing power from one meridian to another.
    a. For the purposes of thickness, a simple cylinder having a power F_C can be
        considered to contribute a "power" F_θ in an oblique meridian θ degrees from the
        cylinder axis: $F_\theta = F_C\sin^2 \theta$.
    b. The total power F used in 4. above is the sum of the sphere F_S and cylinder power
        contribution in the meridian of interest: $F = F_S + F_\theta$

D. *MRP position*
    1. The MRP is placed at the monocular PD for each lens so it is centered laterally at the
        pupil center.
    2. If there were no other considerations, the MRP would likewise be located vertically at
        the pupil centers.
        a. When lenses are designed to reduce aberrations, however, they are designed to
            provide best image quality when the optic axis of the lens passes through the
            center of rotation of the eye.
        b. If the frame held the spectacle lenses in a vertical plane, the optic axis would pass
            through the center of rotation when the OC is in front of the pupil.
        c. However, the fronts of modern frames are tilted so the bottom of the lens is held
            closer to the cheeks than the top.
            (1) The optic axis is tilted away from horizontal.
            (2) This is termed positive pantoscopic angle or tilt.
        d. For each 2° of positive pantoscopic tilt, the OC should be lowered 1 mm from the
            center of the pupil so the optic axis will pass through the center of rotation.

E. *Base curve selection*
    1. The lens power required in the prescription can be provided in a countless number of
        combinations of lens shapes (Appendix 1.III.C); however, the quality of the image
        when the periphery of the lens is used varies considerably from one shape to another.
        a. The best shape for low and moderately powered ophthalmic lenses is the
            meniscus form, with the concave surface toward the eye.
        b. For higher-powered plus lenses, the best shape becomes plano convex with the
            plane surface toward the eye, while for higher-powered minus lenses, the plano
            concave shape with the concave surface gives better performance.

      c. For very high powers, a biconvex form (for plus) or biconcave (for minus) is sometimes used for best optics, with the more concave (or less convex) surface toward the eye.

      d. Whatever its shape, an ophthalmic lens performs better optically with the more concave (or less convex) surface toward the eye.

      e. The meniscus lens form has a mechanical advantage apart from the optics: having a concave surface toward the eye provides more clearance for the eyelashes.

2. It is impossible to design a single lens for which all aberrations are corrected for all viewing distances, for all angles of viewing through the lens, and for all stop distances (rear surface of lens to center of rotation of the eye).

      a. Priorities are set in lens design to reduce the aberrations that cause the most image degradation.

      b. In the early twentieth century, lens manufacturers aimed to improve image quality either by eliminating one of the aberrations (e.g., oblique astigmatism) or by reducing several of the aberrations to tolerable levels for a particular viewing distance, viewing angle, and stop distance.

      c. Later in the century, computers made it possible to minimize the focus error for several working distances, stop distances, and viewing angles in the lens design.

3. Lens designs result in base curve selection charts that group lens powers together with the base curve best suited to minimize focus error.

      a. The base curve determines the shape of the lens; the calculations for all other curves are based upon it.

      b. Although a different base curve might produce absolutely the best image for each different lens power, it is not economically feasible to produce and stock such a vast array of base curves.

      c. Instead an assumption is made about the maximum focus error which can be tolerated in the lens, and a base curve is assigned to a group of lens powers for which that shape will produce focus errors smaller than the tolerance level.

          (1) The focus error tolerance might be on the order of $0.01 - 0.1D$.

          (2) Steep base curves are difficult to mount in frames, so the base curve may be modified slightly from that which is the most desirable optically, especially if the frame is metal.

4. ANSI Z80.1-1987 for ophthalmic lenses does not require that lenses meet any particular standard for off-axis performance; that is, the finishing laboratory is not required to provide any particular base curve to the optometrist unless it is specifically requested.

      a. The optometrist has the responsibility to be sure that the lens ordered will provide a quality image both on and off axis.

      b. The optometrist has several options to ensure that an appropriate base curve is used.

          (1) The Rx can be ordered from a laboratory that uses semifinished lens blanks from a reputable lens manufacturer that provides base curve selection charts for the laboratory to follow.

          (2) Alternatively, the base curve can be specified by the optometrist using charts published by lens manufacturers or using charts published in the literature.

              (a) Fry[1] has provided a chart of recommended base curves for lenses made of ophthalmic crown glass (summarized in Table 8-4).

              (b) Davis[2] has published charts of recommended base curves for lenses made of hard resin and PC, with separate charts for three different stop distances.

5. The base curve may be modified from that recommended by lens selection charts to meet other goals, such as controlling spectacle magnification.

Table 8-4. Recommended Base Curves for Glass Lenses (adapted from Fry GA. The optometrist's role in the use of corrected curve lenses.

Lens Power (spherical equivalent)	Base Curve
> + 6.40D	+12.50D
+ 4.39–+6.40D	+10.50D
+ 1.45–+4.39D	+ 8.50D
− 2.11–+1.45D	+ 6.50D
− 5.88–−2.11D	+ 4.50D
−10.50–−5.88D	+ 2.50D
> −10.50D	+ 0.50D

Source: J Am Optom Assoc 1979; 50:561–562.

F. *Lens-induced phorias*
1. When phorias are measured through lenses with the eyes viewing away from the OCs of the lenses, the net resultant prism induced through the lenses will change the phoria from its true value.
    a. Net resultant base out (BO) prism, while used to correct eso, creates exo; that is, the phoria through BO prism will be increased in the exo direction (or less eso).
    b. Net resultant base in (BI) prism, while used to correct exo, creates eso; that is, the phoria through BI prism will be increased in the eso direction (or less exo).
    c. Net resultant base up (BU) prism, while used to correct a hypo deviation, creates a hyper; that is, the phoria through BU prism will be increased in the hyper direction (or less hypo) for the eye before which the BU prism is held.
    d. Net resultant base down (BD) prism, while used to correct a hyper deviation, creates a hypo; that is, the phoria through BD prism will be increased in the hypo direction (or less hyper) for the eye before which the BD prism is held.
    e. Net vertical prism will not occur when the power in the vertical meridian is the same in both lenses, unless the eyes are at different levels as during a head tilt, hyperorbit, or nonleveled lenses.
2. Phorias induced by off-center lenses occur when testing is done through lenses in the phoropter which are not centered in front of the patient's eyes.

G. *High-plus lenses*
1. High-plus lenses, required to correct high amounts of hyperopia and aphakia, present special problems in lens design.
    a. Center thickness increases significantly in high-plus lenses, resulting in several undesirable side effects.
        (1) The shape factor of spectacle magnification (see Appendix 1) increases with increased center thickness, adding to the magnification from the power factor due to the plus power.
            (a) Everything appears enlarged to the patient; while this is usually considered a disadvantage, it can help improve visual acuity for visually impaired patients.
            (b) The patient's face and eyes appear enlarged through the lenses to an observer.
        (2) The increased lens volume which accompanies increased center thickness causes increased weight, a major problem of high-plus lenses.
    b. A rather large prism effect exists at the edge of a high-plus lens.
        (1) The prism effect at the edge of a plus lens has its base oriented toward the optic axis of the lens.
            (a) Images seen through the periphery of the lens are displaced more peripherally than the corresponding objects (Figure 8-9).

230   Ophthalmic Optics

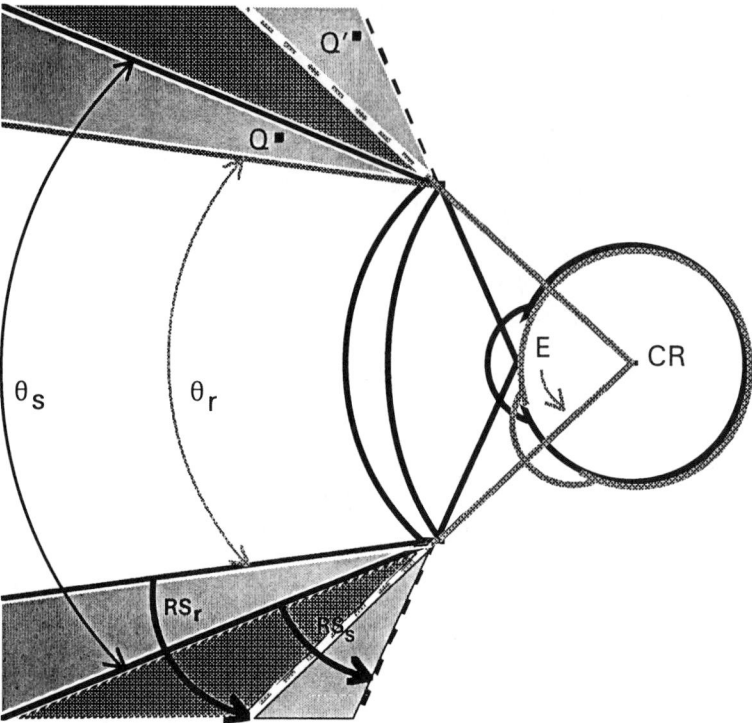

Figure 8-9.   Field of view through a plus lens. With the eye stationary (solid lines), rays from the periphery of the lens enter the center of the entrance pupil E, the field of view through the lens is θ_s, and a ring scotoma RS_s exists around the periphery of the lens. If the eye rotates behind the lens (hatched lines), rays from the periphery pass through the center of rotation of the eye CR, the field of view is θ_r, and a ring scotoma is present which is less peripheral than that for the stationary eye.

        (b)   An image Q′ seen through the edge of the lens corresponds to an object Q located closer to straight ahead.

        (c)   Objects seen outside the periphery of the lens remain unchanged in location.

    (2)   The prism effect causes several adaptations for the patient.

        (a)   The field of view through the lens is smaller than if the lens were not there because the prism moves the image peripherally.

            i.   The size of the field of view through the lens depends upon whether the eye is stationary or rotating.

           ii.   When the eye is stationary, the entrance pupil E is the reference point for the field of view, and the field of view is θ_s.

          iii.   With the eye rotated to point the fovea at the object, the center of rotation CR is the reference point for the field of view, and the field of view is θ_r.

          iv.   As shown in Figure 8-9, $\theta_s > \theta_r$.

           v.   An object Q that lies within the stationary field of view but not in the rotating field of view is seen peripherally with the stationary eye but disappears when the eye rotates to view it foveally.

          vi.   This phenomenon of an object seeming to appear and disappear with eye movement is known as the jack-in-the-box phenomenon.

        (b)   A ring scotoma exists around the periphery of the lens.

           (i)   Objects located within the scotoma are not visible either through the lens or around it.

        (ii)   The location of the ring scotoma is more peripheral for the stationary eye than for the rotated eye, though there is some overlap (darker hatched area in Figure 8-9).

    (c)   As the head rotates, the objects hidden in the scotoma suddenly jump into view either through the lens or around it, contributing to the jack-in-the-box effect.

  c.   The patient experiences a "swimming" sensation when the head rotates due to the BI prism effect of the plus lens increasing the speed with which objects seem to move in the direction opposite to the head movement.

  d.   The eyes must rotate more when looking at a peripheral object through the plus lens than without the lens due to the BI prism.

  e.   Significant BO prism can be induced when the patient reads with the lines of sight inside the OCs of the lens, resulting in increased convergence demand.

  f.   The effects of aberrations are exacerbated in high-powered lenses; aberrations such as spherical aberration and distortion, which are not as important in low powers, cause significant image degradation in high powers.

  g.   The highly curved front surface acts as a convex mirror reflecting images from a wide field.

2.   The optometrist can assist the patient greatly by carefully designing the plus lens and frame to meet the following criteria:

  a.   Center thickness should be as small as possible to reduce both weight and spectacle magnification.

  b.   Vertex distance should be as small as possible to decrease spectacle magnification and increase field of view.

  c.   Aberrations should be minimized.

3.   These specific guidelines should be followed for frame selection and fitting.

  a.   Frame should be small and symmetrical.

    (1)   FPD ≤ PPD + 2 mm.

        (a)   A small frame minimizes decentration.

        (b)   This in turn reduces the required lens blank diameter, decreases center thickness, and reduces peripheral prism effects.

    (2)   ED ≤ A + 2 mm.

        (a)   A symmetrical lens should be used, avoiding pilot shapes.

        (b)   This helps reduce required blank diameter, thereby decreasing center thickness.

    (3)   The guidelines above, referred to as the MED principle (minimum effective diameter), are illustrated in Figure 8-10.

  b.   The frame should allow as short a vertex distance as possible to reduce spectacle magnification.

  c.   The frame should have pantoscopic tilt to help reduce vertex distance.

  d.   It is especially important that the OC of the lens be placed 1 mm below the pupil center for every 2° of pantoscopic tilt.

    (1)   Optical performance will be optimized; the image degrades quickly if the vertical position of the OC is not properly specified.

    (2)   Ideally the frame should fit so the pupil center is 3–4 mm above the GC so the OC can be placed very near the GC to minimize vertical decentration and yet satisfy the OC-pupil relationship.

4.   Several different lens forms are available for high plus to reduce center thickness and decrease prism effects at the edge.

  a.   A full field aspheric lens has a front surface that is aspherical rather than spherical.

    (1)   An aspheric surface becomes flatter toward the periphery.

        (a)   The radius of curvature gradually increases from the center to the edge of the lens.

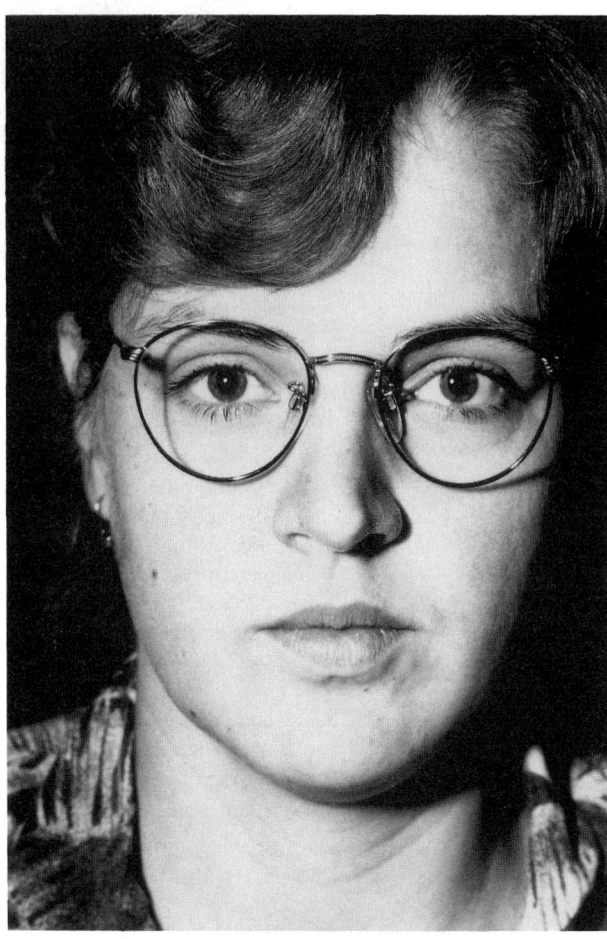

Figure 8-10.   A frame to be used with high-plus lenses should be small and symmetrical so the eyes are close to the geometrical center of the lens and little decentration is necessary.

        (b)   The number of diopters of change in surface power from center to edge is often denoted by "drop"; "4 drop" indicates the power of the front surface is 4.00 D less plus at the edge than at the center.

        (c)   Aspheric surfaces are usually made of several annuli of different radii of curvature which are blended together so the transition areas are invisible.

        (d)   Some aspheric surfaces are part of a conic section, such as an ellipse or a parabola.

    (2)   Full field implies that the surface power extends across the entire lens surface, distinguishing it from some of the other lens types to be described.

    (3)   Advantages

        (a)   Decreased center thickness with accompanying decrease in SM.

        (b)   Decreased weight.

        (c)   Decreased peripheral aberrations.

        (d)   Decreased peripheral prism effects (less power in periphery).

        (e)   Decreased adaptation problems.

        (f)   Improved cosmesis.

        (g)   Wider useful field of view.

    (4)   Disadvantage—increased cost.

    (5)   Aspherics should be considered for lenses in the 4.00–8.00D range and are definitely the lens of choice for powers greater than +8.00D.

       (6)   High-index aspherics are also available (e.g., PC and 1.6 plastic); the high index reduces the center thickness even further.

       (7)   The vast majority of aspherics are plastic; glass aspherics are rare.

   b.   A lenticular lens has a central optical zone ("bowl") with the prescribed power surrounded by a much thinner carrier portion having much less power (e.g., plano).

       (1)   The carrier portion is not useful for viewing; its purpose is to allow the high-plus portion to have a smaller diameter.

       (2)   The diameter of the optical zone is commonly 40 mm, but some manufacturers decrease the bowl size with increasing power.

       (3)   The front surface of the optical zone may be spherical or aspherical (aspheric lenticular).

       (4)   Advantages

          (a)   Center thickness is reduced, resulting in less weight and less spectacle magnification (SM).

          (b)   Diameter is reduced, resulting in smaller peripheral prism effects.

       (5)   Disadvantages

          (a)   Cosmesis is poor due to the obvious appearance of the bowl.

          (b)   Field of view is reduced because of small optic zone diameter.

          (c)   The ring scotoma is closer to the center of the field.

   c.   In a blended lenticular lens, the junction between the optical zone and the carrier is blurred so it is much less visible.

       (1)   The optical zone may be either spheric or aspheric.

       (2)   The characteristics are the same as for the lenticular lens except the cosmesis is markedly improved.

5.   High-index materials are advantageous for high-plus lenses because the center thickness is reduced; however, the lens may be heavier depending upon the material used.

   a.   Virtually all high-index plastics have specific gravities very close to or significantly less than that of CR-39®.

       (1)   Lenses made of high-index plastics will be thinner and usually lighter (or at least no heavier) than CR-39® lenses.

       (2)   They will always be both thinner and lighter than ophthalmic crown lenses.

       (3)   Table 8-5 shows a comparison of center thicknesses and weight for lenses of various plus powers made from several lens materials, the characteristics of which are listed in Table 8-3.

   b.   All high-index glasses, however, have significantly larger specific gravities than either hard resin or ophthalmic crown glass.

       (1)   Even though lenses made of high-index glass will be thinner than hard resin lenses, they will be significantly heavier for all powers.

       (2)   High-index glass lenses will always be thinner than ophthalmic crown lenses, but will be heavier than ophthalmic crown lenses for lens powers less than +6.00D (for 1.7 index lenses) and for lens powers less than +8.00D (for 1.8 index lenses).

6.   In the past, aspheric surfaces have been used for high-plus (e.g., greater than +7.00D), but recently several lens designs have been produced for low-plus as well.

   a.   The use of aspheric surfaces allows flatter base curves to be used for low-plus lenses without sacrificing quality of the optical image.

   b.   Flatter base curves result in thinner lenses and more pleasing cosmetic appearance.

   c.   In high-index lenses, where chromatic aberration can be troublesome, the overall image quality is improved through aspheric surfaces, by correcting or reducing marginal astigmatism and curvature of field.

       (1)   Since chromatic aberration is principally a tangential aberration, the overall blur in the lens is reduced in the tangential meridian if the tangential power error is reduced to zero through the aspheric surface.

Table 8-5.   Thickness and Weight Comparisons for Plus and Minus Lenses Made of Various Materials

Power	Edge Center Thickness (ET)/(CT) Weight (WT)	CR-39	Crown Glass	Spectralite	HIRI	High X	Polycarb	PolyThin	1.6 Hyper-Index Plastic	1.66 Bi-Concave Aspheric	1.7 Glass	1.8 Glass
−18	ET	—	—	—	25.5	26.5	23.1	22.6	21.9	15.1	16.1	13.6
	WT	—	—	—	78.3	75.1	72.7	69.3	78.9	64.0	144.3	143.6
−14	ET	18.5	17.1	17.0	15.7	15.7	15.0	14.5	14.6	12.0	12.0	10.5
	WT	70.2	128.0	60.3	57.7	55.0	54.5	51.1	59.8	52.8	115.1	117.2
−10	ET	12.1	11.5	11.3	10.8	10.7	10.4	9.9	10.2	9.0	9.1	8.1
	WT	51.0	94.4	44.4	43.2	41.1	41.1	37.7	45.3	41.8	91.7	95.0
−6	ET	7.9	7.6	7.3	7.2	7.2	6.9	6.4	6.7	—	6.2	5.5
	WT	36.3	67.7	31.5	31.3	29.7	29.9	26.5	32.6	—	68.4	71.5
−2	ET	4.0	3.9	3.8	3.7	3.7	3.7	3.2	3.5	—	3.4	3.2
	WT	22.1	41.8	19.6	19.5	18.8	19.1	15.7	20.9	—	45.4	49.7
Plano	ET/CT	2.0	2.0	2.0	2.0	2.0	2.0	1.5	2.0	—	2.0	2.0
	WT	14.8	28.4	13.8	13.6	13.0	13.4	10.3	15.1	—	33.6	38.1
+2	CT	3.7	3.6	3.5	3.5	3.4	3.4	—	3.3	—	—	2.9
	WT	20.5	38.8	18.4	18.2	17.4	17.7	—	19.5	—	—	45.5
+6	CT	7.3	6.9	6.6	6.4	6.3	6.3	—	6.0	—	—	4.9
	WT	33.6	61.9	28.0	27.3	26.0	26.9	—	28.1	—	—	61.3
+10	CT	10.7	10.3	—	—	—	8.9	—	8.7	—	—	6.9
	WT	46.1	85.2	—	—	—	34.4	—	37.5	—	—	78.1
+14	CT	14.9	14.2	—	—	—	—	—	—	—	—	9.0
	WT	64.2	117.5	—	—	—	—	—	—	—	—	98.4
+18	CT	19.5	18.7	—	—	—	—	—	—	—	—	11.3
	WT	86.0	160.0	—	—	—	—	—	—	—	—	123.7

Edge (ET) and center (CT) thickness in mm. Weight (WT) in g/pair (28.35 g = 1 oz). Calculations based upon a 60-mm round lens.
Minus Rx calculations at 2.0 center thickness; Poly-thin at 1.5 mm.
Plus Rx calculations based upon following minimum edge thickness: +2.00D at 1.8 mm; +6.00 at 1.4 mm; +10.00 and above at 1.0 mm.
Where boxes are blank, appropriate front bases curves are not currently available.
Used by permission of Walman Optical Company.

     (2)   The ASL™ Aspheric lenses in PC and in Spectralite™ by Sola and the Cosmolit™ lens in hard resin by Rodenstock are examples of aspheric lenses available in low-plus powers.

     (3)   Table 8-6 lists many of the aspheric lenses available together with their characteristics, while Table 8-7 shows comparative weight and thickness data for several powers.

  7.   Antireflection coatings effectively reduce the reflections from the front surface.

Table 8-6.   Characteristics of Aspheric Lenses

Name/Manufacturer	Material/Design	Index of Refraction	Power Range
ASL™ Polycarbonate/Sola Optical	Polycarbonate/aspheric	1.586	−10.00D to +4.00D
Aspheric Profile®/Gentex	Polycarbonate/aspheric	1.586	+3.00D to +8.00D
Bristolite™/Bristolite Consulting & Development, Inc.	Plastic/semi-aspheric	1.498	+2.00 to +10.00D
Cosmolit™/Rodenstock	Plastic/aspheric	1.500	Pl to +12.00D
Hyperal™/Silor	Plastic/aspheric	1.498	Pl to +9.00D
Hyper Aspheric 1.6/Optima	Plastic/aspheric	1.597	−15.00D to +10.00D
RLX-Lite/Signet Armorlite	Plastic/aspheric	1.560	+0.50 to +8.50D
ASL Spectralite™/Sola Optical	Plastic/aspheric	1.537	−8.00 to +6.00D

Modified from *Listing of Aspheric Lenses* by Walman Optical Company.

H.   *High-minus lenses*
   1.   High-minus lenses used to correct high amounts of myopia also present special problems.
      a.   Edge thickness increases significantly in high-minus lenses.
         (1)   The large edge thicknesses are distressing to the patient because they call attention to his/her "eye problem."

Table 8-7.   Center Thickness (CT) and Weight (WT) Comparison for Aspheric Plus Lenses

Material		+2.00	+6.00	+10.00
ASL™ PC	CT	2.3	—	—
	WT	11.2		
Aspheric Profile®	CT	2.4	4.7	—
	WT	12.6	19.1	
Bristolite™	CT	2.2	5.8	9.0
	WT	10.2	25.6	37.2
Cosmolit™	CT	2.5	6.1	9.2
	WT	13.4	26.8	37.4
Hyperal™	CT	2.4	5.7	—
	WT	13.0	24.4	
Hyper Aspheric 1.6	CT	2.4	5.0	8.2
	WT	13.6	23.2	37.0
RLX-Lite	CT	2.3	5.7	—
	WT	10.8	23.6	
ASL Spectralite	CT	2.6	6.2	—
	WT	13.0	28.1	

CT in mm, WT in g/pr; based on 60-mm round lens with 1.0-mm edge thickness. Blanks indicate powers not available.
Modified from *Aspheric Thickness and Weight Comparison Plus Power* by Walman Optical Company.

      (2)   The increased lens volume which accompanies increased edge thickness causes increased weight, though not as much as for high-plus lenses.

      (3)   If the lens is decentered, the edge away from the direction of decentration becomes thicker; e.g., if the lens is decentered in, the temporal edge grows thicker.

    b.   Spectacle magnification decreases due to the minus power factor and the relatively small center thickness.

      (1)   The patient sees everything minified, reducing acuity.

      (2)   The patient's face and eyes appear smaller through the lenses to an observer.

    c.   Images of the edge which are internally reflected by the two lens surfaces cause distracting concentric rings of reflections to appear near the edge of high-minus lenses.

    d.   The prism effect at the edge of a high-minus lens has its base away from the optic axis of the lens.

      (1)   Images seen through the periphery of the lens are displaced more centrally than the corresponding objects.

      (2)   The image seen through the very edge of the lens corresponds to an object located farther away from the center of the visual field.

      (3)   Since objects seen outside the periphery of the lens are not affected by prism, the objects near the edge of the lens are overlapped by the images seen through the edge of the lens, causing a ring of diplopia around the lens.

    e.   The flat front surface (plano base curve) used for high-minus lenses acts as a plane mirror, reflecting large images approximately the size of the objects.

2.   The frame should be selected to minimize edge thickness.

    a.   Keep the eyesize small so FPD $\leq$ PPD + 2 mm to reduce decentration.

    b.   Use symmetrical shapes so that ED $\leq$ A + 2 mm and oblique dimensions are reduced.

    c.   Avoid metal frames and semirimless frames which provide little camouflage for the edge; plastic eyewires not only help conceal the edge, but also help reduce the rings of reflection.

3.   The lens should be designed to reduce or conceal edge thickness.

    a.   High-index materials allow a flatter rear surface curve.

      (1)   Flatter curves decrease edge thickness.

      (2)   Table 8-5 compares the edge thickness and weight for several minus powers.

    b.   Materials such as PC, which have high impact resistance, provide necessary impact resistance with thinner center thicknesses.

      (1)   Center thicknesses as small as 1.5 mm ("polythin"), or even 1.0 mm, can be used, further reducing edge thickness.

      (2)   Figure 8-11 shows the difference in edge thickness for a hard resin minus lens with a 2-mm center thickness (left lens) and a PC "polythin" lens of the same power (right lens).

      (3)   A side effect of increasing the index and decreasing center thickness is that the spectacle magnification is further decreased.

    c.   Edges should be rolled, meaning that the sharp edges of the edge are removed, decreasing thickness.

    d.   Hide-a-bevel should be used.

      (1)   In hide-a-bevel, the bevel is placed near the front surface of the lens rather than closer to the center.

      (2)   The bulk of the edge is positioned behind the eyewire, concealing it.

4.   Lens treatments should be used to reduce reflections.

    a.   Edge coats can help blend the edge into the eyewire, camouflaging it.

    b.   Antireflective coatings minimize the rings of reflections as well as the external reflections from the front surface.

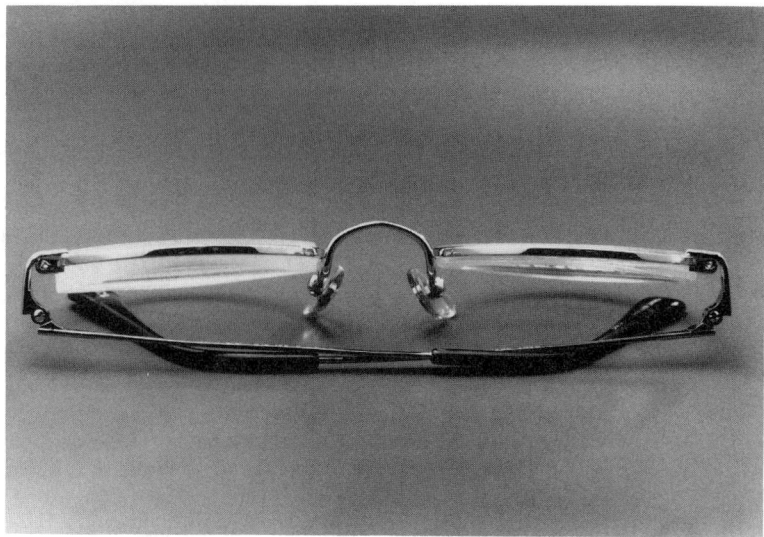

Figure 8-11.   The left lens is a hard resin minus lens with a 2-mm center thickness. The right lens, made of polycarbonate with a 1.5-mm center thickness, has significantly reduced edge thicknesses.

I. Aniseikonia
1. Ideally the sizes of the images transmitted from the retinas of the two corrected eyes to the occipital cortex should be equal (iseikonia), aside from normal differences caused by the position of an object closer to one eye than the other.
2. Aniseikonia (unequal image sizes) can be caused by several factors.
    a. Anatomical factors such as unequal receptor spacing and neural processing can cause unequal images.
    b. Optical aniseikonia is induced by the refracting components, including the components of the eye (inherent) and the spectacle or contact lenses used to correct the ametropia.
3. When anisometropia is present, the lens with the greater plus (or lesser minus) power will form a larger image, as the power and shape factors of the spectacle magnification equation predicts.
    a. The greater the vertex distance, the greater the difference between the image sizes from the correcting lenses, so a contact lens creates less difference than a spectacle lens.
    b. The fact that one spectacle image is larger than the other is not necessarily undesirable; if the retinal image for that eye when uncorrected is smaller than that for the other eye, the spectacle magnification is helpful.
        (1) In axial ametropia, the more hyperopic (or less myopic) eye forms the smaller image, so spectacle magnification is potentially helpful.
            (a) Relative spectacle magnification, which compares the corrected retinal image size to that of an emmetropic standard eye, is one when an axial ametropia is corrected with a spectacle lens in the primary focal plane of the eye (Knapp's law).
            (b) Other anatomical factors, such as receptor spacing, may change this theoretical relationship, so contact lenses may actually become the correction of choice.
        (2) In refractive ametropia, the uncorrected retinal image size is the same for all ametropias, so unequal spectacle magnification is undesirable.
            (a) Contact lenses are preferable to spectacle lenses for refractive ametropias to minimize spectacle magnification.

(b) If spectacles are necessary in refractive anisometropia, the frame should allow as short a vertex distance as possible; equal center thicknesses and equal base curves should be used to reduce differences in spectacle magnification.

4. If aniseikonia is suspected, but measurement is not possible, a clinical rule of thumb is to assume 1% aniseikonia for each diopter of anisometropia, with spectacle magnification needed in the more myopic eye.

 a. The shape of the lens not needing magnification should be changed to decrease its spectacle magnification as much as possible before increasing the magnification in the more minus eye.

 b. Increasing the center thickness increases spectacle magnification whether the lens power is plus or minus as long as the base curve is positive.

 c. To increase spectacle magnification in a plus lens, using a steeper base curve is preferred to increasing center thickness; for a minus lens, using an increased center thickness is preferred to increasing the base curve.

 d. Once a new center thickness (t_n) has been chosen, the following equation can be used to determine the new base curve (F_{1n}) needed to achieve the required correction for aniseikonia (A, expressed in terms of magnification): $F_{1n} = (n_n/t_n)[(A-1) + (t_o/n_o)F_{1o}](1/A)$ where n_n = the new index of refraction if it is changed, n_o = the original index of refraction, t_o = the original center thickness, F_{1o} = the original base curve.[3]

 (1) For example, assume a +2.00D lens made of ophthalmic crown glass has a base curve of +6.25D and a center thickness of 3.2 mm, and that in order to increase the spectacle magnification by 2% a center thickness of 5.5 mm is used.

 (2) The new base curve is $F_{1o} = (1.523/.0055)[(1.02 - 1) + (.0032/1.523)(+6.25)](1/1.02) = +8.99D = +9.00D$.

 e. An alternate method for determining the base curve and center thickness is to use the nomogram in Figure 8-12.

 (1) The nomogram has shape magnification along the left side, front curve along the right side, and center thickness diagonally across the center.

 (2) A front curve and center thickness for the lens not requiring magnification (the lens having more plus or less minus) is chosen to minimize shape magnification.

 (a) A straight edge is used to connect the front curve and center thickness.

 (b) The shape magnification for the lens is the intersection of the straight edge with the shape magnification column.

 (3) The magnification required in the more minus lens to compensate for aniseikonia is added to the shape magnification determined for the other lens to obtain the shape magnification necessary in the more minus (less plus) lens.

 (4) A straight edge is placed on the shape magnification column at the required shape magnification.

 (a) The intersection of the straight edge with the other two columns gives combinations of center thickness and front curve which provide the necessary magnification.

 (b) A combination is chosen that is practical for lens fabrication.

5. When an anisometropic minus prescription is encountered, the edge thicknesses may be considerably different.

 a. It is tempting to use a 1.0- or 1.5-mm center thickness with a high-index material such as polycarbonate or 1.6 for the more minus lens in order to make the edge thicknesses of the two lenses more comparable.

 b. However if the patient is without complaints, such a design must be used cautiously, as it will further reduce spectacle magnification on top of the reduction already attributable to power magnification in the more minus lens.

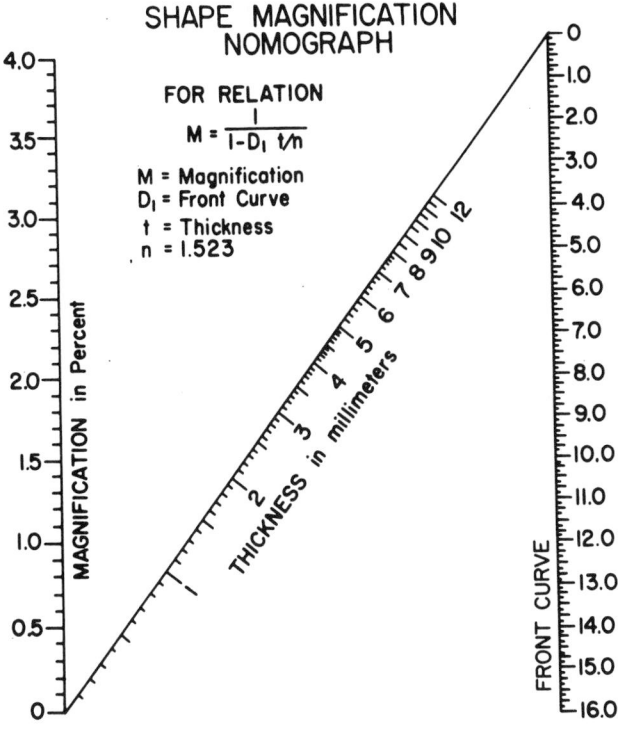

SHAPE MAGNIFICATION NOMOGRAPH

FOR RELATION

$$M = \frac{1}{1-D_1\, t/n}$$

M = Magnification
D_1 = Front Curve
t = Thickness
n = 1.523

MAGNIFICATION in Percent

THICKNESS in millimeters

FRONT CURVE

Figure 8-12.   Shape magnification nomogram. The shape magnification (left column) for a particular lens shape is found by laying a straight edge connecting the front curve (right column) and center thickness (center diagonal). The intersection of the straight edge with the left column is the shape magnification for a lens made of ophthalmic glass. (Used by permission of Polasky M. *Aniseikonia Cookbook II*. 2nd ed. Columbus: The Ohio State University, 1990.)

V. Multifocal Lenses

A. *Definition*

1. A multifocal lens has more than one power and provides the patient with the convenience of multiple powers without the necessity of more than one lens.

2. The powers may be separated with visible borders, as in traditional lined bifocals and trifocals, or they may merge gradually into one another, as in the progressive addition lens.

B. *Bifocals*

1. Bifocals consist of two powers, with the major portion of the lens usually having the power for clear distance vision and the segment portion having the power for a near task such as reading.

   a. The power through the segment is always spherical power "added" to the distance Rx and is referred to as the "add."

   b. For example, suppose the bifocal power for the right eye is written -4.50 -1.50×180 with a $+2.00D$ add (Figure 8-13, top half).

      (1) The total power for the patient when reading through the segment is $(-4.50 +2.00) -1.50 \times 180$, or $-2.50 -1.50 \times 180$.

      (2) This is the power to be written for a "reading only" Rx when a single-vision lens is provided for near work (Figure 8-13, lower half).

2. The base curve of a bifocal is the power of the distance part of the surface on the side of the segment.

   a. Since most segments are on the front surface, the base curve is usually positive.

   b. The toric surface of a spherocylinder lens is always on the side opposite the segment.

      (1) Since most segments are on the front, the toric surface is usually on the rear surface.

      (2) For a rear surface segment, a front surface toric is used.

Rx	Sphere	Cylinder	Axis	Prism	Add
OD	-4.50	-1.50	180		+2.00
OS	-3.75	-1.00	175		+2.00

Remarks: Bifocal Rx

_____,O.D.

Rx	Sphere	Cylinder	Axis	Prism	Add
OD	-2.50	-1.50	180		
OS	-1.75	-1.00	175		

Remarks: Single vision Reading only Rx

_____,O.D.

Figure 8-13. Top figure shows a written prescription for a bifocal. Lower diagram shows a reading-only Rx written for the same prescription.

3. Bifocals can be grouped in several different ways, according to the material from which they are made or according to form.
    a. Bifocals are available in plastic and in glass.
        (1) The segment surface(s) of a glass bifocal is (are) ground.
        (2) The segment surface of a plastic bifocal is molded.
    b. Bifocals can also be grouped according to whether they are fused or one-piece in form.
4. The distance and segment parts of fused bifocals are made from two different glass materials (Figure 8-14a).
    a. Fused bifocals are not made from plastic because of the likelihood that the high temperatures necessary for fusing will cause surface distortion.

a)   b)   c)

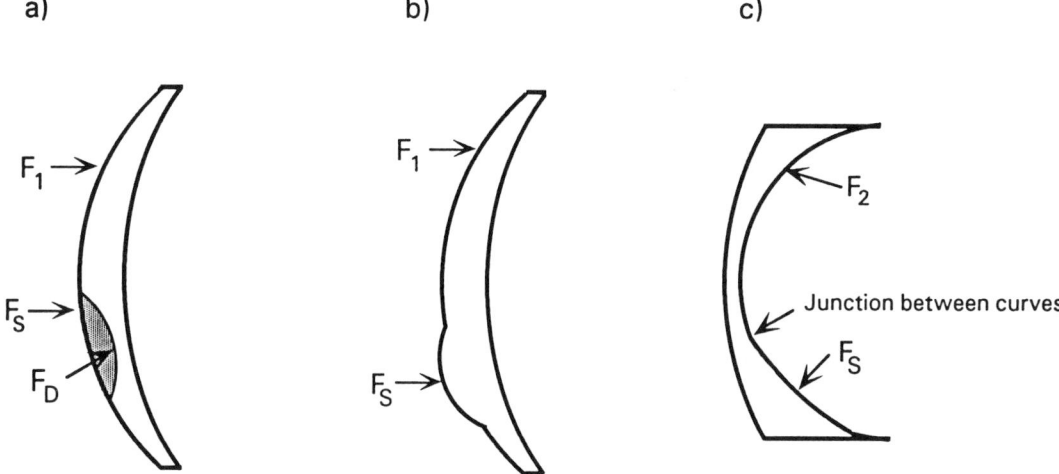

Figure 8-14. Three types of bifocals are viewed in cross section: (a) fused bifocal, (b) front surface one-piece bifocal, (c) rear surface one-piece bifocal. F_1 and F_2 are the front and rear surface powers respectively of the distance lens, F_S is the front surface power of the segment, F_D is the rear surface power of the fused segment.

       b. Fused bifocals currently available all have the segment on the front surface, and the base curve of the lens is the power of the distance part of the front surface.

       c. In a fused bifocal the segment fits into a depression which is ground into the front surface of the distance lens.

          (1) The segment is made from glass having a higher index of refraction than the distance lens.

          (2) The rear surface of the segment, ground parallel to the depression curve, is placed into the depression, and the lens is heated to softening so the segment is fused into the distance lens.

          (3) The front surface of the segment is ground to the same radius of curvature as the front surface of the distance lens.

             (a) The surface feels smooth across the junction between the distance and segment portions.

             (b) If no junction is felt at the edge of a segment, the bifocal is fused, and the lens must be made of glass.

       d. The power of the add F_A is given by two factors: $F_A = (F_S - F_1) + F_D$ where F_1 is the power of the base curve (front surface power of the distance part), F_S is the power of the front surface of the segment in air, and F_D is the power of the rear surface of the segment which is bounded in front by segment material and behind by distance lens material.

  5. In one-piece bifocals, the distance and segment parts of the lens are made from the same material, either plastic or glass.

       a. One-piece bifocals have the segment either on the front or the rear surface, and the base curve of the lens is the power of the distance part on the same surface as the segment.

       b. In a one-piece bifocal, the add is created by changing the curvature of the segment.

          (1) In a front surface segment, the curvature of the segment is steeper than the distance portion; the increased plus of the front surface gives the segment its "add" power (Figure 8-14b).

          (2) In a rear surface segment, the curvature of the segment is flatter than the distance portion; the decreased minus power of the rear surface gives the segment its increased plus power (Figure 8-14c).

(3)   The junction between the segment and the distance lens is perceptible to touch.

c.   The power of the add F_A for a one-piece bifocal depends upon one factor, the difference between the powers of the distance and near portions on the side of segment.

(1)   For a front surface one-piece: $F_A = F_S - F_1$, where F_1 is the power of the front surface of the distance part and F_S is the power of the front surface of the segment.

(2)   For a rear surface one-piece: $F_A = F_S - F_2$, where F_S is the power of the rear surface of the segment and F_2 is the power of the rear surface of the distance portion of the lens.

6.   To understand the optical effects of a bifocal, it is convenient to consider the segment to be a separate spherical lens added to the distance lens.

a.   The segment has its own optical center (seg OC), which represents the point of zero prism in the segment lens.

(1)   The distance from the top of the segment to the seg OC depends on the segment shape, and ranges from zero to 19 mm.

(2)   The maximum width of the segment is at the level of the seg OC.

(3)   When the seg OC is below the top of the segment, the segment contributes BD prism at its top.

(a)   The amount is dependent both on the power of the add and the distance from the top of the segment to the seg OC, according to Prentice's rule.

(b)   The sudden introduction of BD prism at the upper edge of the segment causes an abrupt upward displacement (toward the apex of

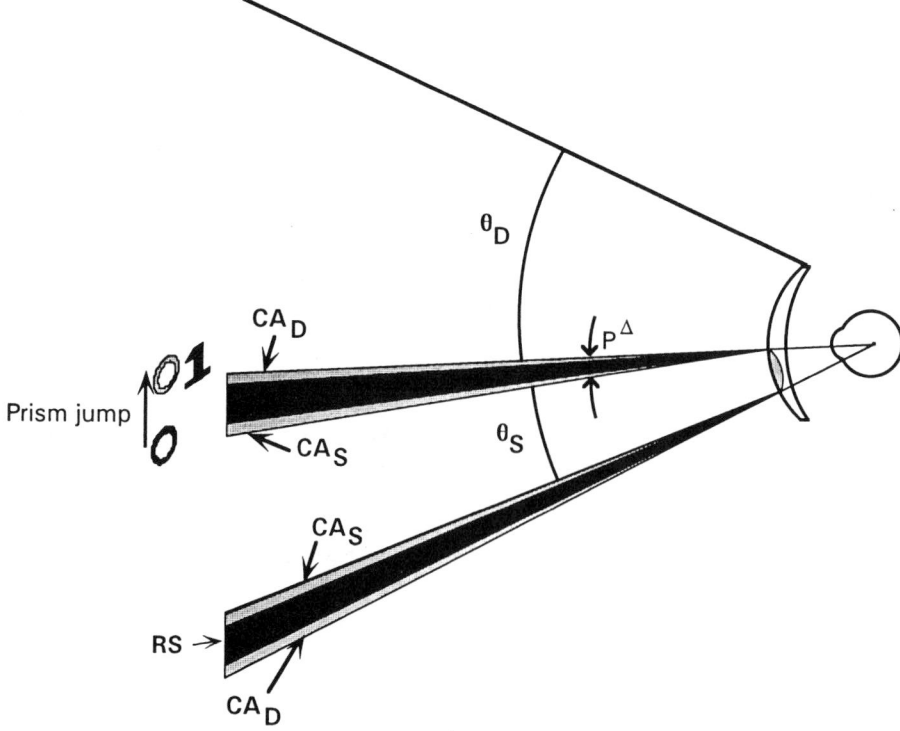

Figure 8-15.   Field of view through a bifocal. θ_D and θ_S are the fields of view through the upper distance lens and segment, respectively. Objects viewed through the upper edge of the segment, such as the dark "O", are displaced upward through an angle P, the prism jump. A ring scotoma RS is present at the periphery of the segment. CA_D and CA_S are the confusion areas for the distance and segment portions of the lens, respectively.

the prism) of the image seen through the segment (Figure 8-15).

    i.   This phenomenon is termed prism jump or bifocal jump.

    ii.   The displacement is similar to the displacement which occurs at the edge of any plus spectacle lens.

    iii.   A ring scotoma is present around the periphery of the segment just as for a plus lens.

(c)   As the eye descends from the distance lens into the segment, several image changes are noted.

    i.   In Figure 8-15, the number "1" is the lowest object which is seen through the distance lens.

    ii.   The image of the "0" is the uppermost character seen through the segment.

    iii.   The image of the "0" is displaced upward through an angle P^Δ, the prism jump caused by the edge of the segment.

    iv.   If the pupil were small enough to transmit only one ray at a time, the "1" would be seen immediately before and separate from the "0".

    v.   The ring scotoma is the area between the "1" and the object "0" (dark).

    vi.   With a normally sized pupil, however, a small area exists at the edge of the segment where rays from both the top of the segment and from the distance lens pass into the pupil.

    vii.   This is a confusion area where diplopia is present due to simultaneous images of different objects through the distance lens and segment.

    viii.   Outside the absolute ring scotoma is the confusion area CA_D for the distance lens, in which objects will be seen simultaneously with images from the segment.

    ix.   Inside the ring scotoma is the confusion area CA_S for the segment, in which objects will be seen simultaneously with images from the distance lens.

    x.   Objects in the ring scotoma are seen neither through the distance lens nor through the segment.

    xi.   The width of the areas of confusion and the ring scotoma and the amount of prism jump depends on the distance from the seg OC to the top of the segment, so segment styles with the seg OC close to the top edge have reduced effects.

(d)   The diplopia at the top of the segment can be bothersome, so patients must be taught to rotate their eyes far enough into the segment to avoid the effects at the edge.

7.   Bifocals are available in several shapes and sizes.

   a.   The round segment has its seg OC at its geometrical center, and is available in both fused or one-piece (Figure 8-16a).

    (1)   The original round segment, the "kryptok," was a flint glass segment set in an ophthalmic crown distance lens.

    (a)   The diameter was nominally 22 mm.

    (b)   Due to inexact manufacturing, the fusion process often resulted in poor optics.

    (c)   The use of flint glass, with its low constringence and high chromatic aberration, further degraded the image.

    (2)   An advantage of the round segment is its relative invisibility because the segment thickness tapers to zero at the edge of the segment.

    (3)   The major disadvantage is that the maximum diameter for reading is 11 mm below the top of the segment, at the level of the seg OC.

a)   b)   c)

d)   e)   f)

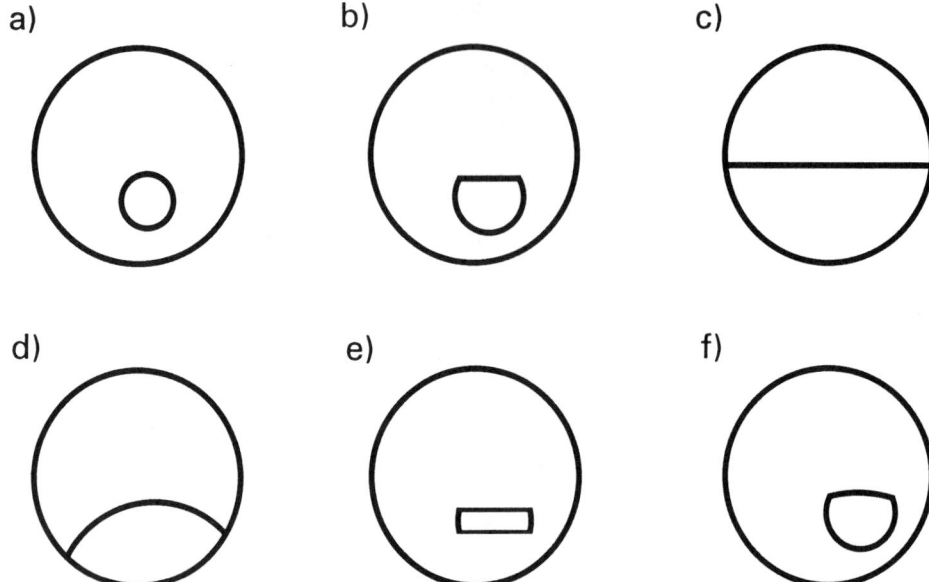

Figure 8-16. Bifocal segment shapes from the front: (a) round, (b) flat top, (c) straight across (full), (d) hemispheric, (e) bar or ribbon, (f) curved top.

(4)   The round bifocal is available in both glass and plastic.
    (a)   Glass round bifocals are either fused or one-piece.
        i.   The fused segments are front surface.
        ii.   The one-piece are either front or rear surface (B style).
    (b)   The term "kryptok," though originally applied to a fused 22-mm round bifocal, is used more generically today to refer to any round 22-mm segment, fused or one-piece.
(5)   Round segments are available in 22-, 24-, 25-, and 28-mm diameters.
b.   The flat-top or D style bifocal, the most commonly used bifocal, is essentially the lower two thirds of a round segment with the upper curved portion removed (Figure 8-16b).
(1)   A major advantage is that the seg OC is located only about 5 mm (varies 0.5–1.0 mm among manufacturers) below the straight top of the segment.
    (a)   The eye has to travel only 5 mm below the top of the segment to the maximum segment width at the level of the OC.
    (b)   Since the top of the segment is placed very close to 6 mm below the pupil center in primary gaze, the total excursion of the line of sight to look through the level of the seg OC is about 11 mm, the average normal reading level as measured by Fry and Ellerbrock.[4]
    (c)   When the eye is at the normal reading level and looking through the seg OC, there are no vertical prism effects from the segment.
        i.   The patient experiences the same prism effects as encountered in a single-vision distance Rx.
        ii.   This perhaps eases adjustment if the patient has previously worn single-vision glasses.
    (d)   The amount of prism jump is smaller for the flat top than for a round segment because of the decreased distance from the top of the segment to the seg OC.
(2)   A disadvantage is that the top of a flat-top segment is thicker than the top of a round segment, so it is more visible.

(3) Flat-top bifocals are available in both glass and plastic.
   (a) Glass flat-top bifocals are fused.
   (b) First a round segment is made by fusing a piece of the high-index glass to be used for the segment with a piece of the glass used for the distance lens.
   (c) The two pieces are fused with a straight horizontal boundary between them.
   (d) The rear surface is ground to the necessary radius of curvature and a depression of the same radius is ground into the distance lens.
   (e) The segment is placed into the depression and the lenses heated to the softening point so the glasses fuse together.
   (f) The upper part of the segment, made of the distance lens glass, fuses imperceptibly into the distance lens, leaving the higher-index segment with a flat top.
   (g) The front surface is ground onto both the distance lens and the segment so both have the same radius of curvature.
   (h) If a finger is moved across the boundary between the segment and the distance lens, the edge of the segment is not felt because of the identical radii of curvature.
(4) Plastic flat-top bifocals are molded onto the front surface of the lens.
   (a) The segment has a shorter radius of curvature than the distance lens.
   (b) The segment bulges out from the distance lens and can be felt with the finger.
(5) Flat-top bifocals are available in the following widths:
   (a) Ophthalmic crown: 22, 25, 28, and 35 mm.
   (b) 1.70 or 1.80 high-index glass: 25 and 28 mm.
   (c) Hard resin: 22, 25, 28, 35, and 45 mm.
   (d) PC: 25, 28, and 35 mm.
   (e) 1.56 plastic: 28 and 35 mm.
   (f) 1.60 plastic: 28 mm.

c. The straight-across (Executive type, E style, or full segment) bifocal has a flat top which extends across the entire width of the lens (Figure 8-16c).
   (1) It is referred to as a monocentric lens because the optical centers of the distance and near lens are coincident at the top of the segment.
   (2) One major advantage of the straight-across bifocal is the width available for near tasks.
      (a) It has the maximum width possible from any segment, making it desirable for many patients who spend significant amounts of time doing nearpoint work, especially work spread out on a desk.
      (b) Since the maximum width is available at the top of the segment, the eyes need not drop far into the segment, so differential prism effects from the distance powers in the vertical meridians of the two lenses are minimized.
   (3) Prism jump and scotoma are eliminated at the top of the segment, but a confusion area remains due to two powers at the segment line.
   (4) A major disadvantage is the weight of the lens caused by the extra center thickness required by the combination of the ledge and the steeper curve of the front surface of the segment.
   (5) Another drawback is the absence of distance power in the lower part of the lens, making the lens inappropriate for people who are very mobile and use the lens only occasionally for near work.

d. The hemispheric bifocal represents the top half of a large circular segment (Figure 8-16d).
   (1) These segments are one-piece, with the segment on the front surface for all plastic hemispherics and some of the glass hemispherics, and the segment on the rear surface for the other glass hemispherics.

(2) Segment widths of 38 or 40 mm are available.
  (a) The seg OCs are located 19 and 20 mm from the tops of the 38- and 40-mm segments, respectively.
  (b) The 38-mm rear surface glass segment was originally manufactured as the Ultex A, and 38-mm segments are still called by this name today.
(3) The hemispheric is one of the few lenses available with a rear surface segment, which means the base curve is minus as well.
(4) Prism jump at the top of the segment is the largest of any of the segments due to the large distance from the top of the segment to the seg OC.
(5) Adequate width for reading is provided well above the level of the maximum width at the seg OC; often the seg OC is not even in the lens itself, depending on the depth of the frame.

e. The ribbon (R) and bar (B) segments are the middle part of a round 22-mm fused segment, having the top and bottom removed (Figure 8-16e).
(1) The ribbon segment is 14 mm deep by 22 mm wide.
(2) The bar segment is 9 mm deep by 22 mm wide.
(3) These segments are available in glass only and are useful for patients who need only a small reading area for occasional spotting and desire maximum area for distance vision.

f. The curved top segment (C or P style) has a slightly curved top which is a balance between the round- and flat-top bifocals (Figure 8-16f).
(1) In hard resin, segment diameters of 25, 28, and 40 mm are available, while in glass a 24-mm segment is available.
(2) The slight curvature makes the top of the segment somewhat less abrupt and less visible than the flat top, while at the same time the maximum width for reading is higher than the round segment.

g. The shapes and sizes of bifocals listed above are not all available in every power or material.
(1) Most bifocal styles are available in add powers up to 3.50–4.00D adds.
  (a) Straight across (E style) segments usually have a maximum add power of 3.00D, since higher adds become very heavy.
  (b) Some of the less commonly used or newer segment types are available in lesser add ranges.
  (c) The styles of segments available in very steep or very flat base curves, such as those needed for high plus or high minus, are limited.
(2) The number of different segment styles available in newer or lesser used materials, such as high-index plastics and glasses, is much more restricted.
(3) As a material is used more widely, the variety of segments available increases; for example, there is a greater number of segment styles and sizes available in PC now than when it was first introduced.
(4) High-power adds are required for patients with low vision or special needs.
  (a) Some flat-top bifocals are available in adds up to 6.00D.
  (b) Certain round and hemispheric bifocals are available in adds as high as 20D.
(5) The lab or *Lenses* (Frames Data, Inc., 2 Park Plaza, Suite 900, Irvine, CA 92714 1994) should be consulted before promising a patient a bifocal in a less common style, power, or material.

h. Special bifocals are available for unusual needs.
(1) Cemented segments can be provided by many laboratories by special order.
  (a) The segment is made separately from the distance lens.
  (b) The front surface curvature of the segment matches the rear surface curvature of the distance lens.
  (c) The segment is cemented onto the rear surface of the distance lens.

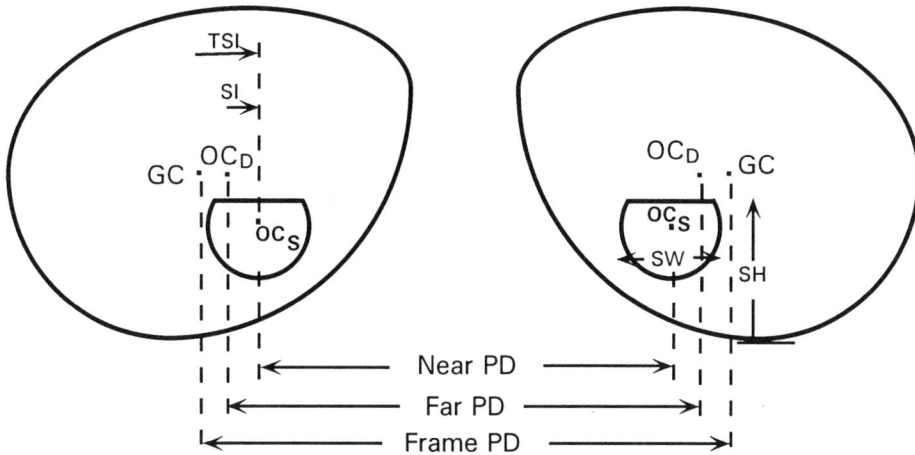

Figure 8-17.   Size and location of a bifocal segment: OC_D = distance optical center, OC_S = segment optical center, GC = geometrical center, SI = seg inset, TSI = total seg inset, SW = seg width, SH = seg height.

        (d)   The add can be provided in a wide range of powers and the position custom designed.

    (2)   A Ben Franklin style bifocal can also be custom made, fashioned after the original bifocal designed by Benjamin Franklin in or around 1785.

        (a)   The distance lens above and the segment below are two separate lenses cemented together at a straight boundary.

        (b)   The appearance is much like a one-piece straight-across type bifocal.

        (c)   Very high adds can be provided.

        (d)   The lens is subject to breaking at the junction.

8.   The position of the segment in the lens is specified horizontally by the seg inset and vertically by the segment height (Figure 8-17).

   a.   Seg inset is the horizontal distance from the distance OC to the vertical line through the seg OC.

    (1)   The seg OCs are normally placed in front of the eyes when they are converged for the nearpoint distance.

        (a)   The seg inset (SI) for each segment is then given by: SI = MDPD − MNPD, where MDPD and MNPD are the monocular distance and near PD's respectively.

        (b)   If the monocular PDs are equal, the seg inset for each lens is simply: SI = (DPD − NPD)/2.

        (c)   With the segment in this position, there is zero horizontal prism from the segments, but prism may be induced at nearpoint from the distance lens, since the eye is looking away from the distance OC.

    (2)   The seg may at times be positioned differently to induce horizontal prism from the segment to offset prism from the distance lens at nearpoint.

   b.   Total seg inset (TSI) is the horizontal distance from the GC of the lens to the seg OC.

    (1)   TSI = Decentration + SI.

    (2)   TSI = FPD/2 − MNPD.

    (3)   If the monocular near PDs are assumed to be equal, TSI = (FPD − NPD)/2.

   c.   The seg height is the distance from the bottom horizontal line of the box around the lens (boxing system) to the top of the segment.

    (1)   This can be difficult to measure directly when the lowest point on the

lens bevel is near the temporal edge of the lens and the segment is near the nasal edge of the lens.

(2) The vertical position of the segment can also be specified through seg drop, the distance from the GC of the lens to the seg top.

9. Selection of the type and size of bifocal depends on several factors.

    a. The D style is most commonly used because of the convenience of position of its widest part.

    b. The round segment can be used if the patient is concerned about the appearance of the bifocal, while a C style is a compromise between the round and the D segments.

    c. The size of the segment is a function of the time spent using the segment.

        (1) Patients who use the segment primarily for spotting rather than for long-term near work will be satisfied with a smaller 22- to 25-mm segment which allows maximum distance lens area.

        (2) Patients who spend much time using the segment and who must scan a large near area, such as a desk or drafting table, will benefit from a larger 28-, 35-, or 45-mm segment, or perhaps even a full segment.

Clinical Alert

The first-time bifocal wearer must be carefully instructed in its use to avoid adaptation problems.

a. Upper lens is for distance viewing with eyes and head straight ahead.

b. When climbing stairs, tilt head down to look over the bifocal rather than through it.

    (1) It is sometimes more necessary to warn experienced bifocal wearers with higher adds about stairs and curbs than first-time wearers.

    (2) The add power for first-time wearers is often low enough that the stairs can be seen clearly enough through the segment, while for higher adds this is no longer true and habits must be broken.

c. For reading, several factors must be emphasized.

    (1) Keep the reading material lower and closer to the body than normal.

    (2) Rotate the eyes down into the segment, keeping the head essentially straight ahead. DO NOT rotate the head down.

    (3) Place the reading material at the expected working distance, typically 16 inches, but shorter for adds higher than 2.50D.

    (4) If the segment line seems to be in the way, move the chin up slightly and rotate the eyes farther down, positioning the near task so it is in view through the segment.

    C. *Blended bifocals*

        1. A blended bifocal ("invisible bifocal") is a round one-piece front surface bifocal (Figure 8-18b).

        a. The junction at the edge of the segment between the front surface of the distance lens and the more highly curved segment is smoothed (blended) to lessen its visibility.

        b. Blended bifocals in hard resin are available from several manufacturers, with segment sizes ranging from 22 to 28 mm.

        c. Younger Optics makes a glass blended bifocal with a 22-mm seg diameter.

        d. When the lens is held in front of graph paper, the blended area is apparent as a zone of distorted squares.

        e. Specular reflection of an overhead light off the front surface of the lens also makes the blended area apparent.

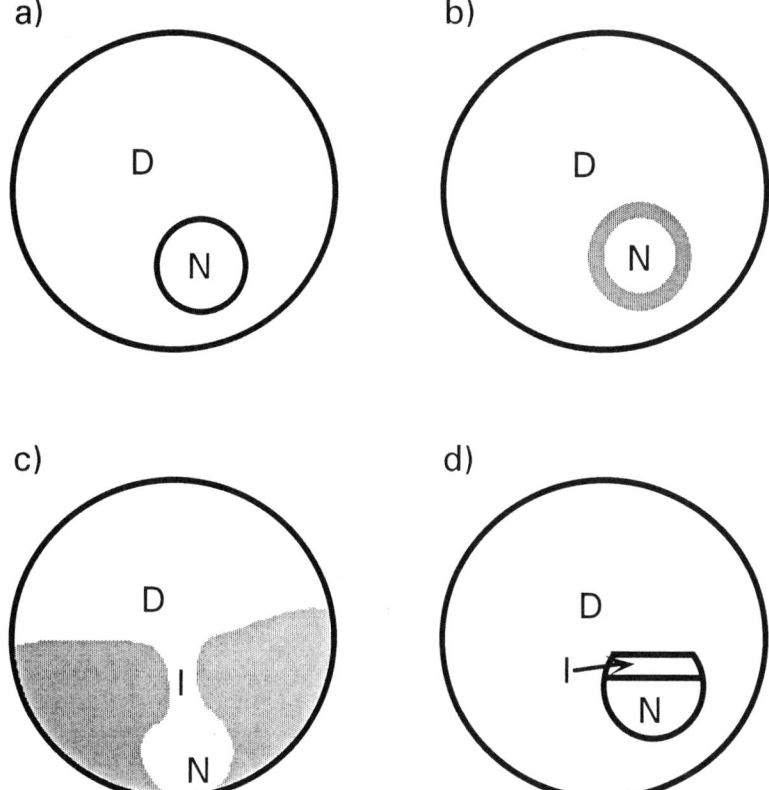

Figure 8-18. Usable areas through multifocals: (a) standard "lined" round bifocal, (b) blended bifocal, (c) PAL, (d) standard "lined" flat top trifocal. D is the area for distance vision, I is the area for intermediate vision, N is the area for near vision. The gray areas in (b) and (c) are areas blurred by aberrations.

      f.   Advantages of blended bifocals

          (1) The reduced visibility of the segment is preferred by patients who are reluctant to have others see that they wear bifocals.

          (2) The lower corners of the distance lens are free of distortion, unlike the progressive addition lens (PAL), so distance vision is not impaired in the lower part of the lens as much as for a progressive lens.

      g.   Disadvantages of blended bifocals

          (1) The actual usable reading area is lessened by the unusable blended zone of blur around the segment (Figure 8-18b).

              (a) The width of the usable area decreases as the add power increases.

              (b) The blur at the top of the segment is particularly disturbing as the eyes must cross this boundary during the change from distance to near vision.

          (2) The blended zone does not provide focus for intermediate distances as a PAL does.

      h.   When a "no-line" or "invisible" bifocal is desired, the progressive lens is prescribed far more frequently than the blended bifocal (Figure 8-18c).

D. *Trifocals*

      1. Trifocals consist of three powers and are in essence bifocals with a third power added to focus intermediate distances (Figure 8-18d).

         a. The add power in a bifocal focuses at a particular near distance, with or without supplemental accommodation.

b. In beginning presbyopia, a significant amount of accommodation remains and the add power is low.

c. Objects between infinity and the nearpoint plane are seen clearly through either the distance lens or the segment by using the remaining accommodation.

d. The amplitude of accommodation eventually becomes small enough that a range of intermediate distances including arm's length is blurred whether the distance lens or segment is used.

e. An additional segment, focused for the intermediate distance, is needed if the patient complains of blur at arm's length.

2. The power of the intermediate add is usually 50% of the near add, although 40%, 50%, 60%, 66%, 70%, and 74% adds are also available for special needs.

a. Trifocals are not usually needed until the bifocal add for near reaches approximately 1.75–2.00D, as the following shows.

(1) If a patient has a 2.00D add, he or she uses 0.50D of accommodation while viewing through the segment at 40 cm; if half the amplitude of accommodation is in reserve, the amplitude is 1.00D.

(2) Assume the patient is fully corrected for distance, has 0.50D of accommodation to use comfortably, has ±0.25D depth of field, and has a 2.00D near add. What is the total range of distances which are apparently clear through the distance lens and through the add?

(a) The far or distant limit of the range of apparently clear vision through the distance lens (F_d) is given by adding (1) any error in the distance lens (E), such as when the patient is wearing an old Rx which has not been updated (zero in this example), (2) the dioptric equivalent of the most distant edge of the depth of field ($-D$), and the least amount of accommodation possible (A_{min}) (see Figure 8-19).

i. $F_d = E + (-D) + A_{min}$

ii. The far limit is $0 + (-0.25) + 0 = -0.25D$.

iii. The far edge of clear vision through the distance lens is at infinity; the $-0.25D$ depth of field term is of no help in this case.

(b) The near limit of apparently clear vision (N) for sustained viewing through the distance lens (N_d) is obtained by considering any error in the distance lens (E) and by using maximum comfortable accommodation (A_{max}) and the near limit of the depth of field ($+D$).

i. $N_d = E + (+D) + A_{max}$.

ii. In the example, the near limit through the distance lens is $N_d = 0 + (+0.25D) + 0.50D = +0.75D$.

iii. The near limit through the distance lens is $1/+0.75D = 1.33$ m = 133 cm in front of the lens.

(c) The far or distant limit (F) of the range of apparently clear vision through the near lens (F_n) depends on the same factors as the far limit through the distance lens except for the extra plus power through the add (Add).

i. $F_n = E + Add + (-D) + A_{min}$.

ii. $F_n = 0 + 2.00D - 0.25D + 0 = +1.75D$.

iii. The far limit through the add is $1/1.75D = 0.57$ m = 57 cm.

(d) The near limit (N) of the range of apparently clear vision through the near add (N_n) depends on the same factors as the near limit through the distance lens except for the extra plus power through the add (Add).

i. $N_n = E + Add + (+D) + A_{max}$.

ii. $N_n = 0 + 2.00D + 0.25D + 0.50D = +2.75D$.

iii. The near limit through the add is $1/2.75D = 0.36$ m = 36 cm.

(e) The total range of clear vision extends from infinity to 133 cm through the distance lens and from 57 to 36 cm through the segment, so the interval from 57 to 133 cm is blurred.

(f) If a 50% intermediate segment were added in a trifocal ($+1.00D$

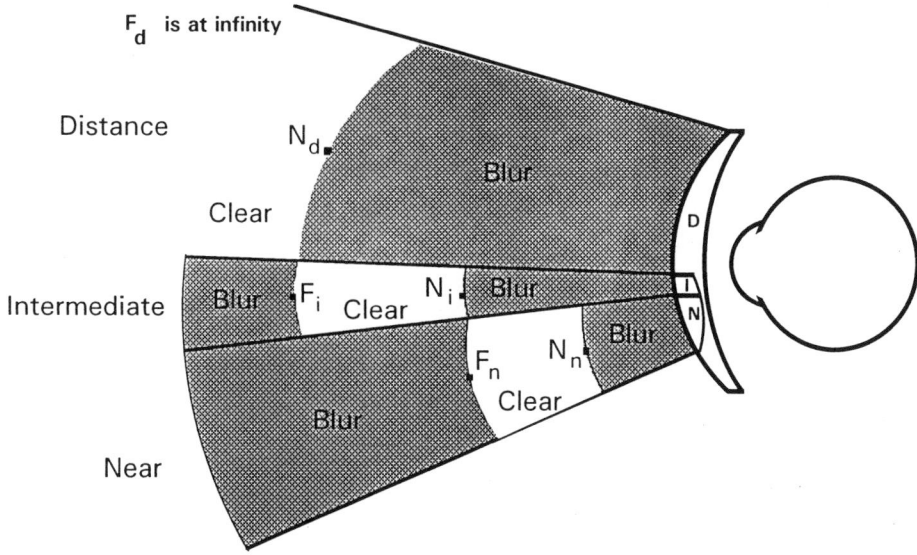

Figure 8-19. Ranges of clear vision through trifocal. F and N are the farthest and nearest points which are apparently clear through a particular segment of the lens. F_d and N_d are the extreme points for the distance lens D; F_n and N_n are the extreme points for the near segment N, the only segment present in a bifocal. In a trifocal, the intermediate segment I is added with the extreme points of clear vision F_i and N_i, respectively. Shaded areas represent areas of blur.

add), the range of clear vision through the intermediate segment would extend from 57 to 133 cm, filling in the gap left by the distant and near power (Figure 8-19).

    i. $F_i = E + \text{Add} + (-D) + A_{min}$.

    ii. $F_i = 0 + 1.00D - 0.25D + 0 = +0.75D$.

    iii.   The far limit through the intermediate is $1/0.75D = 1.33$ m $= 133$ cm.

    iv. $N_i = E + \text{Add} + (+D) + A_{max}$.

    v. $N_i = 0 + 1.00D + 0.25D + 0.50D = +1.75D$.

    vi.   The near limit through the intermediate add is $1/1.75D = 0.57$ m $= 57$ cm.

3. Trifocal sizes are designated by two numbers, such as 7 × 28.

    a.   The first number, 7 in this case, is the depth of the intermediate segment, the distance from the top to the bottom of the intermediate.

    b.   The second number, 28 in this case, is the largest horizontal width of the near segment.

4. Virtually every bifocal style is available in a trifocal.

    a.   Round trifocals come in a 7 × 22 × 36 hard resin and in a front surface one-piece 8 × 34 × 50 glass.

        (1)   The first number is the width of the trifocal annulus surrounding the near power.

        (2)   The second number is the horizontal width of the near segment.

        (3)   The third number is the total horizontal width of the trifocal segment.

    b.   Flat-top or D segments are available in hard resin, glass, and PC.

        (1)   Ophthalmic crown glass segments are made in 6 × 22, 6 × 28, 7 × 23, 7 × 25, 7 × 28, 7 × 35, 8 × 25, 8 × 28, 10 × 25, 10 × 28, 10 × 35, and 14 × 35.

        (2)   High-index 1.7 and 1.8 glass trifocals are made in 7 × 25, 7 × 28, and 7 × 35 in laminated form.

        (3)   Hard resin trifocals are available in 7 × 25, 7 × 28, and 8 × 35.

        (4)   Polycarbonate D trifocals are available in 7 × 28.

c. Straight-across (E-style) trifocals are made in hard resin with a 7- and 14-mm intermediate height and in ophthalmic crown with a 7-mm intermediate height.
d. Hemispheric bifocals (Ultex style) are available in ophthalmic crown and in hard resin.
    (1) Ophthalmic crown segments include a rear surface one-piece 8 × 32 × 50 × 24 and a front surface one-piece 8 × 32 × 50 × 25.
    (2) The hard resin Ultex style is a front surface 8 × 32 × 50.
    (3) The first three numbers are the same as for the round trifocal, and the last is the maximum seg height.
e. A 6 × 22 ribbon seg is made in ophthalmic crown glass.
f. Curved-top (C-style) trifocals are available in a 7 × 24 ophthalmic crown segment and in a 10 × 40 hard resin segment.
g. Other more specialized trifocal configurations are available for occupational needs.
    (1) An inverted flat-top segment, mounted in the top of the distance lens for overhead near tasks, is available combined with a trifocal in standard position below.
    (2) An inverted flat-top segment, a round segment, or full segment in the upper part of the lens is available together with a similar bifocal segment in the lower part.

5. The top of a trifocal segment is usually placed at the lower margin of the pupil.
    a. In this position, the top of the near segment, typically 7 mm lower, is approximately 3–4 mm below the limbus (assuming a 4-mm diameter pupil and 12-mm corneal diameter).
    b. Positioning the trifocal much lower than the lower pupillary margin makes it difficult for the patient to use the near segment.
    c. Use of an intermediate depth greater than the typical 7 mm to increase the area available for arm's length viewing also forces the near segment down to a less convenient position.
6. The horizontal position of a trifocal is specified through seg inset in the same manner as bifocals.

E. *Progressive addition lenses*
1. A progressive addition lens (PAL) provides a gradual and continuous power change from the distance power in the upper part of the lens to the near addition in the lower part.
    a. It is the most commonly used of the "no-line" or "invisible" bifocals.
    b. Unlike the blended zone of the blended bifocal, however, the transition in the PAL between the distance power and the near power is usable for intermediate distances.
        (1) The transition zone is termed the progressive corridor or channel.
        (2) The usable width of the progressive corridor is relatively narrow, limited by unwanted cylinder on either side (Figure 8-18c).
    c. The gradual increase in plus power from the distance power to near power is achieved through a continuous increase in the curvature of the front surface.
        (1) A series of spherical or aspherical horizontal curves with different radii of curvature are smoothly merged into one another so the radii of curvature decrease from the top of the lens to the bottom.
        (2) The unwanted astigmatism in the periphery of the lens is a direct result of the fact that if the curves are joined smoothly together with error-free power in the center of the lens, they cannot be joined free of error in the periphery because of the differing radii of curvature.
        (3) The amount of unwanted cylinder is directly related to the rate at which the power changes along the progressive corridor. As the power changes more rapidly, the following results are found:
            (a) A greater amount of unwanted astigmatism is found in the periphery, and the error-free width of the corridor becomes narrower.

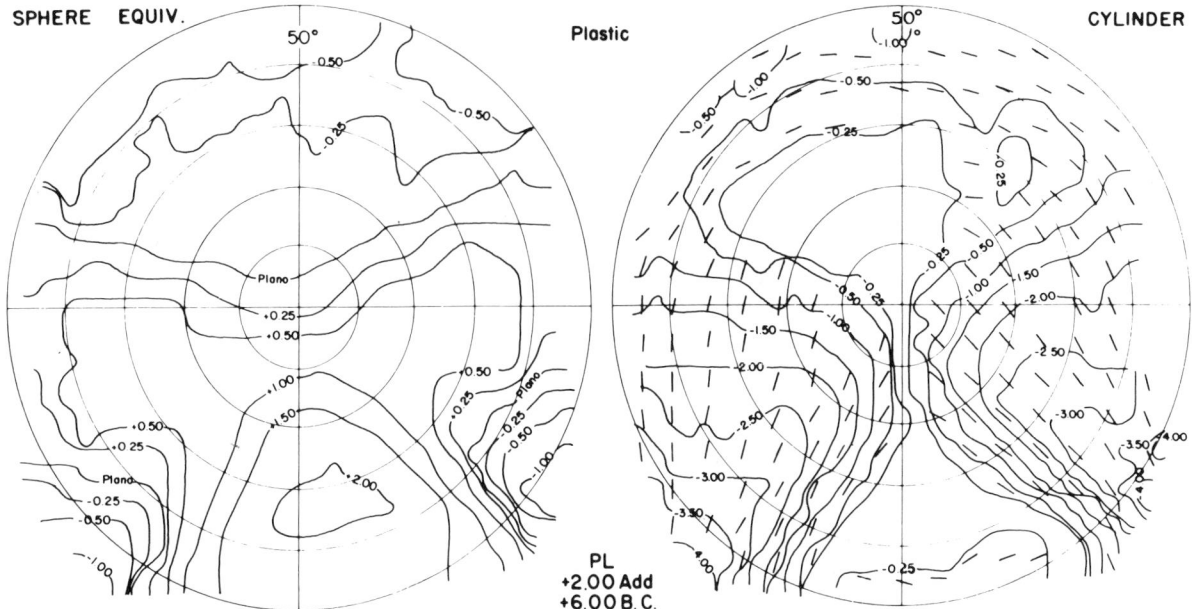

SPHERE EQUIV.   Plastic   CYLINDER

PL
+2.00 Add
+6.00 B.C.

Figure 8-20. Isosphere (left) and isocylinder (right) plots for a PAL. Each line on the plot to the left connects points on the lens for which the spherical equivalent of the unwanted power in the lens is the same as labeled. Each line on the plot to the right connects points in the lens having equal powers of unwanted cylinder. (Used by permission of Sheedy JE, Burian EM, Bailey IL, Borish IM. Optics of progressive addition lenses. *Am J Optom Physiol Opt* 1987;64:90–99.)

        (b)   The length of the corridor becomes shorter, and less depression of the eyes is required to reach the reading area.

        (c)   The vertical extent of the corridor having the requisite power to clear a particular intermediate distance is reduced, making the lens less suitable for intermediate distances.

    (4)   The amount of unwanted cylinder across the lens surface is represented in an isocylinder plot with lines connecting points having equal amounts of unwanted cylinder (Figure 8-20).[5]

    (5)   If the power changes at the same rate along the entire corridor, the width of the corridor is fairly constant until it reaches a more constant reading area where the width increases if the rate of change slows to give more constant power.

    (6)   If the rate of power change varies, being rapid at the top and slower at the bottom, the corridor is narrow at the top and wider at the bottom.

    (7)   The areas of unwanted power and cylinder cause blur, distortion, and a "swimming" sensation as the eyes move across the periphery of the lens.

        (a)   The amount of these undesirable optical effects depends on the amount of the unwanted power and its distribution across the lens.

        (b)   The orientation of the axis of the unwanted cylinder may also be important to the severity of the optical effects, with horizontal and vertical axes being less destructive than oblique.

        (c)   The patient's acceptance of the lens depends at least partially on the level of tolerance to the optical effects.

  2.   A fundamental difference in designs among PALs is the way in which the unwanted astigmatism is distributed throughout the lens.

    a.   Early designs and some current designs reserve the upper part of the lens for error-free distance power and a relatively large error-free area in the lower part of the lens for reading power.

        (1)   Large amounts of unwanted cylinder are induced in the remaining inferior nasal and inferior temporal portions of the lens.

(2) This type of design is termed a "hard" PAL.

(3) The progressive corridor is short and narrow.

b. Other current designs which have enjoyed commercial success allow some unwanted cylinder to encroach into the upper periphery of the lens and into the near area.

    (1) By spreading the cylinder throughout more of the lens, the maximum amount of cylinder found anywhere in the lens is lessened, decreasing the harshness of the periphery of the lens.

    (2) This type of design is termed a "soft" PAL.

    (3) The length of the corridor is more variable among soft designs, though generally it is longer than for a hard lens.

        (a) The longer the corridor, the wider it becomes and the less unwanted cylinder is produced.

        (b) However, as mentioned earlier, the longer the corridor, the more the eyes must be depressed to reach the reading area.

    (4) A helpful, though crude, analogy is to consider the amount of unwanted cylinder to be a fixed volume of sand that can be piled into corners of a sandbox or spread more evenly and thinly across a greater area of the sandbox.

c. In all PALs, whether hard or soft, an increase in the add power will have the following effects:

    (1) The amount of unwanted astigmatism increases.

    (2) The width of the error-free progressive corridor decreases.

d. It is still not known what attributes of the lens are most conducive to patient acceptance.

    (1) Some lens manufacturers produce two different designs, one soft and one hard, in an effort to allow for different patient preferences.

    (2) The conventional wisdom in the industry, judging from advertisements, is that soft designs may be more readily accepted by first-time bifocal wearers than hard designs.

        (a) First-time bifocal wearers usually have the advantage of a low add, which minimizes the unwanted cylinder, making adaptation easier.

        (b) Harder designs, with larger reading areas, may be more easily accepted by patients who are already wearing a traditional bifocal and are accustomed to a larger error-free reading area, provided they can adapt to the cylinder concentrated in the periphery.

        (c) If a patient is already adapted to a particular type of PAL, a change in design should be recommended only with a compelling reason and extreme caution.

e. Performance characteristics of PALs have been presented in a variety of formats.

    (1) The most commonly used are diagrams of isospherical equivalent lines and isocylinder lines (Figure 8-20).

        (a) The isospherical equivalent lines diagram consists of lines drawn across the face of the lens which connect points in the lens having the same spherical equivalent error.

        (b) The isocylinder lines represent points in the lens having equal amounts of unwanted cylinder.

        (c) Each diagram typically shows lines representing 0.50D steps of power change.

        (d) The width of the progressive corridor is often taken to be the distance between the two 0.50D isocylinder lines on either side of the corridor.

    (2) Isocylinder diagrams represent a useful method of comparing objectively the optical performance of various PALs, but it remains difficult to predict a particular patient's reaction to a particular lens based solely on such information.

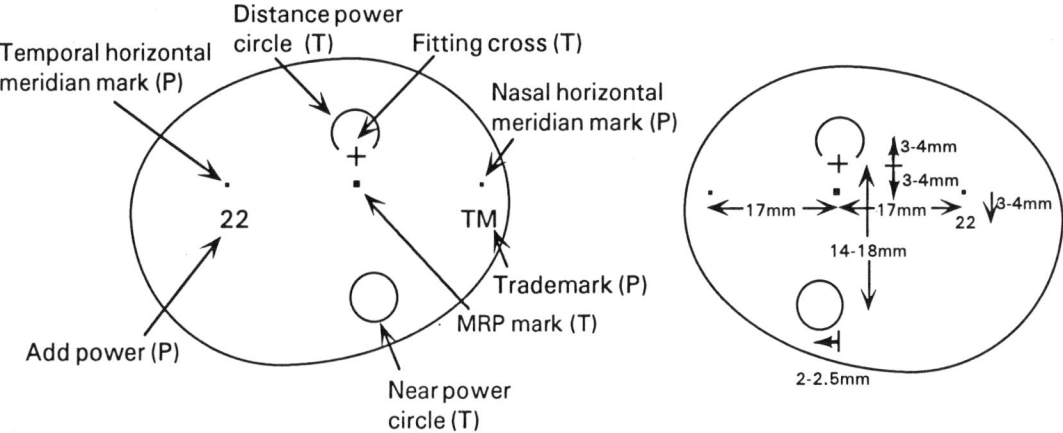

Figure 8-21. Markings on a PAL. Permanent markings are labeled with a P, temporary markings with a T. The fitting cross should be centered in the patient's pupil. Markings are labeled for the right eye while typical distances between markings are given for the left lens.

        (3) Despite the uncertainty in predicting whether a particular PAL is appropriate for a particular patient, the practitioner can prescribe most PALs with reduced risk because most manufacturers guarantee that if their PAL is unsuccessful it will be replaced with a traditional bifocal at no additional cost.

   3. Because of the ever-decreasing radius of curvature toward the bottom of the front surface of the PAL, the bottom edge of the lens is significantly thinner than the top.

     a. In an effort to equalize the top and bottom edge thicknesses and thus reduce overall lens thickness, some PALs are surfaced with equal amounts of BD prism on each lens.

     b. Since equal amounts are surfaced onto each lens, the resultant vertical prism induced is zero between the two eyes.

     c. In effect, the OCs of the lenses are raised for minus lenses and lowered for plus lenses.

     d. When the PAL is verified on a lensometer, the BD prism will be measured if no other vertical prism has been prescribed.

   4. When a PAL is returned from the laboratory in finished form, it has two sets of markings on it, temporary and permanent (Figure 8-21).

     a. The temporary markings are visible marks to assist in verifying the power of the new PAL and in dispensing the lens.

       (1) The fitting cross marks the spot on the lens which should be located at the center of the pupil.

         (a) The fitting cross does not usually mark the distance MRP, which most commonly lies 2–4 mm below the cross.

         (b) The progressive corridor begins at, or shortly below, the fitting cross.

         (c) The fitting cross should be fit 2 mm above the center of the pupil for lenses with long progressive corridors, such as the Varilux Infinity, or where frame slippage is anticipated.

       (2) The distance power circle is located above the fitting cross.

         (a) The distance power in the lens is found by centering this circle on the lens stop of the lensometer.

         (b) Distance power is not measured lower than this because the upper part of the corridor will blur the mires.

         (c) Distance power measured away from the distance power circle in the upper lens is open to error from unwanted astigmatism.

    (3)   The horizontal meridian through the MRP is denoted temporarily in some manner, such as with dashed lines.

        (a)   A dot 3–4 mm directly below the fitting cross and along the horizontal meridian marks the MRP or the functional MRP when thinning prism is present.

        (b)   The functional MRP is the point in the lens with the proper resultant prism between the two lenses, even though the addition of thinning prism makes the gross prism in one lens wrong according to the prescription.

        (c)   Prism in the prescription should be verified at this dot; a blurred mire in the lensometer from part of the corridor is not critical to the measurement of prism.

    (4)   The near power circle is located within the reading area and is generally 14–18 mm below and 2–2.5 mm nasal to the fitting cross.

        (a)   The add is found by taking the difference in front vertex power readings through the distance and near power circles.

        (b)   If the add is measured away from the near power circle, it is open to error from unwanted astigmatism bordering the near area.

    (5)   The temporary markings are removed with an alcohol swab after the lenses have been verified upon their arrival from the laboratory and after the finished pair of glasses has been adjusted to the patient's face to ensure the fitting cross is positioned properly.

  b.   The permanent markings are partially visible markings etched into the lens surface for future reference when the lens is to be identified, verified, or refitted.

    (1)   Two dots, circles, or other similar markings, separated by 34 mm, mark the horizontal meridian.

    (2)   The power of the add is etched 3–4 mm under the temporal dot, often with no decimal point, and sometimes with the second decimal place dropped, as in the case of the Varilux Infinity where "22" denotes an add of 2.25D.

    (3)   Additional information is often found under the nasal dot.

        (a)   A trademark or other symbol identifying the lens may be 3–4 mm below the nasal dot.

        (b)   A number identifying the index of refraction may also be located here, as in the case of the Infinity made from 1.6 plastic where a "6" is etched alongside the trademark.

    (4)   The permanent markings are easy to locate on some lenses but quite difficult on others.

        (a)   On some lenses they are readily visible under normal illumination.

        (b)   On other lenses the markings are fluorescent and can be found using a UV light, such as a Burton lamp, as long as the lens has not been UV coated.

        (c)   Sometimes the markings are so faint they can only be detected by looking at an image of a light source reflected specularly off the lens.

           i.   Viewing the edge of the reflected light source against a dark background is often helpful.

           ii.   Viewing the reflected image off the concave surface of the lens to create a larger, "softer" image is sometimes useful.

           iii.   The lens should be clean when looking for the markings.

        (d)   Occasionally, if the lens has been heavily tinted or coated, the markings may be impossible to find.

        (e)   If the lens has been decentered significantly, the nasal dot may have been cut off in the edging process.

        (f)   The "MRP" of the lens is midway between the two dots in the horizontal meridian.

        (g)   Once the permanent dots have been found, they can be marked and used to restore the temporary markings onto the lens using templates supplied by the manufacturer.

(h) If templates are not available, the "MRP" can be marked at the midpoint between the two dots, the fitting cross 2–4 mm above the "MRP," the center of the distance power circle about 8 mm above the "MRP," and the center of the near power circle about 14–16 mm below and 2.5 mm nasal to the "OC."

(i) If the permanent dots cannot be located, use a lensometer to find the point on the lens with the prescribed amount of prism.

    i. This is the MRP which should be midway between the two permanent dots, so the position of the dots can be estimated and the remainder of the markings replaced.

    ii. If the lenses have thinning prism, this method will be complicated by the overlying equalizing prism in each lens.

(5) Table 8-8 lists the permanent markings that are found on several of the more common PALs.

5. Appropriate selection and proper adjustment of the frame are critical to success with a PAL.

a. The vertical depth from the center of the pupil to the point in the frame directly below should be at least 22–24 mm.

b. Frames with small vertical dimensions or nasal cuts, such as pilot shapes, should be avoided.

c. A frame should be chosen that allows a short vertex distance and a pantoscopic tilt of 10°–12° to maximize the field of view through all areas of the lens.

6. The position of the center of the patient's pupil is specified to the laboratory to indicate where the fitting cross should be placed.

a. Monocular PDs, taken with a pupillometer for maximum accuracy, specify the horizontal position.

b. The vertical height from the tangent to the lowest point in the lens to the pupil center can be measured several ways, with the patient's eyes straight ahead.

(1) The least accurate is to use a millimeter ruler to measure the height to the pupil directly (Figure 8-22a).

(2) The use of a marking pen to mark the position of the center of the pupil is more accurate.

(a) The observer's eye must be carefully aligned in front of the patient's eye to avoid parallax errors.

(b) Once it is confirmed that the mark is at the pupil center, the glasses can be removed and the vertical height to the mark measured.

(3) A plastic seg measure can be placed in the lower eyewire of the frame and the position of the pupil measured directly with the millimeter scale built into the seg measure (Figure 8-22b).

(4) A small hole can be punched into two pieces of opaque or translucent tape and the holes positioned on the lenses of both eyes so that the patient can see a distant object through both simultaneously (Figure 8-22c).

(a) When alternate covering of the eyes confirms simultaneous viewing of the object with both eyes, the positions of both pupils have been determined.

(b) Marking the pupil centers simultaneously minimizes the effects of head movements.

(5) It is imperative that the patient wear exactly the same frame size that will be ordered when the vertical height is taken.

(6) It is critical that the monocular PDs and vertical height be measured with utmost care and accuracy for optimum PAL performance.

7. If the eyes must be depressed too far to reach the reading area, the add power

Table 8-8. Identifying Markings on Progressive Addition Lenses

Manufacturer/lens	Identifying Mark (under nasal circle)	Horizontal Meridian Nasal and Temporal Markings	Add Power
American Optical		Circles	Yes
Omni Pro (HR)	PRO		
Truvision (HR) (decentered)	AO+		
Truvision (G,HR,PGX)			
Truvision Omni (HR,G,PGX,PBX)	AOB		
Truvision Omni (PC)	AOB nasal π (pi symbol) under add		
Truvision Prima (HR)	AOB nasal P under add		
Truvision Technica (HR)	AOT under nasal T under add		
Ultravue	None		No
Hoya			
Hoyalux 3 (1.56 plastic)	H3—looks like (−)3	Circles	Yes
KBco	None	Circles	
Solaris (gray No. 1 polarized)			
Optima	Inverted Italic v	Broken circles	Yes
Progressive Z (1.60 plastic)			
Orcolite	None	Triangles pointing nasally	Yes
Line Free (HR,PC,Trans)			
Pentax		Small dots	No
Zoom (HR)		Ps	
Zoom (HI)		APs (almost looks like Rs)	
Polarlite	None	Circles	Yes
Progressive M (Polarized HR and 1.56)			
Rodenstock	R		Yes
Progressiv R (HR,G,PGX)		Circles	
Progressiv S (HR,1.6G, Colormatic1.6)		Squares	
Seiko	None	Horizontally elongated S nasal and temporal	Yes
P-6 (HR)			
Selex	None	Circles	Yes
Polarex Pro			
Signet-Armorlite		Plus signs (+)	Yes
Elegance (HR,RLX Plus)	None		
Elegance (RLXLite HI)	SA		
Silor			Yes
Super No-Line (HR,G,PGX)	S	Squares	
Adaptar (HR,1.6P,Trans,G, PGX)	III	Diamonds	
Adaptar (1.6)	III6	Diamonds	

(*continued*)

Table 8-8.   (*Continued*)

Manufacturer/lens	Identifying Mark (under nasal circle)	Horizontal Meridian Nasal and Temporal Markings	Add Power
Sola		Yes	
		Nasal and temporal	
XL (HR,PC)	XL	Football-shaped Ss	
XL (PGX)	XL	Circles	
VIP (HR)	None	Football-shaped Ss	
VIP (G,PGX)	S	Circles	
VIP (PC)	VIP	Football-shaped Ss	
VIP Gold (1.54 Spectralite)	VG	Football-shaped Ss	
Varilux		Circles	Yes (2 digits)
Infinity (G,HR,PGX,Trans)	e		
Infinity (1.6G,1.6P)	e6		
Plus (HR)	V	Broken circles	
Plus (PC)	VP		
Plus (G,PGX,PBX)	V15		
Readables (HR)	Triangle		
Overview (HR)	V		
Vision Ease	Overlaping ve	Triangles pointing up	Yes (2 digits)
Delta (HR,G,PGX)			
Unison		U on horizontal meridian	
CV		C on horizontal meridian	
X-Cel	None	Circles	Yes (on HR
Freedom (HR,G)			only)
Younger	None	Cirlces	No
10/30,CPS (HR)			
Zeiss	None	Incomplete squares with	Yes (2 digits)
Gradal (HR,G,Umbramatic SB and SR)		diagonal lines inside	

HR = conventional hard resin plastic, HI = high index, G = glass, PC = polycarbonate, 1.6G = 1.60 index glass, 1.6P = 1.60 index plastic, Trans = Transitions, PBX = Photobrown extra, PGX = Photogray Extra

should not be increased in an effort to raise the desired power to a more accessible position in the lens.

    a. Raising the desired add in this manner places it higher in the progressive corridor where the width of the corridor is reduced.

    b. Instead, the fitting cross should be fit higher (at the expense of the patient tilting his or her head down for distance viewing) or another PAL with a shorter corridor should be used.

VI. Tints and Coatings

   A. *Definitions*

     1. Tints and coatings are applied to a lens to protect the eye, protect the lens, improve visual comfort, improve visual performance, or improve the appearance of the lens.

     2. Absorptive tints and absorptive coatings absorb parts of the electromagnetic spectrum (specifically, ultraviolet [UV], visible, and infrared [IR]) either selectively or uniformly.

       a. Absorptive tints can be used in plastic or glass lenses.

         (1) The most common method of tinting plastic lenses is to apply a dye to the surface of the lens by dipping it into a hot dye bath (surface tinted); these dyes do not adhere to glass lenses.

(a)

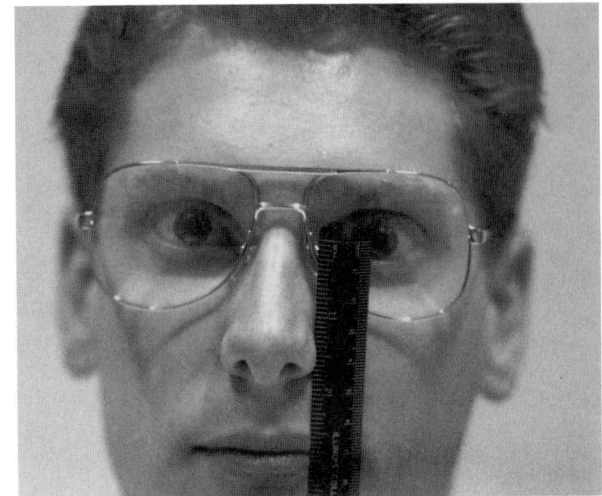

(b)

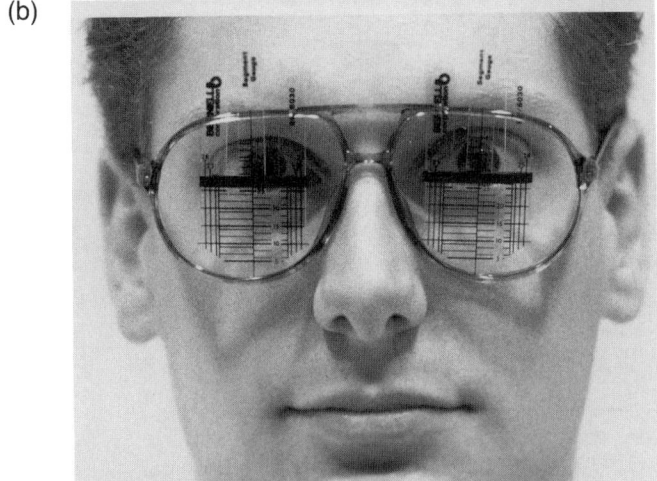

(c)

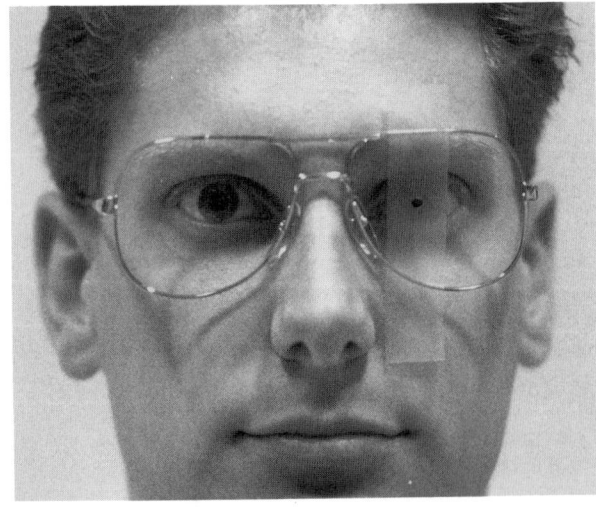

Figure 8-22.   Methods of measuring pupil center height for fitting PALs: (a) Direct measurement with a PD rule, the accuracy of which can be improved by making a mark on the lens at the pupil center for measurement with the frame removed; (b) plastic seg measure with its tip at the lowest point in the eyewire; (c) a piece of tape with a small viewing hole to locate the line of sight.

(2) Glass lenses are tinted by the addition of inorganic metallic oxides to the molten glass matrix when the ingredients are combined (matrix tinted).

(3) A few plastic lenses are also matrix tinted, with the tint throughout the plastic lens material.

    b. Another method of changing the absorption of glass lenses is through the application of absorptive coatings to the lens surfaces through the use of vacuumcoating.

3. Other coatings can be applied to the surfaces of glass and plastic lenses.

    a. Scratch-resistant coatings (SRC) for plastic lenses increase the scratch resistance of these softer lens materials.

    b. Antireflection coatings (ARC) applied to the surfaces of glass or plastic lenses decrease the amount of light reflected from the surfaces while increasing the amount of light that is transmitted.

    c. Mirror coatings significantly reduce light transmission through the lens.

    d. Edge coatings used on high-minus lenses reduce the intensity of internal reflections of the lens edge which cause the concentric rings characteristic of high minus.

4. The transmitted light is the fraction of the light incident onto the front surface of the lens that emerges from the rear surface.

    a. Some of the light is lost by reflection at each of the two surfaces.

(1) Fresnel's law of reflection states that for light incident normal to the surface, the fraction of light reflected r is given by $r = (n' - n)^2/(n' + n)^2$, where n' is the lens index of refraction and n is the index of refraction outside the lens.

(2) For example, at each surface of an ophthalmic crown lens in air, the fraction of light reflected is $r = (1.523 - 1)^2/(1.523 + 1)^2 = 0.043 = 4.3\%$.

(3) The fraction transmitted through the surface is $T = 1 - r = 1 - 0.043 = 0.957$.

    b. Some of the light is lost by absorption within the lens material.

(1) Lambert's law of absorption states that layers of a medium which have equal thicknesses absorb equal fractions of the light incident upon them.

(2) If α is the fraction absorbed by a lens having a center thickness of 1 mm, then the fraction T_m transmitted by the medium is $T_m = 1 - \alpha$.

(3) If a lens made of the same material has a 2-mm center thickness, then the fraction transmitted is $(T_m)^2$.

(4) If the lens has a thickness of 2.6 mm, the amount transmitted is $(T_m)^{2.6}$.

(5) The total fraction of light transmitted through the ophthalmic crown lens having a 2.6-mm thickness is $T^2 T_m^{2.6}$.

(6) For absorptive tints within the lens matrix, the fraction of incident light that is transmitted is thickness dependent.

    (a) The amount of light transmitted varies from the center of the lens to the edge as the thickness changes.

    (b) This is not the case for surface-tinted lenses, in which the transmission is constant from center to edge.

    c. The transmission properties of a lens throughout the UV, visible, and IR spectra are illustrated by means of the transmission curve.

(1) The percentage or fraction of light transmitted as measured by a spectrophotometer is plotted as a function of wavelength.

    (a) Figure 8-23a shows the transmission curves for ophthalmic crown glass, hard resin, and PC, and a high-index plastic.

    (b) Figure 8-23b shows the transmission curves for a brown No. 2 sun lens in several materials:

      i. A glass lens for which the tinting material is throughout the lens.

      ii. A glass lens coated on the surface.

      iii. A hard resin lens tinted on the surface.

      iv. The transmission properties are similar for this tint except in the IR, where the hard resin has considerably greater transmission, and in the UV, where the coated glass lens transmits

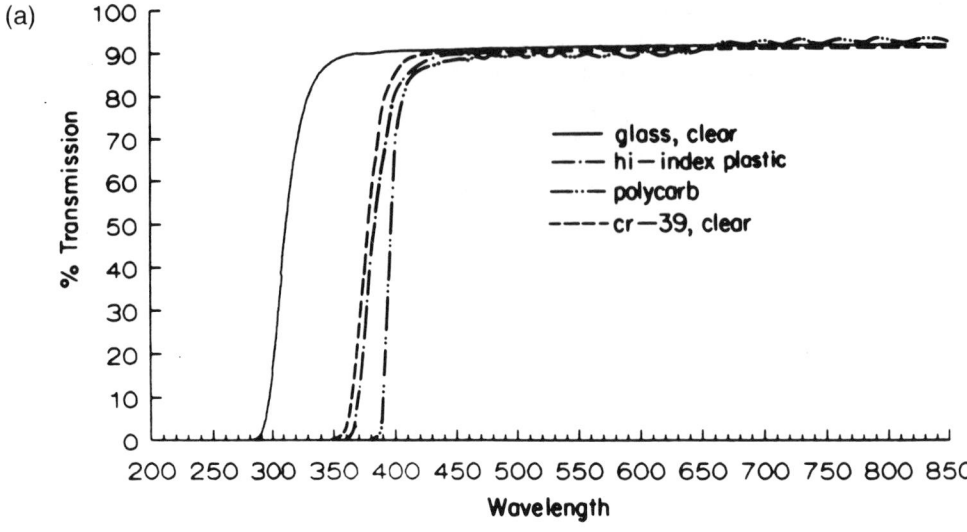

(a)

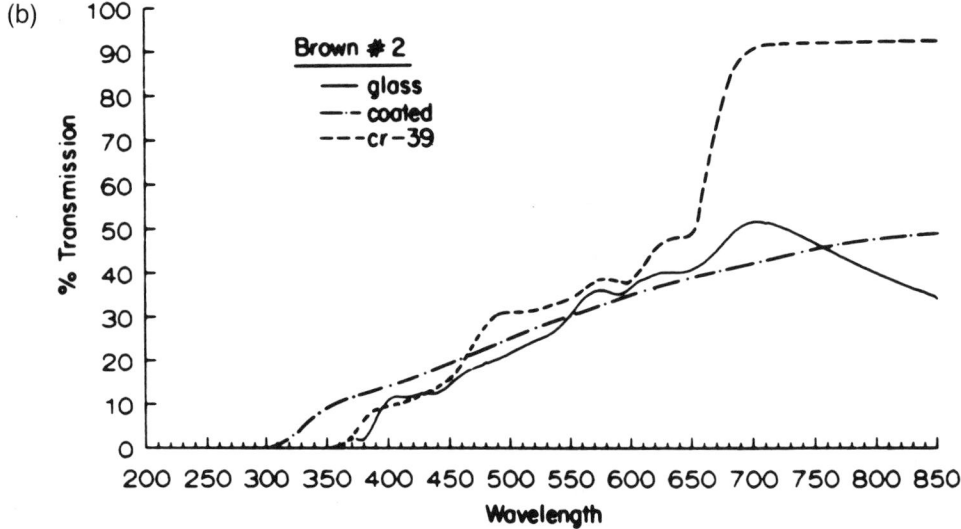

(b)

Figure 8-23.   (a) Transmission properties of four clear ophthalmic lens materials. (b) Transmission properties of a brown No. 2 sun lens in three different types of lenses. (Used by permission of Lee GK. Tints and coatings. In: Sheedy JE, ed. *Problems in Optometry. Environmental Optics. Vol. 2(1).* Philadelphia: J.B. Lippincott Company, 1990:164.)

considerably more UV than the matrix glass lens or the tinted hard resin lens.

(2) A transmission curve is the only way to know exactly the transmission characteristics of a lens.

   (a) It is not possible to infer the transmission properties of a lens based solely on its color.

   (b) For instance, a lens may appear green because it transmits monochromatic light in the green portion of the visible spectrum or because it transmits blue and yellow which combine to appear green.

5. Luminous transmittance denotes the total amount of light transmitted, with relative weighting given to the various wavelengths of the visible spectrum according to the luminosity function.

   a. Wavelengths in the yellow-green near 555 nm, the peak of the photopic luminosity function, are weighted with more significance than the ends of the

visible spectrum (blue and red) because the eye is more sensitive to the yellow-green in photopic conditions.
- b. Some lenses, such as the NoIR™ lenses, give information about transmission in terms of both total transmission (purely energy related) and luminous transmission.
6. Tint densities are customarily denoted through the use of a number or letter, with a higher number or letter indicating a darker tint (less transmission).
- a. Separate labeling systems are used for cosmetic tints and sunlens tints, with a 2.0- or 2.2-mm thickness and 555-nm wavelength commonly assumed.
  - (1) Approximate cosmetic tint transmissions: No. 1, 87%–88%; No. 2, 80%–85%; No. 3, 70%–75%.
  - (2) Approximate sunlens transmissions: No. 1, 65%; No. 2, 50%; No. 3, 35%.
- b. As plastic lenses have become more common with dyes which can be conveniently applied in a continuum of densities, the meaning of these numbers has become less predictable.
  - (1) Many offices have tinted lens samples labeled 1, 2, and 3 which have been generated with the office tinting unit without comparison to any objective standard.
  - (2) Plastic tint samples fade with time, changing the meaning of a particular tint number in a specific office.
  - (3) Finishing laboratories that tint plastic lenses learn from experience with particular offices how dark a tint is desired when a particular number is ordered.
  - (4) When a tint is being ordered from a laboratory that is unfamiliar with one's tinting preferences, a sample sent with the order is desirable.
7. The transmission of a lens is sometimes presented in terms of its optical density (OD), which is reciprocally related to the transmission.
- a. $OD = \log_{10}(1/T)$.
  - (1) If $T = 1.00$ (100% transmission), OD is 0.
  - (2) If $T = 0.10$ (10% transmission), OD is 1.0.
  - (3) If $T = 0.01$, (1% transmission), OD is 2.0.
  - (4) Each unit increase in OD means a tenfold decrease in the transmission of the lens.
- b. ODs are additive.
  - (1) If two lenses are placed together, one having an OD of 0.03 and the other having an OD of 0.02, the OD of the combination is $0.03 + 0.02 = 0.05$.
  - (2) The transmission of the combination can be found from the definition of OD:

$$0.05 = \log(1/T)$$
$$10^{0.05} = 1/T$$
$$1.12 = 1/T$$
$$T = 0.891$$

8. Shade numbers are used to identify transmission properties of lenses used for protection in industry, particularly those used during welding.
- a. Shade number = $(7/3)(OD) + 1$.
- b. $OD = (3/7)$(shade number $- 1$).
- c. Shade numbers range from 1.5 to 14, with shade numbers less than 5 intended for those exposed to welding but not actually welding themselves.
- d. Shade numbers 5 and larger are for welders, with the higher numbers for heavier duty welding with higher amperage and higher light outputs.

B. *Glass tints*
1. For years the staple of the industry before the arrival of the plastic lens, glass lenses were tinted by the addition of metallic oxides to the glass melt.
- a. Different manufacturers use slightly different "recipes," so if a glass lens must be matched in color, the new lens must be ordered from the same manufacturer.

        b. Certain "brand names" labeling glass tints became associated with the manufacturer, some of which still remain.
  (1) American Optical: Calobar—green; True-Color—gray; Hazemaster—yellow; Cosmetan—brown.
  (2) Bausch & Lomb: Kalichrome—yellow.
  (3) Shuron: Neutrex—gray.
  (4) Vision Ease
    (a) Striking Yellow—yellow.
    (b) Vision Ease labels many of its other tints very simply, such as Gray No. 1, Gray No. 2, Tan No. 1.
  c. Typically no more than three transmissions are available in a particular color.
  d. Since the tint is throughout the lens material, the density is thickness dependent.
    (1) A high-minus glass matrix tinted lens is lighter in the center and darker at the edges.
    (2) Since the transmissions associated with a particular tint density are based on a thickness of 2 or 2.2 mm, any part of the lens which is significantly thicker will be darker than the assumed transmission implies.
  2. A second means of coloring glass lenses is through surface coating.
    a. Coatings are applied in high-temperature vacuum chambers in which the metallic oxides are vaporized onto the concave surface of the lens.
    b. Increased density is obtained by increasing the thickness of the coating.
      (1) A gradient coating, varying in density from the top of the lens to the bottom, can be generated by varying the thickness of the coating.
      (2) For a solid coating, the density is constant across the lens surface, so there is no variation with lens thickness, as with a matrix-based tint.
    c. Vacuum coating is done almost exclusively on glass lenses.
      (1) It is possible to vacuum coat plastic lenses, but lower temperatures are required to avoid warpage.
      (2) The ease of surface tinting plastic lenses with dyes minimizes the need for vacuum coating, which is more expensive and time consuming.
    d. Disadvantages of a color coating include
      (1) A coated lens is subject to scratching; it can be stripped and then recoated.
      (2) Surface reflections from the metallic oxide coating are distracting.
        (a) An ARC is often combined with the color coating to reduce the reflections.
        (b) The ARC has a scratch-resistant coating that helps protect the color coating.

C. *Plastic tints*
  1. By far the most common method for tinting plastic lenses is through the application of dye to the surface.
    a. The dye solution is heated to 190–205° (F) and the lens is dipped into the bath for a length of time varying from a few seconds to several minutes.
      (1) A pink No. 1 cosmetic tint requires only a few seconds.
      (2) A No. 3 gray sunlens tint may take 30 minutes or more.
    b. The ions in the dye are attracted to the ions on the surface of the lens and penetrate 3–4 μm below the surface.
    c. A neutralizing solution can be used to remove the dye, making adjustment of the tint density or tint color convenient.
    d. High-index plastics can also be tinted, but the tinting times will be different than for hard resin due to different molecular structures.
    e. SRCs vary in the degree to which the tint can penetrate the surface.
      (1) High-index lenses often are manufactured in semifinished form with nonporous scratch-resistant coatings which the tint cannot penetrate.

(2) When the rear surface is finished, the nonporous coating is removed and may be replaced with a semiporous SRC which is tintable.

(3) When a lens, such as many PC lenses, has a nonporous surface, the lens cannot be tinted as darkly, since only one surface absorbs the tint.

(4) Special care must be taken in tinting lenses with scratch-resistant coatings, since too much heat or too caustic a neutralizing solution will break down the SRC and crazing of the surface will appear.

(5) Tinting a patient's old lenses for sunglasses should be done with caution if the lenses are coated with SRC, since patches of the lens where the coating has worn will tint more darkly.

  f. A variety of factors will cause two lenses left in the bath for the same time to be tinted differently.

(1) Lenses from different manufacturers likely have different molecular structures.

(2) Lenses from the same manufacturer which are from different batches of polymer may tint differently.

(3) A lens from a finished lens blank may tint differently than one from a semifinished blank due to potential differences in polymerization.

  g. With time the tint will fade; UV light, heat, soap, and other agents hasten the process.

  h. Tinting a plastic lens is truly an art, with a continuum of colors possible by dipping the lens in more than one tint.

D. *Clear lenses*

1. Untinted lenses are virtually transparent in the visible spectrum.

  a. Transmission is zero in the UV-C, begins to increase either in the UV-B or the UV-A, and remains fairly constant at maximum transmission through the visible spectrum and into the IR.

  b. The maximum transmission is less than 100% because of the loss of light by reflection at the two surfaces.

2. Ophthalmic crown glass begins transmitting in the UV at approximately 290 nm, so a significant amount of UV is transmitted (Figure 8-23a).

3. Plastic lenses are not inherently effective at absorbing UV, but additives enhance the UV absorption.

  a. Hard resin begins transmitting at approximately 350–360 nm as the result of UV absorbers added to the polymer to help inhibit yellowing of the plastic (Figure 8-23a).

  b. PC begins transmitting at approximately 380 nm as the result of UV inhibitors added to the surface coating (Figure 8-23a).

E. *Cosmetic tints*

1. Cosmetic tints can be obtained in a wide variety of color, including pink or rose, yellow, green, blue, and gray.

2. Cosmetic tints may be used for several reasons.

  a. To blend the lens with the frame.

  b. To reduce the harshness of the clear lens by blending it with the facial coloration.

  c. To improve the appearance of the lens by reducing surface or edge reflections, especially in high myopes, or by reducing the visibility of a segment line.

  d. To reduce glare and/or lens fluorescence in the cataract patient.

  e. To reduce discomfort from ambient lighting.

3. The most common cosmetic tint is the pink or rose tint.

  a. Transmission is reduced slightly in the UV and blue end of the visible spectrum, but in general, transmission characteristics are very close to clear glass or plastic.

  b. Many patients express increased comfort with a pink or rose No. 1 or No. 2 tint, and the prudent decision is not to change it.

F. *Sunlens tints*
1. Sunlens tints significantly reduce the transmission of light, according to the densities listed earlier.
    a. A good general-purpose sunlens for use on bright days should be at least as dark as a No. 3, preferably transmitting 20%–25%.
    b. For special light-rich environments, such as snow skiing, the transmission should be closer to 5%.
2. The most commonly used colors for sunlenses are gray, green, and amber/brown.
    a. Sunlenses in these colors can be made in glass, either matrix-based solid or surface coated, and in plastic with a surface tint.
        (1) In general, the transmission characteristics of the three types of lenses (glass matrix, glass coated, plastic tinted) are quite similar in the visible spectrum, with any differences largely insignificant.
        (2) The plastic lens typically absorbs more effectively in the UV due to the superior absorption of the UV inhibitor in the hard resin.
        (3) The plastic lens absorbs much less effectively in the IR than the glass lenses.
        (4) Figure 8-23b shows the transmission properties of the three types of lens in No. 2 brown.
    b. Perhaps the most popular sun lens color is gray, due to its uniform transmission in the visible spectrum.
        (1) Also termed a neutral density lens, this lens does not cause color distortion, since all wavelengths are attenuated equally.
        (2) Mixtures of iron, cobalt, and nickel are used to achieve the color in the glass lenses.
    c. The transmission curve of the green lens peaks near 550 nm, near the peak of the human photopic luminosity curve.
        (1) The transmission decreases significantly toward the longer and shorter wavelengths in the visible spectrum.
        (2) The green lenses have improved absorption in the UV compared to the gray, though transmission still begins at about 350 nm for the glass lenses.
        (3) Plastic lenses once again have significantly less absorption in the IR compared to the glass lenses.
        (4) There is some color distortion through green lenses, though most patients adapt without difficulty.
    d. The transmission curve of an amber/brown lens shows decreased transmission in the short wavelengths with a gradual increase toward longer wavelengths (Figure 8-23b).
        (1) The attenuation of the blue portion of the visible spectrum lends the lens its amber or brown color.
        (2) These lenses have grown in popularity in recent years due in part to the softer psychological impact of brown compared to the more stark gray or green.
        (3) Another reason for the increased popularity is the decreased transmission in the UV (much like the green) and short visible (blue), which many patients feel enhances contrast and comfort of the lens.
        (4) Again there is some color distortion, particularly in the denser tints.
    e. For patients who desire quite dark tints (approximately 10% transmission or less), glass matrix lenses with an added coating may give superior performance to plastic tints, although a plastic tint can be made quite dense if the lens is left in the dye for several hours.

G. *UV absorbers and minus blue lenses*
1. UV light has been implicated in the progression of degenerative processes in several ocular structures, including the conjunctiva, cornea, crystalline lens, and retina.
    a. The energy of a photon of light is inversely related to the wavelength, so the short visible (blue) spectrum has also come under scrutiny regarding its potential damaging effects.

b. A prudent clinical guideline might be that spectacle lenses should absorb UV shorter than 380 nm under normal circumstances and up to 400 nm (if not 500 nm) under special higher-risk conditions, such as high-altitude skiing, lifeguarding, and aphakic patients.

c. PC with its standard scratch resistant coating absorbs wavelengths shorter than 380 nm, but glass, hard resin, and high-index plastic require additional treatments to provide this level of protection.

    (1) Glass lenses can be treated with a UV-400 coating which absorbs wavelengths shorter than 400 nm and renders the lens faintly yellow.

    (2) Hard resin and high-index plastics can be dipped in UV-absorbing solutions using the same tinting units used for other dyes.

        (a) Depending on the solution, the lens is left in the bath for 1–30 minutes.

        (b) The cutoff wavelength below which all UV and/or visible light is absorbed ranges from 370 to 400 nm depending on the UV solution used.[6]

        (c) The lens should be checked with a reliable spectrophotometer to determine its UV absorbing capacity after the treatment.

        (d) Any other tint treatment of the lens should be applied after the UV treatment to avoid leaching of the tint into the UV solution.

    (3) Some hard resin lenses are made with UV absorbers in the polymer which increase the transmission cutoff to 380 nm.

2. "Minus blue" lenses are lenses that absorb the blue end of the spectrum as well as the UV.

a. These lenses seem to enhance contrast through a mechanism which is unclear.

    (1) One proposed mechanism is reduced light scatter.

        (a) This seems logical, since short wavelengths are scattered more highly by small particles than long wavelengths; absorption of the blue eliminates the greatest sources of scatter.

        (b) However, the particles in many situations, such as water molecules in clouds or fog, are large enough that scatter is not wavelength dependent.

    (2) The contrast enhancement may be due to reduced chromatic aberration leading to increased visibility.

b. Regardless of the mechanism, yellow lenses or "shooting" lenses are heartily endorsed by many marksmen, who maintain that the lenses improve the target visibility, depending on the type of target and its background.

c. Yellow lenses such as the Hazemaster and Kalichrome have steep dropoffs in transmission to zero or close to it for wavelengths shorter than 480–500 nm.

d. "Blublockers" are denser than yellow lenses; the short wavelength cutoff is somewhat longer and the lens appears amber.

e. Corning Optical has a series of photochromic lenses (Corning Glare Control™) which have cutoff wavelengths above 500 nm (see later discussion in section VI.I.2).

f. Younger Optical offers a series of plastic lenses, the Protective Lens Series (PLS), for which the cutoff wavelengths are 530, 540, and 550 nm.

    (1) The tint is throughout the polymer of the lens.

    (2) Though the PLS lenses mimic closely the cutoffs of the Corning Glare Control series, the PLS series is not photochromic.

    (3) Prescription lenses can be made from PLS or they can be provided in clipon form.

H. *IR absorbers*

1. Infrared radiation causes cataract, such as glassblower's cataract, and retinal burns, so IR protection must be provided in environments with large amounts of IR.

2. A few lenses provide IR protection in varying amounts.

a. A glass matrix-based green lens provides fairly good IR protection.

b.   The therminon lens, a pale bluish-green, provides fair IR protection and is helpful for cooks and others exposed to sources of heat such as furnaces and stoves.

c.   NoIR™ lenses are plastic lenses which are available in several colors, including amber and gray-green, and in transmissions as low as 1%.

   (1)   NoIR lenses provide quite good protection from IR and from UV, particularly in the denser tints.

   (2)   NoIR are available only in plano powers, either as goggles for fitting over existing spectacles, as clipons, or as plano glasses.

I.   Photochromic lenses

1.   Photochromic lenses change density in response to the ambient light levels.

   a.   The lens darkens under bright light, such as sunlight, and fades to a lighter density under dimmer illumination, such as indoor lighting.

   b.   The extent of the darkening is dependent upon the UV content of the ambient light, since UV causes more change in density than visible light.

   c.   Both glass and plastic photochromic materials are available.

      (1)   In glass lenses the photochromic property is due to silver halide crystals added to the glass melt.

         (a)   Light which is rich in UV causes the crystals to dissociate and the glass to darken.

         (b)   When the light is removed, the crystals recombine, causing the lens to lighten.

      (2)   Plastic is rendered photochromic through a treatment limited to the surface of the lens.

2.   Corning Glass Works, which makes photochromic glass commonly used in the United States, currently has a family of four crown glass-based full-spectrum photochromic lenses, two 1.6 high-index glass photochromics, and a family of photochromic "minus blue" lenses.

   a.   Crown glass-based full spectrum lenses

      (1)   Photogray Extra® (PGX)

         (a)   PGX is a general-purpose lens with a wide transmission range ranging from 85% in its most faded state to 22% in its darkest state.

         (b)   Transmission is fairly even across the visible spectrum.

         (c)   There is 97% absorption in the UV-A and poor IR absorption.

      (2)   Photobrown Extra® (PBX)

         (a)   PBX is also a general-purpose lens having virtually the same transmission limits as PGX (85% and 25%), but the brown is a warmer color than the gray.

         (b)   Transmission is diminished in the short visible spectrum, especially in the darkened state.

         (c)   There is 98% absorption in the UV-A.

      (3)   Photosun II® (PSII)

         (a)   PSII, designed to provide a darker sunlens than the PGX, has a darkened transmission of 12% and a faded transmission of 40%.

         (b)   The transmission is constant throughout the visible spectrum except for an abrupt increase in transmission for wavelengths longer than 650 nm.

         (c)   UV-A absorption is 98%.

      (4)   Photogray II® (PGII)

         (a)   PGII, designed to provide a lighter cosmetic tint than PGX, has a darkened transmission of 42% and a faded transmission of 87%.

         (b)   The transmission is constant throughout the visible spectrum in both the faded and in the darkened state, though in the darkened state there is an increase in transmission for longer than 650 nm.

         (c)   UV-A absorption is 93%.

      (5) Bifocals are available in these photochromic lenses.
         (a) They are fused on the front surface.
         (b) The segments are made with fusible segment glass which is not photochromic.
         (c) The segment area of a bifocal appears lighter than the rest of the lens.

b. 1.6 high-index photochromics
    (1) PhotoGray 16™.
    (2) PhotoBrown 16™.
    (3) Both 1.6 index lenses perform similarly to their 1.523 counterparts but have the thinness advantage of high-index glass.

c. Photochromic "minus blue" lenses
    (1) Originally named the Corning CPF® lenses, these lenses are now called the Corning Glare Control™ Lenses.
    (2) CPF 450, CPF 511-S, CPF 527-S, CPF 550-S, and CPF 550-XD are all photochromic lenses which begin transmitting wavelengths longer than the wavelength in the names.
       (a) The lenses with the "S" suffix are in the standard series of CPF lenses.
       (b) The 550-XD has the same 550-nm cutoff as the 550-S, but the XD is a darker lens, transmitting less in the rest of the visible spectrum.
       (c) The Glare Control lenses transmit a small, controlled amount of blue in order to reduce color distortion.
    (3) CPF 511-DN and CPF 527-DN are the same lenses as their counterparts in the standard series except that a brown mirror coating is added to the front surface of the lens, which reduces the overall transmission of the lens slightly.
    (4) In the CPF processing, photochromic glass lenses undergo treatment in a hydrogen atmosphere which reduces the silver halide crystals on the surface to elemental silver particles.
       (a) These particles determine the cutoff wavelength below which the transmission is essentially zero.
       (b) The front surface of the lens is refinished to remove the special layer so the activating light rays can enter the lens.
    (5) Patients with eye diseases such as macular degeneration and cataracts find Glare Control lenses improve contrast, performance, and comfort.

3. Photochromic glasses made by Chance Pilkington, Ltd., and by Desag are also used by some lens manufacturers that manufacture the lenses under their own brand names.

4. Several variables modify the darkness of a photochromic glass lens besides the intensity and UV content of the ambient light.
    a. Temperature—photochromic lenses are darker in colder conditions and lighter in hotter conditions, especially when the temperature is above 90°F.
    b. Exposure history—photochromic lenses typically require several cycles of fading and darkening to achieve the greatest range of transmission and fastest speed of change.
    c. Tempering—heat-tempered lenses are darker at higher temperatures and fade more slowly than chemically tempered lenses.
      (1) Chemical tempering gives a wider range of transmissions between fully darkened and fully faded states.
      (2) Chemical tempering gives greater impact resistance than thermal hardening.
      (3) Hardened photochromic glass is not as impact resistant as hardened crown glass, but it is sufficient to pass the drop ball test.

5. Two plastic photochromic lenses are available, the Colormatic® by Rodenstock and the Transitions® by Transitions Optical.
    a. The Colormatic® is light brown when faded and bluish gray when darkened.
    b. The Transitions® is a pale bluish tint when faded and gray-blue when darkened.

    c.   These lenses are cosmetic tints rather than sun lens tints; patients expecting the same performance as photogray extra glass will be disappointed.

    d.   Plastic photochromics have two important disadvantages compared to their glass counterparts.

        (1)   The plastics are more susceptible to the effects of temperature, becoming much darker in cold temperatures and very light in hot temperatures.

        (2)   The plastics tend to lose the capacity to change transmissions after a couple of years.

J. *Polarized lenses*

1.   Polarized lenses selectively remove glare reflected from a horizontal surface.

2.   A layer of polarizing material is enclosed within the glass or plastic lens.

    a.   The polarizing layer is constructed with the molecules aligned in an orderly fashion along one axis.

    b.   This orderly array of molecules has a transmission axis that transmits light waves vibrating in a plane parallel to the axis but absorbs waves vibrating in a plane perpendicular to it.

3.   In order for polarizing lenses to work effectively, the light entering the lens must be plane polarized, that is, vibrating in one plane.

4.   Ambient light from sunlight or indoor lighting is normally unpolarized, randomly vibrating in any of the planes perpendicular to the direction the light travels.

5.   When light is reflected from water, the reflected light is totally plane polarized if the incident light hits the water at an angle of 53° from the normal to the surface (Figure 8-24).

    a.   The reflected light is polarized parallel to the reflecting surface, horizontal in this case.

    b.   For angles of incidence other than 53°, the reflected light is partially polarized; much of the light, but not all, is plane polarized.

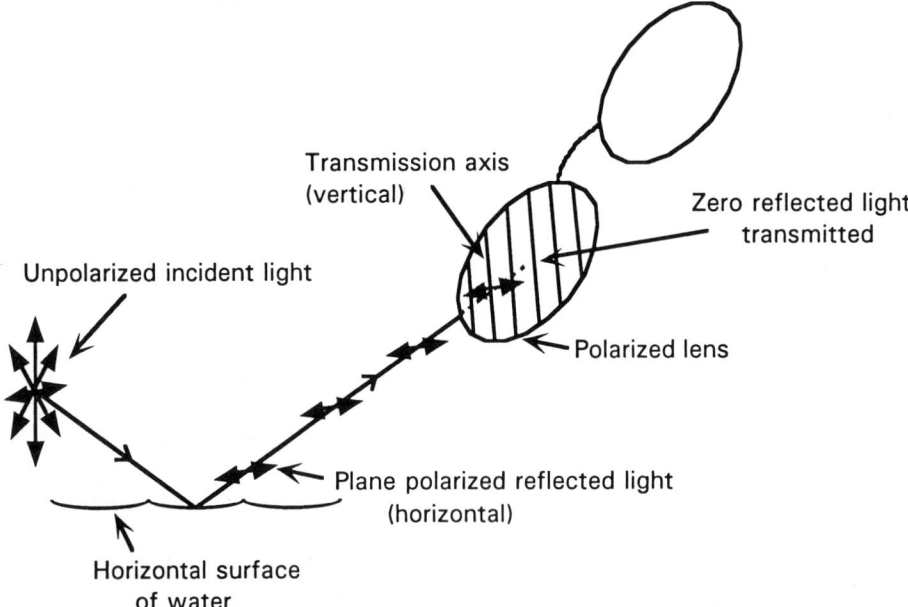

Figure 8-24. Unpolarized light incident on the surface of water at approximately 53° is plane polarized in the horizontal plane. A polarized lens having its transmission axis oriented vertically absorbs all the reflected light, reducing glare from reflective horizontal surfaces.

6. The polarizing layer is oriented in the lens with its transmission axis vertical.
   a. In this position the plane polarized light reflected from horizontal surfaces, such as water, is absorbed and the glare removed.
   b. Light reflected from metallic surfaces is polarized differently than for nonconductors such as water and is not absorbed as effectively.
7. Approximately half of the intensity of unpolarized light is attributable to waves vibrating perpendicular to the transmission axis.
   a. Polaroid lenses therefore attenuate unpolarized light by approximately 50%.
   b. The net result is that the polarizing lens reduces the intensity of unpolarized light by approximately 50% while essentially eliminating glare caused by specular reflection.
8. Polarizing lenses are made in one of two ways, laminated or in-mold.
   a. In the laminated lens, the polarizing layer is bonded between two layers of the lens material.
      (1) Both glass and plastic polarizing lenses are made in the laminated form.
      (2) Because of the differences in expansion coefficients between the polarizing layer and the lens layers, laminated lenses, especially those made from glass, are subject to delamination when temperature changes are abrupt or extreme.
      (3) Laminated lenses cannot be tinted or coated due to the heat during these processes.
   b. The in-mold lenses are fabricated by placing the polarizing layer in the lens mold and pouring the plastic polymer around it.
      (1) The bonding is more stable than for laminated lenses and is less susceptible to heat.
      (2) In-mold lenses can be tinted and coated.
9. Flexing of a polarizing lens will cause it to lose its polarizing efficiency, so care must be taken to avoid conditions under which flexing is likely.
   a. Ultra thin center thicknesses should be avoided.
   b. Lenses must be edged exactly to frame size and shape to avoid tension in the frame.
10. Table 8-9 lists many of the tints and coatings currently available with their main purpose.

K. *Scratch-resistant coatings*
   1. SRCs are applied to plastic lenses to improve their durability under abrasion.
   2. Glass inherently has excellent abrasion resistance and a SRC is not needed.
   3. SRCs for plastic lenses are of two types, inorganic and organic.
      a. Quartz or glass is the primary ingredient in inorganic coatings, with the coating applied through vaporization in a heated vacuum chamber.
      b. The primary ingredient of organic SRC is a siloxane polymer combined with quartz.
      c. Three methods may be used to apply organic SRC.
         (1) The coating may be placed in the glass mold before the lens polymer; during the curing process the coating penetrates into the surface of the lens.
         (2) In the spin process, the coating is applied to the lens surface while it spins, and the lens is then cured by oven or UV.
         (3) In the dip process, the lens is dipped into the coating and then cured by oven, UV, or air.
   4. Care must be exercised to protect lenses with inorganic coatings from conditions of extreme temperature changes.
      a. The great difference in thermal expansion coefficients between the coating and the lens causes the coating to craze or crack under high temperatures.
      b. For this reason, lenses with inorganic SRC cannot be tinted, should not be left in hot environments such as closed cars, and should not be held in the path of hot air in a frame warmer.

5. Inorganic SRCs are typically applied when a lens is returned to have the SRC added.
6. The differences in thermal expansion coefficients are not so great for organic coatings, so lenses can be coated.
    a. If a coating has high scratch resistance, the surface is quite nonporous and not easily tinted.
    b. Easily tinted coatings are softer and more scratch prone.
    c. An organic SRC with a relatively high glass or quartz content may still craze with exposure to too much heat.
7. In-mold SRCs are convenient because they eliminate another step in the lens fabrication, decreasing lens turnaround time.
8. PC and high-index lenses have in-mold coatings applied as a standard feature.
9. Manufacturers have their own formulas for their SRCs, and coatings do not perform equally.
10. The easiest way to identify that a lens has an SRC is to see if water beads on the surface, indicating an SRC is present, though this will not determine whether the SRC is organic or inorganic.

L. *Antireflective coatings*
1. ARCs reduce the intensity of reflections from the surfaces of the lens.
2. Part of the light incident onto a lens is lost by reflection at each surface.
    a. The fraction lost by reflection is proportional to the index of the lens material, according to Fresnel's equations of reflection.
    b. For hard resin, about 4% is lost at each surface, while for 1.6 high-index plastic, 5.3% is reflected at each surface.
    c. Reflections from high-index materials are brighter and more visible.

Table 8-9. Characteristics of Common Lens Tints and Coatings

Tint/Coating	Characteristic
Pink	Comfort (from fluorescent lighting?), cosmesis
Yellow	Reduces scatter, increases subjective brightness, reduces chromatic aberration
Gray	Uniform absorption in visible spectrum No color distortion
Green glass	Good IR absorption
Brown	Psychologically warmer color than gray
UV coating	Absorbs UV-A
Photochromic	Transmission varies with light levels
Corning Glare Control	Photochromic; absorbs UV and blue
Younger PLS	Plastic (nonphotochromic); mimics Glare Control lenses
Therminon glass	Blue-green; increased IR absorption
Didymiun glass	Increased absorption at 589.3 nm for some types of welding
Polarizing lenses	Selectively absorbs light reflected from horizontal surfaces
NoIR	Absorbs UV and IR well
Antireflection coat	Decreases intensity of surface reflections Increases transmission
Scratch-resistant coat	Improves scratch resistance of plastic lens
Edge coat	Reduces graininess of lens edge; may blend with frame

3. Reflected light has several undesirable effects.
   a. Reflected images of objects in front of the lenses, such as light sources, are seen in the lenses by observers.
      (1) The reflected images reduce the visibility of the wearer's eyes.
      (2) This is particularly troublesome to people who perform on stage or do public speaking.
   b. The patient sees reflections in the surfaces of the lens of objects to the rear of the lens.
      (1) Sources of common complaints include lights behind the wearer and the wearer's own eye.
      (2) These reflected images can be distracting and uncomfortable.
   c. Since the reflected images are from a small fraction of the incident light, they will be most noticeable when the source is a bright light and the background is dark.
   d. Light reflected internally between the surfaces of the lens before entering the wearer's eye forms multiple ghost images.
      (1) These multiple images are also most disturbing when formed from a bright source on a dark background.
      (2) Headlights of oncoming cars at night bother many people for this reason.
   e. The light lost to reflection reduces the amount of light transmitted and therefore reduces the intensity of the transmitted images of interest.
   f. Patients wearing glasses for the first time are particularly aware of reflections.
   g. Lens power, base curve, vertex distance, pantoscopic tilt, and face forming (wrapping of the lens to the contour of the brow) all contribute to the position and visibility of the reflections.
4. ARC can be applied as either a single layer or as a multilayer coating.
   a. ARC is based upon the principle of wave interference.
      (1) Figure 8-25 shows an ARC on the rear surface (to the left) of a lens.

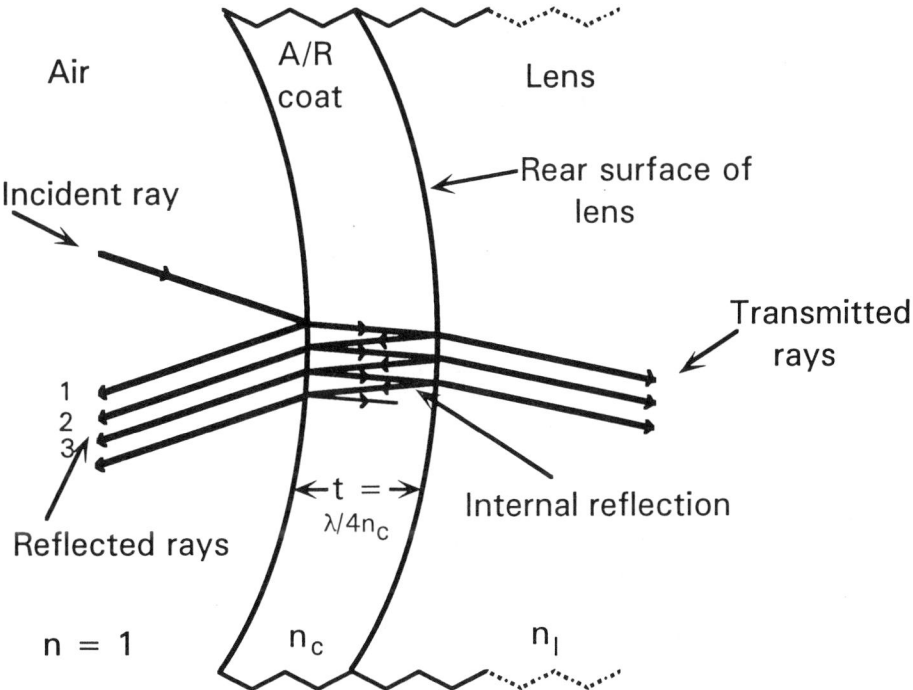

Figure 8-25. Light incident on the rear surface of a lens (lens is to the right) which is coated with an antireflection coating having a thickness of $\lambda/4n_c$. The indices of refraction for the coating and lens are n_c and n_l respectively. Reflected light is internally reflected inside the coating.

(2) Light is reflected from the external surface of the ARC and from the surface between the ARC and the lens.

(3) Some of the light is internally reflected within the ARC, first off the rear surface of the lens, then off the rear surface of the coating.

(4) Multiple waves from consecutive internal reflections emerge to the left from the ARC.

(5) If the path length differences and amplitude relationships among the waves are controlled properly, destructive interference occurs, reducing the intensity of the composite reflected wave to zero.

b. Single-layer coatings must satisfy two criteria to completely eliminate reflections.

(1) The thickness must be one quarter of the wavelength of the light.

  (a) The wavelength must be compensated for the index of the lens.

  (b) The thickness must be $t = \lambda/4n_c$, where λ is the wavelength of the light and n_c is the index of the coating.

(2) In order for the amplitudes to have the correct relationship, the index of the ARC, n_c, must be equal to $n_c = \sqrt{(n_l)(1)}$ where n_l is the index of the lens and 1 is the index of air.

(3) For ophthalmic crown lenses ($n_l = 1.523$), the required index for the ARC is $n_c = 1.23$.

(4) There is no material with an index as low as 1.23 which also has the necessary stability and durability to be a lens coating.

(5) The most suitable candidate is magnesium fluoride.

  (a) Its index is $n_c = 1.38$.

  (b) Magnesium fluoride is commonly used in single-layer ARC.

c. Single-layer ARCs have several shortcomings.

(1) Since magnesium fluoride does not satisfy the amplitude condition, reflections are not eliminated.

(2) Since the thickness of the coating can only satisfy the path condition for one wavelength, all other wavelengths are reflected.

  (a) Normally a wavelength near the middle of the visible spectrum is chosen for the path condition.

  (b) With the middle of the spectrum removed, the remaining blue and red ends of the spectrum combine to give a purplish cast to light reflected from a single-layer ARC.

(3) If the thickness of the ARC is designed to eliminate reflections for light entering perpendicular to the surface, it is not correct to eliminate reflections for light entering at other angles, since the path differences for the multiple reflections depend upon the angle of incidence.

(4) Single-layer ARC can increase transmission from 92% to about 96%.

d. Multilayer ARCs consist of several layers (up to nine or so) of different inorganic materials with the thicknesses adjusted to achieve destructive interference for larger numbers of wavelengths across the visible spectrum.

(1) Quartz is often the first layer vacuum coated onto the lens surface in order to provide a surface to which the remainder of the layers will adhere.

(2) The quartz provides some increased scratch resistance, but the top layer of the coating is often a modified SRC to increase scratch resistance as well.

(3) A multilayer ARC can increase transmission to more than 99%.

e. The quality and effectiveness of any ARC depends upon the coating laboratory's expertise in precisely controlling the thicknesses of the layers.

5. The ARC must be the last lens treatment done.

a. Any tinting must be done first.

(1) It is preferable to tint too dark and neutralize the tint to the proper density to remove tint from the outermost surface of the lens.

      (2) By doing this, the ultrasonic cleaning done prior to vacuum coating will not affect the tint.

      (3) Otherwise the cleaning tends to lighten the tint.

      (4) If the lens must be retinted, the ARC must be stripped first.

  b. SRCs are not necessary with ARC, since most ARCs incorporate some scratch resistance.

      (1) SRC can hinder the adhesion of the ARC.

      (2) SRC must not be added after the ARC.

6. ARC can be applied to photochromic lenses, but the tint will be lighter due to the increased transmission.

7. ARC is helpful on high-minus lenses to reduce the visibility of the concentric rings caused by internal reflection of the edges.

8. One major difficulty of ARC is the tendency for oily films from fingerprints and brows as well as other dirt to be more visible than without the ARC.

  a. Much of this increased visibility is due to the lack of veiling light once the surface reflections have been removed.

  b. Recently ARCs have been introduced with a "hydrophobic" top coating which tend to be easier to keep clean.

M. Other coatings

1. An edge coating is sometimes useful on high-minus lenses.

  a. It reduces the visibility of the internally reflected concentric rings and improves the cosmetic appearance.

  b. Although an ARC is helpful in reducing the visibility of rings seen straight ahead, the edge coating is more useful for the rings observed at more oblique angles.

  c. The combination of edge coating and ARC is often effective.

  d. Edge painting is a somewhat similar technique whereby the edge is painted a neutral gray to achieve the same result.

2. Mirror coatings

  a. Mirror coatings reduce transmission on sunlenses by increasing reflection.

  b. An inorganic coating is vacuum coated onto the front surface.

  c. The mirror coating can be combined with a tint to selectively absorb part of the spectrum in addition to the overall attenuation of the mirror coating.

VII. Prismatic Correction

A. Prism in single-vision lenses

1. When prism is required in a single-vision lens, it can be provided in several ways, through decentration, surfacing, Fresnel prism, or cemented prism.

2. Decentration is routinely used to place the OC of the lens in front of the patient's eye to avoid inducing unwanted prism.

3. When prism is desired, it is sometimes possible to achieve it through decentration, by displacing the OC away from the eye.

  a. The required amount of decentration is easy to calculate for horizontal or vertical prism, if the lens is a sphere or is a spherocylinder with its cylinder axis either horizontal or vertical.

  b. If S_H is the power in the horizontal meridian from the sphere power and C_H is the horizontal power from the cylinder, then the distance h that the OC must be moved from the eye to induce the necessary horizontal prism H is given by Prentice's rule: $h = H/(S_H + C_H)$.

  c. To obtain the total decentration from the GC to the position that induces the necessary horizontal prism, the decentration h is added to the decentration necessary to move the OC from the GC to the eye.

d. For example if the lens power is $-2.00\ -3.00 \times 090$, the frame PD is 72, the patient's distance PD is 64, and 1^Δ BO is required in the right eye, what is the necessary decentration?
   (1) The decentration to move the OC from the GC to the eye is (FPD $-$ PD)/2 $= (72 - 64)/2 = 4$ mm in.
   (2) The decentration to move the OC away from the eye to achieve 1^ΔBO is $h = 1^\Delta/(-2D-3D) = 0.2$ cm $= 2$ mm IN.
   (3) The direction of the 2-mm decentration is IN for BO prism, since the power in the horizontal is minus (Figure 8-26).
   (4) The total decentration is (4 mm in $+$ 2 mm in) $= 6$ mm IN.
e. If S_V is the power in the vertical meridian from the sphere power and C_V is the vertical power from the cylinder, then the distance v that the OC must be moved from the eye to induce the necessary vertical prism V is given by Prentice's rule: $v = V/(S_V + C_V)$.
f. This decentration is added to the decentration necessary to move the OC from the GC to the eye to obtain the total decentration of the OC from the GC to the position which induces the necessary vertical prism.
g. When the cylinder axis is neither horizontal or vertical, the calculation of the decentrations is much more complicated, and it is usually more convenient to order the prism ground in by the lab.
h. Prism by decentration adds no additional cost to the lens as long as a larger, more expensive blank is not required.
i. The amount of prism available by decentration depends on the lens power in the meridian of decentration, the amount of decentration to get the OC to the eye, and the size of the lens blank.
   (1) Relatively high amounts of prism can be achieved from moderate decentrations if the lens power is large.

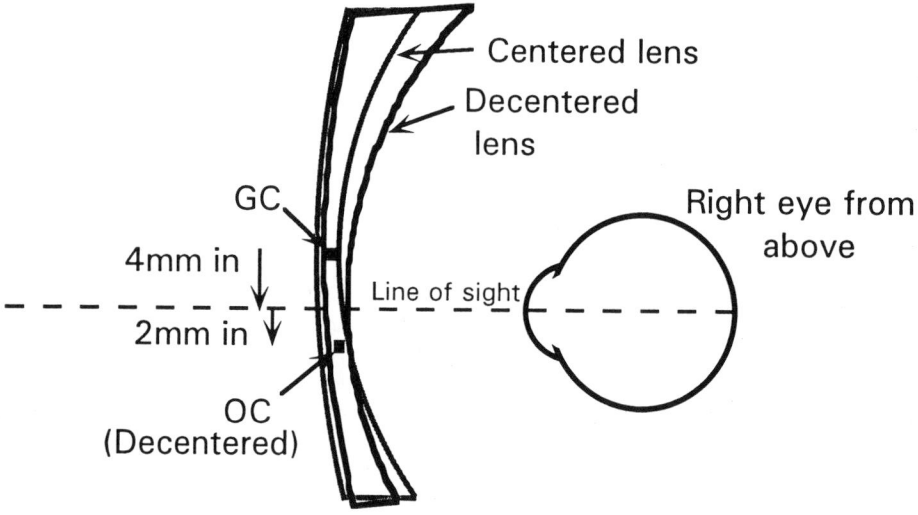

Figure 8-26. Total decentration. The shaded lens represents a centered minus lens with its OC at the GC, having essentially equal nasal and temporal edge thicknesses. The solid lens has been decentered 4 mm in to place the OC in front of the eye and an additional 2 mm in (total of 6 mm) to obtain BO prism. Decentration in for the minus lens causes a larger temporal edge thickness and smaller nasal edge thickness.

  (2) If the prism is achieved by decentering the OC out from the eye, more prism can be obtained because the movement is opposite to the inward decentration which moves the OC from the GC to the eye when the FPD is larger than the patient's PD.

4. Prism by decentration can be divided between the two eyes in several ways.

 a. Equal prism in each eye

  (1) If the powers of the two lenses are equal in the meridian of decentration, equal amounts of prism can be obtained in each lens by equal decentrations, assuming the monocular PDs are equal.

  (2) If the powers are different, equal prism amounts may be obtained by different decentrations, the amount being determined separately for each lens using Prentice's rule.

 b. Equal decentration

  (1) The magnitudes (absolute values) of the powers in the appropriate meridian for the two lenses are added together.

  (2) Using the total power from the two lenses, the decentration is calculated from Prentice's rule.

  (3) The amount of decentration of the OC from the eye is equal for each lens.

   (a) The direction of the decentration is whatever is necessary to contribute to the desired prism direction.

   (b) Two lenses are decentered in the same direction if the powers have the same sign, but in opposite directions if the powers have opposite signs.

   (c) The total decentration for the two lenses may not be the same, however, depending on the direction and amount of decentration to move the OCs to the eyes as the first step in decentration.

  (4) For example, assume the Rx is OD $+1.00 - 3.00 \times 090$, OS $+3.00DS$, with $2^{\triangle}$ BI total prism; the patient's monocular PDs are OD 32, OS 30, and the frame PD is 70 (Figure 8-27).

   (a) To obtain the prism by moving the OCs equal distances from the eyes, the distance is calculated from the absolute values of the powers in the horizontal meridian, 2.00D for the right eye and 3.00D for the left eye.

    i. OC movement $= 2^{\triangle}/(2D + 3D) = 0.4$ cm $= 4$ mm.

    ii. For the right eye, the OC is moved 4 mm OUT from the eye (to obtain 0.4 cm $\times$ 2D $= 0.8^{\triangle}$ BI).

    iii. For the left eye, the OC is moved 4 mm IN from the eye (to obtain 0.4 cm $\times$ 3D $= 1.2^{\triangle}$ BI).

   (b) Although the movements calculated so far are equal, the total decentrations will not be equal because of the differences in direction and the differences in monocular PDs.

    i. Decentration to put the OCs at the eyes is $(70/2) - 32 = 3$ mm IN for the right eye, and $(70/2) - 30 = 5$ mm IN for the left eye.

    ii. Total decentration for the right eye is 3 mm IN + 4 mm OUT = 1 mm OUT.

    iii. Total decentration for the left eye is 5 mm IN + 4 mm IN = 9 mm IN.

    iv. The small decentration for the right eye is easily accomplished, while the decentration for the left eye is borderline, depending on the blank diameters available.

 c. Other combinations of decentrations

  (1) Other combinations of decentrations that result in the necessary prism can be used.

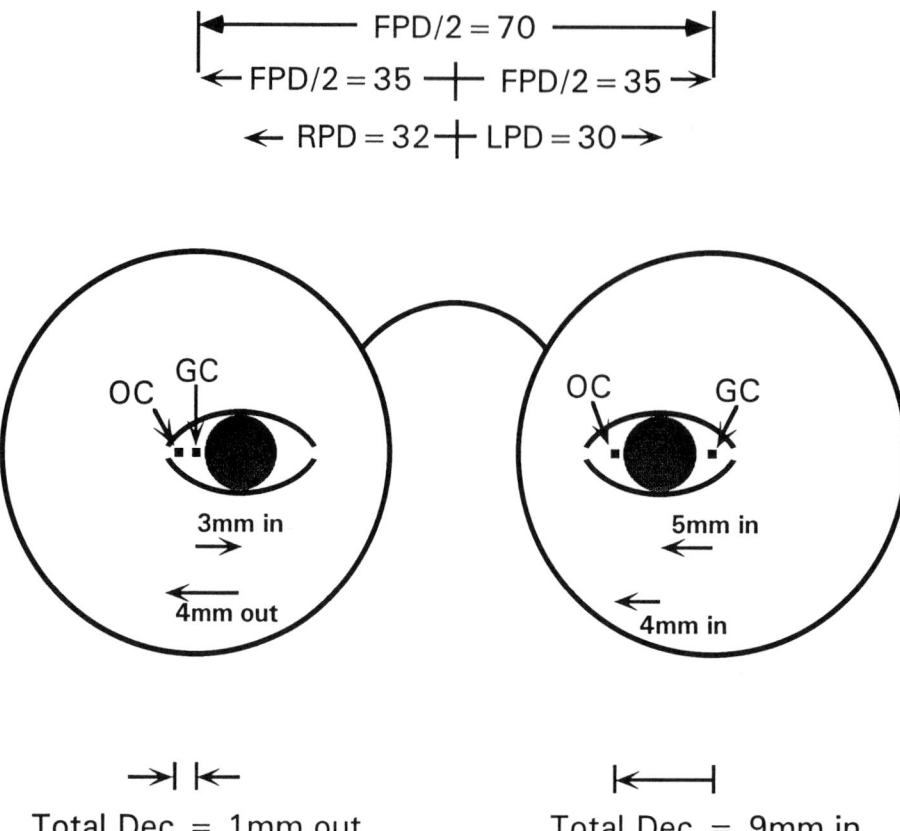

Figure 8-27.   Decentration. Right lens is decentered 3 mm in to place the OC at the eye, then 4 mm out to produce required prism for a total decentration of 1 mm out. Left lens is decentered 5 mm in to place the OC at the eye and another 4 mm in to produce prism for a total decentration of 9 mm in.

(2)   In the previous example, for instance, assume the maximum decentration for the left lens is 7 mm IN.
   (a)   Once the left lens has been decentered 5 mm IN to place the OC in front of the eye, there is 2 mm of decentration IN for prism, resulting in: 0.2 cm $\times$ 3D = 0.6^Δ BI.
   (b)   The remaining 1.4^Δ BI can be obtained from the right lens by moving the OC a distance $1.4^\Delta/2D$ = 0.7 cm = 7 mm OUT.
      i.   The right lens is decentered a total of 3 mm IN + 7 mm OUT = 4 mm OUT.
      ii.   This decentration, which is less than the 7 mm maximum, would be possible.
5.   Prism can also be ground into the lens when the lens is surfaced.
   a.   The semifinished lens is mounted so the rear surface of the lens is generated at an angle to the front surface, resulting in prism.
   b.   Prism generated in this way is optically indistinguishable from prism by decentration.
   c.   The OC of the lens may or may not lie within the physical borders of the lens depending upon the amount of prism.
   d.   Laboratories charge for grinding prism, with higher charges for higher amounts of prism.

  e. It is customary to divide prism between the lenses.

    (1) This equalizes weight and gives a more symmetrical appearance.

    (2) Prism powers less than 2^Δ can be put into one lens without observable differences in the lenses and at a savings of lens grinding costs.

  f. When prism amounts greater than $10–12^\Delta$ are required, grinding is not practical, and alternative methods, such as Fresnel prism or cemented prism, are required.

 6. Fresnel prisms are made from flexible plasticized polyvinyl chloride in powers from 0.5 to 30^Δ.

  a. Tiny prism elements are molded side by side in the surface of the thin membrane.

  b. The use of many tiny prism elements limits the width (apex to base distance) of elements.

    (1) Thickness and weight of the prism are greatly reduced.

    (2) The grooves between adjacent prism elements are visible as parallel lines on the surface of the prism.

  c. The membrane can be cut to any shape, to cover all or part of the lens surface.

  d. The prism is mounted on the rear surface of the lens with water, alcohol, or contact lens wetting solution, and is then held in place by surface tension once the liquid has evaporated.

  e. Fresnel prisms are convenient for testing a prism before incorporating it permanently into the lens.

 7. Cemented prism segments are conventional prisms made of glass or plastic which are cemented to the rear surface of the lens.

  a. The front surface is ground with a curve to match the rear surface of the lens.

  b. Cemented prisms are heavy and thick and have been largely replaced by Fresnel prisms.

 8. When reading is done through a single-vision distance decentered for the distance PD, the lines of sight converge nasal to and below the OCs.

  a. For minus lenses, BI prism is induced; for plus lenses, BO prism is induced.

    (1) Normally the prism is small enough that the patient is not bothered by it.

    (2) If the prism is uncomfortable for the patient, the amount of prism may be reduced by decentering the lens closer to the near PD.

    (3) The change in the decentration risks discomfort during distance viewing, however.

  b. If the powers in the vertical meridian are equal, zero resultant prism is induced.

  c. If there is anisometropia in the vertical meridian, vertical prism is induced.

  d. If the vertical prism causes discomfort, the patient should be instructed to tilt the head down while reading so the lines of sight view through the OCs, eliminating the vertical prism.

B. *Prism in multifocals*

 1. When reading is done through a multifocal, the lines of sight converge and lower to view through the near segment.

 2. If the horizontal prism induced through the distance lens causes discomfort, the inset of the bifocal can be modified to produce compensating prism.

  a. The amount of prism that can be generated by changing the inset of the segment is quite limited.

    (1) The add power is usually 2.50D or less.

    (2) The inset cannot be changed more than a few millimeters without seriously affecting the field of view through the segment, unless large segments are used.

    (3) When the segment is moved, the distance OC is generally moved in the same direction.

b. Sometimes larger amounts of horizontal prism are needed for near through the bifocal.

    (1) Prism segments can be used.

        (a) These are ribbon segments that have prism fabricated into them.

        (b) They are expensive, cosmetically unappealing, and are factory ordered, which causes time delays.

    (2) Fresnel prism can be mounted onto the segment area.

3. When anisometropia is present in the vertical meridian, vertical resultant prism is induced when the lines of sight are depressed to view through the segment.

a. Whereas for a single-vision lens the head can be dropped to view through the OC and avoid vertical prism, the eyes must drop below the distance OC to view through a bifocal segment.

b. If the vertical prism causes discomfort, several options are available to reduce the prism at the reading level.

    (1) The most commonly used treatment is slab off prism (Figure 8-28).

        (a) The lower part of the lens is modified to produce vertical prism.

        (b) For years the surfacing methods used to produce slab off prism resulted in BU prism in the lens with slab off.

            i. The method is known as bicentric grinding because it results in two distance optical centers, one for the upper part of the lens and one for the lower.

            ii. BU prism from slab off compensates for BD prism.

            iii. BD prism is induced in the lens with the greater minus (or less plus) power.

            iv. Therefore conventional slab off is prescribed as BU prism in lens with the greater minus power.

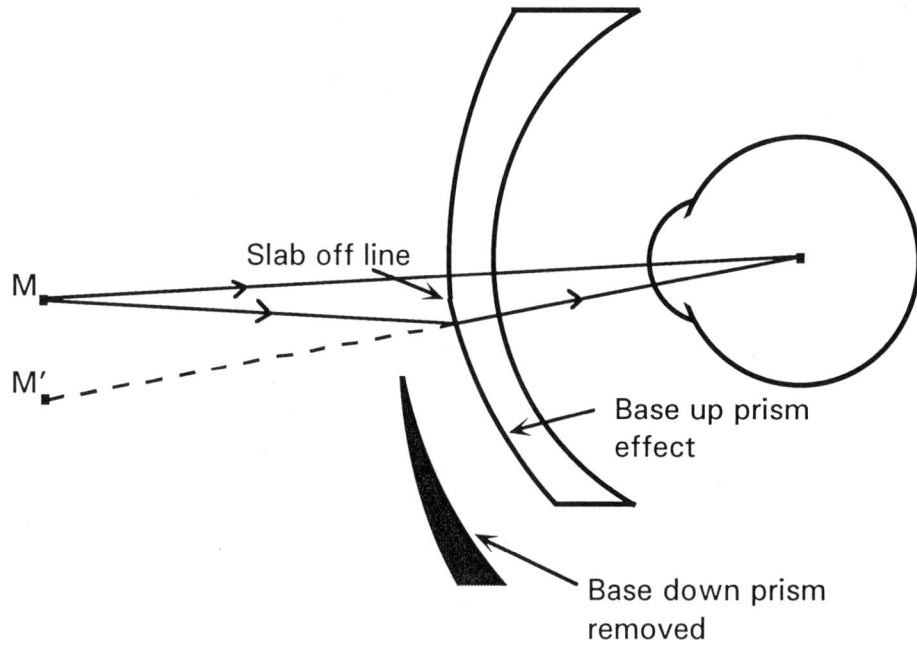

Figure 8-28.   Cross section of a lens with slab off prism. A BD prism component (shaded) is removed from the lens to create traditional slab off, leaving BU prism in the lower part of the lens. The BU prism causes an object M to be displaced downward to M' when viewed through the slab off portion of the lens.

    (2) Within the last few years, molds for plastic lenses have been used in which BD prism is generated.

        (a) This is termed reverse slab off or BD slab off.

        (b) BD slab off is prescribed on the lens of greater plus or less minus.

    (3) Slab off is prescribed in amounts from 1.0 to 6.0$^{\Delta}$.

    (4) The transition line at the top of the slab off is visible and gives the appearance of a full segment lens.

        (a) Slab off is generally used with flat-top bifocals.

        (b) The slab off line is placed at the top of the segment.

  c. R-compensated segments can be used to provide vertical prism in the segments.

    (1) This segment is 14 mm deep, and the seg OC can be ordered anywhere from 4 to 10 mm below the top of the segment.

    (2) By using different seg OC positions for the two lenses, vertical prism is induced.

    (3) The maximum vertical prism is 0.6 times the add power.

    (4) The lower segment OC position is placed in the lens with the greater plus or less minus in the vertical meridian.

  d. Dissimilar segments, having the OCs at different positions from the top of the segments, provide vertical prism in the same way as R-compensated segments.

    (1) Greater amounts of prism can be induced with dissimilar segments than with R-compensated segments because greater differences in segment OC positions are possible.

    (2) The difference in appearance of the two segments is much greater and is cosmetically unattractive.

    (3) One of the greatest OC differences is between a full segment with the OC at the top of the segment and the Ultex A with the OC 19 mm below the top of the segment.

        (a) For this combination the vertical prism is 1.9 times the add power.

        (b) For a 2.50D add, the vertical prism is 4.75$^{\Delta}$.

  e. The OC of the distance lens can be lowered, reducing the vertical prism induced at the reading level but risking increased vertical prism effect for distance viewing.

  f. A reading-only, single-vision Rx can be used to allow the eyes to view through the level of the OCs, eliminating resultant vertical prism.

  g. Contact lenses can be used for distance correction with a single-vision, reading-only Rx or bifocal overcorrection to eliminate anisometropia in the spectacle lens.

VIII. Verification

Before lenses are dispensed to a patient, they must be verified to be sure that all parameters are as ordered.

A. ANSI Z80.1-1987 standard

  1. The American National Standards Institute (ANSI) is a nongovernmental coordinator of voluntary standards development for a wide variety of industries.

  2. ANSI Z80.1-1987 Standard applies to ophthalmic lenses.

    a. First adapted in 1972, the Z80.1 standard was later revised in 1979 and again in 1987.

    b. It represents tolerances recommended by representatives of various groups in the optical and vision care sector.

    c. In certain instances, a laboratory may not meet the standard but the optometrist may decide that greater precision is not necessary.

d. In other instances, the optometrist may suggest that greater precision than suggested by the standard is necessary.
   (1) A good working relationship and communication with the laboratory is necessary.
   (2) The laboratory may agree to greater precision or may determine that it is unreasonable.
e. ANSI Z80.1-1987 is summarized in Table 8-10.

Table 8-10.   Summary of American National Standards Institute (ANSI) Z80.1 1987 Prescription Ophthalmic Lenses—Recommendations

Lens Parameter	Tolerance	Power Range (if applicable)
Sphere power	±0.13D ±2%	0.00–±6.50D >6.50D
Cylinder power	±0.13D ±0.15D ±4%	0.00–2.00D 2.12–4.50D >4.50D
Cylinder axis	+7° +5° +3° +2°	0.12–0.37D 0.50–0.75D 0.87–1.50D >1.62D
Vertical prism	±0.33△ (±1 mm difference in vertical level for higher-power nonprism lenses)	≤3.25D ≥3.37D
Horizontal prism	0.33△ each lens ±1 mm placement error in MRP 0.67△ imbalance for a pair of lenses ±2.5 mm error in MRP separation from specified PD in higher-power lenses	≤3.25D ≥3.37D
Thickness	±0.3 mm (if specified)	
Base curve	±0.75D (if specified)	
Warpage	±1.00D (not applicable within 6 mm of eyewire)	
Segment height	±1 mm of specified height and of each other for pair	
Segment inset	±1 mm of specification	
Impact resistance	Except for lenses listed below, all lenses must be capable of withstanding the drop ball test, whereby a 15.9-mm (5/8 inches) diameter steel ball weighing 16 g (0.56 oz) is dropped 127 cm (50 inches) onto the center of the lens. Laminated, plastic, and raised edge lenses that may be damaged by the test may be certified by the lens manufacturer as conforming to the test requirement or by testing statistically significant samples of the lenses. Certain lenses prescribed for specific visual needs are not suitable for the drop ball test. These lenses should be treated for impact resistance wherever possible, but testing requirements are waived. The lens types include: (1) prism segment multifocals; (2) slab-off prism; (3) lenticular cataract lenses; (4) iseikonics; (5) depressed segment one-piece multifocals; (6) biconcaves, myodiscs, minus lenticulars; (7) custom laminates and cemented lenses.	
Physical quality	Lenses should not have pits, scratches, grayness, bubbles, striae, or water marks visible without magnification in a lighted room against a dark background under an open-shaded 40-watt incandescent lamp with the lens 12 inches from the bulb.	

Table 8-11. Summary of Requirements for Prescription Safety Lenses: American National Standards Institute (ANSI) Z87.1-1989 Standard of Occupational and Educational Eye and Face Protection

Parameter	Requirements
Optical performance	Same requirements as listed in ANSI Z80.1-1987.
Impact testing	Lenses must be capable of resisting the fracture from the impact of a 25.4-mm (1 inch) diameter steel ball dropped 127 cm (50 inches). Prescription lenses, which are likely to experience surface damage at the point of missile contact in this test, may be tested usig an appropriate statistical protocol.
Penetration testing	Prescription lenses are exempt from penetration testing which is required of nonprescription lenses.
Lens thickness	Prescription lenses are not to be less than 3.0 mm thick, except lenses of 3.00D or greater plus power in the most plus meridian must have a minimum thickness no less than 2.5 mm.
Lens marking	Each lens is to be marked distinctly, permanently, and legibly with the manufacturer's monogram. In addition, nonclear lenses are to be marked with the shade number. Special-purpose lenses, such as those used for glassblowing, are to be marked on the surface with an "S" following the manufacturer's trademark. Photochromic lenses are to be marked with a "V" following the trademark.
Frame marking	All major frame components are to be marked with the manufacturer's trademark and with a "Z87" to indicate compliance with the frame requirements of the standard. Frames must also be marked with the A dimension, DBL, and overall length of the temple.

B. *ANSI Z87.1-1989 standard*
   1. Safety glasses, both prescription and nonprescription, are governed by ANSI Z87.1-1989.
   2. The requirements for prescription safety glasses are summarized in Table 8-11.
   3. Prescription safety lenses must meet the following special requirements.
       a. They must be no less than 3.0 mm thick.
           (1) This is for any material, including PC.
           (2) The only exception is for plus lenses 3.00D or greater in the most plus meridian, for which the thickness can be no less than 2.5 mm.
       b. The lenses must pass a more rigorous drop ball test than dress lenses, using a 1-inch diameter steel ball dropped from 50 cm.
       c. The lenses must be permanently marked with the manufacturer's identification monogram.
       d. Special purpose tints are marked with "S" following the monogram, while photochromic lenses are marked with "V."
   4. Safety frames must have all major components marked with the manufacturer's trademark and with "Z87."
   5. Both safety lenses and a safety frame must be used for a pair of glasses to be considered safety glasses.

C. *Lens powers*
   1. The lensometer (focimeter, vertometer) is the instrument most commonly used to measure vertex powers of lenses.
       a. When the power wheel is turned, a target (mire) is moved closer or farther from a standard collimating lens inside the end of the instrument farthest from the observer.
           (1) In the United States, the most common mire consists of two sets of lines perpendicular to each other (Figure 8-29a).
               (a) One line or set of lines is clear when the power of the sphere

a)

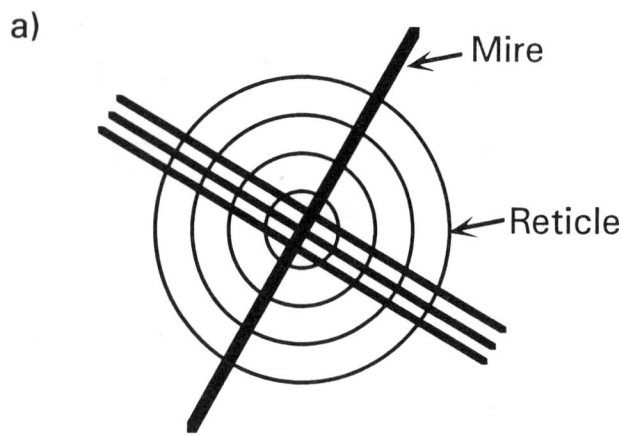

b)

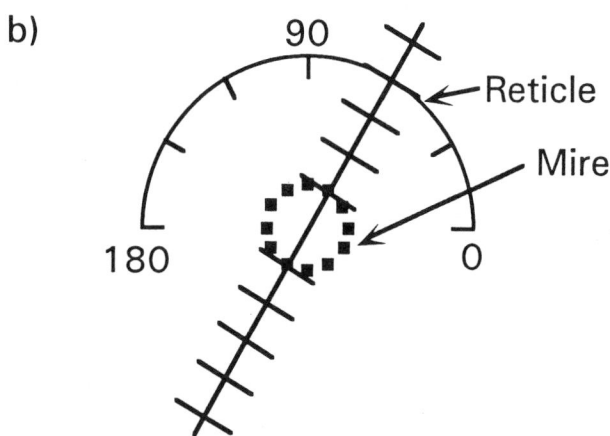

Figure 8-29.   (a) Lensometer target (mire) consisting of a single solid line and a group of three lines perpendicular to the first. (b) A mire consisting of a circle of dots.

meridian of the unknown lens is measured; this set is termed the sphere mire.

(b) The other set of lines is clear when the power reading is taken for the second principal meridian and is termed the cylinder mire.

(2) Less common targets have a circle of dots (Figure 8-29b).

(3) Some instruments have combination targets consisting of the line targets and a circle of dots.

b. An image of the target is viewed by the observer through a telescope which is focused for parallel light.

(1) The telescope has a reticle (cross-hair) within it which is used to measure prism and to sometimes determine the axis of the cylinder.

(2) Before the lensometer is used, the eyepiece must be focused so the reticle is clear to the relaxed eye (no accommodation).

(3) The eyepiece is rotated outward (counterclockwise) until the reticle is blurred and then inward (clockwise) until the eyepiece reticle is first clear.

(4) If the eyepiece is rotated farther inward after the reticle is first clear, accommodation must be used to keep it clear.

a)

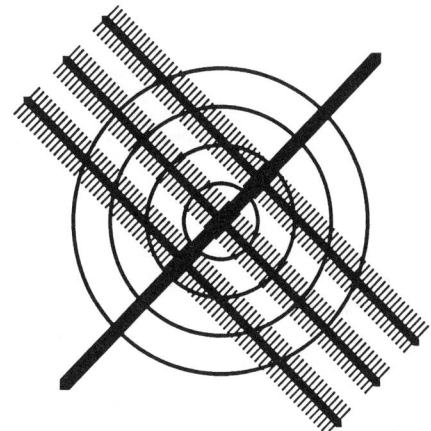

b)

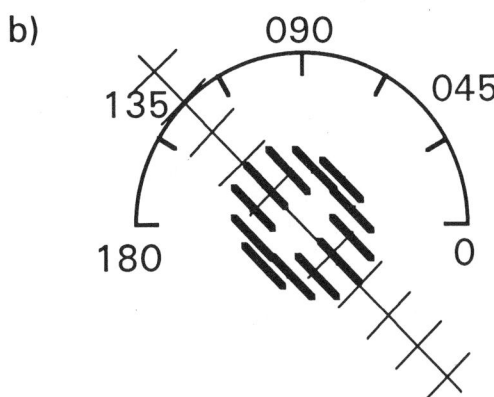

Figure 8-30. (a) Appearance of line mires with the sphere mire properly oriented to be clear at the most plus meridian of the lens. The three cylinder mires are blurred. (b) Appearance of dot mires at the second power reading for the same lens in (a), with the direction of the line segments parallel to the axis meridian of the lens, 135 in this case.

c. When the power wheel is at zero, the mire is at the primary focal point of the collimating lens.
    (1) If the eyepiece is properly focused, the mires and the reticle should both be clear when the power wheel reads zero, with no spectacle lens in the lensometer.
    (2) If this is not the case, the eyepiece should be refocused.
d. When the unknown lens is a spherocylinder, it images a Sturm's conoid complete with two line segments parallel to the principal meridians.
    (1) The lengths of the line segments as well as the dimensions of all other parts of the conoid are proportional to the cylinder power.
    (2) Each point on the mire is transformed into whatever part of Sturm's conoid is in focus through the eyepiece.
    (3) The part of the conoid which is in focus changes as the power wheel is rotated.
    (4) Figure 8-30a shows the power wheel set so that each point in the mire is imaged as a line segment parallel to meridian 045.
e. The direction of the target is changed by rotating the axis wheel.
    (1) A set of the line mires is clear only when aligned parallel to one of the line segments of the conoid.
    (2) As in any Sturm's conoid, the line segment is perpendicular to the meridian in the lens which formed it.

(3) When the mire is rotated so one set of lines is clear, the orientation of the lines is perpendicular to the meridian in the lens for which the power is being measured.

(4) The axis wheel reads the meridian which has the sphere power.

    (a) The sphere mire, which must be clear when the sphere reading is taken, is perpendicular to the direction noted on the axis wheel.

    (b) For example, if the sphere mire is clear when oriented in 045 (Figure 8-30a), the axis wheel will read 135.

    (c) A simple method for determining which set of lines in an unfamiliar lensometer is the sphere mire follows from the foregoing observations: The sphere mire is whichever line(s) is(are) perpendicular to the setting on the axis wheel.

f. To measure the back vertex power of a lens, the rear surface of the lens is placed against the lens stop, whereas to measure front vertex power, the front surface is placed against the lens stop.

g. The following steps are used to measure the back vertex power of a single-vision lens in minus cylinder form.

(1) With the rear surface of the unknown lens against the lens stop, the power wheel is turned far enough in the direction of plus that both sets of lines in the mire are blurred.

(2) The power wheel is turned to reduce plus until one set of mires becomes visible.

(3) The axis wheel is rotated while the power wheel is turned to make the sphere mire perfectly clear.

    (a) When the sphere mire is clear, the power wheel reading is the sphere power and the reading on the axis wheel is the minus cylinder axis.

    (b) If the cylinder mire happens to be focused first, the axis wheel must be rotated 90° to bring the sphere mire into focus.

    (c) If the sphere mire is not focused first at the most plus (or least minus) meridian, the axis will be 90° in error.

(4) Once the sphere power has been read, the power wheel is rotated to less plus (or more minus) until the cylinder mire is clear.

    (a) The power wheel reads the power of the second principal meridian of the lens.

    (b) The cylinder power is the change in power as the power wheel is moved from the sphere mire to the cylinder mire, not the power wheel reading itself.

(5) If both the sphere and cylinder mires come into focus at the same time and remain equally in focus as the cylinder wheel is rotated and the power wheel is adjusted slightly back and forth, the unknown lens is a sphere and only one reading is taken.

h. For lensometers with dot mires, the power wheel is moved from too much plus until the dots are transformed into line segments (Figure 8-30b).

(1) The sphere power is measured at this first position at which line segments are formed.

(2) The sphere wheel is then moved into less plus (or more minus) until the dot targets are transformed into the second set of line segments, which are perpendicular to the first.

(3) The cylinder power is the difference in power wheel readings for the two principal meridians, just as for line mires.

(4) The cylinder axis is determined by using a knob on the eyepiece to rotate the line in the reticle until it is parallel to the second set of line segments (at the second power reading) (Figure 8-30b).

    (a) The direction of the reticle is the axis, 135 in Figure 8-30b, and the direction is read from a protractor scale imaged in the eyepiece.

(b) There is no axis wheel to rotate the mires as in lensometers with line mires.

i. If the power is to be read in plus cylinder form, similar steps are used as for minus cylinder except the power wheel is first rotated from too much minus to the most minus or least plus reading where the sphere mire can be rotated into focus.

j. The add power of a bifocal is defined as the difference in vertex powers between the distance lens and segment on the side of the segment.

k. A front surface bifocal is neutralized as follows.

(1) The distance power of a bifocal prescription is the back vertex power as for a single-vision lens and is measured as outlined above.

(2) The add is measured by turning the lens around so the front surface of the distance part is against the lens stop.

(3) The axis wheel is rotated and the power wheel adjusted until one set of mire lines is clear.

    (a) The power wheel reads the front vertex power of this meridian.

    (b) Only one meridian is necessary, since the add power will be the same for all meridians.

(4) The lens is raised so the front surface of the segment is against the lens stop.

    (a) The power wheel is rotated until the same set of lines is in focus.

    (b) The power wheel reads the front vertex power of the segment in the same meridian that was measured for the distance part.

    (c) The add power is the difference in readings for the two vertex powers.

(5) A clinical shortcut to find the add is often used.

    (a) In this shortcut, the back vertex power through the segment is measured and the difference in back vertex powers is taken to be the add.

    (b) The shortcut is compelling because it requires only one additional measurement (and no modification of the axis wheel) to determine the add.

    (c) The accuracy of the shortcut depends on how closely the back vertex powers of the lens portions match the front vertex powers.

    (d) Back vertex powers will closely match front vertex powers when the lens is relatively thin as in most minus lenses and low-plus lenses.

    (e) If the back vertex power through the segment (the gross power, not the add) is +4.00D or more plus, it is likely that the add calculated from back vertex powers will be too high.

    (f) Note that the high plus can be from either a high-plus distance lens with a low add, or a low-power distance lens with a high add, or from both a high-plus distance lens and a high add.

l. The add for a progressive lens is also defined as the difference in front vertex powers.

(1) The front vertex power (FVP) of the distance lens is measured at the distance power circle.

(2) The FVP of the near portion is measured at the near power circle.

m. The add for a rear surface bifocal is measured by finding the difference between the back vertex powers of the distance lens and segment.

2. The technique of hand neutralization can also be used to verify power in a lens when a lensometer is not available.

a. The change in prism power away from the optic axis of a lens causes an image to move when an object is viewed through the lens.

(1) When a plus lens is moved in front of the eye while a distant object is viewed, the image will move opposite to the lens motion, "against motion."

      (2) When a minus lens is used, the image moves in the same direction as the lens, "with motion."

      (3) When a trial lens of equal power but opposite sign is placed against the lens, the movement is neutralized, i.e., reduced to zero.

      (4) The trial lens is placed against the front surface of the lens to avoid an air gap between the two lenses, so the front vertex power of the unknown is measured.

  b. In a spherocylinder lens, the two principal meridians must be identified and neutralized separately.

      (1) If the lens is oriented so one of the principal meridians is parallel to a distant line object, the image of the line will be parallel to the object.

      (2) Otherwise, the image will appear rotated compared to the object.

      (3) When a principal meridian is identified, any image motion observed while the lens is moved back and forth along the principal meridian is neutralized with a trial lens.

      (4) The other principal meridian is neutralized in the same way while the lens is moved parallel to it.

      (5) The lens powers are put on an optical cross and the prescription taken off in the desired form.

      (6) If the lens is oriented so one of the principal meridians is parallel to a line object, the line image will rotate when the lens is rotated.

         (a) If the image rotates in the same direction as the lens ("with break"), the meridian is the minus cylinder axis.

         (b) If the image rotates in the opposite direction from the lens ("against break"), the meridian is the plus cylinder axis.

3. A lens clock (lens gauge) is used to measure surface powers and can give an estimate of approximate power.

  a. Two fixed legs of the lens clock rest on the surface of the lens with a third moveable leg between them which moves up or down to rest on the surface depending on the curvature.

      (1) The distance between the two fixed legs represents a chord of fixed magnitude.

      (2) The distance the center leg moves up or down from the fixed legs to rest on the surface represents the sagitta.

  b. Through the sagitta equation and single surface power equation, the scale on the lens clock converts the movement of the center leg into a scale of dioptric refractive power.

  c. The scale is generated by assuming that the index of refraction of the lens material is 1.53 and that the lens is in air.

  d. The lens clock is held perpendicular to the lens surface when a measurement is taken (Figure 8-31), and is rotated to different meridians to check for cylinder.

      (1) When cylinder is noted, the meridians of maximum and minimum power are located to identify the principal meridians and the amount of cylinder.

      (2) Care must be taken not to scratch the surface of plastic lenses when the lens clock is rotated.

      (3) Lifting the lens clock off the surface before rotating it will prevent scratching.

      (4) Lens clocks that are advertised to be used with plastic lenses have rounded feet to minimize scratching; they are not calibrated for a plastic material's index of refraction.

  e. The approximate power is obtained by adding the surface powers together.

      (1) The surface powers for hard resin and for ophthalmic crown glass will be close to the lens clock reading.

      (2) When placed on high-index materials, the lens clock will underestimate the true power of the surface.

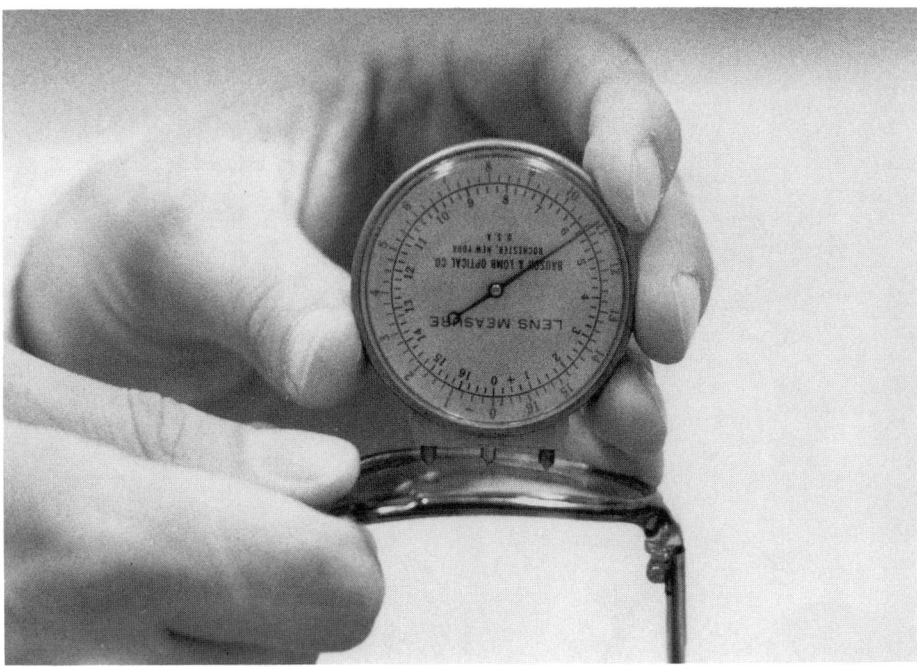

Figure 8-31.   A lens clock placed on a convex front surface of a lens with its legs perpendicular to the lens surface. The reading on the plus scale (for convex surface) is +5.75D to nearest 0.25D.

          (3)   If high-index materials are used, the true power of the lens surface, F_T, is found by modifying the gauge power, F_G, as follows: $F_T = F_G(n_T - 1)/(n_G - 1)$, where n_T is the true index of the lens and n_G is the index assumed by the lens gauge, 1.53.

 D.   *Prism*
    1. The lensometer is used to verify the amount and direction of prism in the lens.
    2. Most lens prescriptions have zero prism, so it must be verified that there is no prism.
       a. With the bottom of the frame resting on the lens platform (stage) of the lensometer, the right lens is placed against the lens stop.
       b. The lens is moved up and down and side to side to center the mire in the reticle.
          (1) The OC of the lens is now located at the lens stop and can be marked with the marking device of the lensometer.
             (a) The marker places three dots in a horizontal line on the lens.
             (b) The center dot is the OC of the lens.
          (2) The OC has zero prism and causes zero displacement of the mire from the center of the reticle.
       c. The left lens is then moved in front of the lens stop without moving the stage.
          (1) The lens is moved from side to side to center the mire horizontally in the reticle, and the OC of the left lens is marked.
          (2) If the mire is at the same vertical level as the center of the reticle, there is zero vertical prism in the lens.
          (3) If the mire is above or below the center of the reticle, the lens has unwanted vertical prism (measurement is discussed below).
          (4) The distance between the OCs marked on the lenses should be the binocular PD.

(5) The distance from the center of the bridge to the OC should be the monocular PD if specified.

(6) The distance from the lowest point on the lens bevel to the OC should be the MRP level that was ordered.

(7) If the horizontal or vertical position of the OCs is different from that which was ordered, the amount of prism induced at each eye can be determined using Prentice's rule.

3. If prism has been ordered, the positions of the MRP as specified to the laboratory through PDs and heights are marked on the lenses.

    a. The MRP mark on the right lens is centered on the lens stop, and the prism is measured by noting the displacement of the center of the mire from the center of the reticle.

        (1) The amount can be measured using the circles or hash marks on the reticle (Figure 8-32).

        (2) Each circle or hash mark represents one prism diopter.

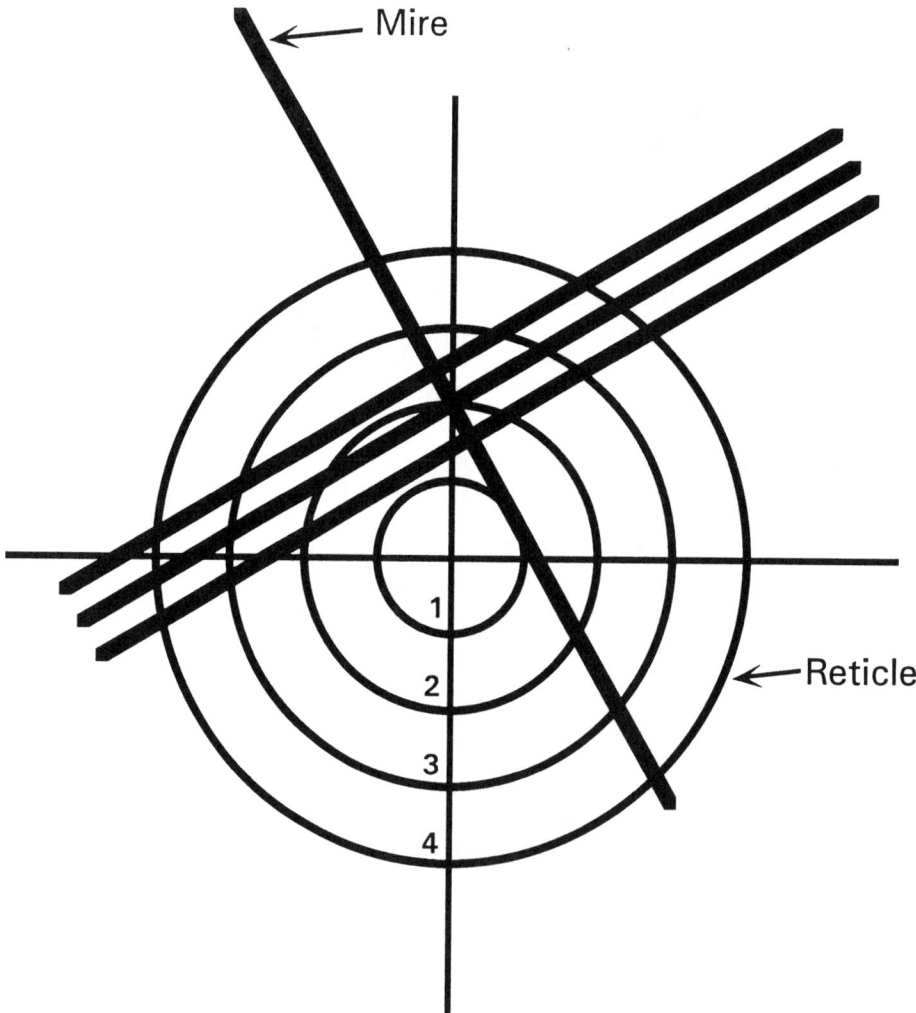

Figure 8-32. Lensometer mire displaced two circles upward from the center of the reticle circles; 2^Δ BU prism is present at point in the lens centered on the lens stop of the lensometer.

(3) The direction of the center of the mire from the center of the reticle is the direction of the base of the prism in the lens.

(4) If the center of the mire is two hash marks above the reticle center, the lens has 2^Δ BU prism, as in Figure 8-32.

(5) If the mire is displaced three circles toward the nose (bridge of the frame), 3^Δ BI is measured.

b. Once the prism in the right lens is measured, the same procedure is followed for the left lens.

c. If the amount of prism is too large to measure with the reticle, a hand-held prism can be held against the lens to neutralize the prism.

d. Some lensometers are equipped with a prism compensator that can be used to measure large amounts of prism up to 15^Δ.

e. If a new patient's current spectacles are being neutralized, the point in front of each eye is marked on the lens, and the steps above are followed to measure any prism.

f. Slab-off prism can be measured with a lens clock.[7]

(1) The first step is to take a reading in the distance portion of the front surface above the slab-off line.

(2) Next a measurement is taken with the center leg of the lens gauge on the slab-off line, one leg above the line and one leg below the line.

(3) The difference between the two readings is the amount of slab-off prism in prism diopters.

E. *Base curve*

1. The base curve is verified with the lens gauge.

2. If the base curve was specified in the order, the lab should supply one within $\pm0.75D$ according to ANSI Z80.1-1987 standard.

3. Warpage in the base curve is also checked by measuring the base curve in several meridians.

a. It is not unusual for the tension from the eyewire or other factors to cause warpage in the lens.

b. As long as the warpage is less than $\pm1.00D$ and does not affect the lens power, it is within the ANSI tolerances.

F. *Lens thickness*

1. Lens thickness is measured with calipers (Figure 8-33).

2. If center thickness has been specified, it should be supplied within ±0.3 mm.

3. On plus lenses the minimum edge thickness should be no greater than necessary to support the lens in the frame with stability.

G. *Lens material, tints, and coatings*

1. The lens material is often difficult to identify exactly, with so many materials now available.

a. Glass lenses can be identified by the added weight of the lens and by the characteristic sharp ring elicited when a metal ring is tapped against the surface.

b. A plastic lens has a duller sound when tapped with a ring.

c. High-index materials are sometimes identified from the brighter reflections from the surfaces.

d. The approximate power of a high-index lens as measured directly with a lens clock is less than the back vertex power of the lens.

2. The lens should be free of defects internally as well as on the surface, including impurities, scratches, nicks, pits, and finishing marks.

3. If the lens has been thermally tempered, the characteristic cross pattern will be seen when the lens is placed in a polariscope.

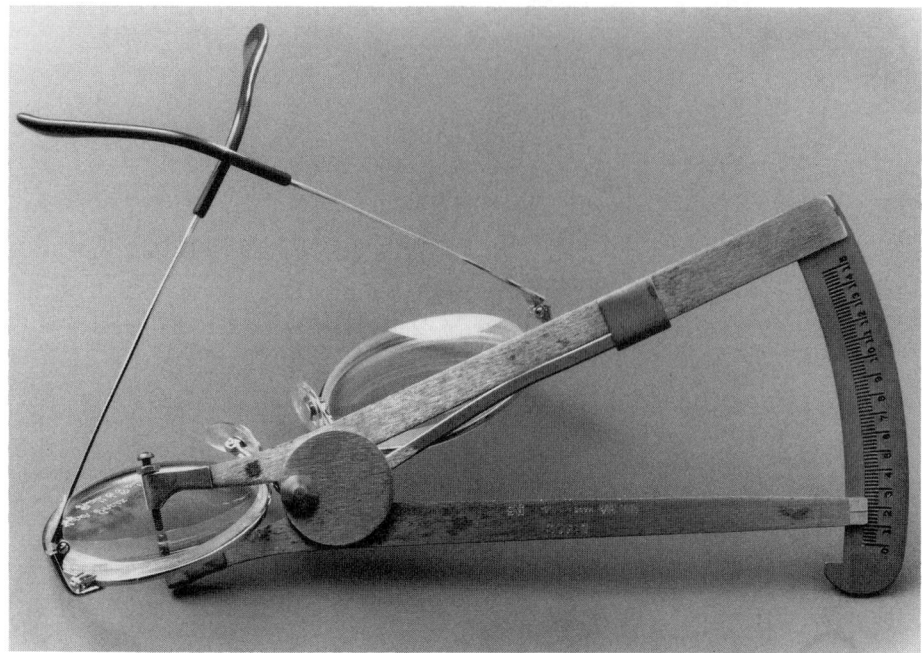

Figure 8-33.   Center thickness of a lens is 1.8 mm as measured with lens calipers.

4. A chemically tempered lens will show a characteristic ring of light when the edge of the lens is placed into a modified polariscope containing glycerin between the crossed polaroids.
5. For glass lenses, the laboratory should provide documentation that the drop ball test was successfully passed.
6. The tint should be proper color and density.
7. An SRC is often detectable by the fact that water will bead on the coated surface.

H. *Multifocals*
1. Segment style, width, height, and inset should be verified.
2. For flat-top lenses, the tops of the segments should be parallel.
3. For progressive lenses, the type of PAL, height of the fitting cross, and monocular distances from the center of the bridge to the fitting crosses should be verified.

I. *Frame*
1. The style, color, eye size, and DBL of the frame are verified.
2. The style and length of the temples are verified.
3. The frame should be examined for blemishes.

References

1. Fry GA. The optometrist's new role in the use of corrected curve lenses. *J Am Optom Assoc* 1979;50:561–562.

2. Davis JK. Prescribing for visibility. In: Sheedy JE, ed. *Problems in Optometry*. Philadelphia: J.B. Lippincott, 1990;2(1):131–155.

3. Remole A. Anisophoria and aniseikonia. Part II. The management of optical anisophoria. *Optom Vis Sci* 1989;66:736–746.

4. Fry GA, Ellerbrock VJ. Placement of optical centers in bifocal lenses. *Optom Weekly* 1941;37:989–996.

5. Sheedy JE, Burian EM, Bailey IL, Borish IM. Optics of progressive addition lenses. *Am J Optom Physiol Opt* 1987;64:90–99.

6. Brown WL, Lee DY. Are all UV-blocking tints for CR-39 lenses the same? *Optom Vis Sci* 1991;68(*Suppl*):184.

7. Peters HB. Measurement of a "slab-off" ophthalmic lens with a lens gauge. *Am J Optom Arch Am Acad Optom* 1949;26:16–18.

APPENDIX 1

Basic Optical Principles

I. Light within an optical material

   A. *With light considered as a wave, wavelength is the distance between two corresponding points on the wavefront.*

   B. *Visible spectrum has wavelengths from 380 to 760 nm, red corresponding to the longer wavelength end of the spectrum and blue to the shorter end.*

   C. *Ultraviolet (UV) has wavelengths from 200 to 380 nm with the following subdivisions:*
      1. UV-A (near) = 320–380 nm.
      2. UV-B (middle) = 290–320 nm.
      3. UV-C (far) = 200–290 nm.

   D. *Infrared (IR) has wavelengths from 760 to 1,000,000 nm with the following subdivisions:*
      1. IR-A (near) = 760–1,400 nm.
      2. IR-B (middle) = 1,400–3,000 nm.
      3. IR-C (far) = 3,000–1,000,000 nm.

   E. *The index of refraction (n) of a material is the ratio of the velocity of light in a vacuum to the velocity in the material.*
      1. Higher index of refraction means light travels more slowly in the material.
      2. Light of different wavelengths travel different velocities (dispersion), with blue light (shorter wavelengths) traveling slower, red faster.
      3. Index of refraction of blue light is greater than that of yellow which in turn is greater than that of red.
         a. Higher index of refraction results in the powers of refracting surfaces being greater for blue than for red.
         b. Chromatic aberration is the change in power of a lens for different wavelengths which results in image blur and/or colored fringes of light at white/dark borders.
      4. The index of refraction used to identify a material is for a wavelength near the middle of the visible spectrum.
         a. The index for 589.3 nm is used in the United States.
         b. For instance, the index used for ophthalmic crown glass, 1.523, is the index for 589.3 nm.

5. Abbe value (optical nu value or constringence) is a measure of the spread of indices of refraction between the two ends of the visible spectrum.
   a. A large Abbe value value (such as 60) means the spread in index is relatively small and chromatic aberration is minimal.
   b. A small Abbe value value (such as 30) means the spread in index is relatively large and chromatic aberration is very significant.

II. Single spherical surface

A. *A single spherical surface (SRS) is the spherical border between two optical materials, such as one surface of a lens which has air on one side and glass or plastic on the other.*

B. *Object rays are those approaching the surface in the first medium, having an index n.*
   1. The vergence of the rays as they enter the surface is $L = n/l$, where l is the distance from the surface to the crossing point of the rays (object point).
   2. Parallel rays from an object at infinity ($l = \infty$) have a vergence of zero.

C. *Image rays are those emerging into the second medium, having an index of refraction n', after refraction from the surface.*
   1. The vergence of the image rays just after emerging from the surface is $L' = n'/l'$, where l' is the distance from the rays to their crossing point (image point).
   2. Parallel rays emerging from a surface have a vergence of zero and head toward an image at infinity.

D. *According to the sign convention, a plus value is assigned to any distance measured in the same direction as light travels, and a negative value is assigned to any distance measured opposite to the direction of light.*

E. *The refracting power F of a surface indicates the amount by which the vergence of the rays is changed by the surface as they traverse it.*
   1. The vergence L of the object rays as they enter the surface plus the surface power F yields the vergence L' of the image rays as they leave the surface: $L' = L + F$.
   2. The physical parameters of the surface determine the magnitude and sign of its refracting power: $F = (n' - n)/r$.
      a. The power of the surface is greater when the difference between the indices of refraction for the two materials surrounding the surface is larger.
      b. The power is greater when the radius of curvature of the surface is shorter.

F. *The primary focal point F is the object point from which object rays diverge or toward which object rays converge when the image rays emerge from the surface parallel to the optical axis (zero image vergence).*

G. *The secondary focal point F' is the image point toward which image rays converge or from which image rays diverge after leaving the surface when the incident object rays are parallel to the axis (zero object vergence).*

H. *The primary focal length f is the distance from the surface to the primary focal point; the secondary focal length f' is the distance from the surface to F'.*

I. *Refracting power is inversely proportional to focal lengths: $F = -n/F = n'/f'$.*

J. *The curvature R of a single surface is $R = 1/r$.*
   1. It is an indication of the shape of the surface but not of the power, since indices of refraction are not considered.
   2. A flat or plano surface ($r = \infty$) has zero curvature and zero power.

K. *The sagitta (or depth) s of a surface having a diameter of (2h) is the distance from the center of the surface to the chord connecting two opposite edges.*
   1. The exact expression for sagitta is $s = r - (r^2 - h^2)^{1/2}$ or $r = h^2/2s + s/2$.
   2. The approximate relationship (when $s \ll r$) is $s \approx h^2/2r$.
   3. The sagitta is important for thickness considerations.

L. *The relationship between surface power* $F = (n - 1)/r$ *and sagitta, using the approximation, is* $s = Fh^2/2(n - 1)$.

III. Lenses

A. *An ophthalmic lens consists of two surfaces separated by a center thickness* t, *with the lens material between them having an index* n_2.
1. The index of the object medium in front of the lens is *n* and the index for the image medium behind the lens is *n'*.
2. For ophthalmic lenses, both object and image media are air, so $n = n' = 1$.

B. *Refracting power (equivalent power,* F_{eq}*) is the amount by which the lens changes the vergence of light rays.*
1. $F_{eq} = F_1 + F_2 - (t/n_2) F_1 F_2$
2. F_1 is the front surface power and F_2 is the rear surface power.

C. *Lenses of the same power may have different shapes, i.e., different* F_1, F_2.
1. Shapes for plus lenses
    a. A biconvex lens has two plus surfaces, not necessarily the same power; an equiconvex lens has two plus surfaces of equal power.
    b. A plano convex lens has one plano (flat) surface and one plus surface.
    c. A meniscus convex (concavo-convex) lens has one plus surface and one minus surface; the magnitude of the plus surface power is greater than that of the minus surface.
2. Shapes for minus lenses
    a. A biconcave lens has two minus surfaces, not necessarily the same power; an equiconcave lens has two minus surfaces of equal power.
    b. A plano convex lens has one plano (flat) surface and one minus surface.
    c. A meniscus concave (convexo-concave) lens has one plus surface and one minus surface; the magnitude of the minus surface power is greater than that of the plus surface.
3. For ophthalmic spectacle lenses, the lens is always oriented so the surface having more plus power is away from the patient's eye.
    a. Aberrations are reduced in this orientation.
    b. Lashes are less likely to rub the rear surface.

D. *The shape of an ophthalmic lens is specified by the base curve.*
1. The base curve is the first surface placed on the lens.
    a. The front surface is almost always spherical.
    b. The unfinished rear surface is ready to accept the spherical or toric surface necessary to provide the back vertex power required in the prescription.
2. The base curve for a single-vision lens is the power of the front surface (F_1).
3. The base curve for a multifocal lens is the power of the distance portion of the surface containing the multifocal.
    a. The surface containing the segment is the first surface applied to the lens.
    b. Since most multifocals are front surface, the base curve will usually be on the front surface.

E. *Vergences for the object and image rays used with the refracting power (designated by* F *or* F_{eq}*) of a lens are measured relative to the principal points of the lens,* H *and* H'.
1. Principal points are a pair of conjugate points which have special properties.
    a. Conjugate points are a pair of object-image points.
    b. If the object is at *H,* the image is at *H'*, having a lateral magnification of +1.
    c. This special property makes them useful for reference points in a thick lens system.

2.   The distance from the front vertex A_1 of the lens to the primary principal point H is given by $A_1H = n_1tF_2/n_2F$.
   a. n_1 is the index for the object medium in front of the lens, and n_2 is the index of the lens.
   b. F_2 is the rear surface power and F is the refracting (equivalent) power.
3.   The distance from the rear vertex A_2 of the lens to the secondary principal point H' is given by $A_2H' = -n_3tF_1/n_2F$.
   a. n_3 is the index for the image medium behind the lens.
   b. F_1 is the front surface power.
4.   The object distance l is measured from the primary principal point H of the lens, and the image distance l' is measured from the secondary principal point H'.
5.   The object ray vergence at H is $L = n/l$.
6.   The image ray vergence at H' is $L' = n'/L'$.
7.   The two vergences are related to refracting power as in a single surface: $F_{eq} = L' - L$.
8.   For spectacle lenses the positions of H and H' are predictably determined by the curvatures of the two surfaces, being positioned closer to the more curved surface.
   a.   For an equiconvex or equiconcave lens, H and H' lie within the lens symmetrically about the center of the lens.
   b.   For a biconvex or biconcave lens, H and H' remain within the lens but are shifted toward the more curved surface.
   c.   For a plano convex or plano concave lens, one principal point is on the curved surface and the other is inside the lens.
      (1)   For a plano convex lens (with the convex surface as the first surface), H is on the curved surface and H' is inside the lens.
      (2)   For a plano concave lens (with the plane surface as the first surface), H' is on the curved surface and H is inside the lens.
   d.   For a meniscus convex (plus lens with one convex and one concave surface), the principal planes continue to move farther from the center of the lens in the direction of the convex surface.
      (1)   In the flatter meniscus convex lenses, the principal points straddle the more curved front surface, with H in front of the lens and H' inside.
      (2)   For more curved meniscus lenses, both lie in front of the lens outside the convex surface.
   e.   For a meniscus concave (minus lens with one convex and one concave surface), the principal planes continue to move farther from the center of the lens in the direction of the concave surface.
      (1)   In flatter meniscus concave lenses, the principal points straddle the more curved rear surface, with H inside the lens and H' behind.
      (2)   For more curved meniscus lenses, both lie behind the lens on the side of the concave surface.

F.   *The primary focal point* F *is the object point from which object rays diverge or toward which object rays converge when the image rays emerge from the rear surface parallel to the optical axis (zero image vergence).*

G.   *The secondary focal point* F' *is the image point toward which image rays converge or from which image rays diverge after leaving the lens when the incident object rays are parallel to the axis (zero object vergence).*

H.   *The primary focal length* f *is the distance from the primary principal point* H *to the primary focal point, and the secondary focal length* f' *is the distance from the secondary principal point* H' *to* F'.

I.   *Refracting power (equivalent power) is inversely related to focal length:* F $= -n/f =$ n'/f'.
   1.   Focal points are located on opposite sides of a lens.
      a.   For plus lenses, F is in front of the lens and F' is behind the lens.
      b.   For minus lenses, F is behind the lens and F' is in front of the lens.
   2.   For a lens in air ($n = n' = 1$), f and f' are equal in magnitude though opposite in sign.

3. Refracting power is useful when it is necessary to do several object-image computations on a thick lens or complex lens system.
    a. The object distance l is measured from H and the object vergence $L = n/l$ is calculated.
    b. The conjugate foci equation $L' = L + F$ is applied to compute the image vergence.
    c. The image distance l' is computed from $L' = n'/l'$.
    d. The time necessary to compute the positions of the principal planes is offset by the time saved by applying the conjugate foci equation once for the entire lens instead of once for each surface.

J. *Front vertex focal length* f_N *is the distance from the front vertex of the lens to the primary focal point.*
    1. Front vertex power (neutralizing power) F_N is inversely related to f_N:

    $$F_N = -n/f_N.$$

    2. $F_N = F_1 + F_2/(1 - tF_2/n_2)$.
    3. F_N represents the power of the lens necessary to neutralize the vergence of light entering the lens when light emerges from the lens with zero vergence (parallel rays).
        a. The front vertex power has the same magnitude as the vergence of light heading toward (or coming from) the primary focal point of the lens.
        b. The sign of the front vertex power is opposite to the sign of the vergence, however.
        c. For example, for a plus lens, F_N is positive, but the vergence of light entering the lens from the primary focal point is negative (diverging).
    4. F_N is used to denote bifocal add powers.

K. *Back vertex focal length* f_V' *is the distance from the back vertex of the lens to the secondary focal point.*
    1. Back vertex power F_V is related to f_V': $F_V = n'/f_V'$.
    2. $F_V = F_1/(1 - tF_1/n_2) + F_2$.
    3. F_V represents the vergence of light emerging from the rear surface of the lens when light entering the lens has zero vergence (parallel rays).
    4. F_V is the power used to denote refractive errors as measured with lenses in a phoropter and to mark the power of ophthalmic lenses.

L. *Approximate power (nominal power, "thin lens power") is an estimate of the power of the lens found by adding the two surface powers.*
    1. The effect of thickness is ignored.
    2. When terms with t are dropped, equations for equivalent power, front vertex power, and back vertex power all reduce to: $F \approx F_1 + F_2$.
    3. If the surface powers are small, t can be relatively large and yet result in a fairly accurate approximate power.
    4. If the surface powers are high, however, as in contact lenses, approximate power will be inaccurate even for relatively small center thicknesses.

M. *The effective power* F_{eff} *of a lens represents the vergence of light at a distance* d *from the rear surface of the lens.*
    1. Light from a distant object which leaves the rear surface of a lens (at plane A) has a vergence equal to the back vertex power of the lens.
        a. At distance d from the rear surface (at plane B), the light has a vergence $F_{eff} = F_V/(1 - dF_V/n)$ where n is the index of the medium in which the light travels behind the lens.
        b. This new vergence is the effective power of the lens in plane B at distance d.
    2. If the original lens (lens 1) is replaced by another lens at plane B, the back vertex power of the new lens $(F_V)_2$ must equal the effective power $(F_{eff})_1$ of the first lens at plane B: $(F_V)_2 = F_{eff} = F_V/(1 - dF_V/n)$.

a. When the spectacle plane is moved closer or farther from the eye, as may occur when a frame change is made, d represents the change in distance.

b. "d" is the vertex distance, the distance from the rear surface of the spectacle lens to the front surface of the cornea, when the effective power at the cornea is desired.

c. "d" is positive when the new lens plane is closer to the eye, as in going from a spectacle lens to a contact lens or in moving the spectacle plane closer to the eye.

    (1) Example: If a $-12.00D$ trial lens corrects the eye at a vertex distance of 16 mm, but the patient's frame places the lens at a vertex distance of 14 mm, what should the power of the spectacle lens be?

    (2) $F_{eff} = F_V/(1 - dF_V/n) = (-12D)/[1 - (+0.002 \text{ m})(-12D)/1] = -11.72D$ or $-11.75D$ (to the nearest 0.25D).

    (3) Note that with the high lens power, even a 2-mm change in distance changes the effective power by 0.25D and must be compensated in the Rx.

d. "d" is negative when the new lens plane is farther from the eye, as in going from a contact lens to a spectacle lens or in moving the spectacle plane farther from the eye.

    (1) Example: If a patient wears a $-3.50D$ contact lens and wants glasses to wear at a vertex distance of 15 mm, what should the power of the glasses be?

    (2) $F_{eff} = F_V/(1 - dF_V/n) = -3.5D/[1 - (-0.015 \text{ m})(-3.5D)/1] = -3.69D$ or $-3.75D$ (to the nearest 0.25D).

    (3) Note that when the distance change is as large as 15 mm, effective power changes must be considered for powers as low as 3.50D.

e. If a plus lens is moved closer to the eye, its effective power at the eye decreases (less plus), whereas if it is moved farther from the eye, its effective power increases.

    (1) Example: Rob wears $+10.00D$ (vertex distance = 14 mm) but reports clearer vision when the glasses are moved down his nose to a vertex distance of 18 mm. What power should be used in the original spectacle plane to give clear vision?

    (2) In this case the starting point for clear vision is with the vertex distance of 18 mm.

        (a) The new plane for effective power is at the 14-mm distance, so $d = +4$ mm.

        (b) $F_{eff} = F_V/(1 - dF_V/n) = +10D/[1 - (+0.004 \text{ m})(+10D)/1] = +10.42D$ or $+10.50D$ (to nearest 0.25D).

f. If a minus lens is moved closer to the eye, its effective power at the eye increases (more minus), whereas if it is moved farther from the eye, its effective power decreases.

Guidelines: Effective Power

Condition	New Lens Power
Plus lenses	
Replace with lens closer to eye	Increased plus
Replace with lens farther from eye	Decreased plus
Move lens farther away from eye for clear vision	More plus in original lens plane
Move lens closer to eye for clear vision	Less plus in original lens plane
Minus lenses	
Replace with lens closer to eye	Decreased minus
Replace with lens farther from eye	Increased minus
Move lens farther away from eye for clear vision	Less minus in original lens plane
Move lens closer to eye for clear vision	More minus in original lens plane

N. *The lateral (transverse) magnification* M_T *of a lens is the ratio of image height* y' *to object height* y.

    1. $M_T = y'/y$.

    2. Lateral magnification can also be expressed as a ratio of object and image vergences: $m = y'/y = L/L'$.

O. *For an ophthalmic lens used with the eye, angular magnification* M_A *compares the image seen through the lens to the object seen without the lens.*

    1. $M_A = \tan \omega'/\tan \omega$.

    2. Angle ω' is subtended at the center of the entrance pupil of the eye by the image formed by the lens.

    3. Angle ω is subtended by the object at the entrance pupil of the eye.

P. *Spectacle magnification (SM) is a special name applied to angular magnification for a spectacle lens when the object is at infinity.*

    1. SM is expressed as: $SM = \tan \omega'/\tan \omega = [1/(1 - tF_1/n_2)] [1/(1 - hF_V)]$.

    2. F_1 is the front surface power, t is the center thickness of the lens, n_2 is the index of refraction of the lens, h is the distance from the rear surface to the entrance pupil of the eye, and F_V is the back vertex power of the lens.

    3. The first factor, $1/(1 - tF_1/n_2)$, is termed the shape factor, while the second, $1/(1 - hF_V)$, is termed the power factor.

    4. If both tF_1/n_2 and hF_V are small compared to 1, SM can be approximated by: $SM \approx 1 + tF_1/n_2 + hF_V$.

        a. The approximation for the general polynomial expansion for $1/(1 - x)$ leads to the simpler form $[1/(1 - x) \approx 1 + x]$.

        b. It is convenient to refer to %SM, defined as: $\%SM = 100(SM - 1) \approx 100(tF_1/n_2) + 100hF_V$.

            (1) A positive %SM means that the retinal image with the spectacle lens is larger than that without the lens.

            (2) A negative %SM means that the retinal image with the lens is smaller than that without the lens.

            (3) In this form of the expression for %SM, the effect of changing one of the variables (e.g., front surface curve F_1) on the image size is easily seen.

            (4) When the base curve is plus, as it is for all lenses except for very high minus, %SM increases for either a plus or minus lens if the base curve F_1 is made steeper (more plus).

            (a) This may also be explained by principal planes movement.

            (b) For a plus lens, increasing the base curve forces the principal planes farther from the rear surface in the direction of the front surface.

            (c) If the back vertex power is kept constant, the back vertex focal length remains constant, but the secondary focal length f' increases and the image of a distant object becomes larger.

            (d) For a minus lens, the same principle holds; steepening the base curve moves the principal planes farther from the front surface toward the steeper rear surface, and the image size increases.

IV. Cylindrical and toric lenses

A. *Cylindrical and toric lenses have power that varies from one meridian to another, in contrast to a spherical lens, for which the power is constant in all meridians.*

    1. On a toric surface the power varies continually from a maximum in one meridian to a minimum in the meridian 90° away.

        a. The meridians of maximum and minimum power are the principal meridians.

        b. A toric ophthalmic lens consists of one spherical surface and one toric surface.

            (1) The toric surface is placed on the rear surface of virtually all modern ophthalmic lenses; years ago it was always on the front surface.

(2) In a multifocal the toric surface is always placed on the surface without the segment, so the toric surface is on the front surface on the rare occasions when a rear surface multifocal is used.

2. A simple cylinder surface is a toric surface which has zero power in one meridian and nonzero power in the other meridians.

   a. It is common, however, for any lens having a toric surface to be termed generically a "cylinder lens."

   b. The axis meridian is the principal meridian which has zero power; the power meridian has maximum power and is 90° away from the axis meridian.

   c. The curvature along meridians between the axis and power meridians is given by $R_\theta = R_C \sin^2_\theta$ where R_θ is the curvature of the intermediate meridian located at angle θ from the axis meridian of the cylinder and R_C is the curvature in the power meridian.

B. *Meridians in an ophthalmic lens are designated by angles from 0 to 180° in a polar coordinate system.*

   1. From the examiner's point of view (facing the patient), zero is to the right for both right and left lenses, while from the patient's point of view, zero is to the left.

   2. 90° is vertically upward and 180° is to the examiner's left (patient's right).

   3. The horizontal meridian is denoted as 180, not 0, by convention.

   4. Designations greater than 180 are not necessary for cylinder axis, since they redundantly identify the same meridians already labeled 180 or less.

C. *Since power varies from one meridian to another in a cylinder lens, light from a point object does not form a point image, but instead forms a series of complex images referred to collectively as the conoid of Sturm.*

   1. The anchors of the conoid are two line segments, one formed at the "image" distance from each of the two principal meridians.

   2. Each line segment is oriented perpendicular to the meridian of the power that formed it (or more accurately, the power that determined its position; see the example that follows.)

   3. If the exit pupil of the optical system is circular, then the "image" seen on a screen at any other position than the two line segments is an oval or ellipse with its major and minor axes parallel to the principal meridians.

   a. The exit pupil is whatever determines the shape and size of the pencil of rays leaving the optical system.

   b. In a system consisting of only one lens, the exit pupil is the rim of the lens.

   c. The "circle of least confusion" (CLC) is a special ellipse having equal dimensions along its two axes and is located at the dioptric midpoint or average dioptric position of the two line segments.

   d. The sizes and shapes of the ellipses formed at various distances from the exit pupil depend on the position of the ellipse relative to the line segments and the CLC.

   4. For a simple cylinder, the line segment formed by the axis meridian (having zero power) is located at infinity when the object is very distant.

   5. Example: A point of light lies 50 cm in front of a toric lens which has powers of +5.00D in meridian 180 (horizontal meridian) and +3.00D in meridian 090 (vertical meridian), the two principal meridians. Find the positions and orientations of the two line segments and the position of the CLC formed by the lens.

   a. Meridian 180 will form a line segment that is oriented vertically (perpendicular to the meridian that forms it) and is located as follows (its data will be identified by subscript "a"):

   $L'_a = L_a + F_a$ $L_a = 1/-0.5 \text{ m} = -2D.$
   $L'_a = -2D + 5D$ $L'_a = +3D.$
   $l'_a = 1/L'_a = 1/(+3)D = +0.33 \text{ m} = +33 \text{ cm}.$

   b. Meridian 090 will form a line segment which is oriented horizontally (in meridian 180) and has the following position (its data are referred to by subscript "b"):

$L_b = 1/-0.5m = -2D$ $L'_b = -2D + 3D = +1D$

$l'_b = 1/L'_b = 1/(+1D) = +1\ m = +100\ cm.$

    c.   The CLC is located at the dioptric midpoint of the two segments: $L'_{CLC} = (L'_a + L'_b)/2 = (+3D + 1D)/2 = +2D.$ $l'_{CLC} = 1/L'_{CLC} = 1/+2D = +0.5\ m = +50\ cm.$

    d.   Between the exit pupil and the CLC, the image of a point object is an ellipse with its longer dimension in the direction of the closer line segment (vertical in this case).

    e.   Farther from the exit pupil than the CLC, the image of a point object is an ellipse with its longer dimension in the direction of the farther line segment (horizontal in this case).

6.   The positions of the line segments, CLC, and the other components of the conoid depend on the vergence of the light from the object as it enters the lens (dependent on the object distance) and upon the powers of each of the two principal meridians of the lens.

    a.   Depending on the signs and relative magnitudes of these values, it is possible for any of the following three situations to exist:

        (1)   Both line segments are real images (formed by converging light from the lens).

        (2)   Both are virtual images (formed by diverging light from the lens).

        (3)   One is real and one is virtual.

    b.   The position of the CLC is always determined from the mean (dioptric midpoint) of the vergences leaving the two principal meridians of the lens.

D.   *Each of the object points in an extended object such as a line or circle (extended object has more than one object point) forms its own Sturm's conoid.*

1.   Consider an object which lies in a plane perpendicular to the axis.

    a.   The distances from the lens to the line segments and CLCs for each of the conoids from all the object points are identical.

        (1)   The line segment closer to the lens in each conoid is the same distance from the lens for each conoid and is oriented the same direction.

        (2)   The dimensions of the components are identical.

    b.   The conoids are displaced from each other because each is centered on its own chief ray rather than on the optic axis, as for the axial object point.

2.   The chief ray is the ray from the object point which passes through the center of the exit pupil.

    a.   If the exit pupil is the edge of the lens itself, then the chief ray passes through the center of the lens.

    b.   If the exit pupil lies away from the lens, the chief ray may not pass through the center of the lens.

3.   A blurred image is created in any plane where a screen is placed.

4.   An apparently clear image occurs in the plane of a line segment of the conoid if the object is parallel to the direction of the line segment.

    a.   In this case each of the line segments formed by adjacent points of the object is aligned to give an apparently clear image.

    b.   For example, if the object is a vertical line and one of the line segments in Sturm's conoid is vertical, then the image of the vertical line object will appear clear when the screen is placed in the plane of the vertical segment.

    c.   On the other hand, the image will be maximally blurred if the screen is placed in the plane of the horizontal line segment.

5.   In the plane of the CLC, all parts of the image appear equally blurred, regardless of the orientation of the object, due to the symmetry of the circular blur circle.

    a.   This blur is generally assumed to be most acceptable to a patient because of the symmetry of the blur for all parts of the object, regardless of orientation.

      b.   The spherical equivalent is the dioptric value that locates the CLC.

      c.   Sph. Eq = Sph + .5 (Cyl). Example: spherical equivalent of $-2.00 -1.00 \times 180$ is $-2.00 + .5(-1.00D) = -2.50$ D.

      d.   The -2.50 D corrects no astigmatism, but places CLC on the retina.

    6.   In the planes of the ellipses, the parts of the object that are aligned parallel to the major axis of the ellipse will appear clearer (though not perfectly clear) than parts of the object that are perpendicular to the major axis of the ellipse.

V. Prism

    A.   *A prism consists of two plane surfaces joined at an angle.*

      1.   The intersection between the two surfaces is called the apical line of the prism.

      2.   The angle between the two surfaces (measured in a plane perpendicular to the apical line) is termed the apical angle (also prism angle or refracting angle).

      3.   A third side to the prism is the base, which lies opposite to the apex.

         a.   The base does not affect the rays passing through an ophthalmic prism.

         b.   The position of the base is used to specify orientation of a prism.

    B.   *A prism changes the direction of light (deviates light) without changing its vergence.*

      1.   Because the vergence is not changed, the image and object are equidistant from the prism.

      2.   Deviation of light causes the image to be relocated.

      3.   When air surrounds the prism, as in virtually all ophthalmic prisms, rays of light are deviated toward the base of the prism.

         a.   For rays diverging from a real object, the image formed by the rays leaving the prism is displaced toward the apex of the prism.

         b.   If the entering rays are convergent, which only occurs for prisms in instruments such as the lensometer, the image is displaced toward the base of the prism.

         c.   For a thin ophthalmic prism (apical angle β less than $10°$), the angle of deviation δ is related to the apical angle by: $\delta = \beta(n' -1)$

            (1) n' is the index of refraction of the prism.

            (2)   The power of the prism has the same units as the apical angle.

         d.   The angle between the ray incident onto the first surface and the ray emergent from the second surface is the angle of deviation δ for the prism.

            (1)   An ophthalmic prism is denoted by its angle of deviation, sometimes termed the prism power.

            (2)   The prism diopter (abbreviated $^\Delta$) is the unit of deviation used for ophthalmic prisms.

            (3)   The power δ of a prism in prism diopters is defined as: $\delta(^\Delta) = x(cm)/X(m)$.

               (a) x is the displacement of a light ray at a distance X from the prism.

               (b)   Displacement x is in centimeters and is measured perpendicular to the incident ray; the distance X is in meters.

            (4)   Degrees are converted to prism diopters using the following: $\delta(^\Delta) = 100 \tan \delta(°)$.

            (5)   For small angles, $1° = 1.75^\Delta$ (sometimes rounded to 2^Δ), but the tangent expression must be used to convert large angles ($>10°$).

    C.   *Prism effects can be induced in ophthalmic lenses by controlling the position at which a patient views through a lens.*

      1.   The optical center (OC), which lies along the optic axis of the lens, is the position in the lens of zero prism.

      2.   The amount of prism δ that a patient experiences while viewing through a lens at a distance d from the optic center of the lens having a power F is given by Prentice's rule: $\delta(^\Delta) = F\ d(cm)$.

         a. F is in diopters, d is in centimeters, and δ is in prism diopters.

b. If the power in the meridian through which the eye views is zero, the prism induced is zero regardless of the distance from the OC.

c. The direction of the base of the prism induced through the lens depends on whether the power in the meridian through which the eye views is plus or minus.

(1) If the power is plus, the base of the induced prism lies toward the optic axis.

(2) If the power is minus, the base of the induced prism lies away from the optic axis.

VI. Mirrors

A. *Mirrors are optical elements that change the direction and vergence of incident pencils of light through reflection.*

1. Spherical mirrors are portions of a spherical surface, having a constant radius of curvature r measured from the surface to the center of curvature C of the surface.

a. A concave mirror has a negative radius of curvature.

b. A convex mirror has a positive radius of curvature.

2. The conjugate foci equation $L' = L + F$ used for lenses applies to mirrors as well, if the following are noted:

a. The index of refraction of the image medium is always the same as that of the object medium, since the medium in front of the mirror serves as both.

b. The direction of light for the image rays is always opposite to the direction for object rays.

c. The sign applied to image distances must be related to the direction of light for the image rays.

3. Primary and secondary focal points are coincident and are located at a distance of half the radius of curvature from the mirror: $f = -f' = r/2$.

4. Reflecting power is related to focal lengths as in the SRS: $F = -n/f = n/f'$, where n' has been replaced with n.

5. Lateral magnification $m = y'/y = L/L'$, or if the object is very distant, the image size $y' = f'$ (tan ω'), where ω' is the angle subtended by the image at the mirror.

B. *Surfaces of ophthalmic lenses, although primarily refracting, also act as reflecting surfaces, creating reflected images that can be distracting.*

1. The size of the image depends on the type of mirror.

a. The convex front surface of a lens forms a convex mirror; the rear surface on a meniscus lens also forms a convex mirror from the observer's point of view.

(1) A convex mirror forms an erect, smaller image from a real object.

(2) Because the image is minified, the field of view represented in the reflected image is increased over other types of mirrors, so more objects will be represented in the image.

(3) The more curved the convex surface, the smaller the image is and the larger the field of view becomes.

(4) Higher plus lenses have steeper convex front surfaces, so images from a wider field of view are seen reflected in the lens.

(5) On a minus lens, the rear surface is steeper than the front surface, while for a plus lens the rear surface is flatter, so images reflected in the two surfaces will differ accordingly in size.

(6) Driving mirrors used on cars and trucks are convex mirrors.

b. From the perspective of the patient, the concave rear surface of a lens forms a concave mirror, with characteristics similar to a shaving mirror.

(1) When a real object is located closer to the mirror than its focal point, an erect, enlarged image is formed.

(2) Patients, particularly myopes with steeper concave rear surfaces, some-

times are disturbed to see enlarged erect reflected images of their own eyes in the rear surface of the lens.

(3) When a real object is located farther from the mirror than its focal point, an inverted image is formed.

c. A plane surface forms a plane mirror.

(1) A plane mirror produces an erect image which is the same size as the real object.

(2) The front surface for certain high-minus lenses is plano; large images reflected from the front surface of a lens indicate a high-minus lens.

2. The intensity of the reflected image depends on the difference in index of refraction between the two media comprising the surface.

a. Fresnel's law of reflection for light incident nearly perpendicular to the surface shows the dependence of the intensity of the reflected image I_r on the index of refraction of the lens: $I_r = I_o(n - 1)^2/(n + 1)^2$.

(1) I_o is the incident intensity.

(2) n is the index of refraction of the lens; it is assumed that air surrounds the lens, so 1 is the index of air.

b. For lenses made of high-index materials, a larger percentage of the incident light is reflected from each surface.

(1) The intensity of the reflected images is larger for high-index materials.

(2) For hard resin lenses, 4.0% of the incident intensity is reflected, while for PC lenses, 5.1% is reflected, a noticeable increase.

VII. Aberrations

A. *The equations for such relationships as object-image positions and magnification which were presented earlier are accurate under the following "paraxial" assumptions:*

1. The object is close to the optic axis.

2. The amount of a surface which is used is limited to a small area close to the axis.

3. When the limitations of these assumptions are exceeded, the image becomes noticeably affected by blur or asymmetry even in its sharpest focus.

4. The polynomial expansion of $\sin \theta = \theta + \theta/3! - \theta/5! + \theta/7! - \ldots + \ldots$ shows the basis for the approximations.

a. All terms in the expansion are necessary to calculate θ exactly.

b. When θ is small (in radian units), however, only the first term is necessary to approximate $\sin \theta$.

c. This approximation underlies the equations discussed earlier (first-order optics).

d. When θ approaches $10°-20°$, the second term must also be used to approximate $\sin \theta$ more accurately (third-order optics).

5. Seidel described five monochromatic aberrations which affect the image when the object is far enough off axis or the area of the lens used is far enough from the axis that the third-order approximation is necessary.

a. Spherical aberration, the first Seidel aberration, affects an axial object point when the lens diameter is increased beyond paraxial limits.

(1) Rays of light entering more peripheral parts of the lens form images at points along the axis which are different from the image point for paraxial rays.

(2) The amount of spherical aberration is significantly decreased by decreasing the diameter of the aperture which limits the diameter of the pencil of rays passing through the lens.

b. Coma, the second Seidel aberration, affects the image of an off-axis point and is sometimes called oblique spherical aberration.

(1) If the surface of the lens is divided into zones of increasing radius,

centered about the optic axis, each zone farther from the axis forms a circle image which is successively farther from the paraxial image.

(2) The term coma originated from the cometlike appearance of the composite image, which has the paraxial image at its apex.

(3) The effect of coma decreases as the object is located closer to the axis and as the aperture of the lens is decreased.

c. Marginal astigmatism (oblique astigmatism, radial astigmatism), the third Seidel aberration, also affects the image of an off-axis object point.

(1) Movement of the object point off-axis (or, alternatively, rotation of the lens) induces cylinder power in the lens.

(2) The image from a spherically powered lens resembles the Sturm's conoid formed by a cylinder lens, having two line images and a CLC.

(3) The distance between the two line segments, which can be used as a measure of the amount of astigmatism induced, increases the farther the object moves off-axis.

(4) If a plane of object points perpendicular to the axis is placed at the axial point M, then each off-axis point forms its own conoid centered on its chief ray.

(5) The plane containing the chief ray from the object point and the optic axis is the tangential plane for that object point; the intersection of the tangential plane with the lens is the tangential meridian.

(6) The plane that contains the chief ray and that is perpendicular to the tangential plane is the sagittal plane; the intersection of the sagittal plane with the lens is the sagittal meridian.

(7) The tangential meridian has a power $F_T = F[1 + (\sin^2 \alpha)/2n]$, where F is the power of the lens, n is the index of refraction of the lens, and α is the angle of obliquity, the angle between the optic axis and the chief ray.

(8) The induced cylinder power has the same sign as the lens power and has a magnitude of $F_S = F_T \tan^2 \alpha$; the axis of the induced cylinder is the sagittal meridian (which is the meridian of rotation if the lens is rotated).

(9) The line segment in the induced conoid which is formed by the tangential meridian is oriented perpendicular to the tangential plane, while the line segment formed by the sagittal meridian is oriented perpendicular to the sagittal plane.

(10) Consider a plane of object points through an axial point M which is perpendicular to the axis.

(a) The surface that contains all tangential line images from all the object points is a paraboloidal surface curved toward the lens.

(b) The paraboloidal surface passes through M′, the axial image of M.

(11) The surface that contains all sagittal line images from the plane of object points described above is another paraboloidal surface which is less curved than the tangential surface and also passes through the axial image point M′.

(12) The tangential and sagittal surfaces are coincident at the axis (at M′).

(a) This indicates there is no astigmatism for the axial point.

(b) The surfaces become farther apart off axis as a result of the increasing astigmatism with distance off axis.

(13) Marginal astigmatism decreases for objects closer to the axis, but it remains unaffected by a decrease in the diameter of the lens aperture.

d. Curvature of field, the fourth Seidel image, describes the form of the image of an off axis once marginal astigmatism has been corrected.

(1) If an extended object, such as a line, lies in a plane perpendicular to the axis and the lens has been corrected for astigmatism, the image of each object point will be a point, but the points will be located on a paraboloi-

dal curved surface which passes through the axial image point predicted from first-order optics.

(2) The curved surface is termed the Petzval surface and has a radius of curvature (for the portion closest to the axis) which is approximated by $r = -nf'$ where n is the index of refraction of the lens and f' is the secondary focal length of the lens.

(3) Curvature of field decreases for objects closer to the axis but is unchanged as the lens aperture decreases.

e. Distortion, the fifth Seidel aberration, describes a variable lateral magnification which affects the image once astigmatism and curvature have been corrected.

(1) In paraxial optics, it is assumed that the lateral magnification produced by a lens is constant for any object height as long as the lens power and object position remain constant.

(2) Once the angle of obliquity exceeds paraxial limits, however, the lateral magnification is different for different object sizes.

(3) Pincushion distortion occurs when the lateral magnification is greater for points that are farther off axis.

    (a) It is characteristic of minus lenses when the limiting aperture is in front of the lens and of plus lenses when the limiting aperture is behind the lens.

    (b) In ophthalmic lenses, used with the pupil of the eye behind the lens, pincushion distortion is characteristic of plus lenses.

(4) Barrel distortion occurs when the lateral magnification is smaller for points that are farther off axis.

    (a) It is characteristic of plus lenses when the limiting aperture is in front of the lens and of minus lenses when the limiting aperture is behind the lens.

    (b) In ophthalmic lenses, used with the pupil of the eye behind the lens, barrel distortion is characteristic of minus lenses.

6. Chromatic aberration (CA) affects image focus when polychromatic light (e.g., white light) passes through a lens or prism.

a. The index of refraction of the lens material is different for each wavelength (dispersion), which causes the lens to have a different power for each wavelength.

b. Short wavelengths have higher indices of refraction, so a lens has higher power for blue than for red light.

c. CA for a lens can be expressed as a difference in focus along the axis (longitudinal CA).

d. It can also be expressed as a blur in the plane of focus of one of the wavelengths.

(1) Rays of the other wavelengths converging toward or diverging from their image foci in other planes cause blur when they pass through the plane of focus for the focused wavelength.

(2) This blur is termed lateral or transverse chromatic aberration (TCA).

e. The amount of TCA is $\text{TCA} = dF_D/v$ where d is the distance from the axis to the position in the lens which is used to image, F_D is the power of the lens for the Fraunhofer D wavelength (589.3 nm), and v is the Abbe value for the lens material.

(1) TCA is noticed by the observer most readily as colored fringes at the borders between black and white.

(2) TCA is greater for lenses of larger diameter, or as a patient rotates the eyes to use a more peripheral part of the lens.

(3) TCA is greater for higher-powered lenses.

(4) TCA is greater for lenses with low Abbe value ν, which is characteristic of many of the high-index materials.

    (a) Patients are more likely to complain of colored fringes with high-index materials.

    (b) It is important that the optical center be placed close to the line of sight in order to minimize the distance d.

APPENDIX 2

Guide to Troubleshooting Problems with Frame Adjustment

Maladjustments and Remedies

Condition	Cause	Remedy
Pads dig into nose evenly		
	Pads too tight	Widen distance between pads
	Temple tension too great	Reduce tension by moving first bend in temple farther back or making temple bend less steep
	Pads too small for weight of glasses	Replace with larger pads
	Pads too hard	Use soft nose pads, nose pad covers over pads, or stick-on foam cushion on pad
	Tender skin	Toughen skin with alcohol or other means
Pads dig into nose unevenly	Pads do not fit flatly on nose	Correct pads to fit flatly on nose
	Front edge of pads cuts nose	Decrease flare (splay) angle
	Back edge of pad cuts nose	Increase flare (splay) angle
	Top of pad cuts nose	Decrease frontal angle
	Bottom of pad cuts nose	Increase frontal angle
	Temple angle greater on one side	Correct temples
One pad only presses uncomfortably into nose	Incorrect pad angle	Correct as above
	Unequal temple spread	Increase temple spread on temple opposite the pad
Spectacles slide down nose	Distance between pads too great	Bring pads closer together; lessen front and splay angles (angling or snipe nose plier)

(continued)

Maladjustments and Remedies (*Continued*)

Condition	Cause	Remedy
	Bridge size too large	Order correct size or shrink bridge; bridge-reducing plier or heat bridge and bend eyewires in (compensate cylinder axis)
	Temple tension too weak or temples too long	Replace with shorter temples or increase tension (first bend at point where ear attaches to head)
	Too much temple spread (temples too wide open)	Add face form. Heat and bend end pieces in. If temples bowed, heat and straighten, then add face form and bend pieces in if necessary
	Incorrect nose pad angle	Change angles to achieve maximum contact between nose pad surface and nose (angling or snipe nose pliers)
	Incorrect frame style for patient	Select smaller, lighter frame to better fit patient's facial, bridge, and nasal structure; some patients have no natural bumps or positioning points on nose to stop bridge.
Lashes touch the lens	Distance between pads too great	Bring pads closer together
	Guard arms on pads too short or too curled	Remove curl and put it farther down the guard arm (half round pliers)
	Temple tension too great or temples too short	Replace temples or reduce tension
	DBL too large	Use smaller DBL. Reduce bridge
	Insufficient pantoscopic angle	Increase pantoscopic angle to bring top half of lenses away from lashes (depending on insertion point of temple to eyewire)
Eyewires touch cheeks	Too much distance between pads	Bring pads closer together
	DBL too large	Shrink bridge; use plastic buildup pads to raise frame
	Pantoscopic temple angle	Reduce pantoscopic tilt
	Lenses too large in vertical dimension	Refit with smaller eye size. Refit with frame having smaller vertical dimension or with bridge farther from top of eyewire
	Guard arms angled improperly	Bend guard arms down and reangle pads
	Lenses too close	Lengthen guard arms and replace curl
Lenses touch brow	Lenses too close	Lengthen guard arms
	Resting point on nose too high	Lower spectacles by raising guard arms and pads
	Too much retroscopic tilt	Reduce retroscopic tilt
Frame sits too low on patient's face	Nose pads too far apart	Reduce distance between nose pads; decrease frontal and splay angles
	Guard arms bent improperly	Bend guard arms down (vertically) and reangle pads vertically
	DBL too large	Shrink bridge with bridge-reducing plier, or heat bridge and rotate eyewires in

(continued)

Maladjustments and Remedies (*Continued*)

Condition	Cause	Remedy
	Improperly fit frame	Choose frame with smaller DBL, more vertical height, or with bridge farther from top of eyewire
One lens higher than the other	Temples not adjusted to ear heights	Correct temples either retroscopically or pantoscopically
	One guard arm and pad lower than the other	Adjust to balance
	Deformed nose	Compensate for difference with guard arm and pad
	Skewed bridge	Heat and realign
	End pieces unequally bent (one bent in more than other)	Heat and equalize the bends
	One lens closer to face than the other (bifocals will appear to have one seg higher than the other)	Equalize temple tensions (spread) on the two sides
	Unequal pantoscopic tilts	Decrease pantoscopic tilt on lower side
Lenses too far from eyes	Pads too close together	Spread pads
	Guard arms too long	Shorten guard arms, placing curl closer to bridge
	DBL too small	Increase DBL using bridge-stretching plier
One lens out farther than the other	Temple tension uneven	Equalize tensions by changing positions of bends and/or angles at ear
	Endpieces uneven	Bend endpiece in on side of closer lens, bend endpiece out on side of farther lens
	Temple bowed	Straighten bowed temple
	Skewed bridge	Heat and align, putting lenses in same plane
	One side of patient's face wider than the other	Widen angle of temple (endpiece bent out) on side of face which is larger
Temples hurt behind ears	Tension too great	Loosen temple tension by changing position of first temple bend or angle of bend
	Uneven pressure	Bend temples to conform to shape of ear, increasing area of temple against head
	Area of contact too small between temple and ear	Use temple tubing to increase size of temple surface
	Temple too short, not conforming to back of head	Replace with longer temples
	Corroded or rough surface	Replace temple
	Temple rides too far out on top of ear and cartilage	Bend tip of temple to correct
	Temple tip rides too far out at base of ear	Bend tip of temple in
Temples press the outer ear	Bend down portion of temple not conformed to head	Conform bent portion temple to head
	Temple tips bent in too much toward head, pushing ears out	Bend temple tips out somewhat to relieve outward pressure at top of bend

(*continued*)

Maladjustments and Remedies (*Continued*)

Condition	Cause	Remedy
Temples press on top of ear	Temple bend too close to front of temple	Place temple bend at top of ear, where ear attaches to head
Temple ends touch outer ear	Temple ends too far out	Bend temple ends to conform to shape of head
Comfort cable digs into bottom of ear	Tip of cable bent in	Bend tip cable out slightly away from head
	Cable too long	Cut cable to stop just short of lower ear lobe; put ball of solder on end to protect
	Cable itself irritates	Place a temple cover (comfort slip) on the cable
Temples are loose	Temple screws loose	Tighten loose screw. Apply clear nail polish to screw to prevent loosening
	Hinge barrels not matched	Press barrels of hinge together with pliers
	Rivet broken	Tighten rivets with anvil and hammer
	Rivet broken	Frame part may require replacement
Bifocal segments cause blurred area	Segments too high	Bend guard arms up and reangle the pads Stretch the bridge (zyl) Increase distance between pads Increase pantoscopic angle Shorten guard arms down and reangle the pads Shorten guard arm by adding more curl
	Segments too low	Bend guard arms down and reangle the pads Shrink the bridge (zyl) Decrease distance between pads Decrease pantoscopic angle Lengthen guard arm by putting curl farther from bridge
Bifocals are uneven	Uneven pantoscopic tilt	Equalize pantoscopic tilt
	Asymmetric vertical positions of patient's eyes	Measure segment heights to conform to position of each eye

Kevin L. Alexander. *The Lippincott Manual of Primary Eye Care*. Copyright © 1995 by J.B. Lippincott Company.

CHAPTER **9**

Contact Lenses

Edward S. Bennett
Vinita Allee Henry

I. Preliminary Evaluation

A. *Purpose*

It is extremely important for the practitioner to perform a comprehensive preliminary evaluation on every potential contact lens patient. This allows the practitioner to determine if the patient is suitable for contact lens wear and also minimizes the risk of future failures or problems otherwise present due to poor patient selection. If the patient is deemed a good candidate, the information obtained during the prefitting examination will assist in determining such factors as lens material, lens design, wearing time, and care regimen and will become the baseline data on the patient from which changes caused by lens wear will be judged.

B. *History*

A good history includes determining the patient's reasons for wanting to wear contact lenses, medical history, and contact lens history (if any).

1. Reasons for contact lens wear
   a. Cosmesis.
   b. Inconvenience of glasses.
   c. Improved vision. Examples include patients with keratoconus, corneal trauma, and corneal distortion.
   d. Sports and recreation. Most athletes, both professional and weekend, benefit from the wider field of vision provided by contact lenses; in addition, problems such as lens fogging or dislocation of spectacles are eliminated.
   e. Occupational considerations. In addition to athletes, individuals in the performing arts benefit greatly from contact lens wear. Contact lenses are contraindicated for patients working in dusty, dirty environments (e.g., coal miners, sanitation workers) where debris and particulate matter may become trapped under the lens. In addition, individuals working around noxious fumes such as laboratory workers and hairdressers are borderline contact lens candidates at best due to the probability of a chemical keratitis and lens surface contamination. Some workers, such as plumbers and automobile mechanics, experience difficulty cleaning all of the dirt and oil from their hands and therefore may be poor candidates. Some individuals (e.g., pilots, flight attendants, video display terminal operators) may work in environments in which dryness is often present or blinking is inhibited. With these individuals, contact lens wear is not contraindicated but may be restricted to daily wear with an aggressive cleaning and rewetting drop regimen.

    f. Specific interests in contact lens wear. Does the patient have a preconceived idea of what kind of contact lens is desired (e.g., disposable, extended wear, bifocal)?

2. Medical history

    a. These symptoms or conditions may contraindicate or restrict contact lens wear:

      (1) Itching, burning or tearing.

      (2) Allergies (seasonal or chronic).

      (3) Sinusitis.

      (4) Dryness of mouth, eyes, or mucous membranes.

      (5) Nocturnal lagophthalmos.

      (6) Convulsions, epilepsy, and/or fainting spells. Individual should be identified as a contact lens wearer.

      (7) Diabetes. Juvenile diabetics, in particular, should be contraindicated. They may have varying degrees of corneal anesthesia with a low rate of epithelial healing and the potential to develop neurotrophic keratitis.

      (8) Collagen-vascular disorders. Patients with rheumatoid arthritis and related collagen-vascular disorders may have Sjogren's syndrome with keratoconjunctivitis sicca and associated tear film abnormalities. In addition, handling difficulties may be present.

      (9) Pregnancy. It is preferable to fit the patient after childbirth when tear film stability would be present.

     (10) Psychiatric treatment. If the patient is on medications to control anxiety, depression, or manic-depressive states, a judgment decision is necessary; but these individuals should not necessarily be discouraged from contact lens wear, especially if contact lenses benefit them visually.

     (11) Thyroid imbalance. For example, in hyperthyroidism, the disturbed metabolism that results in exophthalmos and lack of blinking can make contact lens wear difficult, as there may be an insufficient tear flow to the cornea.

    b. Certain medications can affect contact lens wear, specifically by their effect on the tear film. Patients currently on any of these medications should either be contraindicated as contact lens wearers until medication use is discontinued or placed on a limited wearing schedule and carefully monitored. These medications include:

      (1) Antihistamines.

      (2) Anticholinergics.

      (3) Tricyclic antidepressants.

3. Contact lens history

If the patient is currently wearing lenses or has worn them in the past, it is important to determine why the patient wants a refit, as this may affect the type of (soft or rigid) lens material to be used. The following questions should be asked:

    a. What is (or did) the patient wear? Satisfaction? Symptoms?

    b. Reason(s) for discontinuing wear or desiring to.

    c. Verify parameters (if appropriate).

    d. Care regimen (if appropriate). Satisfaction?

    e. Is there a frequent history of changing lens materials? (Is the patient a "shopper.")

C. *Refractive information*

An evaluation of corneal topography in combination with a careful refraction and subsequent determination of predicted residual astigmatism is imperative in predicting both the lens type and material to be used and the likely future success.

1. Corneal topography

Corneal topographic evaluation is important in determining the appropriate base curve radius to be diagnostically fitted in either a rigid or a hydrogel lens material.

a. Corneal contour

    (1) Corneal Cap (apical zone/apical cap)—equals the central region of the cornea, approximately 4 mm. The average curvature of the corneal cap equals 7.9 mm (42.75D).

    (2) The cornea is spherical centrally with gradual flattening of the cornea from the center to the periphery.

b. Evaluation

    (1) *Keratometer*—the most common instrument for measuring corneal curvature. This instrument averages the curvature values of two points on the cornea separated by approximately 3 mm in both the major and minor meridians. This instrument has the advantages of both ease of use and low expense. However, the disadvantages include:

        (a) Only the central 3 mm of the cornea (approximately 8% of the corneal area) is evaluated.

        (b) It assumes the central 3 mm of the cornea to be spherical, which may not be true. The magnitude of the error is related to the rate of peripheral corneal flattening.

        (c) Inaccuracy with decentered corneal cap.

        (d) Experimenter error.

        (e) Keratometry change may not correspond with refractive change.

    (2) Clinicians should recognize that keratometry represents a starting point for base curve determination, predicted residual cylinder value, etc. However, fluorescein pattern evaluation is most important with rigid gas-permeable lenses (RGPs), while centration, movement, and lens lag are most important with hydrogel lenses.

    (3) Midperipheral/peripheral corneal evaluation. There are several other methods of evaluation which, although more expensive, allow the examiner to obtain more information on the topography of the cornea. These include autokeratometry, photokeratoscopy, and topographic modeling. The latter systems produce a color-coded representation of the curvature of the entire corneal surface (32 rings). The combination of computer technology and photokeratoscopic measurements produces a comprehensive topographic map of the cornea. These methods are especially helpful with patients exhibiting some form of irregular cornea (e.g., keratoconus, corneal warpage syndrome, trauma, etc.).

c. Final analysis

If keratometry is to be the method of choice, it is important to remember that it only represents a starting point. Above all, there is no substitute for a thorough biomicroscopic evaluation of the lens-to-cornea fitting relationship.

2. Refraction

It is important to perform a careful refraction to help in calculating both the lens power and the expected residual astigmatism. Residual astigmatism for spherical soft lens wearers is simply equal to the refractive astigmatism. For calculating the residual astigmatism with rigid lens wear, the following formula should be used:

CRA (calculated residual astigmatism) = refractive astigmatism − keratometric astigmatism

Example: If refraction = $-2.00 - 1.00 \times 180$ and keratometry = 42.00 @ 180; 42.25 @ 090

CRA = $-1.00 \times 180 - (-) 0.25 \times 180 = -0.75 \times 180$.

Typically, if the actual residual astigmatism (ARA), obtained by refracting over a rigid lens, equals 0.75D or greater, a spherical rigid lens is not recommended due to reduced vision. If the ARA equals the CRA in the above case, the best option may be a soft toric lens.

D. *Slit lamp evaluation*

A comprehensive slit lamp examination will play a vital role in determining whether the patient is a good contact lens candidate. The following should be evaluated on a prospective contact lens wearer:

1. External observation

It is important to evaluate the eyelashes and external eyelids for blepharitis, entropion, trichiasis, or other abnormality.

2. Conjunctiva

The bulbar and tarsal conjunctiva should be evaluated for injection, pinguecula formation, or pterygia. The tarsal conjunctiva should be evaluated with fluorescein application and lid eversion using the following scale:

0 = satin

1 = several papillae per millimeter of lid area

2 = papillae equals 0.5 − 1.0 mm in size

3 = Giant papillary conjunctivitis (GPC); papillae are present on all regions of the upper lid; papillae as large as 1 mm or greater are often present along the tarsal fold.

A patient with grade 2 or greater papillary hypertrophy should not wear lenses on an extended-wear schedule. Preferably a rigid lens material or a planned replacement/disposable hydrogel lens material should be fitted.

3. Cornea

Carefully evaluate the following:

a. *Limbal vasculature.* 360° evaluation; documentation of limbal vessel encroachment onto the cornea should be made; ≥ 2 mm encroachment is a contraindication to contact lens wear.

b. *Staining.* Fluorescein application is essential to evaluating a new patient. Any areas of punctate staining should be noted; the existence of coalesced staining may contraindicate fitting. The cause of the staining should be determined. Sequential staining is recommended[1]; preferably one drop of liquid fluorescein can be instilled every 3 minutes for 15 minutes. A second option would be to moisten a fluorescein-impregnated strip with preservative-free saline. Always perform this procedure even if it is likely the patient desires hydrogel lenses. The eye can be thoroughly irrigated a few times to rinse out the dye.

c. *Scars/infiltrates/opacities*—Carefully scan the cornea to determine if any of these conditions exist and document them. Active corneal infection or inflammation (corneal infiltrates, microbial keratitis, etc.) should contraindicate contact lens wear at that time.

d. *Endothelium*—Evaluate for presence of guttata, dystrophies, and polymegethism (changes in endothelial cell size). The presence of an endothelial dystrophy should contraindicate contact lens wear.

E. *Binocular vision status*

1. History

A comprehensive binocular vision history must include the following:

a. Eye trauma.

b. Eye surgery.

c. Strabismus.

d. Binocular vision therapy as a child.

2. Prismatic correction

If base in (BI) or base out (BO) prism is necessary to provide binocularity and relieve asthenopic stress, it must be prescribed in spectacles.

3. Accommodation/convergence

The prepresbyopic moderate to highly myopic patient may experience accommodative problems when switching from spectacles to contact lenses and must be advised that a bifocal add may be required at an earlier age. Convergence is similarly affected. A spectacle-corrected myope has BI prism when fixating at near. A contact lens-corrected myope does not have BI prism when fixating at near and must converge for a given distance. A spectacle-corrected hyperope has BO prism when fixating at near. A contact lens-corrected hyperope does not have BO prism when fixating at near and must converge less for a given distance. Likewise, a contact lens-corrected hyperope will need to accommodate less after switching from spectacles (i.e., the onset of presbyopia is later).

F. *Anatomic measurements*
  1. Corneal diameter
      a. Typically slightly greater than horizontal visible iris diameter (HVID) and ranges from 10 to 13 mm.
      b. Measured with PD stick tilted inward and reading the horizontal scale (Figure 9-1).
      c. This measurement will help determine overall/optical zone diameter of the contact lens.
  2. Pupil diameter
      a. Perform similar to HVID. (Figure 9-2).
      b. Perform under both normal and dim illumination; the latter will help in determining the optical zone diameter of the lens, which should be 1–2 mm larger than the pupil to allow for absence of flare with vertical translation with the blink.
      c. Pupil size (dim illumination)
          (1) Small pupil: <5 mm.
          (2) Medium pupil: 5–7 mm.
          (3) Large pupil: >7 mm.

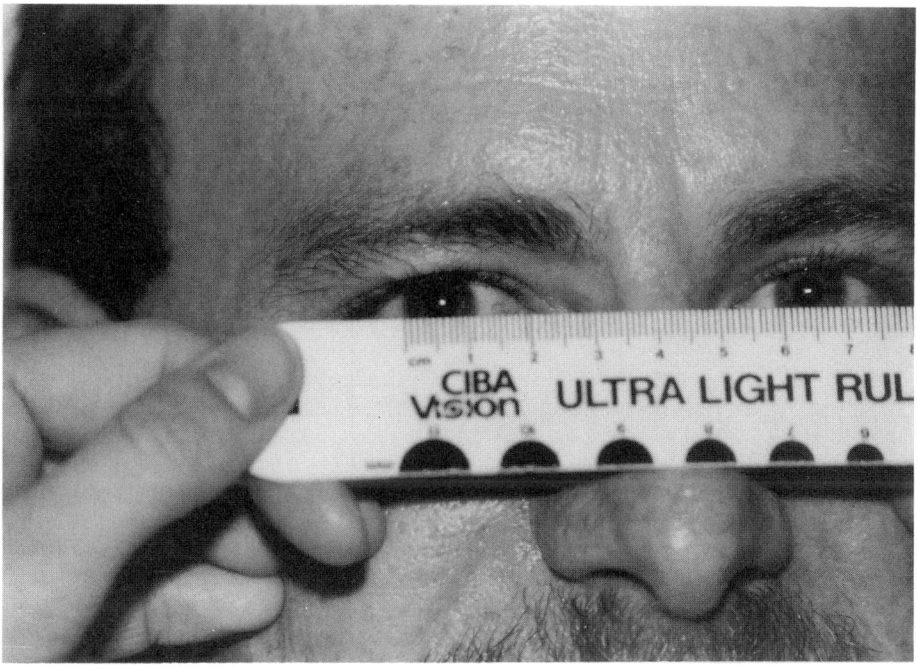

Figure 9-1. How to obtain corneal diameter.

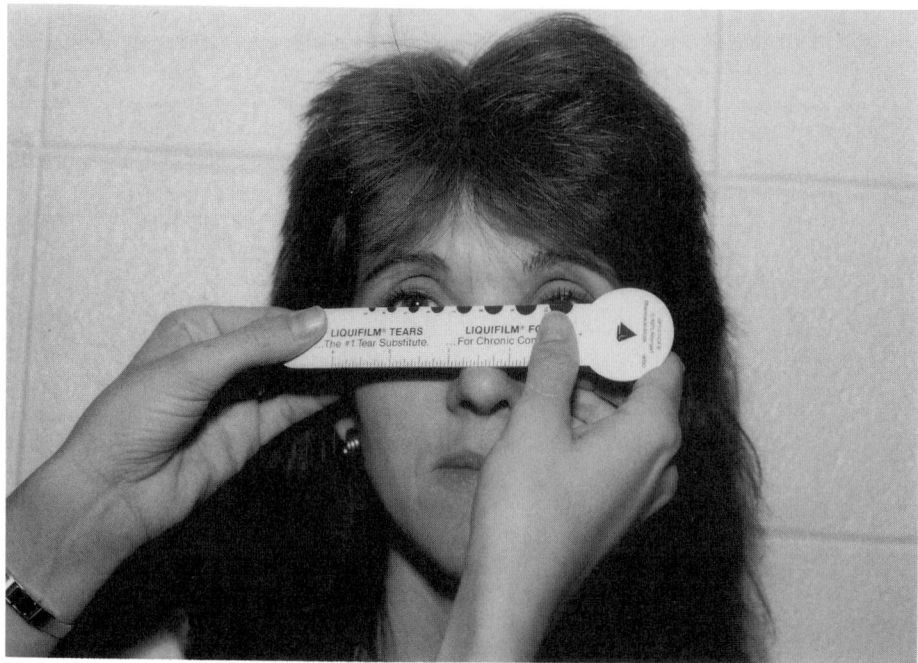

Figure 9-2.   Proper measurement of pupil diameter.

     d. For large pupil sizes, select a large optical zone (>8 mm) or a hydrogel lens with a large optical zone (do not assume all hydrogel lenses have large optical zones!)

  3. Palpebral aperture height

     a. With straight-ahead gaze, this is equal to the vertical measurement of the opening between the upper and lower lids.

     b. Perform with the patient relaxed and looking straight ahead; also note and record the lid-to-cornea relationship (Figure 9-3).

     c. This procedure will help determine type of lens and lens diameter for optimum patient comfort. A patient with an abnormally large palpebral fissure (≥12 mm), will need a large-diameter lens for stability and comfort; likewise, a patient with an abnormally small palpebral fissure (≤9 mm) will require a small-diameter lens.

G. *Lid tension/blink rate*

  1. Lid tension

     a. This is determined via lid eversion; grasping the upper lid between the thumb and forefinger and gently pulling outward will give the practitioner an estimation of the lid tension over the globe.

     b. Tight lids will pull a lens upward; loose lids will displace a lens downward.

  2. Blink rate

     a. A normal rate is 10–15/minute.

     b. Blink rate should be performed without the patient's knowledge; the amplitude and completeness should be noted.

     c. If the patient presents with only 10%–50% completeness of the blink, rigid lenses are contraindicated unless a lid attachment or superior fitting relationship exists after the blink[2]; if the patient is a very infrequent blinker, hydrogel

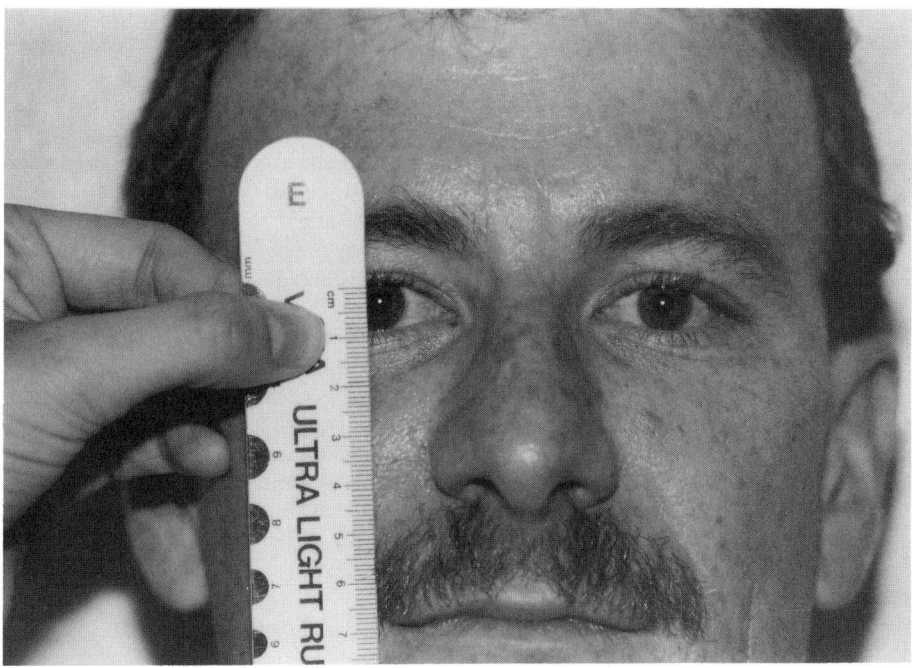

Figure 9-3. Determining the palpebral aperture height.

lenses for social or occasional wear are recommended due to probable lens dehydration and corneal desiccation effects.

H. *Tear film evaluation*

There are several methods to determine whether a patient is a good contact lens candidate or not based on tear quality and/or volume.

1. Biomicroscopic evaluation: two methods
    a. Tear meniscus
        (1) Good test for determining borderline dry eye patient; this enables evaluation of the height and quality of the lower tear prism; if this is not continuous, an aqueous deficiency is present.
        (2) The tear meniscus has an anterior border consisting of a line just behind the meibomian gland orifices. Where the meniscus meets the cornea, a black line exists that represents localized thinning.
        (3) Apply fluorescein over the inferior bulbar conjunctiva about 1–2 minutes before evaluation[2] and observe with cobalt blue and Wratten No. 12 filters. When the meniscus is so thin as to appear as a fine line, it is a significantly unsaturated tear meniscus.
    b. Interference phenomena
        (1) With the patient viewing superiorly, specular reflection, in combination with the high-intensity illumination and high magnification, should be used.
        (2) A spectrum of colored interference patterns of the lipid layer will be observed with this technique. If the lipid layer is insufficient, no interference patterns will be observed.
2. Tear breakup time (tear BUT)
    a. Most widely used test of lacrimal function and a good predictor of contact lens success.
    b. It is equal to the postblink time for dry spots to form in the tear film.

c. Fluorescein is instilled and the cornea is evaluated with a wide slit lamp beam (2–4 mm) under low magnification (10–20×) with the cobalt blue filter; the number of seconds until multiple dry spots form, appearing as dark regions in the green-dyed tear film, is recorded. The patient is instructed to refrain from blinking during this period.

d. An average value is 10–15 seconds, with less than 10 seconds possibly indicative of dry eye.[3] If a patient has a tear BUT equal to 6–9 seconds, a daily wear schedule should be recommended. In addition, the patient should be told that there is borderline dry eye and they may not be able to obtain a comfortable all-day wearing schedule. If the tear BUT is ≤5 seconds, contact lens wear should be contraindicated.

e. Important considerations that could affect results of tear BUT testing:
   (1) Do not manipulate the lids immediately prior to testing.
   (2) Do not use a benzalkonium chloride preserved solution to wet the fluorescein-impregnated strip.
   (3) Have the patient make several blinks prior to performing the test.
   (4) Applanation tonometry should not be performed before this test.
   (5) Repeat the test several times, especially if low values are being obtained.
   (6) Fluorescence is enhanced if a Wratten No. 12 or similar yellow filter is placed over the observation system.

3. Schirmer tear test
   a. Evaluates basal tear secretion and part of the reflex secretion.
   b. A strip of filter paper (5 × 30 mm) is placed slightly temporal over the lower lid with the patient viewing superiorly. The 5-mm notched portion of the strip is placed approximately one-third of the way from the outer canthus in the inferior palpebral conjunctiva. The patient should continuously look upward.
   c. The average is 22.3 mm for normals and 7.6 mm for dry eye patients.[4] >10 mm for 5 minutes or >6 mm for 1 minute is normal. A very high volume of tears, noted by the wetting of the complete strip or most of the strip, may not be valid. An extremely low volume, noted by a very small area of strip coverage (0–4 mm), is usually valid.
   d. This test is typically performed without an anesthetic; in severe dry eye, a topical anesthetic (e.g., proparacaine) can be applied to the lower cul-de-sac to minimize the effects of reflex tearing and to determine the aqueous deficiency (basal secretion test of Jones). The strip should be inserted several minutes after the anesthetic. The difference between this value and that determined without an anesthetic represents an indirect measure of the reflex tear secretion.
   e. Important considerations
      (1) Use low room illumination.
      (2) It is important for the strip to rest in a slightly temporal position so that when the lower lid kicks inward during blinking, contact with the cornea, which may cause excess ocular irritation and reflex tearing, is avoided.
   f. Problems encountered with this test include discomfort and inconsistency or unreliability.

4. Phenol red thread test
   a. Developed by Hamano[5] in Japan, it has been performed on several hundred thousand Japanese subjects.
   b. It utilizes a high-quality 70-mm cotton thread soaked in phenol red dye.
   c. It is performed similar to the Schirmer test; the end of the thread is inserted over the lower lid onto the temporal palpebral conjunctiva while the patient views superiorly. The test is performed for 15 seconds, and the amount of the test strip which has turned red is measured (Figure 9-4).

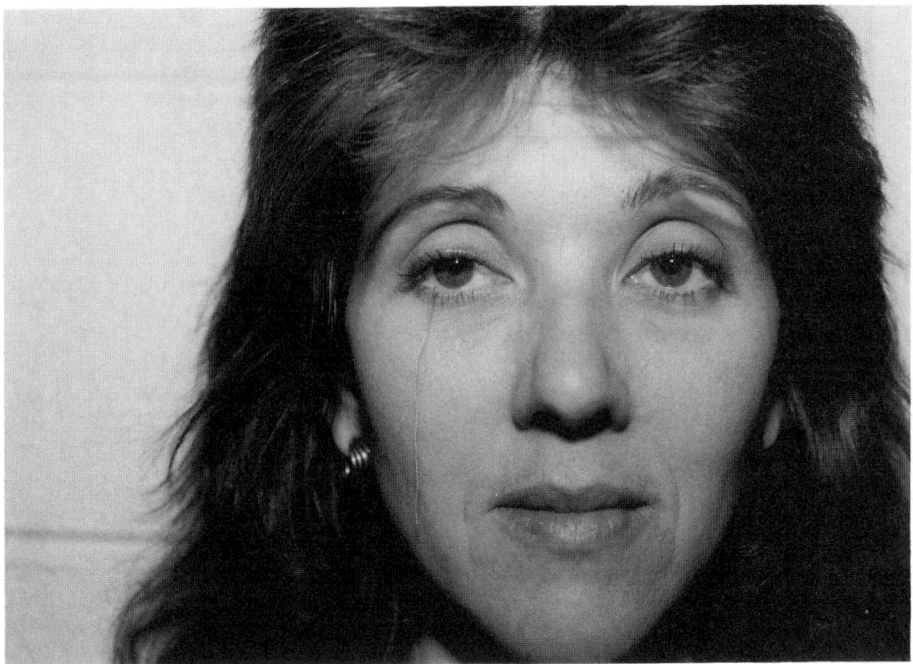

Figure 9-4. The phenol red thread test.

    d.   The average value in Japan has been found to be 16.7 mm; in the United States, this value is equal to 23.9.[6] <9 mm has been diagnostic of dry eye.

    e.   The benefits of this test include
       (1) No anesthesia necessary; minimal discomfort.
       (2) 15-second test time.
       (3) Little reflex secretion.
       (4) More valid than Schirmer.
       (5) Environmental effects such as humidity are minimized due to the short testing time.

    f.   Criticisms include
       (1) Relatively low absorption capacity; individuals may secrete tears at a higher rate than can be absorbed by the thread.
       (2) This test may only measure residual tears in the cul-de-sac, not tear volume.

5. Rose bengal
    a.   Stains dead and degenerated epithelial cells; typically inferior staining is present.
    b.   Beneficial in the diagnosis of keratoconjunctivitis sicca.
    c.   A drop of 1% rose bengal is instilled into the conjunctival sac (or an impregnated strip moistened with an unpreserved saline solution is used); this is followed by irrigation of the external eye with an isotonic saline solution. The amount and location of the red stain will dictate the severity of the condition. Typically in keratoconjunctivitis sicca, the inferior cornea and conjunctiva will exhibit a large amount of staining. It particularly stains dead cells with an intense red color, while cells that are devitalized are stained a weaker color. In marginally dry eyes, the conjunctival surface may stain in a discrete punctate fashion, whereas in pathological dry eye, there is typically a more dense confluent staining with a uniformly intense red color. Typically, the adjacent

triangular sections of the exposed bulbar conjunctiva, both nasally and temporally, will stain. After the patient blinks 3 to 6 times and the excess dye has been washed away by the tears, the eye is examined with white light.

    d. The following grading sequence has been recommended for evaluating this condition[7]:

0 = absence of staining.

1 = staining of $<1/3$ of the cornea.

2 = staining of between $1/3$ and $2/3$ of the cornea.

3 = staining of between $2/3$ and the entire cornea.

4 = staining over the entire cornea.

5 = inferior conjunctival staining.

6. What series of tests should be used?

    a. Tear BUT should be performed for an accurate predictor of contact lens success based on tear quality.

    b. Biomicroscopic evaluation of both the tear prism and the presence of staining should be performed.

    c. A tear volume test, preferably the phenol red thread test due to its short time period and relative comfort, should be performed.

I. Final consultation

1. Evaluation of motivation

A highly motivated patient can often tolerate discomfort and other problems that would be difficult for the patient who has only a marginal motivation. Motivation can be tested by explaining that contact lenses are a health care device and have to be cared for constantly and without error. Patient motivation to wear contact lenses is a twofold desire to see well and to improve appearance; the greater a patient's need for contact lenses, either visual or psychological, the more likely it is that motivation will be high. Other factors to consider include the following:

    a. Satisfaction with spectacles (is the patient only exhibiting a casual interest in contact lenses or "shopping"?)

    b. With a younger child, is it the child who really desires the contact lenses, or is a vanity-conscious parent the only one who desires them? If the latter is true, the child is not ready for lens wear.

    c. If limited wearing time is probable due to, for example, borderline dry eye, does the patient still desire lens wear?

    d. If the patient is overly concerned about fees, discomfort, possible complications, etc., success is unlikely.

    e. If the patient exhibits hypochondriac-like concerns about minor ailments, he or she may not be willing to tolerate the initial discomfort or adaptation associated with contact lens wear. Likewise, if the patient is quite timid, successful contact lens wear is much less probable than with patients who are independent and confident.

    f. If the patient does not agree with the practitioner's recommendations (e.g., rigid gas-permeable lenses [RGPs], not hydrogels; hydrogen peroxide, not chemical disinfection; daily wear only, not extended wear), lenses should not be ordered and careful documentation in the patient's record is required.

    g. If the patient is very concerned with comfort or reacts strongly to RGP wear (e.g., excessive tearing, blinking, and inability to open eyes), hydrogel lenses should be considered.

2. Benefits of RGPs versus hydrogel lenses

A discussion of which lens material is best for a given patient is important. These factors can be considered when discussing this decision with a patient. These factors are summarized in Table 9-1.

3. Comfort

If the patient is very concerned about discomfort, hydrogel lenses should be

Table 9-1. Comparison of RGP and Hydrogel Advantages

RGP Advantages	Hydrogel Advantages
Vision	Initial comfort
Ocular health	Reduced initial chair time
High oxygen transmission	Variable wear
Wettability	Disposability
High astigmatic correction	No foreign body sensation
Ease of care/easier compliance	Athletes
Long-term comfort	Ability to change eye color
Stability/durability	Residual cylinder with RGPs
Reduce myopic progression	
Benefit irregular cornea patient	

considered (assuming the patient is even motivated for contact lens wear in general). If the patient is a high reactor with RGPs during diagnostic fitting (e.g., even after a 15- to 30-minute period, the patient is still tearing and has little desire to gaze straight ahead), hydrogel lenses should be considered.

J. *Suitability*

After obtaining all of this information, the bottom line is: Is the patient a suitable candidate for contact lens wear? Good versus poor candidates are summarized in Table 9-2.

K. *Summary*

Careful patient selection is paramount to successful contact lens wear. If a comprehensive history, preliminary evaluation, and assessment of suitability are performed, it is likely that an accurate decision on the patient's contact lens wearing status can be made. Whether the patient is considered a candidate for contact lens wear or not, being provided with an honest appraisal of probability of successful lens wear will eventually benefit both parties.

II. Optics

The following six topics will be presented:
1. Contact lens power.
2. Lacrimal lens.
3. Prismatic effects.
4. Vergence demands.
5. Accommodation.
6. Magnification.

Table 9-2. Candidates for Contact Lens Wear

Good Candidates	Poor Candidates
High motivated	Unmotivated
High myopia	Dry eye
Hyperopia	Moderate allergies/antihistamine use
Aphakia	Active infection, giant papillary conjunctivitis, coalesced staining
Irregular cornea	Poor hygiene
Refractive anisometropia	Pregnancy
	Binocular vision problem

A. *Contact lens power*

   1. Contact lens as a thick lens

     Although a contact lens is thin compared to other modes of refractive correction, it should be treated as a thick lens using the thick lens formula[8]:

$F_t = F^1 + F_2 - (t/n)F_1F_2$

F_t = equivalent lens refractive power (D)

$F_1 = (n' - n)/r_1$ = refractive power of the anterior lens surface

$F_2 = (n - n')/r_2$ = refractive power of the posterior lens surface

t = center thickness (meters)

n = refractive index of the lens material

n' = refractive index of medium surrounding lens

r_1 = radius of curvature of anterior surface (in meters)

r_2 = radius of curvature of posterior surface (in meters)

$$\begin{array}{ll} n' = 1.49 & F_1 = \dfrac{1.49 - 1.00}{0.0078} \\ n = 1.00 & \\ r_1 = 7.80\text{mm} & = +62.8\text{D} \\ r_2 = 8.40\text{mm} & F_2 = \dfrac{1.00 - 1.49}{0.0084} \\ & = -58.3\text{D} \end{array}$$

$$F_e = F_1 + F_2 \text{ (thin lens)} = +4.50\text{D}$$
$$F_1 + F_2 - t/n\, F_1F_2$$
$$+62.38 + (-)58.3 - \frac{.00025}{1.49} \, (+62.8)(-58.3)$$
$$+4.50 - (-)0.61$$
$$= +5.11\text{D}$$

   2. Front vertex versus back vertex power

     a. Definition

       It is impractical to use the equivalent power of a contact lens as the definition of refractive power, because the position of the principal planes varies with the lens design and the two surface powers. A fixed position to measure refractive power is found by using either front vertex power (FVP) or back vertex power (BVP).

$$\text{FVP} = F_1 + \frac{F_2}{1 - (t/n)F_1} \qquad \text{BVP} = \frac{F_1}{1 - (t/n)F_2} + F_2$$

n = refractive index of the lens

$$\begin{array}{ll} r_1 = 7.2 \text{ mm} & F_1 = \dfrac{1.49 - 1.00}{0.0072} \\ r_2 = 8.5 \text{ mm} & \\ n = 1.00 & = +68\text{D} \\ n' = 1.49 & F_2 = \dfrac{1.00 - 1.49}{0.0085} \\ t = 0.35 \text{ mm} & = -57.65\text{D} \end{array}$$

$$\text{FVP} = +68 + \frac{57.65}{1 - (.00035/1.49) - 57.65}$$

$$= +11.12\text{D}$$

$$\text{BVP} = \frac{+68}{1 - (.00035/1.49)68} + (-)57.65$$

$$= +11.45\text{D}$$

    b.   Measuring FVP and BVP

        FVP—convex surface against lensometer stop

        BVP—concave surface against lensometer stop

    c.   Summary

        (1)   Significant difference in BVP vs. FVP in medium- to high-plus powers.

        (2)   FVP is always less than BVP.

        (3)   BVP is typically used.

2.   Effective power

    a.   Definition

        As a minus lens is brought closer to the eye, its effective power increases, so that refractive power must be decreased to maintain a constant amount of power relative to the eye. As a plus lens is brought closer to the eye, its effective power decreases, so that its refractive power must be increased to maintain a constant amount of power relative to the eye. Effective power is:

        Clinically significant at $\pm$ 4.00D.

        Referred back to the corneal plane.

        Calculated for each meridian.

        (1)   Example 1

Sp Rx: $+6.00 - 2.00 \times 090$
Vertex: 12 mm

Horizontal meridian: $f_{180} = 1/F_{180} = 1/+4D = 0.25 \text{ m} = 250 \text{ mm}$

Vertical meridian: $f_{090} = 1/F_{090} = 1/+6D = 0.167 \text{ m} = 167 \text{ mm}$

Focal lengths = 12 mm less; therefore = 238 and 155 mm

Horizontal meridian: $F_{180} = \dfrac{1}{+0.238 \text{ m}} = +4.20D$

Vertical meridian: $F_{090} = \dfrac{1}{+0.155 \text{ m}} = +6.45D$

Corneal plane Rx: $+6.45 - 2.25 \times 090$ or $+6.50 - 2.25 \times 090$

        (2)   Example 2

Sp Rx: $-4.00 - 2.00 \times 180$
Focal lengths: -262 mm, -179 mm

Horizontal meridian: $F_{180} = \dfrac{1}{-0.262 \text{ m}} = -3.82D$

Vertical meridian: $F_{090} = \dfrac{1}{-0.179 \text{ m}} = -5.59D$

Corneal Plane Rx: $-3.82 - 1.77 \times 180$ or $-3.75 - 1.75 \times 180$

The effective power can also be determined by the following formula:

$$F_c = \frac{F_s}{1 - dF_s}$$

where

F_c = contact lens power
F_s = spectacle lens power
d = distance between the spectacle lens and contact lens in meters

(3) Example 3
Refraction: $-6.50 - 1.00 \times 180$ (12 mm vertex distance); at corneal plane this will equal:

$$\frac{-6.50}{1 - (0.012 \times -6.50)} = -6.03D$$

$$\frac{-7.50}{1 - (0.012 \times -7.50)} = -6.88D$$

Therefore, the spectacle prescription at the corneal plane is equal to: $-6.03 - 0.85 \times 180$ or $-6.00 - 0.75 \times 180$.

b. Summary
(1) In compound hyperopic astigmatism: sphere and cylinder increase.
(2) In compound myopic astigmatism: sphere and cylinder decrease.

B. *Lacrimal lens*
1. Definition
The fluid lens is formed by the precorneal tear film when the contact lens base curve radius (or posterior optical zone) is not equal to the anterior corneal curvature.

Lacrimal lens power = base curve (in diopters) − "K" (i.e., flatter keratometric reading) reading (in diopters).

a. When a lens has been fit steeper than the cornea, a plus lacrimal lens power is created; therefore, a corresponding minus power is necessary in the contact lens.
b. When a lens is fit flatter than the cornea, a minus lacrimal lens is created; therefore a corresponding plus power is necessary in the contact lens.
2. Tear lens powers

Keratometry: 42.00 @ 180, 43.00 @ 090
"On K" = 42.00D BC (8.04 mm)
= O tear lens power (42–42)
1D flatter than K = 41.00D (8.23 mm)
= −1.00D tear lens power (41–42)
1D steeper than K = 43.00D (7.85 mm)
= +1.00D tear lens power (43–42)

a. Predicted contact lens power = spherical spectacle Rx − lacrimal lens power

Rx: $-2.00 -1.00 \times 180$
"On K" = −2.00D
1D flat = −2.00D +1.00D = −1.00D
1D steep = −2.00D −1.00D = −3.00D

b. Final contact lens power = diagnostic contact lens power + over-refraction

Rx: $-2.00 - 1.00 \times 180$
Ks: 42.00 @ 180 43.00 @ 090
Diagnostic lens
BCR: 41.50

CL power: -3.00
OR: $+1.50$
Final CL power =
$-3.00 + (+) 1.50 = -1.50D$

c. Predicted over-refraction = (spectacle Rx − diagnostic CL power) − lacrimal lens power

$$= [-2.00 - (-) 3.00] - (-) 0.50 = +1.50D$$

d. Example: Rx: $-4.00 - 1.00 \times 180$

Step one: Vertex Sp. Rx to cornea (12 mm)
$= -3.81 - 0.91 \times 180$ or
$-3.75 - 1.00 \times 180$

Step two: Predicted OR = Sp. Rx − Dx CLP − LLP
$= -3.75 - (-) 3.00 - (43.25 - 43)$
$= -1.00D$

Step three: Predicted Final CL Rx = Dx CL power + OR
$= -3.00 + (-) 1.00$
$= -4.00D$

C. *Prismatic effects*

1. Definition

    Prism in a contact lens Rx is produced by varying the thickness of a contact lens while maintaining the same front and back surface curvature for proper refractive power. Typically, base down prism is used to stabilize toric and bifocal lenses.

    $$p = \frac{100(n - 1)(BT - AT)}{BAL}$$

    where

    p = prismatic power
    n = RI of prismatic lens
    BT = base thickness
    AT = apex thickness
    BAL = length of base apex line, usually diameter of CL along base-apex line of prism

    If $n = 1.49$
    BT = 0.30 mm
    AT = 0.12 mm
    BAL = 8.8 mm

    $$p = \frac{100(1.49 - 1)(0.30 - 0.12)}{8.8}$$

    $$= \frac{8.8}{8.8} = 1\Delta$$

2. Decentration
   a. *Back vertex power* becomes more plus and less minus as thickness increases toward the base of the prism (Prentice's rule).
   b. *Contact lens decentration on the eye* can induce prism.

$$BVP = F_d$$
$$= \text{prismatic power}$$
$$F = \text{BVP of contact lenses}$$
$$d = \text{decentration of light from optical center (in cm)}$$

Example: Contact lens decenters 2 mm inferiorally

$$F = +5.00D$$
$$= +5.00D \times 0.2 = 1PD$$

   c. *Anisometropia,* as with spectacle correction, can result in prism if contact lenses decenter.

Example

OD +6.00D CL power
OS +2.00D CL power

Both contact lenses decenter 2 mm inferiorly
$F_d = 1.2\ (6 \times 0.2)$ OD $0.4\ (2 \times 0.2)$ OS
difference = 0.8 PD

   d. *Prism contact lenses* typically decenter inferiorally. The total prism power on the eye equals refractive component due to decentration (via Prentice) plus the prism component of the lens.

Example 1

OD contact lens
$F = +6.00D$
1.5 PD base down
decentered 2 mm inferior

$df = 0.2(+6.00) = 1.2$
Total = 1.5 + 1.2 = 2.7 PD

Example 2

If $F = -6.00D$
Total = 1.5 + (−) 1.2 = 0.3 PD

3. Summary
   a. Prism effects from decentration are insignificant at low powers but may be significant at high powers.
   b. Contact lenses typically move similarly on the eye; therefore, prismatic difference is minimal except in high anisometropia.

D. *Vergence demands*
   1. Contact lens benefits versus spectacles
      Contact lenses move as the eyes rotate into different directions of gaze; therefore, many prismatic effects common to spectacles are eliminated.[8] Among these effects are:
      a. Base right and base left prism for bilateral myopia, and base left prism and base right prism for bilateral hyperopia in right and left gaze present with spectacle wear.

   b.   Vergence demand alterations in anisometropia during right and left gaze.
   c.   Vertical prismatic effects in up and down gaze and imbalance in down gaze from anisometropia.
   d.   Increased near convergence demand for bilateral hyperopia and decreased near convergence demand for bilateral myopia.
2.   Contact lens disadvantages versus spectacles
     Difficulty may be experienced by:
   a.   Exophoric binocular myope switched to contact lenses.
   b.   Exophoric hyperope.
   c.   Those benefitting from lateral prism.

E.   *Accommodation*
   1.   Corneal accommodative demand: spectacle wearer
        Accommodative demand is less for a myopic eye corrected by a spectacle lens than for an emmetropic eye. Likewise, a spectacle-corrected hyperopic eye has higher accommodative demand at near than does an emmetropic eye. The reason for this is that the accommodative demand equals the effective power of the spectacle lens power at the corneal plane minus the effective power of the spectacle lens plus near vergence power. For a 40-cm near distance, −2.50D vergence would reach the spectacle lens. The effective power at the corneal plane would, therefore, increase in minus for a myopic lens and decrease in plus for a hyperopic lens.
        An example is provided in Figure 9-5. When viewing a 40-cm object, the ver-

Accommodative Demand: High Myopic Refractive Error

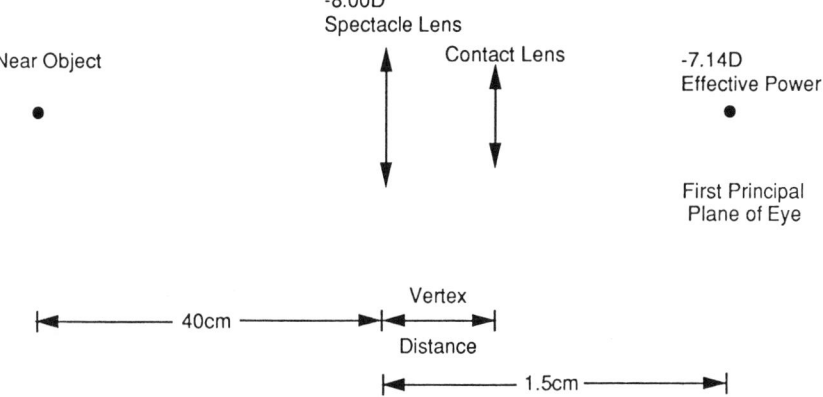

Step One: Vergence of light striking spectacle lens
               = -1/.4 = -2.50D
Step Two: Power leaving spectacle lens = -2.50+ (-)8.00
               = -10.50D
Step Three: Effective Power at First Principal Plane =
               -10.50/1-(.015)-10.50 = -9.07D
Step Four: Accommodative Demand = -9.07 - (-)7.14 = -1.93D
               Emmetropic Accommodative Demand = -(1/.415) = -2.41D

Figure 9-5.   The accommodative demand of a highly myopic spectacle wearer.

gence at an $-8.00D$ spectacle lens is $-2.50D$. The power leaving the spectacle lens is equal to $-10.50D$. The effective power at the cornea (15-mm vertex distance) is equal to $-9.07D$. The effective power for the distance correction ($-8.00D$) is equal to $-7.14D$. The difference between these values is $-1.93D$. This is 0.48D less than the emmetrope who has an accommodative demand equal to $-2.41D$ (1/0.40 m + 0.15 m).

2. Corneal accommodative demand: contact lens wearer
    The contact lens wearer has the same accommodative demand as the emmetrope, as the contact lens is placed at the corneal plane (i.e., 2.41D). Therefore, it has been calculated that the $-4.00D$ spectacle-wearing myope has to accommodate 0.25D more with contact lenses and the $-8.25D$ myope, 0.50D more.[8] This could be significant in the prepresbyopic high myope who desires contact lens wear.

F. *Magnification*
    1. Magnification of correction
        a. Definition.
            Magnification of correction is equal to the ratio of retinal image size of the corrected ametropic eye to the retinal image size of the same eye uncorrected. It can be used to help determine the ratio between retinal image size with contact lenses versus spectacles.

            Retinal image size between CL and spectacle lens can be directly compared:

            $$\frac{\text{CL power factor}}{\text{Spectacle lens power factor}} = 1 - df$$

            d = stop distance of spectacle lens (i.e., vertex + 3 mm)
            F = BVP of spectacle lens

            $$\text{If } d = 15 \text{ mm (0.015 m)}$$
            $$F = -12.00D$$

            $$1 - dF = 1 - 0.015 \times (-)\,12)$$
            $$= 1.18$$
            $$= 18\% \text{ larger retinal image for CL}$$

        b. High myopia
            A significant minification (SM < 1.0) of the retinal image occurs with spectacle correction, which is substantially alleviated when contact lenses are worn. This is due to the increase in retinal image size.
        c. Aphakia
            Magnification = 35% or higher with spectacles, 5%–8% with contact lenses, and 0% with intraocular lenses.
    2. Relative spectacle magnification (RSM)
        a. Definition
            RSM compares the corrected ametropic retinal image to that of a standard schematic eye. The effects of both axial ametropia, in which the refractive error results from axial length factors, and refractive ametropia, in which the refractive error results from changes in the refractive components of the eye, can be evaluated.

            Axial ametropia

            $$RSM = \frac{1}{1 + g(BVP)}$$

where:

RSM = relative spectacle magnification
g = distance in meters from anterior focal point of eye to correcting lens; $g = 0$ if lens is 15.7 mm in front of eye
BVP = back vertex power of lens

Spectacles (−10D)   Contact lenses (−10D)

$$= \frac{1}{1 + 0.002(-10)} \qquad \frac{1}{1 + 0.015(-10)}$$

$$= \frac{1}{0.98} \qquad\qquad = \frac{1}{0.85}$$

$$= 1.02 \qquad\qquad = 1.18$$

$$= 2\% \text{ magnification} \qquad 18\% \text{ magnification}$$

Refractive ametropia
(= SM power factor)

$$\text{RSM} = \frac{1}{1 - d(\text{BVP})}$$

d = stop distance in meters from correcting lens to entrance pupil = vertex distance + 3 mm

BVP = back vertex power of lens

Spectacles (−10D)   Contact lenses (−10D)

$$= \frac{1}{1 - 0.015(-10)} \qquad \frac{1}{1 - 0.003(-10)}$$

$$= \frac{1}{1.15} \qquad\qquad = \frac{1}{1.03}$$

$$= 0.87 \qquad\qquad = 0.97$$

$$= 15\% \text{ minification} \qquad = 3\% \text{ minification}$$

3. Summary

In theory, ametropia of axial origin is best corrected with spectacles and refractive ametropia is best corrected with contact lenses. Typically, the latter situation is present, and contact lenses benefit the high myope by increasing retinal image size and benefit the hyperopic/aphakic patient by minimizing magnification. However, most axial ametropes also perform well with contact lenses.

III.   Rigid Gas-Permeable Materials, Lens Design, and Fitting

A. *Material properties*
1. Oxygen permeability/transmission
   a. Dk (oxygen permeability)—measure of the potential for oxygen transmissibility of a material which is independent of size, shape, or surface condition of the lens.
   b. Dk/L (oxygen transmission)—measure of the predicted amount of oxygen to be transmitted through the lens material and design. It is dependent on the Dk value of the material and lens thickness (typically center thickness for rigid lenses).
   c. EOP (equivalent oxygen percentage)—measure of the amount of oxygen in the tears between the lens and the cornea, determined in vivo; it is a predictor of how much oxygen will reach the anterior corneal surface with a particular lens material and design, the maximum value equaling 21%.
   d. How much oxygen is needed? Research has shown that a Dk/L = 24 (EOP = 10%) should satisfy the daily wear requirements of every patient.[9] A 30-Dk lens with a center thickness of 0.12 mm and a 60-Dk lens with a center thickness of 0.24 mm should satisfy this requirement. However, as corneal deswelling occurs more rapidly with rigid than hydrogel lenses due to the amount of tear exchange, a slightly lower Dk/L should be acceptable in daily wear. With this in mind, RGP lenses can be divided into low Dk (25–50) and high Dk (>50). It is unlikely that a lens material with a Dk < 25 will meet the cornea's oxygen requirements.
2. Surface wettability
   a. This is the ability of the blink to spread tear film mucin across the anterior contact lens surface.
   b. Lenses that dry between blinks before the tear film is refreshed are more prone to deposits. The mucin layer on the surface undergoes chemical changes (i.e., becomes more mucus-like) and surface wettability is reduced. These surface deposits can result in symptoms of blurred vision and redness and possibly result in giant papillary conjunctivitis (GPC).
   c. The goal of any contact lens material is to maintain the mucin layer in an unchanged form for as long as possible.
3. Flexural resistance
   a. The ability of a rigid lens to resist the bending or flexing forces of the lid when a rigid lens is on a toric cornea; otherwise, the lens will flex during the blinking process and fail to correct all of the patient's corneal astigmatism.
   b. Flexure is most commonly experienced with high-Dk materials, thin center thickness, base curve radii fit steeper than "K," and large optical zone diameters.
4. Specific gravity
   a. The weight of an RGP lens at a given temperature divided by the weight of an equal volume of water at the same temperature.
   b. Often compared to water (specific gravity = 1.00), specific gravity values for RGP materials can be divided into low (≤1.10), medium (1.11–1.20), and high (>1.20) values. The lower specific gravity or "lighter" materials are more likely to exhibit good centration characteristics by being more resistant to the forces of gravity.
5. Other properties
   Other properties include the hardness, scratch resistance, and optical quality.

B. *Material types and composition*
1. Fluoro-silicone/acrylate (F-S/A)
   a. Most RGP lenses are F-S/A.
   b. Composition includes
      (1) "Silicone"—silicon as siloxane bonds in side branches of the main carbon-

carbon polymer chain; provides oxygen permeability by diffusion while exhibiting both poor flexural resistance and poor surface wettability.

    (2) Fluorine—provides surface wettability/deposit resistance by promoting tear film interaction with the lens surface; also provides a small amount of oxygen permeability by solubility.

    (3) Methacrylate—conventional non-oxygen-permeable plastic provides stability and surface wettability.

    (4) Wetting agents—such as methylcrylic acid and HEMA enhance surface wettability.

    (5) Crosslinking agents enhance stability and improve machining characteristics.

  c. Benefits of fluoro-silicone/acrylate over previous silicone/acrylate lens materials is the addition of fluorine, which provides enhanced surface wettability and allows for higher oxygen permeability (most F-S/A lens materials have Dk values from 30 to 100).

2. Silicone/acrylate (S/A)

  a. Composition similar to F-S/A with the absence of fluorine.

  b. Little used today as a result of the hydrophobicity (poor wetting nature) of "silicone," especially in high-Dk materials.

  c. Most S/A lens materials have Dk values <30.

3. Polystyrene

  a. Introduced in the 1980s giving low specific gravity and good flexural resistance.

  b. Currently used as the SoftPerm (SBH) material with a styrene-based center (8.0 mm with one peripheral curve) and a 25% water content hydrogel periphery (14.3 mm overall diameter).

  c. Fit similar to an RGP lens material, it is evaluated with Fluorosoft (Holles Lab.), not fluorescein. At minimum, 0.50 mm lag with the blink is recommended.

  d. Primary benefits include initial comfort similar to a hydrogel lens and good centration. Therefore, patients with irregular cornea, including early keratoconus, and "sensitive" patients in need of astigmatic correction will benefit from this lens.

  e. Problems with this lens material include adherence, tearing in the junction between the hydrogel and rigid sections, limited parameters available, cost, and difficulty of lens removal.

4. Silicone elastomer

  a. Provide outstanding oxygen permeability (Dk = 340) and intermediate diameters (11.3 and 12.5 mm).

  b. A viable and popular option for the pediatric aphakic patient who requires excellent oxygen transmission in combination with better initial comfort than provided with RGPs.

  c. Greatest problem is hydrophobic nature of lens surface, which tends to reduce lens life to approximately 6 months.

C. *Material selection*

In selecting the appropriate RGP lens material for a given patient, five categories can be used to make this judgment: (1) refractive error, (2) corneal topography, (3) refits, (4) occupation/hobbies, and (5) age. This information is summarized in Figure 9-6.

1. Refractive error

  a. Due to stability, surface wettability, and lesser center thickness, almost all myopic daily wear patients would benefit from a low-Dk F-S/A. The only exception would be if edema is present with these materials.

  b. Because of the greater center thickness and corresponding reduction in Dk/L, hyperopic patients benefit from high-Dk F-S/A lens materials.

2. Corneal topography

  a. Patients with moderate corneal astigmatism (i.e., ≥1.50D) benefit from the flexural resistance provided by low-Dk F-S/A materials.

RGP Material Selection

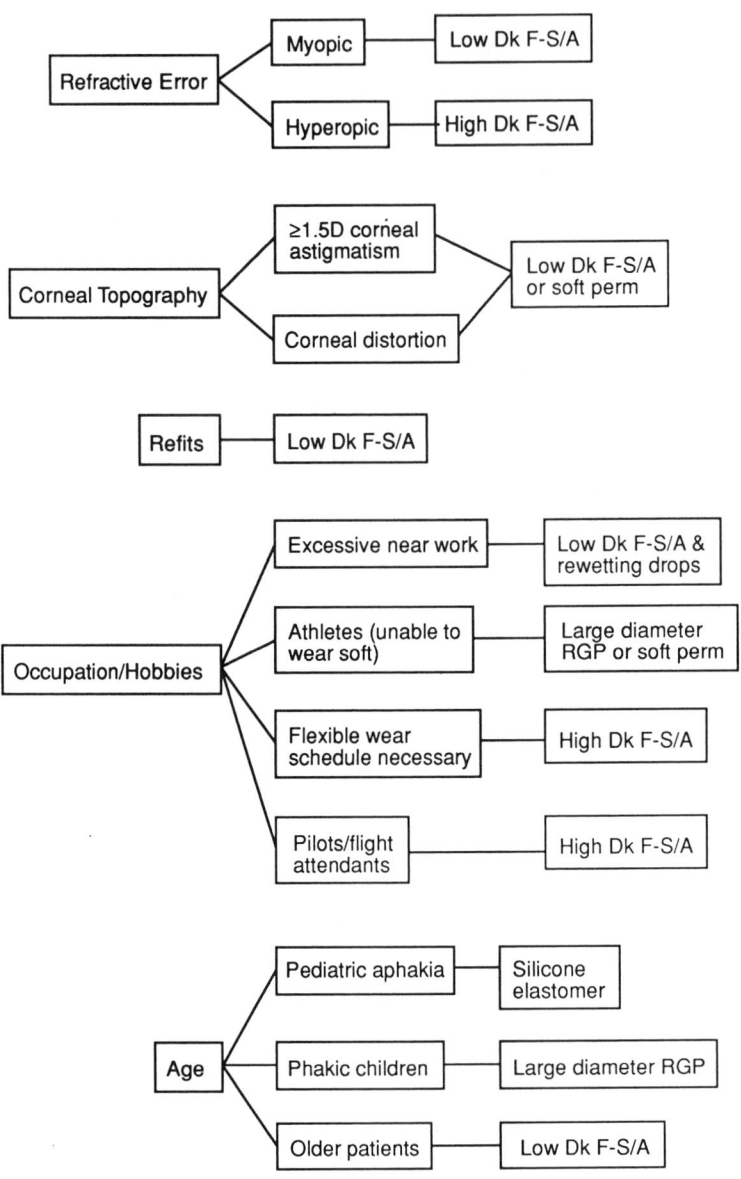

Figure 9-6.   RGP material selection nomogram.

    b.   Patients exhibiting an irregular cornea resulting from trauma, keratoconus, long-term PMMA wear, etc. would benefit from either the stability and flexural resistance provided by low-Dk F-S/A lenses, or the centration and initial comfort properties provided by the SoftPerm lens.

3.   Refits

    a.   Former PMMA and first-generation RGP lens wearers (i.e., <20 Dk) should be refit into low-Dk F-S/A lenses due to the tendency of these individuals to scratch and warp the more flexible high-Dk lenses.

b. Previous hydrogel lens wearers who have experienced deposit-related problems resulting in lid inflammation and/or have frequently torn their lenses would benefit from refitting into any RGP lens material, although, once again, they would benefit from the most wettable material available.

4. Occupation
   a. Individuals performing an excessive amount of near work would benefit from a highly wettable material supplemented by frequent application of rewetting drops, as blinking is typically reduced.
   b. Athletes who are unable to wear hydrogel lenses would benefit from either a SoftPerm lens or a large-diameter RGP lens design.
   c. Individuals who require flexible wear due to extended periods of work (police, nurses, etc.) would benefit from a high-Dk F-S/A lens material.
   d. Pilots and flight attendants, who are often exposed to less than optimum oxygen levels, would benefit from a high-Dk F-S/A lens material.

5. Age
   a. Pediatric aphakes often benefit from a silicone elastomer lens.
   b. Phakic children would benefit from larger RGP lens designs, which would be less likely to dislodge.
   c. Older patients, who typically exhibit a reduction in tear volume, would benefit from a low-Dk F-S/A lens material. This would also be true with a borderline dry eye patient.

D. *Fitting and evaluation*
1. Diagnostic versus empirical fitting
   a. Approximately 50% of all practitioners order lenses empirically (i.e., without application of diagnostic lenses). The practitioner either will design the lenses based on the patient's refractive information or will provide the laboratory with refractive information such that they can design the lenses.
   b. Benefits of empirically designing lenses include
     (1) It eliminates the so-called fitting visit.
     (2) A "used" diagnostic lens will be avoided.
     (3) Use of the manufacturer's fitting guide, which may be just as effective as the best fitting diagnostic lens.
   c. The application of diagnostic lenses, however, has many benefits:
     (1) Fewer reorders, as an optimum lens-to-cornea fitting relationship is often achieved prior to ordering.
     (2) Practitioner confidence in the fitting relationship.
     (3) Patient experiences rigid lens sensation.
     (4) Ability to evaluate vision/residual astigmatism.
   d. A study comparing diagnostic versus empirical fitting found the following benefits of diagnostic fitting[10]:
     (1) Over 50% fewer reorders.
     (2) Greater patient compliance.
     (3) Greater respect and appreciation for the contact lenses; in part, a result of patient confidence in the practitioner as a result of having experienced a successful contact lens fit and had questions answered at the fitting visit.
2. Diagnostic fitting sets/inventories
   a. Fitting sets—several fitting sets would be recommended, including
     (1) 20 lens −3.00D power sets in both low-Dk and high-Dk materials (Table 9-3).
     (2) A +3.00D power fitting set similar to the above in a high-Dk lens material and with a minus lenticular edge design.
     (3) A −8.00D diagnostic set similar to the above in a low-Dk lens material and with a plus lenticular edge design.

Table 9-3.   Recommended Parameters for a 20-Lens Diagnostic Set, Low-Dk RGP Material

	Overall Diameter		9.2 mm	
	Optical Zone Diameter		7.8 mm	
	Center Thickness		0.14 mm	
	Power		−3.00 D	
	BCR (mm)	SCR/W	ICR/W	PCR/W
1.	7.42	8.00/.3	8.80/.2	10.00/.2
2.	7.46	8.10/.3	8.90/.2	10.10/.2
3.	7.50	8.20/.3	9.00/.2	10.20/.2
4.	7.54	8.20/.3	9.00/.2	10.20/.2
5.	7.58	8.30/.3	9.10/.2	10.30/.2
6.	7.63	8.30/.3	9.20/.2	10.40/.2
7.	7.67	8.40/.3	9.30/.2	10.50/.2
8.	7.71	8.50/.3	9.40/.2	10.60/.2
9.	7.76	8.50/.3	9.50/.2	10.60/.2
10.	7.81	8.60/.3	9.60/.2	10.70/.2
11.	7.85	8.60/.3	9.60/.2	10.80/.2
12.	7.89	8.70/.3	9.70/.2	10.80/.2
13.	7.94	8.70/.3	9.70/.2	10.90/.2
14.	7.99	8.80/.3	9.80/.2	11.00/.2
15.	8.04	8.80/.3	9.90/.2	11.10/.2
16.	8.08	8.90/.3	10.00/.2	11.20/.2
17.	8.13	8.90/.3	10.10/.2	11.30/.2
18.	8.18	9.00/.3	10.20/.2	11.40/.2
19.	8.23	9.10/.3	10.30/.2	11.50/.2
20.	8.28	9.20/.3	10.40/.2	11.60/.2

    (4) Keratoconic, bitoric, aphakic, and bifocal diagnostic sets are also recommended and are discussed later in this chapter.

    (5) Representative lens parameters can include the following:
Overall diameter (OAD): 9.2 mm.
Optical zone diameter: 7.8 mm.
Base curve radii: 40.75D (8.28 mm) to 45.50D (7.42 mm) in 0.25D steps.
Periphery: tricurve or tetracurve design.
Center thickness: approximately 0.14 mm for low-Dk and 0.17 mm for high-Dk lenses in −3.00D power.

  b. Inventories—the advantages of a large (100–200) lens inventory are

    (1) Convenience to patient: some individuals can be fit directly from stock; others can receive replacement lenses without delay.

    (2) Lens parameter changes can be made without delay.

3. PMMA versus RGP diagnostic lenses

  a. For maximum success, fit same material as to be ordered due to

    (1) Variation in thickness between materials.

    (2) Variation in other design parameters between materials.

    (3) A high-Dk material may flex more on the eye than a PMMA or low-Dk lens material.

4. Fluorescein application

  a. Description—sodium fluorescein is an organic compound which is inert and harmless to tissue. It is invaluable for assessing the lens-to-cornea fitting relationship.

   b. Application—the strip is wetted with a sterile saline solution and then placed against bulbar conjunctiva with patient viewing inferiorally or superiorally. For optimum fluorescence, use of liquid fluorescein is beneficial.

   c. Methods of observation

     (1) Burton lamp. This is the traditional method of viewing the fluorescein pattern and utilizes a +5.00D lens for magnification. It is inexpensive, easy to use, and provides a large overall field of view.

     (2) Biomicroscope. This method allows the observer to vary magnification, illumination, and slit beam width when observing the fluorescein pattern. The pattern should be viewed under low magnification with a wide (diffuse) slit beam and high-intensity illumination. The cobalt blue filter is required, as it transmits blue light which will activate the fluorescein dye. The use of a Wratten No. 12 (or equivalent) yellow filter over the observation system will enhance the appearance of the fluorescence, which is especially important with ultraviolet-inhibiting lenses.

   d. Pattern evaluation—areas of fluorescein pooling appear green; areas of absence appear dark or black. Several patterns are present and include:

     (1) Alignment fit—can be observed when the lens evenly contours the cornea with light, even pooling; the lens periphery should exhibit a denser green color to indicate more tear exchange at this location. This would be a desirable pattern.

     (2) Apical clearance—can be observed when the lens evenly contours the cornea with a light, even pooling. This can result in midperipheral bearing and seal-off.

     (3) Apical bearing—can be observed when there is direct contact of lens against central cornea. Excessive corneal bearing can result in corneal distortion or warpage.

     (4) Dumbbell—with corneal astigmatism greater than 1D, a dumbbell-shaped pattern can be observed due to lack of lens-to-cornea alignment. Along the steeper meridian of the cornea, the tear layer thickness vaults the cornea with the tear layer thickness increasing toward the lens edge. Along the flatter meridian, the tear layer thickness decreases toward the periphery with bearing typically present paracentrally/midperipherally.

     (5) False fluorescein patterns—can occur in certain cases, including

       (a) A steep base curve radius lens may result in poor tear exchange with a misleading amount of fluorescein centrally due to midperipheral sealoff.

       (b) If the peripheral curve is too steep, peripheral seal-off can occur and the fluorescein pattern will appear to exhibit apical clearance.

       (c) In individuals in whom the fluorescein dissipates quickly, a pseudo-apical flat relationship can result.

       (d) A pseudo-steep pattern can occur in high-minus lenses due to the great edge thickness blocking the fluorescence.

   e. Video education—Table 9-4 provides a list of educational videos on fluorescein pattern evaluation available from the CLMA/RGP Lens Institute Video Library (1-800-343-5367).

5. Author's design/fitting philosophy

   a. Overall/optical zone diameter (OAD/OZD)—depends on the following factors:

     (1) An average OAD/OZD = 9.2/7.8 mm. When a larger lens is desirable, 9.6/8.2 mm; when a smaller lens is needed, an 8.8/7.4-mm lens is recommended.

     (2) Palpebral aperture size—average = 9.0–10.5 mm; if larger, increase OAD; if smaller, decrease OAD.

     (3) Pupil size—OZD should be greater than pupil diameter in dim illumination.

Table 9-4. Contact Lens Manufacturing Association RGP Lens Institute Video Library

Patient Promotional
RGP Lens Care and Handling
Fundamentals of Fluorescein
Keratometry
Lensometry
The Radiuscope
RGP Diagnostic Fitting—Vol I
RGP Diagnostic Fitting—Vol II
RGP Clinical Pearls—Vol I
RGP Clinical Pearls—Vol II
RGP Grand Rounds—Vol I
RGP Grand Rounds—Vol II
RGP Modification
RGP Verification
Building Your Practice with RGPs
Fitting Toric RGPs
Fitting Keratoconus and Irregular Corneas
Clinical Biomicroscopy

Available from Contact Lens Manufacturers Association, 421 King St., Suite 224, Alexandria, Virginia 22314 (800-343-5367).

(4) Refractive power—often need greater OAD with hyperopic than myopic patients for greater pupil coverage with higher mass lens.
(5) Corneal curvature—select larger than average OAD with flatter corneas (i.e., <41D) and smaller than average with steeper corneas (i.e., >45D). A rule of thumb is to select an OZD equal to the base curve radius in millimeters. (i.e., if 7.5 mm BCR, select 7.5 mm OZD)

b. Base curve radius (BCR)—the purpose of the BCR is to optimize the fitting relationship of the lens to the cornea. The BCR to be selected depends on several factors, including the corneal curvature, the observed fluorescein pattern, and the lens-to-cornea fitting relationship. In most cases, with the exception of high astigmats and hyperopic patients, a flatter than "K" ("K" = the flatter keratometric value) BCR is selected. The author's recommended BCR selection is provided in Table 9-5. The BCR should be flattened 0.25D for every increase in OZD of 0.5 mm, and steepened 0.25D for every decrease in OZD of 0.5 mm.

c. Peripheral curve radii/width—typically encompass the outer 20%–35% of the lens. Designs in common use are either tricurve [(i.e., BCR, secondary

Table 9-5. RGP Base Curve Selection Criteria

Corneal Cylinder (keratometry)	Base Curve—Diagnostic Lens
0–0.50 D	0.50–0.75 D flatter than K
0.75–1.25 D	0.25–0.50 D flatter than K
1.50 D	"On" K
1.75–2.00 D	0.25 D steeper than K
2.25–2.75 D	0.50 D steeper than K

curve radius (SCR), and peripheral curve radius (PCR)] or tetracurve [(BCR, SCR, intermediate curve radius (ICR), and PCR].

The peripheral curves are increasingly flatter than the BCR to both contour the cornea and allow good peripheral tear exchange. They, however, serve no optical function. The following design guidelines are recommended:

Small (<9.0 mm)OAD	Large (≥9.0 mm)OAD
SCR/W = BCR + 1.0/0.3 mm	SCR/W = BCR + 0.8/0.3 mm
PCR/W = SCR + 2.0/0.3 mm	ICR/W = SCR + 1.0/0.2 mm
	PCR/W = ICR + 1.4/0.2 mm

    d. Center thickness—the center thickness is greater and the center of gravity more anterior in plus lenses than in minus lenses. A lens that is too thick can result in inferior decentration and a reduction in oxygen transmission. A too-thin lens can result in flexure. Two rules of thumb are important:

    One: Increase center thickness 0.02 mm for high-Dk lens materials.

    Two: Increase center thickness an additional 0.02 mm for each diopter of corneal astigmatism.

It is extremely important to verify center thickness. A recommended center thickness guide is given in Table 9-6.

    e. Edge thickness/design—a thin, tapered, rolled-edge design is desired. As there can be inconsistency in edge quality from manufacturing, careful verification is important. The use of a minus lenticular edge design for all low-minus (≤−1.50D) and plus power lenses is recommended for the benefit of increased lens-to-upper lid interaction. Likewise, a plus lenticular is recommended for all high- (≥−5D) minus power lenses to reduce edge thickness.

6. Aspheric designs

    a. Definition—typically consists of a design that gradually flattens, often at a similar, if not greater, rate than the cornea. Eccentricity, or "e" value, refers to deviation from a circular path with a circle having an eccentricity equal to zero. The cornea has an "e" value of about 0.4. Most single vision aspheric designs have an "e" value between 0.4 and 0.6, which represents an elliptical curve. Presbyopic designs have "e" values as large as 1.0 or greater (termed hyperbolic) to generate a greater plus correction.

    b. Types—there are essentially three designs:

        (1) "Pseudo-aspheric" designs are not true aspheric designs but consist of numerous peripheral curves blended together and typically promoted as "aspheric-like."

Table 9-6. Custom Design RGP Center Thickness Values (in millimeters)[a]

Power (D)	Dk value	
	(20–45)	(45–70)
−1.00	0.18	0.19
−2.00	0.16	0.18
−3.00	0.14	0.16
−4.00	0.14	0.15
−5.00	0.13	0.14
−6.00 and greater	0.13	0.14

[a]Add 0.02 mm per diopter of corneal cylinder.

(2) Spherical optical zone/aspheric periphery.
(3) Aspheric optical zone/aspheric periphery.
c. Advantages and disadvantages include the following:
(1) *Advantages*
(a) Alignment fitting relationship.
(b) Better initial comfort because of absence of peripheral curve (pc) junctions.
(c) Better centration on against-the-rule (ATR) and irregular corneas.
(d) Easier to fit.
(2) *Disadvantages*
(a) Reduced vision.
(b) Variable vision if decentration present.
(c) Verification difficult.
7. Power determination and lens order
a. Once the proper lens design and an optimum lens-to-cornea fitting relationship have been achieved, determination of the final lens power can occur. This is obtained with a comprehensive overrefraction and an understanding of both tear layer optics and vertex distance. The final power simply equals the diagnostic lens power plus the spherical overrefraction value if the BCR is unchanged. This is also illustrated in Figure 9-7. If the overrefraction values

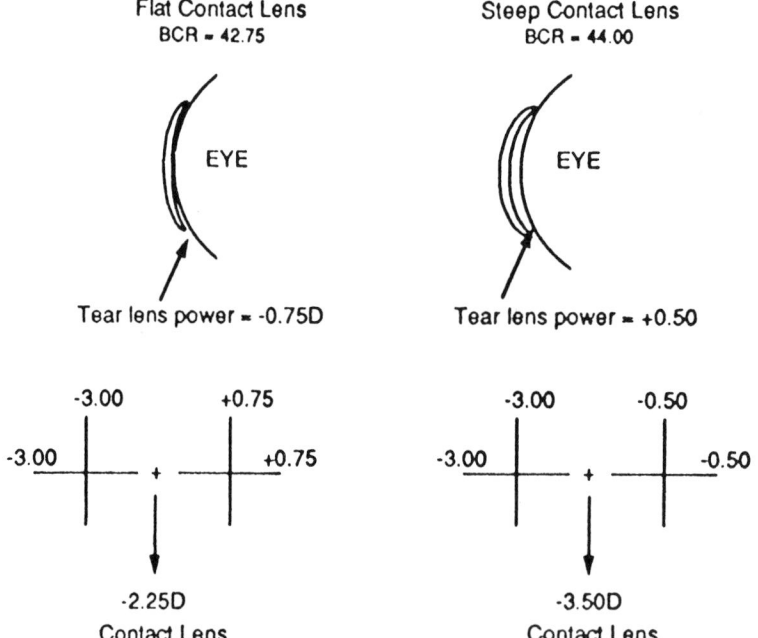

Figure 9-7.   Determining the final lens power considering both vertex distance and tear lens changes.

do not equal the predicted, this could be due to any one or combination of the following:

(1) Inaccurate refraction.
(2) Inaccurate keratometry values.
(3) BCR not as marked.
(4) Lens power not as marked.
(5) Flexure.
(6) Lens decentration.

b. An example of a custom-designed lens based upon a diagnostic fitting in which the predicted powers equaled the final powers ordered is given in Figure 9-8.

University of Missouri St. Louis

University of Missouri-Saint Louis
School of Optometry

Contact Lens Fitting Data

Patient: KREMER (Last) JUDIE (First) M.I. — File # — Date 11/16/93

Keratometry — Average (Low K); Average (High K)
R 42.50 @180; 43.75 @090
L 43.00 @180; 43.50 @090

Current Subjective Refraction
R −7.50 −1.50 × 180 20/20 (@12mm = −6.75 −1.25 × 180)
L −7.75 −0.75 × 180 20/20 (@12mm = −7.00 −0.50 × 180)

Predicted Lenses: Rigid ☑ Soft ☐ Special Design (specify)

	B.C.R.	S.C.R./W	P.C.R./W	Dia.	O.Z.D.	Power	C.T.
R	7.99 (42.25)			9.4		−6.50	
L	7.94 (42.50)			9.4		−6.50	

Diagnostic Lens		#1	#2	#3
B.C./Dia./Power/C.T.	R	7.99/9.4/−6.00/.14	/ / /	/ / /
	L	7.94/9.4/−6.00/.14	/ / /	/ / /
Fluorescein Pattern (H.C.L.) or Over-K readings (S.C.L.)	R	alignment		
	L	pattern OU		
Appearance of Mires (S.C.L.)	R	—		
	L	—		
Position and Lag	R	slightly superior		
	L	c̄ 2mm lag OU		
Retinoscopy (sphero-cyl)	R	−0.50 −0.25 × 090 20/20	20/	20/
	L	−0.25 DS 20/20	20/	20/
Subjective (best sphere)	R	−0.50 DS 20/20	20/	20/
	L	−0.50 DS 20/20	20/	20/

Final Lens Design: Rigid ✓ Soft ___ Laboratory: Mo-Con

	B.C.R.	S.C.R./W	P.C.R./W	Dia.	O.Z.D.	Power	C.T.	Tint
R	7.79	8.80/.3	11.20/.2	9.4	8.0	−6.50	.14	blue
L	7.94	8.80/.3	11.20/.2	9.4	8.0	−6.50	.14	blue

Blend: Medium — Additional information: FP30 + Lenticular Edge OU; ICR/W = 9.80/.2

Student Intern: S. Stolc — Supervising Clinician: E. Bennett

Comments:

Figure 9-8. An example of lens power calculations and design parameters of an RGP patient.

IV. RGP Lens Care and Patient Education

A. *Introduction*

1. Successful care and handling of RGP lenses depends on several factors, including:
    a. Proficiency with handling rigid lenses.
    b. Awareness of the functions of each solution and the importance of performing each function properly.
    c. Several methods of education should be used, including video.
    d. The "do's and don'ts" of contact lens wear must be explained.
2. This section addresses these important factors which, in turn, should result in a greater number of successful patients.

B. *Care regimen*

1. Wetting and soaking—most solutions are multipurpose, typically including wetting and soaking; these solutions have the following functions:
    a. Temporary enhancement of lens surface wettability.
    b. Maintenance of lens in hydrated state, similar to "on eye" situation.
    c. Disinfection.
    d. To act as mechanical buffer between lens, cornea, and lids.
2. These solutions are formulated with preservative and wetting agents.
    a. Preservatives
        (1) Perform the following functions:
            (a) Provide necessary degree of disinfection.
            (b) Do not cause toxicity reactions.
            (c) Avoid adverse surface wettability/lens parameter changes.
            (d) Be compatible with the tear film.
        (2) Preservatives in use today include the following:
            (a) Benzalkonium chloride (BAK)
                i. Quaternary ammonium compound effective at 0.004% against wide range of bacteria and fungi.
                ii. Binds with hydrogels and will cause toxicity reaction.
                iii. May concentrate on surface of S/A lenses, possibly resulting in superficial punctate keratitis.
            (b) Chlorhexidine
                i. Bactericidal and often used in 0.0005% concentration.
                ii. Much greater binding ability to hydrogels than RGPs.
                iii. Often combined with thimerosal or ethylene diaminetetraacetate (EDTA) due to limited effectiveness against yeast and fungi; it has also been relatively ineffective against *Serratia marcescens*.[11]
            (c) Thimerosal
                i. Organic mercurial compound that may cause immediate allergic reactions in mercurial-sensitive hydrogel wearers; it appears to cause only rare reactions in RGP wearers.
                ii. Slow-acting and may be ineffective against *Pseudomonas*.
                iii. Most effective when combined with another preservative such as chlorhexidine.
            (d) EDTA
                i. A chelating agent, not a true preservative.
                ii. Used in combination with a preservative because of synergistic effect against *Pseudomonas*.
            (e) Benzyl alcohol
                i. Originally used as solvent; properties such as low molecular weight, bipolarity, and water solubility make it a viable preservative.

ii. Exhibits good antimicrobial activity and little binding, especially to F-S/A lenses.[12]

(f) Polyaminopropyl biguanide (PAPB)

i. Used in hydrogel solutions (Dymed) due to low sensitivity rate; used in RGP solutions due to effectiveness against *Serratia marcescens.*

ii. As concentrations are 30–50× higher in rigid than in hydrogel solutions, toxicity reactions have been reported.[13]

b. Wetting agents

Use either polyvinyl alcohol or methylcellulose derivatives to enhance lens surface wettability:

(1) Polyvinyl alcohol

(a) Water-soluble and relatively nontoxic to ocular tissues.

(b) Good viscosity-building properties and good spreading ability of the tear film on the lens.

(2) Methylcellulose derivatives

(a) Used successfully in more viscous RGP solutions.

(b) May retard regeneration of corneal epithelium.

C. *Cleaning*

1. Nonabrasive surfactants

a. Nonparticulate detergents to remove lipids, mucoproteinous film, and debris from the lens.

b. Use of digital pressure or friction important to remove deposits.

2. Abrasive surfactants

a. Contain detergents and small abrasive particles to assist in removing adherent debris.

b. Appear to be more effective than nonabrasive cleaners in removing deposits.

c. Particulate matter has become smaller and less abrasive in newer cleaners due to problems such as surface microscratches and lens parameter changes occurring in large abrasive cleaners.[14]

3. Surfactant soaking

a. Has been proven to reduce borderline dry eye patients' symptoms of dryness and fogging.

b. One solution is used for both cleaning and disinfection, which dissolves deposits during soaking, minimizing need for digital pressure.

4. Enzymatic. Used weekly, typically for a 2-hour cycle in combination with saline, enzymes appear to be safe and effective against protein deposits.

5. Laboratory cleaners and solvents

a. Laboratory-approved extra-strength cleaners can be beneficial for occasional in-office cleaning of lenses that have either poor initial surface wettability or mucoprotein deposits that are resistant to daily and weekly cleaning.

b. Unapproved solvents should never be used with RGP lens materials.

D. *Rewetting and relubricating*

These solutions, used while the lens is on the eye, should perform the following functions:

1. Rewet the lens surface.

2. Stabilize the tear film.

3. Rinse away trapped debris.

4. Break up loosely attached deposits.

E. *Dispensing visit*

Patient education *begins* at the dispensing visit. Begin by using fluorescein to evaluate the cornea for staining prior to lens application. Next, insert the lenses and after partial adaptation has occurred (i.e., the patient has stopped tearing and is willing to gaze straight ahead), evaluate the lenses and educate the patient.

1. Lens evaluation
    a. Visual acuity
        (1) If reduced, evaluate with biomicroscopy to rule out poor surface wettability or decentered lens position.
        (2) If biomicroscopy reveals no problems, perform overrefraction.
    b. Overrefraction
        (1) If good visual acuity is present, perform a spherical overrefraction.
        (2) If reduction of one line or more occurs, perform spherocylindrical overrefraction.
        (3) If a spherical overrefraction improves acuity, this power modification can typically be performed in-office. If spherocylindrical overrefraction improves acuity, perform overkeratometry; if toric, lens is flexing.
    c. Slit lamp biomicroscopy
        (1) Important for evaluating lens-to-cornea fitting relationship, movement, fluorescein pattern, and surface wettability.
        (2) Determine if both fluorescein pattern and lens centration are similar to that at the diagnostic fitting visit; if not, recheck center thickness and BCR.
        (3) If poor surface wettability exists, use laboratory cleaner or solvent and rub wetting solution onto the lens prior to reinsertion.
2. Handling
    a. General recommendations
        (1) Frequent reassurance is crucial for the beginning contact lens wearer, as a frequent cause of dropouts is lack of confidence in handling the lenses.
        (2) It is even more—not less—important to ensure successful handling in patients who desire to insert lenses often or whose wearing schedule dictates this (extended wear and disposable lens patients).
        (3) A minimum of three successful insertions and removals is recommended.
        (4) Two visits, closely spaced apart, may be necessary if the patient becomes frustrated and does not initially master successful lens handling.
        (5) Other sources are available for a more comprehensive explanation of how to insert and remove rigid lenses.[15-17]
    b. Insertion
        (1) Patient should use an adjustable mirror.
        (2) Proper lid retraction is important; for right eye, lens should be placed on right index finger. Middle finger of left hand should be placed *underneath* upper lashes to lift upper lid. Middle finger of right hand should be placed *over* lower lashes to depress lower lid.
        (3) Patient should look straight ahead as if looking through the lens; reassurance should be provided that lens will not damage eye.
        (4) The procedure should be performed in reverse for the other eye.
        (5) If patient fails to master insertion, he or she should be instructed to practice touching the eye with a warm drop of water placed on the index finger.
    c. Removal.
        Three methods can be used:
        (1) Method 1
            (a) Place index finger of same hand as eye at the junction of the lateral edge of the lids.
            (b) With eye opened wide, the lids are pulled laterally; at the same time, the patient blinks and the lens should be ejected.
            (c) Many patients cannot use this method because of such factors as loose lid tension, low edge lift lens design, or large overall diame-

ter; therefore, it helps to also teach the patient to remove the lenses with both hands using either method 2 or method 3.

    (2) Method 2

        (a) The middle and index fingers of the same hand as the eye from which the lens is to be removed are positioned centrally over the lower lid; the same fingers of the opposite hand are placed under the lashes of the upper lid.

        (b) Slight pressure of lids against globe is applied, as it is the lid margins that actually eject the lens.

        (c) The lids are then pulled temporally and, while the patient blinks, the lens is ejected.

        (d) If pressure is not applied against the lid margin and/or the fingers are not placed over the lashes, the lids will evert and there will be insufficient pressure to result in ejection.

    (3) Method 3

        (a) This is similar to method 2 except that a vertical, not lateral, motion is used.

        (b) The fingers are positioned as in method 2; the lower lid is pushed superiorly and the lens is ejected.

  d. Recentration

        (a) It is important to demonstrate how to recenter a decentered rigid lens, as this is a common adaptation problem with new RGP lens wearers.

        (b) Location of a decentered lens can be determined with a mirror or by placing the finger gently over different regions of the lids.

        (c) When the lens is found, the patient should first look away from the lens (i.e., temporally, if the lens is nasal). The index finger of the same hand as the eye should be placed on the opposite side of the lens; when the patient then looks toward the lens, it should reposition onto the cornea.

3. Cleaning

  a. Cleaning with a surfactant cleaner should be performed immediately after removal to prevent mucoprotein deposits from drying onto the lens surface.

  b. Cleaning should be performed carefully in the palm of the hand, not between the fingers, which can result in warpage.

  c. Patients should be instructed as to the complications resulting from improper or inadequate cleaning (i.e., reduced vision, redness, giant papillary conjunctivitis, etc.) and only use recommended product(s).

  d. Patients should be instructed to clean the left lens as thoroughly as the right; otherwise unilateral deposit-related complications can result (left lens syndrome).

  e. Weekly 2-hour cycle enzymatic cleaning may be desirable, especially with borderline dry eye and extended-wear patients.

4. Care regimen

  a. Every product in the care kit provided to a new RGP wearer should be explained to the patient.

  b. If any alternative solutions are acceptable, this information should also be included.

  c. To enhance compliance, patients should be asked to name their solutions at progress evaluation visits.

  d. Patients should be advised to soak their lenses in the disinfecting solution at night for the following reasons:

    (1) Disinfection.

    (2) Enhanced surface wettability.

(3)   Maintenance of hydrated state.

(4)   Minimizing the effects of lens damage resulting from dry, dirty case.

e.   Patients should be warned not to use tap water or saliva for wetting or rewetting RGP lenses; tap water also cannot be used for disinfection. Although rare, the sight-threatening *Acanthamoeba* keratitis has been associated with improper tap water use with RGPs. If used at all, tap water should only be used to rinse off the cleaner prior to disinfection at night.

f.   Patients should also be warned not to "top off" their disinfection (i.e., instead of totally replacing the disinfection solution each night, a few drops of new solution are added to the old; therefore, contamination is likely).

g.   The lens case is also very important and should be deep-welled to hold sufficient solution, have a ribbed or holed well to minimize suction, and easily differentiate right from left lens. The case also represents a location for microorganisms that can be difficult to kill, as they may encapsulate themselves in a glycocalyx biofilm. This can be minimized by:

(1)   Washing the case every morning with a toothbrush and warm water, rinsing the water off with saline, and then allowing it to air dry.

(2)   Replacing the case on a regular basis (every 3–6 months).

5.   Scratches

a.   Every patient should be warned about the surface softness of RGP lenses.

b.   Lenses should be handled over a towel or soft tissue.

6.   Foreign-body particles

a.   Instruct patient that foreign particles can be irritating to the eye.

b.   If the particle is present only momentarily, the lens can be removed and rewetted; if persistent, the practitioner should be notified.

7.   Cosmetics

a.   Cosmetics can be the cause of lens surface deposition.

b.   Cosmetics should be applied after lens insertion.

c.   Cosmetics recommended for contact lens wearers are usually acceptable, especially if they are water soluble and contain very few fragrances or fillers.

d.   Mascara with "lash builders" can flake and cause injury to the cornea.

e.   Eyeliner should only be applied to the outer lid margin to eliminate contact with the meibomian glands.

f.   Any cream or oil that is used on the face or hands can be transferred to the lenses, resulting in discomfort and blurred vision. Lanolin-containing skin creams or soaps are particularly liable to result in poor surface wettability. The use of bar soaps or optical-compatible hand soaps is recommended.

8.   Adaptation

a.   Patients should be told about individual variation in adapting to lenses, although how they reacted to the initial lens sensation should provide a hint as to the length of the adaptation period.

b.   Often this period is 10–14 days.

c.   Patients should be reassured that comfort will gradually improve.

d.   Normal symptoms such as lens awareness (especially when viewing superiorly), mild redness, and slight photophobia should be explained; in addition, abnormal symptoms such as pain and persistent tearing should also be mentioned; pain and discomfort should never be described as normal symptoms.

e.   A typical wearing schedule would be the following:

Days 1 and 2: 4 hours

Days 3 and 4: 6 hours

Days 5 and 6: 8 hours

Days 7 and 8: 10 hours

Days 9 and 10: 12 hours

f.   Progress visits can be scheduled at 1 week, 1 month, 3 months, and 6 months after dispensing. Regular 6-month evaluations should then be recommended.

Table 9-7.   Checklist for RGP Patient Instruction Manual

1. Composition, benefits, and applications of an RGP lens
2. Insertion, removal, and decentration
3. Cleaning techniques
4. Normal and abnormal adaptation symptoms
5. Importance of adhering to prescribed wearing schedule
6. Causes of reduced wear (*e.g.*, colds, hay fever, medications)
7. Importance of using the recommended care regimen (not saliva or nonrecommended brands); alternative acceptable solutions
8. How to minimize loss and surface damage
9. Benefits of a spare pair of lenses or spectacles
10. Swimming and showering
11. Cosmetic use
12. Caring for lens case
13. Visit schedule
14. Fee and refund policy
15. Service agreement and insurance
16. Office telephone number
17. Doctor's home telephone number

9. Educational methods
    A four-step process is recommended for successful patient education: (1) written, (2) oral, (3) video, and (4) reinforcement.
    a. Written
        (1) A comprehensive instruction manual providing the information given in Table 9-7 should be presented to the patient.
        (2) It should be written in layman's language and be easy to read.
        (3) It can also have a patient agreement form which provides such information as refund policy and care regimen (Figure 9-9). This should be signed in duplicate by the patient for medicolegal considerations.
        (4) The assistant can discuss the most important information with the patient and encourage questions.
        (5) The manual should preferably be printed professionally or by a desktop publishing system; Anadem Publications, Inc. (P.O. Box 14385, Columbus, OH 43214) has such a manual complete with graphics and available on diskette if the practitioner desires to continually update the material.
    b. Oral. This is more important than the written as the patient will respond well to comprehensive oral instructions reinforcing proper care and handling.
    c. Video
        (1) An excellent method of reinforcing oral and written instructions is video.
        (2) A generic rigid lens patient education video is available from the CLMA/RGP Lens Institute Video Library.
    e. Reinforcement
        (1) Important care instructions should be reviewed with the patient at *every* follow-up visit.
        (2) The following questions should be asked:
            (a) What solutions are being used (i.e., are they the same as dispensed?)
            (b) How often are the lenses being cleaned?
            (c) What method is being used for cleaning?
            (d) What is the current condition of the lens case (encourage the patient to bring case with them)?
            (e) Does the patient have any questions?
        (3) Always carefully document in the patient's record any evidence of noncompliance with recommended care instructions.

STATEMENT BY PATIENT   **(File Copy)**

This is to certify that on _____, 19__ I received instructions in the proper methods of insertion, removal, use and care of my contact lenses. Having proved myself to be competent enough to carry out the above instructions, the contact lenses were given to me. I realize that success with contact lenses cannot be guaranteed and that any refund will be subject to the policy outlined below.

_____   _____
Patient's Signature   Student Clinician's Signature

                    _____
                    Instructor's Signature

The solutions prescribed with these _____ contact lenses are:

wetting and rinsing _____

soaking/disinfectant _____

cleaning _____

enzyme cleaner _____

storage case _____

other _____

IN CASE OF EMERGENCY:

Phone: 1. University of Missouri-St. Louis, Optometry Clinic, 553-5131
               during school hours.
            2. Student Clinician evenings or weekends (in the case that you
               require assistance and cannot reach anyone at the clinic)

                              _____

                              _____

REFUND POLICY:

Patient discontinued within 60 days from dispensing......$100.00 of contact lens **fees** paid is refunded

        After 60 days.. no refund applies

REPLACEMENT POLICY:

        Class A...single $ 50   pair $ 85
        Class B...single $ 65   pair $ 115
        Class C...single $ 80   pair $ 135
        Class D...single $100   pair $ 175

Your contact lens is Class A B C D and no refund applies after _____

Follow-up Visits are suggested every 6 months after the initial 120 day period.
The Standard fee for a follow-up visit is $16.00. A comprehensive eye examination should be performed every two years.

FEE AND COSTS ARE SUBJECT TO PERIODIC REVISIONS

Figure 9-9.   An example of a patient agreement form.

(4)   This may be the most important step of the four-step education process. It has been found that patients who are not provided with reinforcement of their care instructions are at 8 to 10 times greater risk for contamination of their care regimen.[18]

V.   RGP Problem Solving

The purpose of this section is to provide diagnostic and management information for three common problems/challenges: (1) reduced vision, (2) corneal desiccation, and (3) refitting.

A.   *Reduced vision*
A reduction in vision as compared to the best spectacle-corrected visual acuity is

Cause   Vision Loss Via   Diagnosis

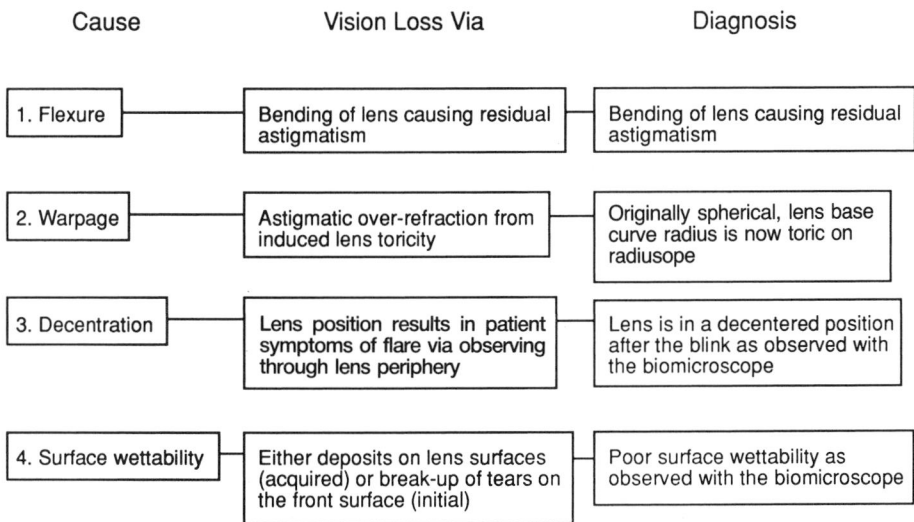

| 1. Flexure | Bending of lens causing residual astigmatism | Bending of lens causing residual astigmatism |

| 2. Warpage | Astigmatic over-refraction from induced lens toricity | Originally spherical, lens base curve radius is now toric on radiusope |

| 3. Decentration | Lens position results in patient symptoms of flare via observing through lens periphery | Lens is in a decentered position after the blink as observed with the biomicroscope |

| 4. Surface wettability | Either deposits on lens surfaces (acquired) or break-up of tears on the front surface (initial) | Poor surface wettability as observed with the biomicroscope |

Figure 9-10. A nomogram showing causes of reduced vision with an RGP lens wearer.

typically the result of (1) flexure, (2) warpage, (3) decentration, or (4) poor surface wettability (Figure 9-10).

1. Flexure
    a. Description
        (1) Results from surface forces during the blink process that induce a certain amount of toricity within the lens.
        (2) Causes include a steep fitting relationship, reduced center thickness, large optical zone diameter, and material flexibility.
        (3) Diagnosed by performing keratometry over the patient's lenses, preferably during diagnostic fitting; the values obtained should be spherical; the presence of any toricity in this measurement is typically the result of flexure. If toricity is present, patients will typically report asthenopic complaints indicative of inadequate astigmatic correction.
    b. Management
        (1) The most important change, unless it compromises the fitting relationship, would be to flatten the BCR by, at minimum, 0.50D if a steep fitting relationship exists.
        (2) Increasing the center thickness by 0.02 mm per diopter of corneal astigmatism is beneficial; however, this change should only be considered if option one is not possible, as the increased lens mass may compromise the fitting relationship.
        (3) Other secondary, but effective, management options include reducing the optical zone diameter of the lens by, at minimum, 0.03 mm or changing materials (typically from a higher to a lower Dk).
2. Warpage
    a. Description
        (1) Differs from flexure in that toricity is permanent; toricity is present when the BCR is verified with a radiuscope and it is acquired over time, whereas flexure is present immediately upon diagnostic fitting.
        (2) Primary cause is the application of excessive digital pressure during the cleaning process; it is caused by cleaning between the fingers, not in the palm of the hand, especially in former PMMA wearers who are not accustomed to warping their more rigid former material.

    b. Management

        (1) Routinely verify the BCR at all patient progress evaluation visits; therefore, if a small increase in toricity is detected, the patient can be properly educated before further change.

        (2) Educate all patients, *especially* former PMMA wearers, to clean the lenses carefully in the palm of the hand.

        (3) If warpage persists, changing to a lower Dk material and, possibly to a "hands-off" system (e.g., Hydramat, PBH) is recommended.

3. Decentration

    a. Induced problems

        (1) Corneal desiccation.

        (2) Corneal warpage.

        (3) Poor corneal alignment.

        (4) Reduced vision.

    b. Causes

        (1) Decentered corneal apex.

        (2) An unusual corneal topography.

        (3) Lid characteristics.

        (4) A less than optimum lens design.

        (5) The specific lens material.

    c. Evaluation

        (1) If keratometry is the only option for corneal curvature evaluation, lens design and, particularly, fluorescein pattern evaluation, become very important.

        (2) Inferior, superior, and lateral decentration will be discussed.

            (a) Inferior decentration

                i. An "On K" to "Flatter than K" fitting relationship appears to be preferable to steep fitting designs, especially in minus powers, unless a superior positioned upper lid is present.

                ii. Center thickness should be kept at a minimum; it has been found that increasing center thickness typically has only a slight effect on oxygen transmission but can have a large effect on lens mass and, therefore, centration characteristics.[19]

                iii. The effect of using a minus lenticular edge design to "lift up" a plus or low-minus power lens is beneficial, as is the use of the "lid attachment" lens design with an anterior positioned edge (e.g., Fluorocon 9.5-mm diameter lens from PBH).

                iv. If the aforementioned options are unsuccessful, consideration can be given to changing to a lower-specific-gravity material.

            (b) Superior decentration. The opposite type of changes is indicated, including the use of a thinner edge design and a steeper base curve radius. In addition, a larger overall diameter design may be beneficial.

            (c) Lateral decentration

                i. Often results from a decentered corneal apex, a flat lens, or an against-the-rule astigmatic patient. In the latter case, the lens tends to move more in a lateral motion tending to follow the steeper corneal meridian.

                ii. Some options have enjoyed limited success, including selecting a larger overall diameter or a steeper BCR. However, a viable alternative is to fit an aspheric lens design; in particular, a progressive or bi-aspheric lens design. Management of rigid lens decentration is provided in Figure 9-11.

RGP LENS DECENTRATION

POSITION	CAUSES	MANAGEMENT
INFERIOR	1. High center thickness (CT) 2. Too thin or thick edges 3. High specific gravity material 4. Corneal topography 5. Loose lid tension	1. Verify CT; use manufacturer thickness guide 2. + lenticular for > -5.00D - lenticular for < -1.50D/all plus powers 3. Lid attachment design 4. Lower specific gravity 5. Flatter BCR
SUPERIOR	1. Thick edge 2. Flat BCR 3. Thin CT 4. Corneal topography 5. Tight lid tension	1. Steeper BCR 2. Thicker CT 3. Thinner edge design
LATERAL	1. ATR Astigmatism 2. Decentered corneal apex	1. Aspheric lens design 2. Larger OAD 3. Steeper BCR

Figure 9-11.   Management of RGP lens decentration.

4. Poor surface wettability

Poor wettability can be divided into (1) initial and (2) acquired.[20]

a. Poor initial wettability

(1) Causes. Poor initial wettability is almost always a manufacturing problem and could result from

(a) Too much heat build-up during the manufacturing process.

(b) Poor polishing techniques.

(c) Improper or old diamond used for cutting.

(d) Residual pitch polish left on the lens surface.

(2) Diagnosis. This problem is typically diagnosed from the appearance, not of a film, but of a breakup of the tear film on the lens during biomicroscopic evaluation.

(3) Management

(a) This problem can often be prevented by presoaking the lenses for a minimum of 24 hours prior to dispensing in the recommended soaking solution.

(b) If compromised wettability still persists, the lens can be conditioned by rubbing wetting solution onto the surface using the same technique as when cleaning the lens.

(c) If the wettability is still not optimum, a compatible laboratory cleaner (e.g., The Boston Laboratory Cleaner, Polymer Technology Corporation) or solvent (e.g., FluoroSolve, Paragon Optical, Inc.) can be used.

(d) As a final procedure, light surface polishing of the lens can be performed, although this is rarely necessary.

b. Acquired poor surface wettability

The more commonly experienced problem is acquired mucoprotein film or haze on the anterior lens surface. Typically this occurs over a time period of several weeks to several months. The thick filmlike appearance is easily diagnosed by biomicroscopy.

    (1)   There are several causes, including poor tear quality, improper blinking, inadequate compliance, use of improper solutions, foreign contaminants, and surface scratches.

    (2)   Patients having a borderline tear quality should be placed on an aggressive care regimen including daily use of either an abrasive cleaner or a surfactant cleaner, supplemented both by weekly enzymatic cleaning and by rewetting drops several times each day. Patients should be educated about the importance of cleaning the lenses thoroughly *immediately* after lens removal, followed by placement in the appropriate soaking solution. Patients should also be advised to wash their hands thoroughly with a non-lanolin-containing hand soap prior to handling their lenses, as hand creams and other substances on the hand can adhere to the lens surface and compromise wettability.

    (3)   To clean a heavily deposited lens in the office, the aforementioned laboratory cleaners or solvents should be used. In addition, if scratches or deposits are present on the surface of the lens, a light polish should be beneficial.

    (4)   Finally, if all else fails, changing from an S/A to an F-S/A material or from a high-Dk to a lower- (25–50) Dk F-S/A material should improve deposit resistance.

B. *Corneal desiccation*
    1. Description
       a. Corneal desiccation or "3 and 9 o'clock" staining refers to the drying or dehydration of the peripheral cornea.
       b. This is a very common lens-induced complication, occurring in over 50% of patients wearing rigid contact lenses.[21]
       c. Initially, and in most cases, the desiccation consists of isolated punctate stains. However, in certain cases the staining can coalesce with engorgement of the adjacent conjunctival blood vessels. In most severe cases, peripheral corneal thinning occurs with ulceration, neovascularization, and scarring (Figure 9-12). If symptoms are present, they are typically dryness and redness.

    2. Management
       Factors to consider in the management of corneal desiccation include the lens material, lens centration, edge lift, and tear film stability.
       a. Lens material. A low-Dk F-S/A material may be optimum for reducing desiccation; if severe desiccation persists, a hydrogel material may be necessary.
       b. Lens centration. A superior positioning lens tucked underneath the upper lid is important in minimizing the incidence of moderate to severe cases of corneal desiccation. This position allows the lid and lens edge interaction to be at a minimum; therefore, interference with the normal blinking pattern is reduced. To minimize this problem, the same design principles mentioned in the decentration section (V, A, 3) of this chapter apply.
       c. Edge lift.
          (1)   Edge lift is a controversial parameter. It is important to avoid excessive edge lift designs to reduce the peripheral tear volume, to decrease the gap between the lid and the cornea, and to minimize the potentially compromising effect on the blink caused by the interaction between the upper lid and the lens edge.
          (2)   A tricurve or tetracurve design with a peripheral curve width no greater than 0.3 mm and a peripheral curve radius no flatter than 11.0 mm is recommended.
          (3)   An aspheric design may be advantageous because of better alignment of the posterior surface with the cornea.

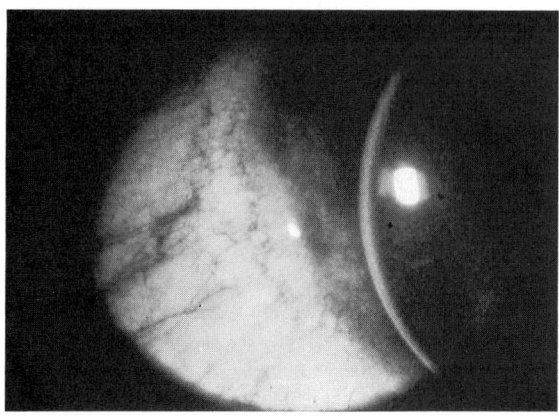

Figure 9-12. Corneal desiccation resulting in peripheral neovascularization and scarring.

    (4)   If the edge lift is too low, however, peripheral sealoff can result, possibly causing both staining and vascularization.

  d. Tear film stability. As the interblink interval is typically 4–6 seconds, patients should have a minimum tear BUT of 5 seconds to be fitted with contact lenses. Patients with low to borderline tear quality fit with rigid lenses typically will have subjective symptoms of dryness accompanied by corneal desiccation due to evaporation of the tear film over the peripheral cornea. The use of rewetting drops, as much as every hour, will help somewhat in increasing the number of hours of daily lens wear.

C. *Refitting into RGPs*

There are numerous cases in which patients can benefit by refitting from another lens material into RGPs. This includes PMMA and hydrogel lens wearers.

1. PMMA into RGP

  a. Why refit PMMA wearers? Even in the absence of symptoms, the PMMA wearer should be refit into an oxygen-permeable lens material. The cornea needs an oxygen level of approximately 10% (equivalent to an oxygen transmission value of 24 Dk/L) to avoid corneal swelling in the daily wear situation.[9] Therefore, with a comprehensive evaluation, it is very likely that any one or a combination of the following hypoxia-related complications will be present with PMMA lens wear:

    (1)   Central corneal clouding (CCC). A circumscribed region of epithelial edema that appears as a grayish haze against the dark background of the pupil when sclerotic scatter/split limbal illumination with biomicroscopy is used. Although the patient ordinarily experiences acceptable visual acuity with contact lens wear, vision is usually unsatisfactory through spectacles.

    (2)   Edematous corneal formations (ECFs). These are subepithelial arborized or dendritic-appearing formations located in the central cornea.

    (3)   Polymegethism. Alteration or variation in endothelial swelling which is best observed during biomicroscopy with a parallelepiped using high magnification and illumination.

    (4)   Corneal warpage syndrome. Prolonged corneal edema can result in corneal distortion with unpredictable keratometry and refractive changes in as many as 30% of long-term PMMA wearers.[22]

  b. Patient consultation

    (1)   Discuss benefits of RGP lenses, including oxygen permeability, ability to see through spectacles, and ocular health; in addition, mention the possibility of dryness and initial sensation of RGPs.

        (2) Audiovisuals including photographs or video presentations presenting PMMA-induced problems are beneficial.

        (3) Be cautious in refitting PMMA wearers into soft, as they are accustomed to the vision and durability provided by a rigid lens; if the patient is very motivated, be sure to gradually wean him or her off the PMMA and obtain refractive stabilization. It is possible the patient will become more astigmatic during this process.

    c. Refitting strategy

        (1) It is important to perform a comprehensive evaluation of the patient while the patient is *still wearing his or her lenses,* preferably for several hours. This will allow observation of the amount and types of corneal edema and the level of difficulty in determining the refractive and keratometric values.

        (2) The most effective strategy is to immediately refit the patient into RGP lenses *without loss of wearing time.* This has the benefits of limiting excessive refractive change and enhancing patient satisfaction. If there is minimal or no corneal compromise, the patient can be refit with no change in wearing time. If severe distortion is present, the patient should reduce wearing time to the minimum number of hours possible. The patient should be advised to return for a visit in 1 week, at which time much improvement in mire quality, postrefraction visual acuity, and corneal integrity is usually present and the patient can be refit. The patient should never be told to remove the lenses "cold turkey" for any length of time prior to refitting due to the possibility of large and unpredictable refractive changes.

    d. Lens material and design

        (1) Low- to medium-Dk (i.e., 25–50) lens materials are recommended, as they provide greater rigidity, which results in both less corneal sensitivity and less refractive change during the stabilization period when compared to higher-Dk materials. In addition, former PMMA wearers appear to experience warpage-related problems with high-Dk RGP lenses. If clinical signs of hypoxia continue with RGP lens wear, the patient can later be refit into a higher-Dk material.

        (2) Next determine whether to fit the patient based on the refractive findings or to simply duplicate the PMMA lens measurements (assuming a good lens-to-cornea fitting relationship exists) in an RGP lens material. The latter method has been proven to be quite successful; however, there is merit in using the refractive findings obtained immediately after PMMA lens removal as the baseline values for diagnostic fitting purposes if the clinical signs of corneal warpage syndrome are absent or minimal. It is important to consider the decreased surface wettability and greater flexibility compared to PMMA when fitting and designing RGP lenses. It is not uncommon to select a flatter BCR, larger diameter, steeper peripheral curve (decreasing edge clearance), and increased center thickness lens design as compared to PMMA in an effort to optimize performance.

    e. Prescribing spectacles. On the average, noncorneal warpage syndrome patients will need about 3 weeks for refractive stabilization to occur before spectacles can be prescribed. Corneal warpage syndrome patients should be told it may take as long as several months.

2. Hydrogel into RGPs

    a. Why refit into RGPs?

        (1) Giant papillary conjunctivitis associated with hydrogel lens wear.

        (2) Reduced vision from uncorrected refractive astigmatism, surface deposits, and/or a poorly fitting soft toric lens.

        (3) Other reasons include persistent edema, infiltrative keratitis, neovascularization, and difficulty in handling the larger-diameter lenses.

b. Patient consultation
   (1) As with PMMA wearers, hydrogel lens wearers need to be educated regarding the benefits of RGPs.
   (2) If the hydrogel lens wearer is *not* experiencing any symptoms or clinical signs but is simply inquiring about RGPs (e.g., a friend may be wearing them successfully or perhaps he or she is simply interested in what's new), realistic expectations about the initial lens sensation and adaptation period need to be provided. In most cases these patients should not be refit unless motivation is *extremely* high.

c. Refitting procedure
   Unless severe corneal compromise or lid inflammation is present necessitating hydrogel lens removal, these patients can be refit and gradually increase RGP lens wear while simultaneously decreasing hydrogel lens wear. The refitting is similar to that for a new patient, with the exception that even more encouragement than usual is necessary during the adaptation ("awareness") phase.

VI. Fitting and Evaluation of Hydrogel Lenses

Hydrogel lenses, also referred to as soft or hydrophilic lenses, are appealing to many patients as a result of both the immediate comfort provided by these materials and the availability of specialty lenses (e.g., cosmetic tinted lenses, disposable lenses); however, hydrogel lenses are not a viable option for all patients. A comprehensive preliminary evaluation will provide the practitioner with information that will be the key to selecting the type of contact lens suitable for each particular patient.

A. *Material selection*
   1. Water content. Most hydrogel lenses have water contents between 38% and 79%. They can be divided into low (up to 50%), medium (50%–60%), and high (greater than 60%) water contents. Typically, low-water-content lenses are worn on a daily wear basis, and medium- to high-water-content lenses are worn on a flexible- or extended-wear basis. Very thin, low-water-content lenses may also be worn on a flexible- or extended-wear basis.
   2. Manufacturing methods. Hydrogel lenses can be spin cast, lathe cut, cast-molded, or a combination of these procedures.
   3. Lens classifications. The major categories of hydrogel lenses are: (1) daily wear, (2) flexible/extended wear, (3) planned replacement/disposable, (4) tints (visibility, enhancing, and opaque), (5) torics, and (6) bifocals.
   4. Refractive error. Spherical hydrogel lenses are most commonly available in powers of approximately −10.00 to +4.00D. Most toric hydrogel lenses are available in cylinder powers of −0.75 to −2.00D. For those patients with a greater refractive error, there are lens materials available in specialty powers, such as high-plus, aphakic, high-minus, and high-astigmatic powers. Typically, spherical refractive errors and low astigmats will be the best candidates for hydrogel lens wear. These patients will be able to achieve acceptable visual acuity with a spherical or toric hydrogel lens.
   5. Deposit-prone patients. Patients who experience frequent depositing on lenses, even when using a rigorous care routine, would be best fit in a glycerol methacrylate material (e.g., CSI, PBH) or a program such as planned replacement or disposable lenses.
   6. Marginal dry eye. Low- to medium-water-content lenses and thicker lenses (0.10–0.14 mm) are preferable, as these lenses dehydrate less rapidly than thin or high-water-content lenses. Lens lubricants/rewetting drops may also benefit these patients.

B. *Patient evaluation*
   1. Ocular/systemic conditions. Factors that contraindicate contact lens wear of any type are inflammation or disease of the anterior segment and any systemic disease

that can be complicated by contact lens wear and pregnancy. Factors contraindicating hydrogel lens wear include irregular corneas (e.g., keratoconus, ocular trauma), radial keratotomy, chronic allergies, chronic antihistamine use, and giant papillary conjunctivitis.

2. Occupation/hobbies. Occupations with tasks that include exposure to fine particles of dust or mist are not suitable for contact lens wear unless the recommended protective eyewear, such as safety goggles, is worn. Many people with particular occupations or hobbies may be benefitted by contact lens wear, for example, athletes, actors, models, and politicians. Contact lenses are beneficial because they both improve cosmesis and eliminate the need for constantly wearing spectacles which may decrease the field of view, fog up with precipitation changes, slide down, or break. Hydrogel lenses are preferable for athletics as they are more difficult to dislodge than RGP lenses. Occasionally, patients desire lenses to wear just for hobbies, such as tennis or basketball, or just for social occasions to improve their appearance. These part-time wearers would best be fit with hydrogel lenses, as adaptation to lens wear takes little time. Caution should be taken by these patients in storing lenses for long periods of time. Lenses should be disinfected weekly and prior to wear, and the storage solution should be frequently changed to prevent contamination and dehydration. Likewise, caution should be taken not to overwear the lenses when they have not been worn for a long period of time.

3. Age. Children fit with a hydrogel lens may experience difficulty inserting the large-diameter lens. A few lenses are available in smaller diameters (e.g., 12 mm), which will aid in lens insertion. A visibility tint or a cosmetic tint is beneficial to presbyopic patients when handling, inserting, and removing the lens. There are no age limitations as to when contact lenses may be appropriate for children and teenagers. The child's motivation and sense of responsibility are the best indicators as to when contact lenses might be suitable.

4. Patient hygiene and compliance. Poor patient hygiene and noncompliance are contraindicators for hydrogel contact lens wear. Hydrogel lenses are more prone to deposits, and hydrogel lens-wearing patients are more susceptible to infections than RGP patients due to the characteristics of the lens. Extra care is required to keep the lenses clean and disinfected.

C. *Lens selection and evaluation: new patient*

Lenses are available in varying powers, BCRs, diameters, thicknesses, water contents, and tints. To select the lens for the patient, first determine the categories in which the patient is most interested: daily wear lenses, extended-wear lenses, planned replacement, disposable lenses, tinted lenses to enhance or change the eye color, bifocal lenses, toric lenses, or a combination of these. Although lenses may be fit empirically, the ability to fit diagnostic lenses is beneficial to both the patient and the practitioner. If a large enough inventory of hydrogel lenses is available, the patient can be dispensed lenses the same day.

1. Base curve radius. Hydrogel contact lenses will typically be available in two to four BCRs or sagittal depths. A good guideline for initial BCR selection is to select the middle BCR provided (or the flatter BCR or sag value if only two BCRs are provided) for average keratometry readings (41.00–45.00D). Likewise, if the keratometry readings are steeper than 45.00D, the patient can be initially fit with the steeper BCR or greater sag value. If the keratometry readings are flatter than 41.00D, a flatter BCR or smaller sag value can be selected. If the initial lens is too tight, a flatter BCR should be attempted; if the lens is too loose, a steeper BCR can be fit. In an acceptable fit, the hydrogel lens will center well over the cornea and exhibit approximately 0.5–1 mm movement. A tight lens will exhibit less than 0.5 mm movement, often producing conjunctival drag. A flat lens will move more than $1\frac{1}{2}$–2 mm, often moving partially off the cornea. Lens decentration and edge

lift may also be present. A method called the "push-up test" may be used to judge if the lens is truly tight or just exhibiting minimal movement. This test is performed by gently pushing on the inferior edge of the lens with the lower lid; a tight lens resists movement, whereas an acceptable lens will move when nudged with the lower lid.

2. Lens diameter. The overall diameter of the hydrogel contact lens is selected to obtain 360° corneal coverage. The appropriate diameter needed can be obtained by measuring the horizontal visible iris diameter (the diameter across the iris from limbus to limbus) and adding 2 mm. Ideally the lens will extend onto the sclera, at minimum, 0.5 mm in all directions. Lenses are customarily available in diameters of 13.8–15.0 mm; however, there are a few manufacturers who produce smaller or larger diameters. If the lens decenters, a larger than predicted overall diameter may be needed to provide adequate coverage.

3. Power. The power of the lens is based on the predicted power and a refraction over the diagnostic lens. The predicted power of the lens is determined by the patient's spectacle prescription which is vertexed back to the corneal plane if the prescription is greater than ±4.00D. If the patient has a spherocylindrical prescription with a low amount of astigmatism, it may be necessary to use the spherical equivalent to predict the patient's contact lens prescription. The final prescription should be equal to that achieved by the best sphere overrefraction plus diagnostic lens power or a close compromise between the predicted power and the overrefraction plus diagnostic lens power.

4. Center thickness. Typically, a center thickness of a −3.00D lens will be approximately 0.08 mm. The greater the minus power, the thinner the lens; likewise, the more plus power, the thicker the lens. A thicker lens (e.g., 0.12 mm) is easier for the patient to handle, and thinner lenses (e.g., 0.035 mm) with low water content are used for extended or flexible wear; however, many manufacturers currently provide their standard daily wear lenses in 0.05- to 0.07-mm thicknesses for low-minus powers. These are durable enough for the average patient, and the thicker lenses (e.g., 0.12 mm) may be reserved for those patients with handling and durability problems.

5. Evaluating lens fit. After the hydrogel diagnostic lens is selected, the lens should be inserted and allowed to settle 10–15 minutes. Visual acuity, overrefraction, lens movement, centration, and coverage should all be evaluated to determine the lens fit.

6. Lens parameters to specify on order. BCR or sag value, overall lens diameter, power, name of lens, manufacturer name, tint, and possibly center thickness.

D. *The contact lens examination: existing wearer*
1. Hydrogel lens evaluation
   a. Case history. The patient should be questioned about symptoms, complaints, wearing schedule, solutions used, and lens care.
   b. Wearing time. The hydrogel lens should be comfortable and be able to be worn 12–16 hours daily or up to 7 days for extended wear, if not worn for sports or social occasions only.
   c. Procedures to perform at examinations. A routine follow-up examination should include visual acuity, overrefraction, biomicroscopy with and without lenses, keratometry with and without lenses, and subjective refraction without lenses.
   d. Visual acuity. Should be 20/25 or better in most cases with lens correction.
   e. Lens fit. The hydrogel lens will exhibit good centration, complete corneal coverage extending, at minimum, 0.5 mm onto the sclera, and move 0.5–1 mm on the blink. In addition, examine the lens condition for defects and/or deposits.
   f. Frequency of exams. After dispensing the lenses, evaluations should be per-

formed on a routine basis to ensure that complications do not occur. Follow-up visits for daily wear can be scheduled at 1 week, 1 month, and 3 months after dispensing and every 6 months thereafter. Follow-up visits for extended wear can be scheduled at 1 week of daily wear and 24 hours, 3 days, 1 week, 2 weeks, 1 month, 3 months, and 6 months after first wearing the lenses for extended wear and every 3 months thereafter.

2. Ocular examination after lens removal
   a. Cornea and conjunctiva. These structures should be inspected for changes resulting from edema (e.g., striae, microcysts, polymegethism), neovascularization, limbal engorgement, and injection.
   b. Fluorescein evaluation. It is important to evaluate the lids and the cornea with fluorescein at every visit to monitor any subtle changes that may occur with long-term hydrogel lens wear. Care must be taken to rinse the fluorescein from the eye with saline or have the patient wear spectacles for 2–4 hours afterwards to prevent staining of the lens.
   c. Lid eversion. The upper and lower lids should be everted to monitor signs of giant papillary conjunctivitis.

VII. Hydrogel Contact Lens Care and Patient Management

A. *Patient compliance*
   1. Factors affecting compliance
      a. Care system. Systems are perceived by the patient as too costly, complex, or time consuming.
      b. Patient factors. Sloppy habits, laziness, confusion, taking shortcuts, mixing and matching solutions, deleting steps (e.g., daily cleaning, disinfection).
      c. Patients should be cautioned to consult with their practitioner prior to changing any solution in their regimen. At each progress visit, have patients explain their care routine to the practitioner or the staff member to ensure that the care regimen is still appropriate.
      d. Good intensive patient education, reinforcing the education at each visit, and frequent evaluations to monitor lens wear will aid in maintaining patient compliance.

B. *Patient education*
   1. Educational materials
      a. Written information in the form of a patient handbook that discusses insertion and removal, care and handling, solutions, wearing schedule, emergency phone numbers, and consequences of noncompliance.
      b. Videotapes that discuss insertion and removal, lens care, and handling.
      c. Posters or photo albums of complications that may result from noncompliance to emphasize care.
   2. Educational environment
      a. Patient education should be treated as important, to impart the seriousness of good lens care to the patient.
      b. Adjustable mirrors, large counter space, adequate lighting, a sink that closes, and fresh cases and solutions should be provided for the patient to practice insertion, removal, and lens care.
      c. The person who is educating the patient should be knowledgeable about lens care and handling.
   3. Hydrogel lens insertion
      a. Place the lens on the index finger. The index finger should be dry, as the lens will stick to the finger instead of the eye if the finger is too wet.
      b. While holding the lids apart with the third finger of each hand, the lens may be placed on the sclera as the patient looks up or directly on the cornea as the patient looks straight ahead into a mirror.

    c. It is recommended that patients become accustomed to a routine of always inserting and removing the same lens first; for example, the patient always inserts the right lens first and removes the right lens first.

4. Determining hydrogel lens inversion

    a. Determining hydrogel lens inversion may be accomplished by one of the following methods:

        (1) Method 1. The lens is placed upright on the index finger and viewed from the side. A lens which is right-side out will appear bowl-shaped, whereas one which is inverted will appear more like a saucer with the edges flared out.

        (2) Method 2. The "taco test" is another method of determining if a lens is inverted. In the "taco test," the lens edges are pushed together. If the edges curl toward each other, like a taco, the lens is correct. On the other hand, if the edges curl out, the lens is inverted.

    b. An inverted lens may result in slightly reduced vision, excessive lens movement, and/or flaring out of the edges from the sclera. If the patient observes any of these symptoms, he or she may suspect an inverted lens and try inserting the lens the other direction to determine if this corrects the symptoms.

5. Hydrogel lens removal

    a. The lids are held apart with the third finger of each hand.

    b. Place the index finger directly on the cornea and slide the lens onto the sclera as the patient looks up.

    c. The lens is gently pinched off the sclera with the fingerpads of the thumb and index finger. Caution should be taken that the lens is not pinched directly off the cornea, as this may result in a corneal abrasion. The fingernails should not be used to pinch the lens off, as this may result in fingernail tears in the lens.

6. Hygiene

    a. Hands should be washed prior to handling lenses to remove bacteria, lotions, oils, cosmetics, etc.

    b. The lens case should be rinsed with saline and air dried between uses. Cases should be replaced every 3 months.

    c. Solution bottles should be clean, capped, and unexpired. The tip of the solution bottle should not come in contact with the lens or hand. Fresh solution should be used daily.

B. *Lens care*

1. Disinfection

    a. Thermal disinfection requires storing the hydrogel lenses in a thermal unit which exposes lenses to temperatures of approximately 80°C for approximately 20 minutes to disinfect the lenses. It is an effective method of disinfection; however, tear film components may become baked onto the lens, producing deposit-related complications. Lenses with more than 55% water should not be disinfected with heat.

    b. Chemical disinfection uses chemical preservatives. This is a popular type of disinfection because of the relatively few steps required. Some chemical preservatives may cause sensitivity reactions in patients (e.g., thimerosal); however, the newest preservatives (e.g., Polyquad and Dymed) appear to be less toxic. Chemical disinfection may be used on all types of lenses and has little effect on lens life. It takes a minimum of 4–6 hours for a chemical disinfecting cycle.

    c. Oxidative disinfection with 3% hydrogen peroxide solution is also used to disinfect lenses. Depending on the product, it will require one or two steps to perform disinfection and neutralization/dilution of the hydrogen peroxide. This is a safe, effective, and preservative-free method of disinfection. It may be a more confusing method of disinfection for some patients. If the patient fails to neutralize the hydrogen peroxide prior to lens insertion, the acidic hydrogen peroxide will produce a mild to moderate punctate keratitis. The patient will experience stinging, moderate to severe discomfort, and injection. Oxidative disinfection can be performed in as little as 20 minutes to as long as 12 hours.

2. Saline. Saline solution is necessary to keep the hydrogel lens in a hydrated state. Saline is not toxic to the eye and is a sterile solution used to rinse lenses free of foreign matter, in addition to its use in dissolving enzyme tablets. Distilled water should not be used, as it is not necessarily sterile or pure. Saline is not capable of disinfecting hydrogel lenses and should not be used as a substitute for disinfecting solution. Saline is available in preserved and unpreserved solutions. Unpreserved saline is available in aerosol containers, unit vials, and salt tablet formulated saline. *Salt tablet formulated saline should never be used.* There is no benefit to homemade saline and there are many risks, primarily the risk of *Acanthamoeba* keratitis. Patients should not be allowed to continue the use of homemade saline and careful documentation is required if the patient refuses to follow your advice.

3. Surfactant cleaners

   a. Surfactant cleaners should be used after lens removal each day to prevent deposits on the lens surface. Deposits will be removed more easily initially upon lens removal rather than waiting until after disinfection. The lens should be placed in the palm of the hand with a few drops of cleaner and rubbed gently back and forth for 20–30 seconds.

   b. The lens should be thoroughly rinsed after cleaning and prior to lens disinfection. Disinfection is greatly enhanced when the lens is cleaned and rinsed.

   c. Surfactant cleaners are available as nonabrasive and abrasive cleaners. Patients prone to deposits benefit from the use of abrasive cleaners such as Opticlean, Opticlean II, and Opti-Free daily cleaner (Alcon Laboratories). MiraFlow (Ciba Vision) is an excellent cleaner for patients with a tendency toward lipid deposits, as the ingredient isopropyl alcohol dissolves lipids.

4. Enzymatic cleaners

   a. Enzymatic cleaners are to be used at minimum once a week to break down peptide bonds, allowing protein to be rubbed off mechanically.

   b. The proper sequence to follow when enzyming hydrogel lenses is surfactant cleaning, rinsing, enzymatic cleaning, rinsing, and disinfection.

   c. Soaking time varies from 15 minutes to 2 hours. Daily wear lenses may be left in an enzyme cleaner overnight; however, disinfection should be performed after enzyming.

   d. There are four unique enzyme cleaners that combine two steps in one: (1) ReNu Thermal Enzymatic Cleaner (Bausch & Lomb), which can be placed directly in the case and used during thermal disinfection; (2) Ultrazyme (Allergan Optical), which is dissolved in hydrogen peroxide combining the enzymatic and disinfection steps; (3) Enzyme Plus (Pilkington/Barnes-Hind), which combines the surfactant and enzyme in one step; and (4) Opti-Free Enzymatic Cleaner (Alcon Laboratories), which combines enzymatic cleaning and disinfection in Opti-Free in one step.

5. Lens lubricants/rewetting

   a. Lens lubricants are used directly in the eye with or without lenses.

   b. The use of lens lubricants or rewetting drops is optional; however, they may be beneficial in cases of dry eyes, foreign body sensation, irritations, and for morning and evening use in extended wear.

   c. Patients should not substitute artificial tears, RGP lens lubricants, or ophthalmic medications for hydrogel lens lubricants, as the preservatives are not necessarily compatible with the hydrogel lens materials, with the possible result being lens discoloration and/or toxic reactions.

VIII. Hydrogel Troubleshooting

A. *Patient care*
   1. Thorough, ongoing patient care may prevent future complications associated with hydrogel contact lens wear. Symptoms elicited and clinical signs observed signal contact lens-related conditions that should be eliminated or monitored prior to severe complications.
   2. Frequent follow-up evaluations, every 6 months for daily wear patients and every 3 months for extended-wear patients, are recommended to monitor the contact lens patient.

B. *Symptoms*
   1. Reduced vision may be related to the lens, the prescription, or the cornea.
       a. Lens deposits. When the lens becomes deposited with protein or lipids, the patient may complain of foggy or hazy vision. Diagnosis is obtained by observation of the lens with the biomicroscope, although excessive debris may be noted without the use of magnification. Daily use of a surfactant cleaner and weekly use of an enzymatic cleaner should improve lens cleanliness; however, in severe cases the lens will have to be replaced.
       b. Incorrect prescription. Reduction in Snellen visual acuity will be noted if the patient is wearing an incorrect lens prescription. An overrefraction should be performed to determine if the lenses have been switched or if the prescription is inadequate. A pinhole visual acuity measurement will determine if the reduction is refractive or possibly pathological in nature. New lenses must be ordered with the correct prescription or, if switched, each lens should be placed in the appropriate eye.
       c. Uncorrected refractive astigmatism. The flexibility of a hydrogel lens limits its ability to effectively correct astigmatism. Individuals with 0.75 to 1.00D of refractive astigmatism may begin to experience symptoms of decreased visual acuity while wearing spherical hydrogel lenses, especially if they perform extensive near tasks. Overrefraction with placement of the appropriate cylinder in the phoropter will improve visual acuity, allowing the patient to determine the acceptability of the compromised vision. Astigmatic correction may be obtained with a toric hydrogel, a rigid lens, or a spectacle overcorrection.
       d. Toric lens rotation. Lens rotation, either subsequent to each blink or as a result of persistent mislocation, may be a cause of reduced visual acuity in astigmatic patients. Individuals who exhibit astigmatism at an oblique axis are more prone to have lens rotation as compared to with-the-rule and against-the-rule astigmats. Slit lamp examination of the toric lens will determine whether the lens is stable, with adequate centration and movement, or whether excessive rotation occurs after each blink. A refraction performed over the patient's current contact lenses or diagnostic lenses may be beneficial in determining the appropriate power and axis to order for the patient. Excessive lens movement may require a steeper base curve or larger overall diameter to reduce rotation and improve visual acuity. Increasing the amount of prism in prism-ballasted lenses and/or changing to a different design (e.g., truncated, slab-off, thin-zone designs) may also be beneficial. The option of refitting the patient into spherical RGP lenses may also be considered in challenging cases, if the individual's corneal toricity accounts for the majority of the refractive astigmatism.
       e. Defective lenses. Characteristics of defective lenses include both damage (scratches, tears, nicks, holes) and poor optics. Both may contribute to irritation, discomfort, and reduced visual acuity. Biomicroscopy will demonstrate the source of the problem if a lens is damaged. Careful examination of the

lens edge may be necessary to locate a nick or small tear. The absence of improvement in visual acuity with an overrefraction may be indicative of poor optics, necessitating lens replacement. Lens replacement is undoubtedly the most effective method of handling defective lenses.

f. Lens inversion. A common complaint, especially with new hydrogel lens wearers, is difficulty with lens inversion. Individuals wearing thin lenses often exhibit frustration in determining whether the lens is right side out prior to insertion. Mild irritation may be noted due to the increased movement of the lens. Examination of the lens edge with the biomicroscope will reveal stand-off from the bulbar conjunctiva and excessive movement. Patient methods of determining lens inversion have been discussed previously in patient education. Removal of the lens, accompanied by correct orientation, will resolve any decrease in visual acuity or irritation noted by the patient.

g. Visual reduction with contact lenses and spectacles. A reduction in visual acuity, apparent with both contact lens and spectacle correction, may be indicative of a more serious complication. Removal of the contact lenses and inspection of the cornea and conjunctiva is imperative in determining the cause of the decreased visual acuity. Some physiological factors that may influence vision with hydrogel contact lens wear include corneal abrasion, corneal edema, corneal staining, increased mucus production resulting from giant papillary conjunctivitis, "myopic creep" resulting from edema, or a pathological condition unrelated to contact lens wear.

2. Discomfort. When a hydrogel contact lens wearer experiences discomfort, the lens should be removed immediately. If the discomfort persists, the patient should be educated to contact his or her practitioner immediately. Further biomicroscopic evaluation of the cornea, both with lens wear and upon removal, will aid in determination of the source of the discomfort. In addition, corneal staining evaluation with fluorescein application is important.

a. Discomfort upon lens insertion. If discomfort occurs upon insertion, the source is most likely either a torn lens, a sensitivity to the solutions used, or (if applicable) the prism ballast of a toric lens.

b. Discomfort after lens removal. Typically, discomfort present after the lens is removed is due to problems related to the cornea and should be considered an ocular emergency. Corneal abrasions, ocular infections, corneal ulcers, or other ocular problems may be causing the pain. Fluorescein evaluation is important in determining the extent of the corneal disturbance.

c. Constant discomfort with lens on. When the discomfort of hydrogel lenses is constant, the source of the discomfort may be a tight lens, corneal edema, or lens deposits (assuming a torn lens has been ruled out). Biomicroscopy and fluorescein evaluation will aid in determination of the cause. A tight lens may be managed by altering the lens parameters, either by flattening the BCR or by decreasing lens diameter. For a patient experiencing edema-related symptoms, a change to a lens with higher oxygen transmission, whether hydrogel or RGP, will be beneficial. A deposited lens may be replaced with a clean, new lens to alleviate the symptoms. Educating the patient on proper care of hydrogel lenses may decrease lens deposits.

d. Immediate discomfort after a period of lens wear. The most frequent cause of immediate discomfort is a trapped foreign body (e.g., dust, cosmetic particles). This discomfort should be eliminated by removing the lens and rinsing it with saline. A large foreign body may cause a corneal abrasion; therefore, if the pain continues it is important that the patient be seen immediately. A deposited lens, especially jelly bumps or a contaminated lens, may result in discomfort that increases as the period of lens wear increases. A torn lens may also cause immediate discomfort; however, typically the discomfort is noticed upon lens insertion. A deposited or torn lens will require lens replacement.

3. Burning. Burning and stinging are most often related to contact lens solution sensitivity, failure to neutralize the hydrogen peroxide disinfection solution, or inadequate rinsing of the lens after either surfactant or enzymatic cleaning. Reinforcement of appropriate lens hygiene at each visit is beneficial in maintaining patient compliance and avoiding unnecessary irritation. Irritation with continued use of a chemical disinfecting system may indicate hypersensitivity or toxicity to the preservative. A generalized stippling is indicative of a toxic or hypersensitivity reaction, and if severe enough, may elicit tearing and photophobia, as well as decreased visual acuity. Patients with a preservative sensitivity may achieve success with the use of a preservative-free, hydrogen peroxide disinfecting system (e.g., Ultracare-Allergan). Reviewing cleaning and disinfection procedures at each visit may assist in alleviating solution-related discomfort associated with the use of inappropriate care techniques.

4. Dryness. A contact lens patient may present with symptoms of dryness, scratchiness, and/or "gritty" feeling eyes. This may be a result of the patient's poor tear quality and/or quantity. A complete blink approximately every 5 seconds is also required to spread the tear film over the cornea.

   a. Patient factors. The patient should be questioned about any medical conditions, such as Stevens-Johnson syndrome (mucin deficiency), pregnancy (increase in tear viscosity), or Sjogren's syndrome (aqueous deficiency). Medications that may alter the tear film are antihistamines, anticholinergics, anti-anxiety agents, phenothiazines, and oral contraceptives.

   b. Environmental factors. The occupational environment, for example, working near heat and air-conditioning vents, may exacerbate dryness symptoms. Air currents from automobile vents may also cause discomfort. Long-term computer use may cause a decreased blink rate, resulting in symptoms of dryness.

   c. Treatment. Lens lubricants will provide short-term relief for these patients. Blinking exercises, conscious complete blinks, computer breaks, and vent deflectors may also relieve the dryness. More extensive measures to increase wearing time and alleviate dryness might include using a humidifier or saline soaks (hydrogel lenses are removed and soaked in saline 3–5 minutes prior to reinsertion). Patients exhibiting dryness should be fit with low-water, thick hydrogel lenses to prevent dehydration of the lens. Limited wearing time, punctal occlusion, or even discontinuation of contact lens use may be necessary if other treatment methods fail.

5. Excessive lens movement. Excessive hydrogel lens movement may be due to a deposited lens, an inverted lens, a dehydrated lens, or a lens that has too flat a base curve. Observation of the lens with the biomicroscope will aid in a differential diagnosis.

6. Foggy or hazy vision.

   a. Foggy or hazy vision through a hydrogel contact lens may be due to a coated lens or to corneal edema. A common symptom elicited from patients is the appearance of halos around lights. Clinical signs of either a contaminated lens or corneal edema may be observed with a biomicroscope. The patient may be questioned on his or her care procedures and wearing times. Poor lens hygiene or improper care will result in a contaminated or coated lens. Overwear of the lens may result in corneal edema.

   b. Treatment. In cases of a contaminated or coated lens, visual acuity will improve with replacement of the lens. The patient may need to utilize an abrasive cleaner, increase the number of enzymatic cleanings per week, change the disinfection method, replace the contact lenses more frequently, or switch to an RGP material. Patient education on proper cleaning and disinfection techniques will help prolong the life of the contact lens. In the case of corneal edema, removal of the contact lens and exposure of the cornea to air will result in a reduction in the amount of corneal edema. Switching a patient to a higher-water-content lens and/or a thinner lens while maintaining the patient on a daily wear schedule will help reduce the level of edema.

C. *Clinical signs*
   1. Staining. Fluorescein evaluation is important to monitor corneal integrity with hydrogel contact lens wear. Fluorescein must be rinsed from the eye with saline or lens wear discontinued for approximately 2 hours after the use of fluorescein in a hydrogel wearer to prevent discoloration of the lens; consequently, its application is often neglected during routine examination. A high-molecular-weight fluorescein, fluorexon, may be used with hydrogel lenses without risk of discoloration; however, fluorescence is reduced as compared to fluorescein strips and many conditions may go undiagnosed.
      a. Causes of staining
         (1) Infection.
         (2) Mechanical trauma (e.g., damaged lens, removal trauma).
         (3) Lens deposits.
         (4) Trapped foreign body.
         (5) Desiccation.
         (6) Hypoxia.
         (7) Solution sensitivity.
      b. Treatment
         (1) Staining as a result of infection is an ocular emergency and requires the appropriate treatment and follow-up care required. Obviously, lens wear should be discontinued until the infection and results of the infection are cleared up.
         (2) A damaged or deposited lens should be replaced. Reeducation on care, handling, insertion, and removal may be necessary if the trauma from damage, deposits, or removal is due to careless lens care or handling.
         (3) In cases of hypoxia or desiccation, the lens should be replaced by another lens made of material that provides greater oxygen (thinner and/or increased water content) in the case of hypoxia and less lens dehydration (thick, low-water-content lens) in the case of desiccation. Rewetting drops may also be helpful in cases of desiccation.
         (4) When debris is trapped on the lens, the lens should be removed, cleaned, and rinsed prior to reinsertion. Depending on the severity of the staining, the patient may require further treatment and discontinuation of lens wear.
         (5) Solution sensitivity may result from noncompliant lens care, such as not thoroughly rinsing the cleaner or enzyme off, or incomplete neutralization of hydrogen peroxide disinfection. The care system should be reviewed with the patient to correct these mistakes. A patient using a chemical disinfection system, especially those containing thimerosal or chlorhexidine, may be sensitive to the preservative. The patient should be changed to a different disinfection method, such as a chemical disinfectant containing polyquad or Dymed, or a nonpreserved system.
   2. Corneal edema
      a. Clinical evaluation. Corneal edema related to hydrogel lens wear is typically generalized or diffuse. The biomicroscope and the pachometer are most useful in evaluating hydrogel-related corneal edema.
      b. Clinical signs
         (1) Striae. Posterior folds in Descemet's membrane resulting from a minimum of 6% swelling. They can be observed by indirect illumination at the central stroma with a parallelepiped beam, high illumination, and high magnification. If several striae are present, this is an indicator that

higher oxygen transmission is required, either by using a new material or by reducing wearing time.

(2) Microcysts. Epithelial microcysts often result after several weeks of extended wear. Possessing a semiopaque vacuole-like appearance, they can be observed using a similar biomicroscopic technique as striae. If numerous (>25), the patient should temporarily discontinue contact lens wear. The microcysts typically come to the surface and then stain prior to resolving.

(3) Endothelial changes. The endothelial cell size and shape can become less uniform with contact lens wear. These changes are especially apparent with long-term PMMA lens wear and hydrogel extended wear. Endothelial cell size and uniformity is best evaluated with specular reflection.

(4) Progressive increase in myopia (myopic creep). Chronic low-level hypoxia can result in an increase in myopia in hydrogel lens wearers, notably in extended wear. If the patient experiences a reduction in vision, a refraction should be performed.

c. Management. When hydrogel-related corneal edema is observed, the following options should be considered:

(1) Changing the lens material to one that will provide greater oxygen transmission (thinner and/or higher-water-content hydrogel lens).

(2) Ensuring that the fit is optimum.

(3) Refitting the patient in an RGP lens material to provide greater oxygen transmission.

(4) Decreasing the wearing time. Depending on the severity of the corneal edema, lens wear may be discontinued until the clinical signs have resolved.

3. Injection

a. Generalized injection. may or may not be related to hydrogel contact lens wear.

(1) Possible lens-related causes

(a) Corneal hypoxia.

(b) Tight lens.

(c) Solution sensitivity.

(d) Trapped foreign body.

(e) Deposited lens.

(f) Damaged lens.

(g) Ocular complications related to the above conditions.

(2) Non-lens-related causes

(a) Allergic, viral, or bacterial conjunctivitis.

(b) Related to other ocular or systemic conditions.

(3) To differentiate the cause of the injection, perform a thorough case history, including questions such as: When was the injection initially observed? Does it continue after the lenses are removed? Is the injection of recent or chronic occurrence? Are the eyes irritated, burning, or itching? Is there any discharge and if so, what type: mucous, watery, or stringy? Was there an occurrence that preceded the injection, such as change in solutions, swimming, lack of sleep, illness, traumatic injury, or foreign body? Based on the case history, the elimination of causative factors, and a thorough evaluation with the biomicroscope, the diagnosis may be made.

b. Lens-related generalized injection. Moderate to severe injection of the eye at any time should be treated as an ocular emergency due to the risk of corneal ulcers and infection. Patients may present with mild injection due to a variety of factors (environment, dryness, etc.); however, if the injection is acute with no known cause, a thorough evaluation is necessary to rule out serious conditions.

    (1) Symptoms of lens-related injection: Typically occurs upon insertion or after lens wear, and will improve as lens wear is discontinued. Immediate injection with burning on insertion will most likely be related to a solution sensitivity (preservatives, improper solution use). Management of injection resulting from solution sensitivity requires changing the care system or reeducating the patient on the proper use of the solutions. As the wearing time increases over a period of a day with daily wear or over a period of days with extended wear, corneal hypoxia, a tight lens, or a deposited or damaged lens may result in a generalized injection. Evaluation with the biomicroscope will determine the cause. Management requires replacing the lens or refitting to improve the fitting relationship and/or oxygen transmission of the lens.

    c. Non-lens-related injection. If the hydrogel lens is fitting properly, nonpreserved solutions are used, the lens is clean and new, and the injection continues after the lens wear is discontinued, evaluate the eye for other causative factors. A simple case history may elicit the cause, such as allergies, dryness, lack of sleep, trauma, cigarette smoke, etc. Further evaluation with the biomicroscope with and without fluorescein will aid in diagnosing the problem. Some patients present with mild injection on a consistent basis, which may be improved by lens lubricants.

4. Corneal vascularization. Vascularization of the normally avascular cornea is a serious complication of contact lens wear. Typically vascularization occurs in hydrogel contact lens wearers as a result of a tight lens fit, limbal compression, corneal edema, extended wear, or overwear.

    a. Stages. Three stages occur in the process of corneal vascularization secondary to contact lens wear.

        (1) *Stage 1:* filling of preexisting limbal capillary plexuses.

        (2) *Stage 2:* new vessel growth which extends from the limbal arcades toward the central cornea.

        (3) *Stage 3:* sprouts canaliculize and form "true" vessels and may occur at any depth within the cornea.

    b. Management. Contact lens management of corneal vascularization may involve a reduction in wearing time, changes in the fitting relationship, a change in lens design, and/or a change in lens material in an attempt to increase oxygen transmission to the cornea. Individuals on an extended-wear schedule may switch to daily wear, whereas daily wear patients may reduce their number of hours by removing the lenses during less critical times (e.g., after work or on weekends). A tight lens-to-cornea fitting relationship, causing a constriction in venous return, may need to be loosened. Selecting a thinner lens design in the same material or selecting a higher-water-content lens material without significantly increasing lens thickness will increase oxygen transmission. Extended-wear patients may find it necessary to switch to a daily wear schedule or a medium- to high-Dk RGP material to control corneal vascularization. In cases of severe vascularization, permanent lens removal may be necessary to promote vessel regression.

D. *Specific conditions related to hydrogel contact lenses*

1. Giant papillary conjunctivitis. This condition is also called contact lens related papillary conjunctivitis and may be abbreviated as GPC or CLRPC. The development of GPC has been noted in both rigid and hydrogel contact lens wearers; however, it is more common in hydrogel wearers.

    a. Signs and symptoms. Clinical symptoms and signs commonly accompanying this condition include conjunctival hyperemia, excess mucus, giant papillae on the upper tarsal conjunctiva, increased contact lens movement, itching, lens deposits, reduced wearing time, and contact lens intolerance. Lid ever-sion, accompanied by fluorescein staining, is essential in the early diagnosis of GPC and should be performed on all contact lens patients prior to fitting and at each subsequent visit.

b. Etiology. The papillary reaction of the upper tarsal conjunctiva in GPC has been most often attributed to both an immunological response to, and a mechanical irritation from, surface deposits on the contact lens. The allergic reaction results from the presence of antigens (denatured proteins, lipids, foreign material, etc.) on the surface of the lens. Improper and poor cleaning habits and infrequent replacement of the contact lens contribute to the initia-tion and exacerbation of the disease process.

c. Treatment. Many cases of GPC may be remedied by early intervention. In the early stages of GPC, most symptoms should be alleviated by regular surfactant and enzyme cleaning. Surfactant cleaning is essential and should be performed daily or upon lens removal prior to disinfection. If symptoms persist with daily cleaning, an abrasive cleaner or more frequent cleanings are recommended. Weekly enzymatic cleaning is essential in maintaining a relatively deposit-free surface; biweekly or even more frequent enzyme cleaning may be beneficial in cases of GPC. The introduction of both disposable and planned replacement contact lenses will likely assist in decreasing the number of patients presenting with clinical signs and symptoms of GPC. Switching to a rigid lens may also be considered because of its better surface wettability properties. In severe cases, lens wear may be discontinued until the clinical signs disappear. At that time, lens wear may be cautiously reinstated, with emphasis on lens cleanliness, frequent lens replacement, and reduced wearing time. Medical intervention may be necessary in cases of GPC not abatable by previously mentioned techniques. With the discontinuance of cromolyn sodium production (Opticrom, Fisons Corp.), the treatment has become even more challenging to the practitioner. Fluorometholone 0.10% (1 drop in each eye four times daily for 1 week, tapered by 1 drop each week for 3 weeks) and Suprofen (Alcon Laboratories, Inc.) may be effective in reducing both clinical signs and symptoms of the condition. Other nonsteroid anti-inflammatory (NSAID) drugs may be effective as well.

2. Contact lens associated superior limbic keratoconjunctivitis (CL-SLK)

a. Etiology. Factors that may contribute to this condition are sensitivity to thimerosal-preserved solutions, hypoxia due to the lens wear and upper lid coverage, mechanical irritation from the contact lens, and immunological response to environmental antigens adhering to lens deposits.

b. Symptoms
    (1) Blurred vision.
    (2) Lens discomfort/intolerance.
    (3) Photophobia.
    (4) Tearing.
    (5) Itching.
    (6) Burning.

c. Clinical signs
    (1) Affects the superior cornea and conjunctiva.
    (2) Conjunctival chemosis and injection.
    (3) Micropannus.
    (4) Corneal infiltrates.
    (5) Epithelial thickening.
    (6) Corneal haziness.
    (7) Superficial punctate staining of the cornea and conjunctiva.

d. Treatment. The contact lens should be removed until all clinical signs and symptoms, except vascularization, have resolved. The patient will detect a noticeable difference within days; however, it may take weeks to months to resolve the clinical signs. Ocular lubricants may relieve the irritation of the upper lid on the superior bulbar conjunctiva and cornea. Steroid-antibiotic combinations may be required in severe cases.

e. Lens wear after CL-SLK. After resolution, the patient may be able to wear hydrogel lenses again if nonpreserved care systems (i.e., heat disinfection, hydrogen peroxide with nonpreserved solutions) are used. To reduce the chance of lens deposits and hypoxia, a lens that provides greater oxygen transmission (e.g., an extended-wear lens worn on a daily wear basis) and that is resistant to deposits or is replaced frequently (e.g., CSI-T, frequent replacement/disposable lenses) is advised. The wearing time should be kept at daily wear with possibly a further reduction in wearing time, for example, weekend wear, 3 days daily wear/1 day off, 8-hour days, etc. The patient may also be refit with RGP lenses, which will provide decreased diameter, increased resistance to deposits, and increased oxygen transmission. Regardless of the lens modality, the patient should be monitored closely to prevent exacerbation of the condition.

IX. Verification and Modification

The purpose of this section is to discuss verification of both rigid and hydrogel lenses and modification of rigid lenses.

A. *Verification*
1. Base curve radius
   a. Description.
      The base curve radius (BCR) is one of the most important rigid lens parameters to verify, as it affects the lens-to-cornea fitting relationship. Verification of a hydrogel BCR is very difficult to perform in-office, and therefore the BCR is generally not measured.
   b. Equipment.
      The most commonly used method of determining the BCR of a rigid lens is the radiuscope or radiusgauge with the concave lens mount. There are other methods of measuring BCR in saline that may be more accurate but also are more expensive or complicated.
   c. Purpose.
      Verification of the rigid lens BCR should be performed before dispensing and periodically throughout lens wear to ensure that the lenses have the BCR that was ordered and that the lens is not warped. Soaking the rigid lenses for 12–24 hours in an approved disinfecting solution is necessary to determine if the lens, after hydration, is still within tolerance. Verification of a hydrogel BCR is necessary only when the BCR is unknown or the BCR given on the vial appears inaccurate based on evaluation of fit on the eye.
   d. Procedure for determining the BCR of a rigid lens with a radiuscope/radiusgauge
      (1) A small amount of water should be placed in the depression of the lens mount.
      (2) The lens should be clean and dry and placed in this depression, concave side upward. Caution should be taken not to submerge the entire lens or allow any fluid on the concave surface, as this will result in an inaccurate reading or a poor-quality image.
      (3) The lens mount should be centered and positioned so that a small green beam of light can be observed reflected in the lens. The aperture selector should be in the large aperture position at the back of the instrument.
      (4) When viewed in the oculars, the real and aerial images will be observed as a spoke or star pattern. The real image will appear at the lower end of the scale at approximately zero and will be centered; however, the aerial image will be located approximately 6–9 mm on the scale and may not

be centered. This aerial image should be centered and the lens mount should not be moved again before setting the instrument at zero and taking a reading. Note that between the two images, the light filament will be observed.

(5) Upon obtaining a clear, sharp spoke pattern of the real image at the lower end of the scale, the needle should be placed on zero. This can be accomplished by using the knob located at the left side of most radiuscopes and the back of most radiusgauges. The manual provided with the instrument should provide this information.

(6) The objective should be adjusted with the coarse adjustment knob to obtain a clear sharp focus of the aerial image. As the scale increases in value, the light filament will be observed prior to viewing the aerial image. The BCR will be the reading taken from the zero point to the clear, sharp focus of the aerial image.

(7) The BCR is read off the millimeter scale to the nearest hundredth. The millimeter scale is located in the ocular of the radiuscope and on a clock dial at the back of the radiusgauge. For example, a typical BCR would be recorded as 8.20 mm.

(8) If the needle of the instrument will not position at zero when the real image is in focus, the nearest whole number should be used. This whole number will be added or subtracted from the final reading. For example, if the real image is in focus at +1.0 and the final reading is 7.0 mm, the BCR is 8.0 mm.

(9) If the lens has a toric surface or is warped, the spokes of the aerial image will not all be in focus at the same time. First, one spoke will come in sharp focus; this will represent the steepest curve. The spoke 90° away from the first spoke will next come in focus, and this is the flatter curve.

2. Front convex radius

   a. Description. The convex surface radius should be measured to determine if a rigid lens is front toric or bitoric. This is not necessary with hydrogel lenses.

   b. Equipment. The equipment is identical to that used for measurement of a base curve radius except that the convex lens mount is used.

   c. Procedure. The procedure is similar to determining BCR except that the real image is now the upper image and the aerial image is the lower image. The needle should be set at the nearest whole number when the real image is in focus. When the aerial image is in focus, the number is read from the scale and subtracted from the whole number. For example, if the real image is in focus at 8.00 mm and the aerial image is in focus at 1.00 mm, the resulting front curve radius would be 7.00 mm.

3. Lens power

   a. Description. Back vertex power verification with the lensometer is typically the method by which power is determined for contact lenses.

   b. Equipment.
      A lensometer is used to determine the power of a contact lens. Most lensometers have a contact lens accessory device that can be placed on the lens stop to aid in more accurate measurements. A wet cell may be used with the lensometer when determining the power of a hydrogel lens.

   c. Purpose.
      The power of a contact lens is important when verifying that the correct lens power has been received, when determining the power of a diagnostic lens so a final lens power may be ordered, and to ensure that the patient does not change the rigid lens power by the use of abrasive lens cleaners. Verifying the hydrogel lens power on the vial is sufficient prior to dispensing.

   d. Procedure
      (1) The method is similar to that used to verify spectacles.

(2) Tilt the lensometer into a nearly vertical position.

(3) The lensometer should be adjusted for the individual user prior to verifying the lens power as specified in the instrument manual.

(4) The rigid lens should be clean and dry. The hydrogel lens surface should be blotted dry on a lint-free tissue or cloth or placed in saline in a wet cell.

(5) The lens is placed concave side against the lens stop of the lensometer and the power drum is adjusted until a clear image is achieved. If a clear image is not achieved with the hydrogel lens, remove the lens for cleaning and try again.

(6) Caution should be taken not to flex the lens.

(7) The power of the lens is read off the power drum. When using a wet cell, the power found must be multiplied by a correction factor to determine the actual lens power. This correction factor is different depending on the water content; however, it is approximately 4.6. A small degree of inaccuracy will cause variance in the powers found; therefore, exact determination of a hydrogel power, especially in the wet cell, may be difficult.

(8) To measure prism on a rigid contact lens, the lens must be centered with the concave side against the lens stop. The reticule inside the ocular consists of concentric black rings designating 1–5 prism diopters. If the center of the target was on the first concentric ring of the reticule, it would correspond to 1 prism diopter. Prism is primarily used in front toric lenses to reduce rotation.

(9) Toric lenses will yield a spherocylindrical power. Front toric lenses should be rotated on the lensometer until the prism in the base down direction. The resulting power will be recorded in a spherocylindrical notation. In toric lenses with no prism, such as bitorics and back torics, the power is not recorded in the spherocylindrical form, but as the values found in each meridian. The Tori-Check (General Ophthalmic, Park Ridge, Illinois) is a device which aids in orientating a hydrogel toric lens for power determination.

4. Center/edge thickness
   a. Description.
     Verifying this parameter in rigid lenses is important for flexure, oxygen transmission, comfort, and lens position.
   b. Equipment.
     A dial gauge is the most frequently used method of determining rigid lens thickness; however, radiusgauges have a thickness gauge incorporated into the instrument. A radiuscope is the most frequent method of determining the center thickness of a hydrogel lens.
   c. Procedure for determining the center thickness of a rigid lens
     (1) Position the lens on the gauge (centered for center thickness and at the edge for edge thickness).
     (2) Lower the plunger onto the lens.
     (3) The thickness is read directly off the gauge; for example, if the needle is on 23 then the thickness is recorded as 0.23 mm.
   d. Procedure for determining the center thickness of a hydrogel lens
     (1) The radiuscope mires should be focused on a microscope slide and zero the scale at that point.
     (2) The hydrogel lens is placed on the slide convex side down, having the radiuscope beam reflected from the center of the contact lens.
     (3) The radiuscope microscope is then moved up until the back surface mire image is clearly in focus. Be sure to focus on the surface image and not the aerial image. The reading on the scale is the center thickness of the contact lens.

5. Inspection of the lens edge
    a. Equipment. Stereomicroscope, projection magnifier, edge profile analyzer.
    b. Purpose. The shape and condition of the lens edge is perhaps the most important factor in providing patient comfort.
    c. Procedure
        (1) Palm test—Place the lens concave side down in the palm of the hand and gently push it across the palm. A good edge will glide easily and feel smooth. A poor edge will feel scratchy, show resistance to movement, and may make an audible scratchy sound. Use this method in combination with one of the edge profile methods.
        (2) Projection magnifier—projects a magnified image of the lens allowing inspection of the edges. The lens can be positioned so as to view the lens from both straight ahead and profile positions.
        (3) Edge profile analyzer—an attachment for the radiuscope which provides a profile of the edge.
        (4) Stereomicroscope—provides a highly magnified view of the lens edge.
6. Linear dimensions
    a. Description. Overall diameter (diameter of lens from edge to edge), optic zone diameter (central lens diameter between peripheral curves), and peripheral curve widths may be verified. The junction blend of the peripheral curves on a rigid lens may also be determined.
    b. Equipment. A measuring magnifier is the most commonly used piece of equipment; however, a projection magnifier may be used. A PD stick, V-channel gauge, or dial gauge may be used to determine overall diameter. In addition, a wet cell may be used with a hydrogel lens.
    c. Procedure
        (1) The lens is placed on the measuring magnifier and held up to a background light source. By positioning the lens on the scale, the diameter, optic zone diameter, and peripheral curve widths can be easily measured. If a wet cell is used, the wet cell should be placed against the measuring magnifier scale with the hydrogel lens concave side down. If the wet cell is not used, the hydrogel lens should be blotted dry on a lint-free tissue. Do not distort or flatten the hydrogel lens on the reticule.
        (2) Rigid lenses may have a bicurve (base curve and peripheral curve), a tricurve (base curve, secondary curve, and peripheral curve), or a tetra-curve (base curve, secondary curve, intermediate curve, and peripheral curve) peripheral curve design.
        (3) The measuring magnifier may need to be moved back and forth slightly in the light source to determine where the rigid lens curve exists and the type of junction blend. The junction of the peripheral curves is very easy to distinguish with a light blend, less easy to distinguish with a medium blend, and very difficult to distinguish with a heavy blend.
7. Surface inspection
    a. Equipment. Stereomicroscope, projection magnifier, biomicroscope, and measuring magnifier; for hydrogel lenses a phase contrast microscope may also be used.
    b. Purpose. Examination of the rigid lens surface may reveal surface scratches, cracking/crazing, residual pitch, deposits, and film. Examination of the hydrogel lens may reveal deposits, rust spots, tears, and surface defects.
    c. Procedure. The lens is viewed, while being held under the stereomicroscope and well illuminated, in the beam of the biomicroscope either on or off the eye; the lens is projected onto the screen of the projection magnifier in a frontal view; or the lens is viewed with the measuring magnifier. The magnification may not be high enough with the measuring magnifier to reveal small surface defects. Phase contrast microscopes are quite expensive; however, this is an excellent way to observe highly magnified deposits on a hydrogel lens.

    B. Modification

      1. Why modify
   a. Increase office efficiency by not sending lenses out to laboratory.
   b. More convenient to the patient.
   c. Higher success rate and practitioner satisfaction with RGP lenses; more control over lens design and fitting relationship.

      2. Equipment (Table 9-8)
   a. Unit
      (1) Should be large enough to provide a deep-welled bowl to minimize splash during procedure.
      (2) If possible, use an adjustable spindle speed unit; the use of a speed greater than 1000 RPM may result in heat-induced damage to the lens surface.
   b. Accessory tools
      (1) Most modification accessory tools are typically included with the unit; if not, it is important to purchase tools with the same taper size as the unit.
      (2) Accessory tools include the following:
         (a) Brass or diamond-impregnated radius tools for peripheral curve flattening or blending (brass only).
         (b) Sponge tools (flat, cone, and edge) for front surface polishing, back surface polishing, and edge polishing.
         (c) Spinner for front surface polishing and repowering.
         (d) Suction cup holder for mounting the lens.
         (e) The aforementioned verification equipment including a radiuscope, edge analyzer, lensometer, and a 7× or 10× magnifier.
   c. Polishing compounds
      (1) Decrease heat buildup and should be used liberally during the modification procedure; they contain surfactants to lubricate and cool the lens during the procedure and a mild abrasive to erode lens material.

Table 9-8. A Partial Listing of Modification Equipment Suppliers

Conforma Laboratories 4705 Colley Ave. P.O. Box 2693 Norfolk, VA 23508 804-423-5807 800-533-4084 (VA), 800-426-1700 (Nat'l)	P.O. Box 988 Mesa, AZ 85201 602-892-7601 800-528-8279
Davison Chemical Supply Co. Chattanooga, TN	Polychem, Inc. 4218 Howard Ave. P.O. Box 289 Kensington, MD 20895 301-564-1180 800-492-6820 (MD), 800-638-6880 (Nat'l)
Kontur Kontact Lens Co. 200 S. Garrard Blvd. Richmond, CA 94804 415-235-5225 800-227-1320 (Nat'l), 800-772-2421 (CA)	
	Valley Contax 1310 Coburg Rd. P.O. Box 7727 Eugene, OR 97401 503-344-1310 800-452-2525 (OR), 800-547-8815 (Nat'l)
Marlin Industries 18635 Ventura Blvd. P.O. Box 284 Tarzana, CA 91356 818-344-9051 800-423-5926 (Nat'l), 800-472-2020 (CA)	
	Vigor Optical Co. 53 West 23rd St. New York, NY 10010-4275 212-807-3801 800-221-5140 (Nat'l)
Paragon Optical, Inc. 947 E. Impala Ave.	

(2) Polishes may be premixed (e.g., Fluoro-Shine, Sil-O2-Care, Boston Polish) or in powder form to be mixed with water (e.g., X-Pal).

3. Procedures

Prior to performing any modification procedure, it is important to obtain the original specifications of the lens in case the lens is damaged during the modification process. Procedures to be performed include peripheral curve fabrication and blending, edge polishing, surface polishing, and repowering. Diameter reduction is not recommended due to the possibility of heat-induced damage to the lens surface. The performance of these procedures will be mentioned briefly; for a more comprehensive and dynamic overview of how to modify RGP lenses, the modification video listed in the aforementioned CLMA/RGPLI Video Library is recommended. In addition, attending a hands-on workshop, either sponsored by an organization or associated with a local Contact Lens Manufacturers Association (CLMA) laboratory, will be beneficial.

a. Peripheral curve fabrication

(1) Peripheral curve flattening will increase tear exchange, eliminate peripheral bearing, and reduce sealoff; blending the junction between two peripheral curves will increase tear exchange, lens movement with the blink, and initial comfort.

(2) Typically, the radius tool is covered by velveteen or similar material; as most tool sets have radii from approximately 7.6 to 12.00 mm, if flattening of the peripheral curve is desired, either an 11.00-mm or a 12.00-mm radius tool is typically selected. One of three methods is recommended:

(a) Method 1. The lens is attached to the suction cup concave side out and the suction cup is held toward the bottom for greater control (Figure 9-13). The lens is held vertically to the radius tool and rotated in a figure-eight design. The lens should be inspected every 5–10 seconds.

(b) Method 2. The lens is held at a 30° angle to the vertical with a suction cup and the entire outer edge of the lens is in contact with the covered tool at all times. The suction cup is rotated slowly and

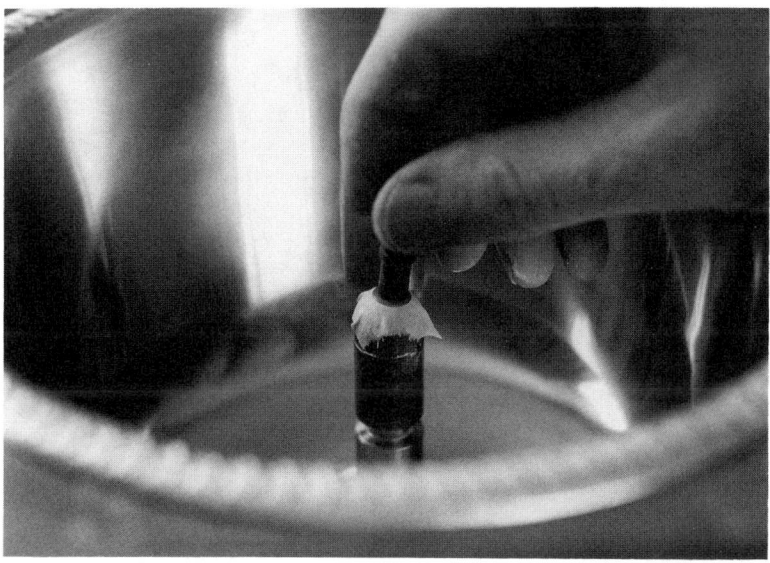

Figure 9-13. Application of a peripheral curve using the figure 8 method.

evenly with the fingers in the opposite direction of the spindle rotation until the curve has been applied.

    (c) Method 3. The lens is attached to a spinner and held at a 45°–60° angle. This positions the lens slightly off center with regard to the radius tool. The lens must be spinning at all times to minimize any degradation of optical quality.

   (3) In all three procedures, polish must be applied almost continually to avoid heat-induced scratches or defects of the posterior surface. It is especially important to be very cautious when modifying the peripheral curve radius of a high-Dk material.

   (4) When blending the junctions between two peripheral curve radii, select a tool with a radius between the two curves to be modified while also compensating for the approximately 0.2 mm added to the radius tool by the pad covering the tool. For example, when blending between an 8.80-mm and an 11.00-mm radius, select a 10.20-mm tool for blending minus 0.2 mm for the pad; this equals a 10.00-mm tool. A 10-second medium blend is most common, although a 5-second light blend or a 20-second heavy blend can also be applied.

  b. Edge polishing/shaping

If the edge is defective, as determined by verification, several methods are possible for modifying this important lens parameter.

   (1) Method 1. One common method of edge polish is to use a sponge tool (Figure 9-14). The lens is mounted on a suction cup with the concave surface out. The sponge should be thoroughly moistened with water and placed on the spindle. With the suction cup held vertically to the sponge tool, the lens is pushed into the central hole of the sponge and moved up and down in the sponge for a minimum of 30–60 seconds. Polish should be liberally applied.

   (2) Method 2. A flat pad covered with velveteen is often used for edge polishing and shaping (Figure 9-15). The lens is attached to a suction cup or spinner convex side out, and with the end of the tool pointing toward the center of the pad, the edge of the lens is lowered gently onto

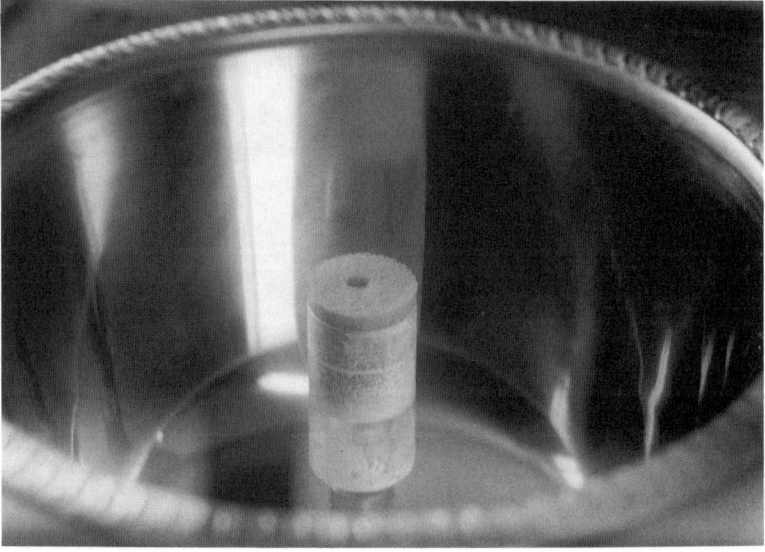

Figure 9-14.   Using a flat sponge with a central aperture for edge polishing.

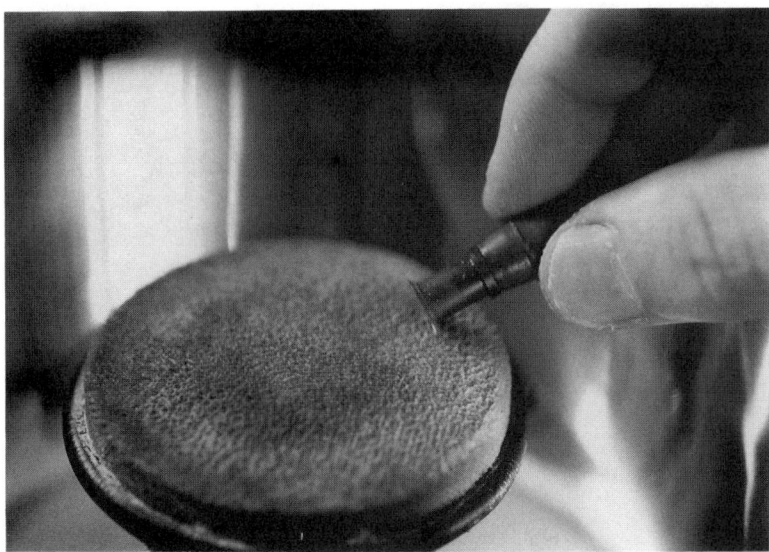

Figure 9-15.   A flat velveteen-covered pad for edge polishing.

the pad about two-thirds of the way out from the center. When the edge of the lens touches the rotating flat pad, the lens is moved across the pad. If a spinner is used, it should be allowed to rotate with the drum for about 15 seconds at a time. When using the suction cup, the lens should be rotated with the fingers in a counterclockwise direction as it is moved across the surface of the pad. This procedure may take up to a few minutes depending upon the bluntness of the edge.

(3)   Method 3. An anterior or CN bevel may be added to the lens edge to decrease the edge thickness or bluntness. This procedure is also beneficial in lowering a high positioning lens. This is most commonly achieved with the use of a 90° cone tool. The lens is mounted to a suction cup so that the convex surface faces the cone tool. A square piece of velveteen or similar material with a corner removed (e.g., 25%) is placed within the tool so that it conforms to the cone surface. The lens is then placed within the cone while it rotates and is gently rocked forward and backward and left and right to a slight degree. Polish is liberally applied and the lens should be evaluated about every 10 seconds until the desired thickness and shape is achieved. This should be followed by one of the aforementioned polishing procedures.

c.   Surface polishing

(1)   Convex surface. The newer RGP lens materials are typically softer and easier for patients to scratch, which is typically accompanied by difficult-to-remove surface deposits. The patient will often complain that the lens is fogging up due to accumulation of debris in the scratches and the subsequent surface filming. These scratches can be polished very easily without damaging the lens surface.

(a)   Method 1. The lens is mounted to a suction cup convex side out and centered reasonably well by visual inspection. A flat sponge tool is used, which is wetted thoroughly and then saturated with polish. Once the tool is rotating, polish is frequently applied and the lens is placed halfway between the center and the edge of the sponge. The lens should be held at a 45° angle and rotated in a direction opposite to the rotation of the tool (Figure 9-16). The lens

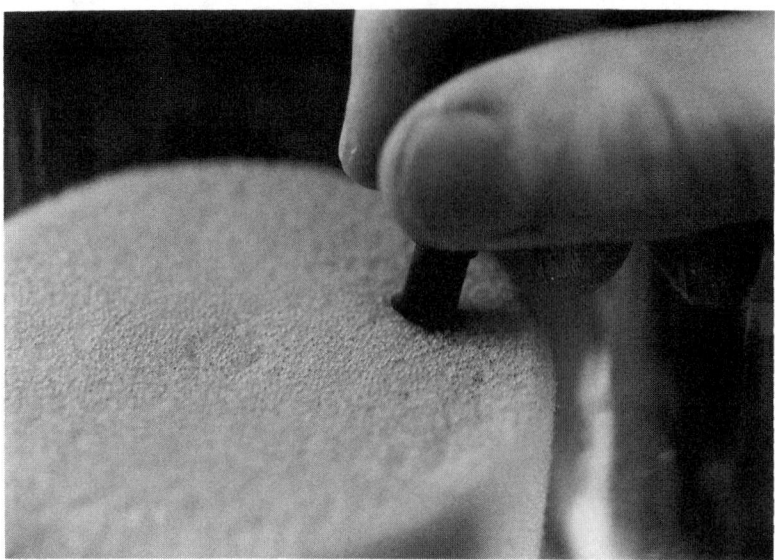

Figure 9-16.   The use of a flat sponge tool for polishing the front surface of an RGP lens.

should be removed every 15 seconds to evaluate both the surface and the optical quality with a lensometer.

(b)   Method 2. Very light scratches and surface deposits may be removed adequately using one of several available hand-polishing pads. Typically, the front surface of the lens is rubbed into the pad, which has been presoaked with polish. Prolonged polishing, however, may result in small microscratches.

(2)   Concave surface. Although it is rare for the posterior surface to become scratched, it is not uncommon for deposits to adhere because of either insufficient lens movement or inadequate patient cleaning. These deposits may contribute to lens adherence to the cornea during extended wear.

(a)   Method 1. To polish the concave surface, the lens is mounted to a suction cup concave side out. A cone-shaped sponge premoistened with water is placed on the spindle. After the spindle is rotating, polishing compound is added and the suction cup is tilted slightly, with the lens placed just off the center of the sponge. With the lens depressed into the sponge, the suction cup is rotated with the fingers opposite the rotation of the spindle for 10–15 seconds. This may be repeated, if necessary, after inspection.

d.   Repowering. A significant advantage to fitting RGP lenses is the ability to modify the power of the lens in-office to provide an immediate improvement in the patient's visual acuity. This is also very cost-effective in comparison to ordering a new lens.

(1)   Adding minus

(a)   Method 1. Minus power addition is much more common than plus. An unconventional but effective method is to use a Dr. Scholl's medium toepad on a specially manufactured plexiglas tool (made by Howard Brown, Indiana University School of Optometry, Bloomington, IN).[23] The toepad is wetted with water and polish and mounted on the spindle. As the toepad rotates, the lens (mounted convex side out) is positioned perpendicular to the toepad approximately 1 to 1.5 cm from its apex (Figure 9-17). As the

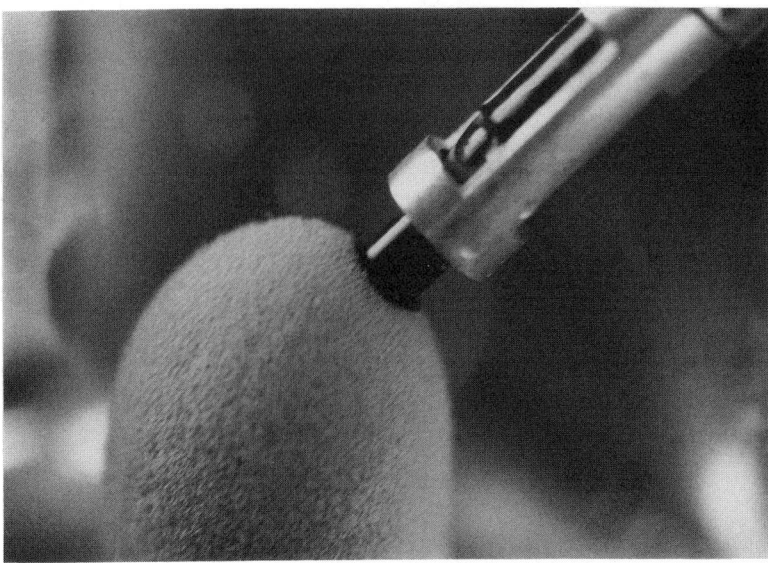

Figure 9-17.   The proper method of adding minus power using a toepad tool and spinner.

lens rotates, apical thickness is reduced faster than peripheral thickness and a flatter front curvature is achieved, resulting in increased minus power. The power should be monitored every 10–15 seconds.

(b)   Method 2. A traditional method of adding minus power utilizes a flat velveteen-covered drum tool or flat sponge. The lens is attached to the suction cup (or spinner) convex side out approximately $1/2$ inch inside the peripheral edge (Figure 9-18). The principle behind this method is that the periphery of the flat tool spins faster than the center. Barely touching the surface, the lens is

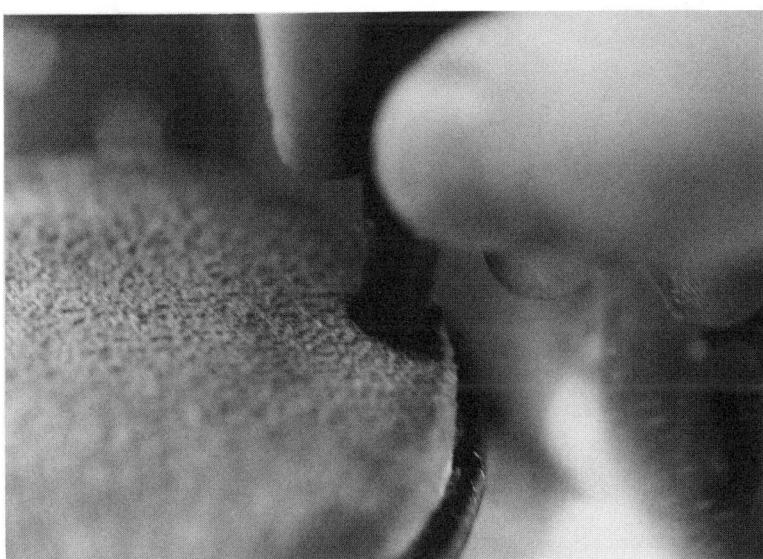

Figure 9-18.   The use of a velveteen-covered pad and suction cup for adding minus power.

rotated against the motion of the tool. As a few revolutions can increase the minus power by 0.50D (the practical limit to maintain optical quality), the optical quality should be evaluated several seconds after the procedure is initiated.

(2) Adding plus

    (a) Method 1. The toepad and spinner can be used in a similar manner as with adding minus power. However, once the spinner is rotating, the angle of the spinner and lens should be lowered until approximately one-half to one-third of the lens is in contact with the toepad, then the spinner should be torqued out of vertical alignment with the toepad so that only the periphery of the lens is in contact with the toepad. Plus power is being added as material is being removed from the periphery of the lens and not the center. It is more time-consuming to add plus power, however, and 0.50D is the practical limit.

    (b) Method 2. The drum tool or flat sponge tool can be used to add plus power as well. The lens is placed at the center of the tool (not the periphery) and is rotated with the fingers or with the spinner against the rotation of the pad. Since the drum speed of rotation is zero at its center, more lens material is removed from the lens edge. As with minus power, no more than 0.50D should be added.

IX. Summary

This chapter has attempted to provide a concise clinical approach to contact lens material selection, lens design, fitting, care, and problem-solving. For fitting specialty designs (e.g., torics, bifocals, and keratoconic lenses), the author's text *Clinical Manual of Contact Lenses* is recommended.[24] As contact lens materials change frequently, it is important not only to read texts and published articles but also to attend continuing education courses, particularly those which are video-aided, in an effort to supplement your contact lens education.

References

1. Korb DR, Herman JP. Corneal staining subsequent to sequential fluorescein instillations. *J Am Optom Assoc* 1979;50:361–367.

2. Josephson JE. Chapter 4: Examination of the anterior ocular surface and tear film. In Stein HA, Slatt BJ, Stein RM. *Fitting Guide for Rigid and Soft Contact Lens,* ed 3. St. Louis: CV Mosby, 1990:39–50.

3. Bennett ES, Gordon JM. The borderline dry-eye patient and contact lens wear. *Contact Lens Forum* 1989;14(7):52–74.

4. Nelson PS. A short Schirmer test. *Optom Monthly* 1982;73:568–569.

5. Hamano T, Mitsunaga S, Kotani S, et al. Tear volume in relation to contact lens wear and age. *CLAO J* 1990;16:57–61.

6. Sakamoto R, Bennett ES, Henry VA et al. The Phenol Red Thread Tear Test: A cross cultural study. Poster presented at the Annual Meeting of the American Academy of Optometry, December 1992, Orlando, FL.

7. Zuccaro VS. Rose bengal: A vital stain. *Contact Lens Forum* 1981;6:39–43.

8. Benjamin WJ. Chapter 14: Visual optics of contact lens wear. In: Bennett ES, Weissman BA, eds. *Clinical Contact Lens Practice*. Philadelphia: J.P. Lippincott, 1991:1–42.

9. Holden BA, Mertz GW. Critical oxygen levels to avoid corneal edema for daily and extended wear contact lenses. *Invest Ophthalmol Vis Sci* 1984;25:1161.

10. Bennett ES, Henry VA, Davis LJ, Kirby S. Comparing empirical and diagnostic fitting of daily wear fluoro-silicone/acrylate contact lenses. *Contact Lens Forum* 1989;14(3):38.

11. McLaughlin R, Barr JT, Rosenthal P, et al. The new generation of RGP solutions meets increasing demands. *Contact Lens Spectrum* 1990;5(1):45–50.

12. MacMillian TF, Benjamin WJ. Cleaning and storage of rigid contact lenses prior to dispensing. *J Am Optom Assoc* 1992;63:333–342.

13. Begley CG, Weirich B, Benak J, Pence NA. Effects of rigid gas permeable contact lens solutions on the human corneal epithelium. *Optom Vis Sci* 1992;69:347–353.

14. Carrell BA, Bennett ES, Henry VA, Grohe RM. The effect of rigid gas permeable lens cleaners on lens parameter stability. *J Am Optom Assoc* 1992;63:193–198.

15. Mandell RB. Chapter 12: Lens care and storage. In: *Contact Lens Practice*. 4th ed. Springfield, IL: Charles C. Thomas, 1988:326–351.

16. Bennett ES. Chapter 4: Rigid lens care and patient education. In: Bennett ES, Henry VA. *Clinical Manual of Contact Lenses*. Philadelphia: J.P. Lippincott. 1994.

17. Bennett ES, Grohe RM. Chapter 25: Lens care and patient education. In: Bennett ES, Weissman BA, eds. *Clinical Contact Lens Practice*. Philadelphia: J.P. Lippincott, 1991:1–14.

18. Wilson L, et al. Contamination of contact lens cases and solutions. *Am J Ophthalmol* 1990;110:193–198.

19. Hill RM, Brezinski SD. The center thickness factor. *Contact Lens Spectrum* 1987;2(10):52.

20. Grohe RM, Caroline PJ. RGP non-wetting syndrome. *Contact Lens Spectrum* 1989;4(3):32–44.

21. Henry VA, Bennett ES, Forrest JF. Clinical investigation of the Paraperm EW rigid gas permeable contact lens. *Am J Optom Physiol Opt* 1987;64:313–320.

22. Rengstorff RH. The Fort Dix Report: Longitudinal effects of contact lenses. *Am J Optom Arch Am Acad Optom* 1965;42:153–163.

23. Morgan BW, Bennett ES. Chapter 27: Modification. In: Bennett ES, Weissman BA. *Clinical Contact Lens Practice* Philadelphia: J.P. Lippincott, 1991:1–19.

24. Bennett ES, Henry VA. *Clinical Manual of Contact Lenses*. Philadelphia: J.P. Lippincott. 1994.

CHAPTER **10**

Binocular Vision Problems

John R. Griffin
Graham B. Erickson

This is a brief overview of the anomalies of binocular vision. Emphasis is on detection and diagnosis; however, basic clinical approaches in vision therapy are presented that are appropriate for the primary eye care practitioner. The Suggested Readings at the end of this chapter are a resource for more detailed coverage of diagnosis and therapy.

I. **Case History of Strabismus**

The clinician should ask questions that help establish a diagnosis of strabismus. Information is needed regarding the time of onset, mode of onset, frequency of onset, contributing factors, and previous treatment. Relevant questions to patients (or parents of infants and children) are listed below.

Strabismus Case History

When was the eyeturn first noticed?
Which eye turned?
Was it always the same eye that turned?
Was the turning all the time or only part of the time?
If part time, was the eyeturn associated with a particular time of day, viewing distance, position of gaze, or particular activity?
Was the turning in, out, up, or down?
Did the eyeturn appear suddenly or gradually?
Was it a result of injury or other health problems?
Has the eyeturn become better or worse since the onset?
If the eyeturn has changed, was it in the magnitude and/or frequency?
Were there any symptoms associated with the eyeturn, e.g., double vision?
Was any treatment given? If so, when did it begin? What kind of treatment?
How long did it last? What were the results of treatment?
Is there a family history of an eyeturn?
What are the main concerns, e.g., cosmetic appearance only?

II. **Strabismus in Primary Gaze**

Both objective and subjective testing should be done when strabismus is suspected. These tests, when corroborated by a case history, provide the diagnosis of the deviation of the visual axes.

Clinical Alert

For all baseline data, any existing ametropia must be optically corrected. In addition, all testing should be performed at both far (6 m) and near (40 cm).

A. *Objective tests*
1. Direct observation
   Guidelines
   a. Purpose. Assessment of cosmesis.
   b. Equipment. None.
   c. Procedure. Observation of intermittency, eye dominance, unilateral versus alternating strabismus, changes in magnitude with varying gaze position and fixation distance, presence of abnormal head posture, and the cosmetic appearance of the deviation under ordinary conditions in true space (i.e., out of instruments).
   d. Results. Obvious ocular deviation, head tilt, or lid abnormalities may direct further testing.

Clinical Alert

Epicanthal folds may cause a nonstrabismic individual to appear to be esotropic. Also abnormal head posture is suggestive of nonconcomitancy.

2. Hirschberg test
   Guidelines
   a. Purpose. Refinement of direct observations (more sensitive).
   b. Equipment. Penlight or transilluminator.
   c. Procedure. The patient fixates the penlight which is in the midline at eye level, from approximately 75 to 100 cm, while the examiner's sighting eye is directly behind the penlight.
   d. Results. The relative position of each corneal light reflex is assessed in relation to the center of each pupil. For example, temporal displacement of a light reflex indicates esotropia (negative angle kappa). (Figures 10-1 and 10-2 for clarification.) Each millimeter of relative displacement of the light reflex represents approximately 22^Δ of strabismic deviation.

Clinical Alert

The presence of anatomical factors such as corectopia (displaced pupil) may affect the estimated magnitude of the deviation.

3. Brückner test
   Guidelines
   a. Purpose. Detection of an angle of strabismus less than 5^Δ.
   b. Equipment. Direct ophthalmoscope.
   c. Procedure. At approximately 75 to 100 cm, the direct ophthalmoscope light is directed toward the patient's nose so that both eyes are illuminated simultaneously. The examiner observes the fundus reflex of each eye to determine if the brightness is equal.
   d. Results. If a strabismus is present, the deviating eye will appear to be brighter than the fixating eye. This test is often sensitive to strabismic angles as small as 1^Δ.

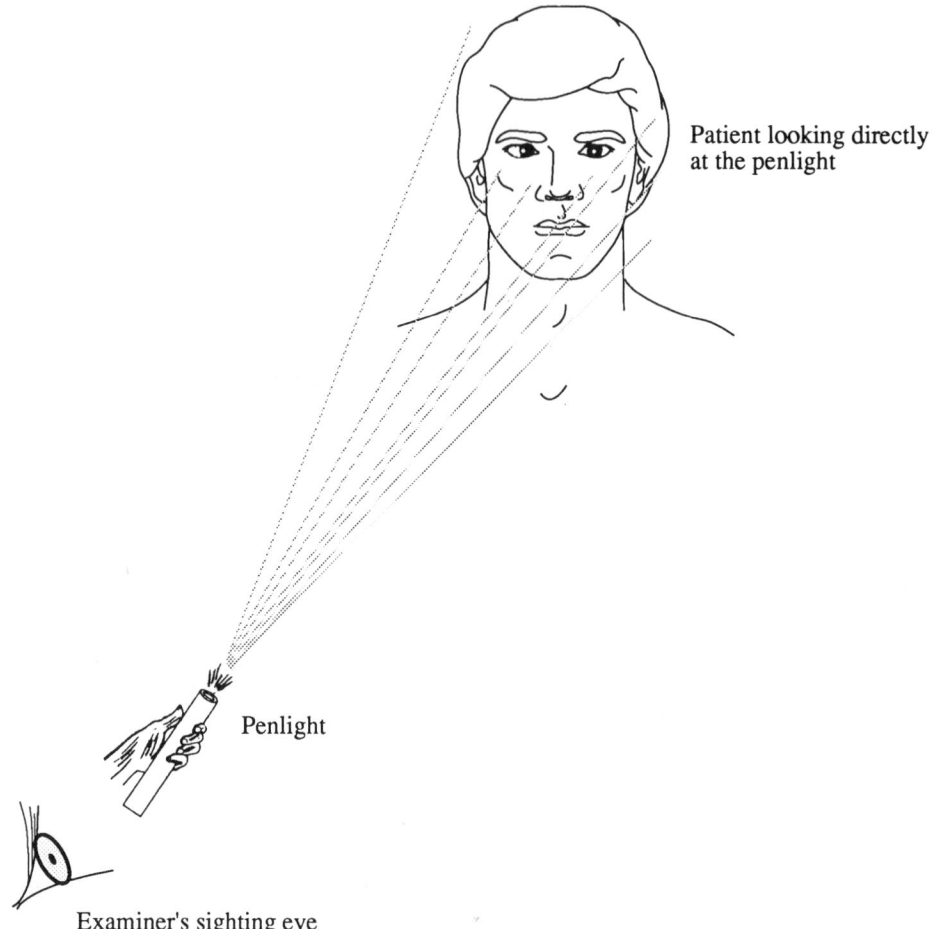

Patient looking directly at the penlight

Penlight

Examiner's sighting eye

Figure 10-1.   Hirschberg test. Objective view of patient with esotropia of the right eye.

Clinical Alert

Anisometropia will also cause a relative brightness difference of the fundus reflexes. Also, the Brückner test may be unreliable because of anisocoria, pigmentary differences, and other factors.

---

4. Unilateral cover test
    Guidelines
    a. Purpose. Determination of heterophoria versus heterotropia, unilateral versus alternating strabismus, intermittent versus constant strabismus, eye dominancy, direction of the deviation, and estimation of the magnitude of strabismus.
    b. Equipment. Occluder, detailed fixation target (to control for accommodation).
    c. Procedure. The occluder is introduced before one eye as the unoccluded eye is observed for any movement. This is repeated several times, allowing adequate time for refixation after each occlusion. This sequence is also performed for the other eye (Figure 10-3).

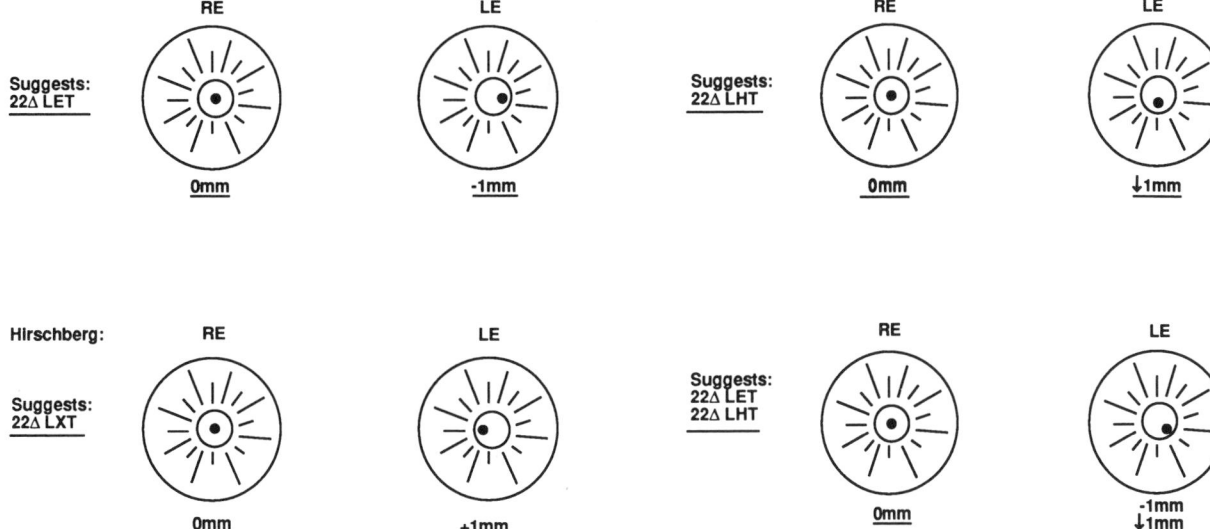

Key: **Reflex displacement is recorded in millimeters with the appropriate sign,**

i.e., nasal displacement is (+), temporal (-), vertical up (↑) or down (↓).

Figure 10-2.   Examples of Hirschberg test results.

d.   Results. An inward movement of the unoccluded eye indicates exotropia. An outward movement indicates esotropia. Hypertropia is indicated by a downward movement. The examiner estimates the magnitude of the deviation based on the amount of movement observed. The strabismus is unilateral if only one eye is observed to move. In an alternating strabismus, movement may occur with occlusion of either eye; however, the dominant eye will move (deviate) less frequently. Constant strabismus is suggested when movement is observed every time the fixating eye is occluded. The unoccluded eye is not expected to move in cases of heterophoria.

Clinical Alert

A "sympathetic" movement of the unoccluded eye may occasionally be observed in large heterophoria. In such cases, the examiner should look at the eye behind the occluder to see the eye moving to its dissociated posture.

---

5.   Alternate cover test
     Guidelines
     a.   Purpose. Measurement of the angle of deviation of the visual axes (whether heterophoric or heterotropic).
     b.   Equipment. Occluder, detailed fixation target, prisms (loose prisms or prism bar).
     c.   Procedure. Following the unilateral cover test, each eye is alternately occluded at a rate of approximately 2 seconds per occlusion, maintaining dissociation of the vision of each eye. The examiner estimates the magnitude of the

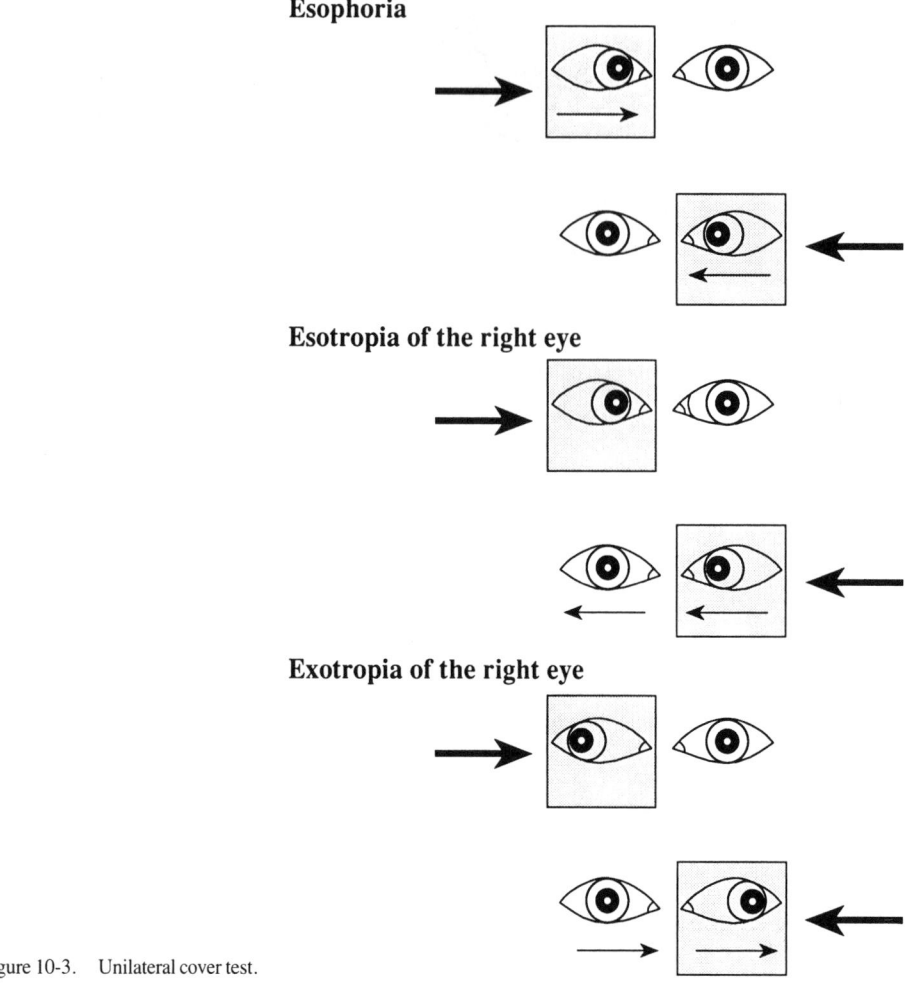

Esophoria

Esotropia of the right eye

Exotropia of the right eye

Figure 10-3.   Unilateral cover test.

deviation, in prism diopters, based on the amount of eye movement observed. A neutralizing prism of approximately the estimated magnitude is placed between the occluder and the deviating (nondominant) eye, as determined previously by the unilateral cover test. (Figure 10-4.) The occluder is then switched to the other eye while the examiner closely watches for any movement of the eye behind the prism. Neutrality is reached when there is no movement behind the prism. Further refinement can be accomplished by bracketing, i.e., with prism powers that slightly under- and overcorrect the deviation. This procedure is repeated with the prism before the other eye.

d. Results. Base-out prism neutralizes an eso deviation; base-in neutralizes an exo deviation; and base-down neutralizes a hyper deviation.

Clinical Alert

The presence of eccentric fixation affects the measurement of the angle of deviation. For example, a nasal eccentric fixation will cause an eso deviation to be measured smaller than the true magnitude.

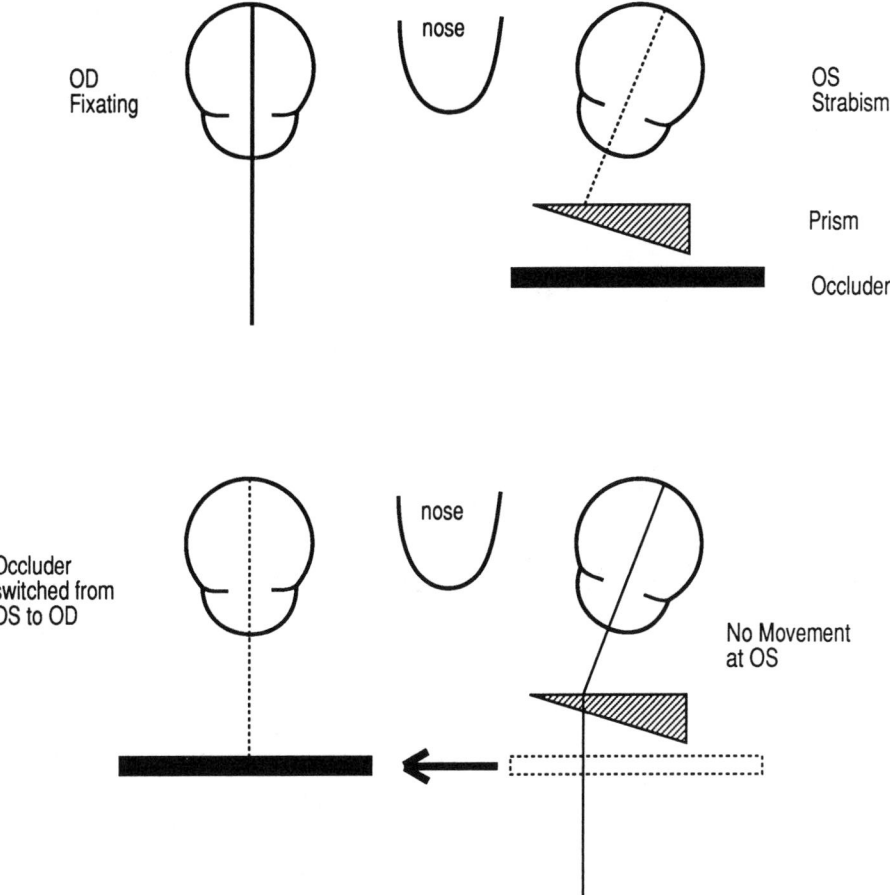

Figure 10-4.   Illustration of procedure for the alternate cover test.

6.   Four base-out prism test
    Guidelines
    a.   Purpose. Objective detection of a very small angle of strabismus.
    b.   Equipment. 4^Δ loose prism, detailed fixation target.
    c.   Procedure. The patient is asked to fixate the target while the examiner quickly places the prism in a base-out orientation before the suspected deviating eye. The examiner observes both eyes for any movement. The procedure is then repeated with the prism before the other eye.
    d.   Results. If there is no strabismus present, a slight convergence movement will be observed (Figure 10-5). If there is strabismus, however, there will be no eye movement observed when the prism is placed before the deviating eye (assuming central suppression of that eye); but when the prism is placed before the fixating eye, a version movement will be observed (Figure 10-6).

Clinical Alert

In most cases of normal binocular vision, the examiner will observe a version movement of the patient's eyes before there is a convergence response. The direction and magnitude of a strabismic deviation is not measured with this test.

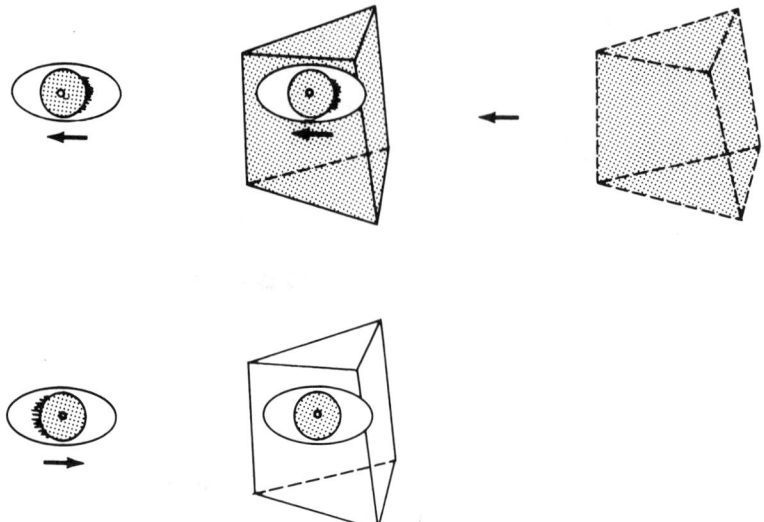

Figure 10-5.   Nonstrabismic response on the four base-out prism test.

B.   *Subjective tests*
1.   Maddox rod test
Guidelines
a.   Purpose. Determination of the direction and magnitude of the subjective angle of deviation.
b.   Equipment. Maddox rod, penlight or transilluminator, prisms.
c.   Procedure. The Maddox rod (clinically most often rods) is placed with its axis at 180° (rod horizontal) before the fixating eye while the patient fixates the penlight held in the midline at 40 cm. If suppression does not interfere, the patient should simultaneously see a vertically oriented red streak of light and the white fixation light. The patient is asked to report the position of the red streak in relation to the white fixation light. The examiner places the estimated amount of neutralizing prism before the eye with the Maddox rod;

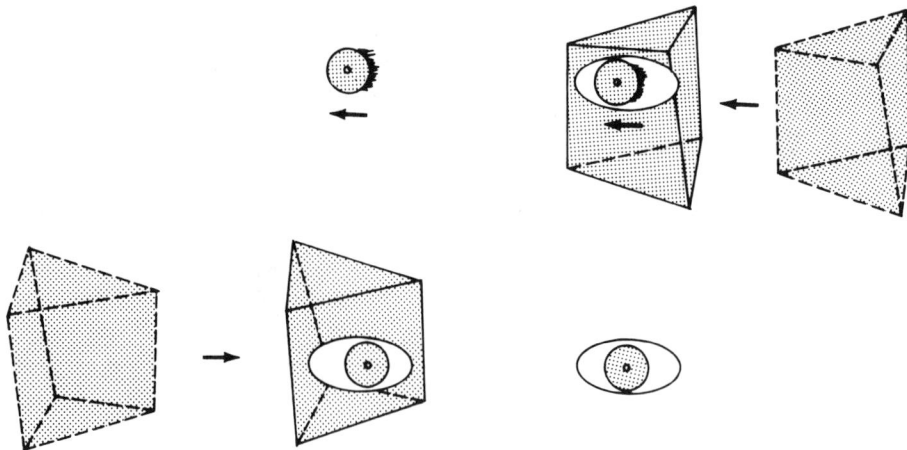

Figure 10-6.   Example of the response on the four base-out prism test of a patient with esotropia of the right eye.

neutrality is reached when the red streak is perceived to be exactly in the center of the fixation light. This procedure is repeated with the fixation light at 6 m.

d. Results. If the red streak passes directly through the fixation light without prisms, no deviation is presumed, since the subjective angle is zero. A heterophoria or heterotropia will cause the red streak to be displaced in a direction specific to the direction of the deviation. For example, an "uncrossed" (eso) deviation is present when the Maddox rod is held before the right eye and the streak is perceived to be to the right (patient's) of the fixation light. In a "crossed" (exo) deviation, the red streak would appear to be to the patient's left of the fixation light. If a right hyper deviation is present, the red streak is seen below the fixation light, and base-down prism must be introduced before the right eye to neutralize the vertical deviation.

Clinical Alert

This test does not differentiate between a heterophoria and a heterotropia. Also, the presence of anomalous correspondence (ARC) will affect the results of this test.

---

2. Red lens test
    Guidelines
    a. Purpose. Determination of the direction and estimated magnitude of the subjective angle of deviation.
    b. Equipment. Red lens, penlight or transilluminator, prisms.
    c. Procedure. The patient is asked to look at the white light held in the midline at 40 cm. The red lens is introduced before the normally fixating eye. (Figure 10-7.) Assuming suppression is not interfering, the patient should report seeing either a fused (pink-colored) light or diplopic lights (a red and a white light). If the patient sees two lights, the examiner should inquire where the white light is located in relation to the red light. The estimated amount of neutralizing prism is then placed before the eye without the red lens; neutrality is achieved when the two lights are fused into one. Bracketing of the responses is recommended for accuracy of the magnitude measurement, as well as providing information on the patient's sensory-motor fusion ability. (Good sensory-motor fusion is indicated if a pink light is still reported when either a base-in or a base-out prism of additional power is introduced.) This procedure is repeated at 6 m.
    d. Results. A fusion response indicates no manifest deviation; however, a heterophoria or intermittent strabismus may be present, but compensated for, if there is adequate sensory-motor fusion. When two lights are reported, the direction of the deviation is related to the position of the red light, as when interpreting results of the Maddox rod test.

Clinical Alert

The presence of anomalous correspondence (ARC) will affect the results of this test.

---

3. Von Graefe method
    Guidelines
    a. Purpose. Measurement of the subjective angle of deviation of the visual axes.

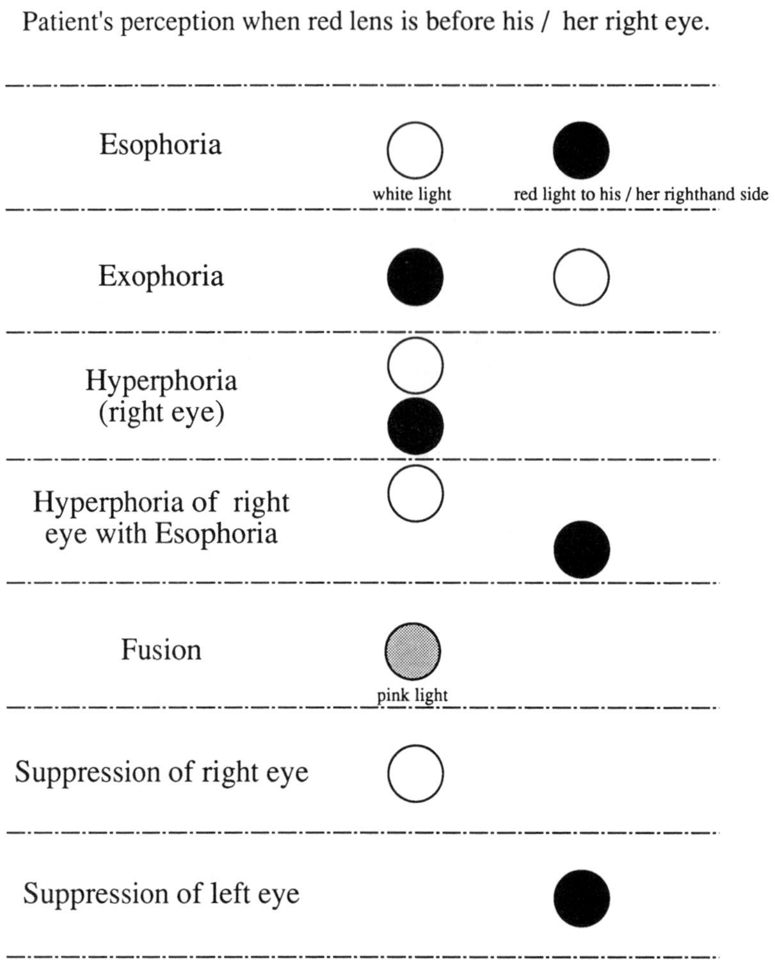

Patient's perception when red lens is before his / her right eye.

Esophoria

white light   red light to his / her righthand side

Exophoria

Hyperphoria
(right eye)

Hyperphoria of right
eye with Esophoria

Fusion

pink light

Suppression of right eye

Suppression of left eye

Figure 10-7.   Red lens test.

b. Equipment. Phoropter, nearpoint acuity card, farpoint acuity chart.
c. Procedure. The following is a suggested clinical method. At 40 cm, the patient fixates (through the phoropter) a vertical line of threshold acuity letters on a nearpoint acuity card. Risley prisms are placed before both eyes, 6^Δ base-up before the left eye and approximately 14^Δ base-in before the right eye. The patient should observe two columns of letters, the top one being to the left of the bottom ("uncrossed" diplopia), provided the deviation is (1) eso, (2) ortho, or (3) less than 14^Δ of exo. If suppression is a problem so that only one column is perceived, the examiner should "flash" the right eye with an occluder (allowing only brief exposures) while attempting the measurement. The patient is instructed to watch the bottom target (keeping the letters clear) and respond when the top column appears to be directly above the bottom one as the examiner slowly rotates the Risley prism of the right eye to decrease the amount of base-in power. To determine the presence of a vertical deviation, a horizontal row of threshold-sized letters is displayed with the patient attending to the top row of letters. The vertically oriented Risley prism over the left eye is then rotated until the patient reports that the rows are in horizontal alignment. This procedure should be repeated at 6 m, but with a

single letter target that is larger than threshold. Responses should be brack-
eted for increased accuracy.

d. Results. The magnitude of the deviation is read directly in prism diopters
from the Risley prism scale. The direction of the prism orientation indicates
the direction of the deviation. For example, base-out prism neutralizes an eso
deviation.

Clinical Alert

This test will not differentiate a heterophoria from a heterotropia. Results are
also invalidated by anomalous correspondence (ARC).

C. *Variables of the deviation*

1. Concomitancy. Concomitancy (clinically often referred to as "comitancy") is
determined by evaluating the magnitude of the deviation in various positions of
gaze. This is discussed in detail in section III.

2. Frequency. Frequency of the deviation is determined mainly by the objective
tests discussed throughout this section. However, subjective reports of diplopia
are also very beneficial in the estimation of the strabismus. A daily journal by the
patient helps document the frequency of diplopia, as well as objective reports
from others (family and friends) who notice the strabismus on a cosmetic basis.
This documentation also allows assessment of other variables such as direction,
laterality, and possibly causative factors (e.g., fatigue). With testing and this
documentation, the clinician is able to judge whether the strabismus is constant
(100% of the time) or intermittent (deviation manifest between 1% and 99% of
the time). The less frequent the strabismus, the better is the prognosis for functional cure (discussed in the section entitled "Strabismus Prognosis").

3. Direction. The deviation can be horizontal, vertical, torsional, or any combination of the three directions (Table 10-1). This variable will have a strong impact
on the prognosis (discussed in section V).

4. Eye laterality. Laterality of the deviation is determined by using the objective
tests discussed in this section. For example, the unilateral cover test will differentiate whether the deviation is unilateral or alternating. The examiner should make
the judgment in the case of alternating strabismus whether it is essential (habitual) or forced (conscious effort required by the patient to effect alternation).

5. Eye dominancy. This is most easily assessed by sighting tests such as the hole-in-
the-card test. With both hands, the patient holds a card with a small hole in its
center. The patient sights a distant fixation target through the hole as the card is
held at arm's length, and each eye of the patient is occluded to determine the eye
preferred for fixation. This method is necessary in cases of heterophoria, or
latent intermittent strabismus, since there is no observable manifest deviation.

Table 10-1. Direction of Deviation

Horizontal	Vertical	Torsional
Eso	Hyper	Incyclo
Exo	Hypo	Excyclo

The deviation may be mixed, e.g., esotropia and hypertropia.

The objective tests discussed in this section also help determine the dominant eye. On subjective tests, as a rule, the nondominant eye is the suppressing eye.

Clinical Alert

In cases of extraocular muscle paresis, the dominant eye may sometimes be affected. In such cases, the deviation is larger than if the nonaffected eye is fixating (because of Hering's law of equal innervation).

---

6. Magnitude. The magnitude of the deviation is assessed with the alternate cover test and with the subjective tests discussed in this section. This is an important prognostic measurement (prognosis is usually less favorable with increased magnitudes).
7. AC/A. This is the accommodative-convergence to accommodation ratio. Objective measurements of the angle of deviation (whether strabismic or phoric) can be made at far (6 m) and near (40 cm) with the alternate cover test. From these two measurements, a far-near AC/A can be calculated:

$$AC/A = IPD + 0.4 \, (H_n - H_f)$$
$$IPD = \text{interpupillary distance in centimeters}$$
$$H_n = \text{angle of deviation at near}$$
$$H_f = \text{angle of deviation at far}$$

Note: Exo is $(-)$ and eso is $(+)$
For example, if an exo deviation is 5^Δ at far and 10^Δ at near:

$$AC/A = 6 + 0.4 \, [-10 - (-5)]$$
$$AC/A = 4^\Delta/1 \, D$$

Clinical Alert

This is only a calculated representation of the true AC/A, which is the change in accommodative vergence associated with the change in accommodative response at a fixed distance (usually a laboratory measurement). Due to proximal effects when measuring from far to near, the calculated method often results in a slightly higher ratio than the true AC/A. This is especially so when comparing the calculated ratio with the clinical gradient method for estimating the AC/A.

---

8. Variability. The magnitude of the deviation for any test distance may change from one time to another, e.g., from day to day. It is not unusual to measure a difference in magnitude up to 5^Δ in subsequent examinations. This may be attributable either to examiner measurement error or to physiologic variability. Significant changes in magnitude, however, may be due to several factors, such as the influence of medication, alcohol, fatigue, and emotional stress. Also, any pathologic or neurologic factors (e.g., cerebral palsy) that affect the magnitude should be accounted for. The concern of most patients is the effect of variability on cosmesis.

Clinical Alert

Variability pertains to the primary position of gaze, and should not be confused with the factor of nonconcomitancy, which causes variation in the magnitude from one gaze position to another.

9. Cosmesis. The main concern of many strabismic patients is their cosmetic appearance. An esotropic patient's cosmesis is adversely affected by one or more of the following factors: (a) negative angle kappa (corneal light reflex temporal to center of pupil) of the fixating eye, (b) wide nasal bridge, (c) epicanthal folds, (d) small interpupillary distance, (e) wide face. Conversely, an exotropic patient's cosmesis is adversely affected by (a) positive angle kappa (corneal light reflex nasal to pupillary center), (b) narrow nasal bridge, (c) lack of epicanthal folds, (d) large interpupillary distance, (e) narrow face.

Clinical Alert

Prisms incorporated in spectacle lenses may exacerbate the cosmetic appearance of the strabismus. For example, base-out prisms will exaggerate the appearance of esotropia. The examiner should be sensitive to the patient's cosmetic concerns when prismatic spectacles are considered as a treatment option.

---

10. Diagnostic examples. Variables of the deviation are put together to form a diagnostic statement of the strabismic deviation.
    a. Example 1. Concomitant, constant, unilateral, right esotropia of 25^Δ at far and near, 6/1 AC/A, nonvariable deviation, and fair cosmesis.
    b. Example 2. Concomitant, intermittent (30% of the time at far, 5% at near), unilateral, right exotropia of 25^Δ at far and 15^Δ at near, 10/1 AC/A, basic deviation varying approximately 8^Δ from day to day, and poor cosmesis when deviation is manifest at far.
    c. Example 3. Concomitant, constant, alternating (left eye preferred), esotropia of 15^Δ at far and near, 6/1 AC/A, nonvariable deviation, and fair cosmesis. (Complete diagnoses with additional variables will be discussed later, along with appropriate prognoses.)

III. Action of the Extraocular Muscles and Concomitancy

A. *Action of extraocular muscles and description of diagnostic action fields (DAFs)*
There are six extraocular muscles (EOMs) per eye. In the primary position, the medial rectus is for adduction, the lateral rectus for abduction, the superior rectus for supraduction and incycloduction, the inferior oblique for supraduction and excycloduction, the inferior rectus for infraduction and excycloduction, and the superior oblique for infraduction and incycloduction.

The eye can be moved to DAFs whereby the individual action of each EOM is isolated. For example, if the right eye is abducted approximately 25°, the only elevating muscle is the superior rectus. When the eye is in the upward and outward position, the integrity of

Table 10-2. Diagnostic Action Fields of Extraocular Muscles

Eye Position	Right Eye	Left Eye
Right Gaze	Lateral rectus	Medial rectus
Left Gaze	Medial rectus	Lateral rectus
25° right gaze and up	Superior rectus	Inferior oblique
25° left gaze and up	Inferior oblique	Superior rectus
25° right gaze and down	Inferior rectus	Superior oblique
25° left gaze and down	Superior oblique	Inferior rectus

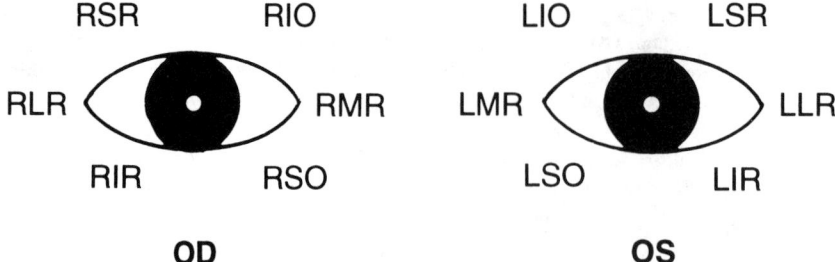

Figure 10-8.   Position of the diagnostic action field of each extraocular muscle.

the superior rectus muscle can be assessed. The DAFs for each eye are given in Table 10-2 (Figure 10-8 for illustration).

Clinical Alert

Theoretically, the oblique muscles should be adducted 57° for pure vertical action; similarly, the vertical recti should be abducted 23° (see Figure 10-9 for clarification). Since 57° of adduction is clinically impractical, a compromise of approximately 25° in either direction allows for sufficient magnitude of horizontal excursion in the assessment of the four cyclovertical muscles of an eye.

B.   *Monocular testing (ductions)*
   Guidelines
   1.   Purpose. To assess the integrity of the EOMs.
   2.   Equipment. Fixation target (e.g., penlight), occluder.

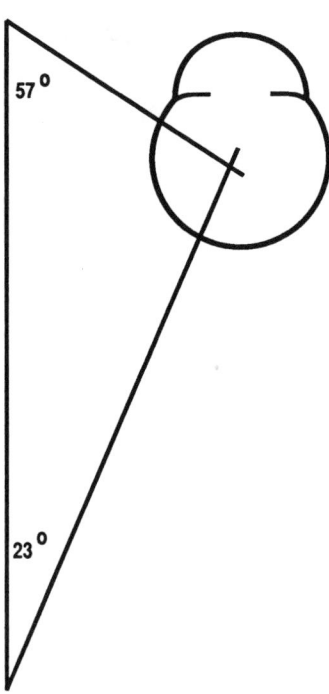

Figure 10-9.   Top view of the right eye in the primary position of gaze illustrating the principal incycloduction effect of the superior oblique and the principal supraduction effect of the superior rectus.

3. Procedure. The DAF of each EOM is assessed by having the patient monocularly (one eye occluded) fixate a penlight target in the six diagnostic positions of gaze. For example, the right superior rectus (RSR) is tested by having the patient look up at the penlight which is approximately 25° to his or her right. This is done either as a pursuit eye movement or a saccadic movement from primary position to the diagnostic position of gaze.

4. Results. An underaction of an EOM is indicated when there is an insufficient excursion into the diagnostic position of gaze. Underactions may be due to mechanical restriction, paresis (partial paralysis), or paralysis.

Clinical Alert

Underactions due to mechanical restrictions are fast, but the excursion is insufficient. On the other hand, a mildly paretic EOM does not always cause a noticeable underaction, but the velocity of the saccade from the primary position to the diagnostic position of gaze is abnormally slow.

C. *Binocular testing for concomitancy*

If the deviation remains the same in all positions of gaze, it is concomitant (clinically often called "comitant"). If the deviation is different by 6$^\Delta$ or more in one or more positions, it is considered to be nonconcomitant (may be referred to as "noncomitant" or "incomitant"). A possible exception may be in the case of "A" (relatively more eso in upgaze) or "V" (relatively more eso in downgaze) patterns in which up and down gaze magnitudes may slightly exceed this criterion. Clinicians do not generally consider mild "A" or "V" patterns to be nonconcomitant deviations.

Nonconcomitancy is either nuclear or infranuclear (i.e., below the nucleus of III, IV, or VI) in etiology, due to the following reasons: (a) a disease of one or more EOMs causing dysfunction (least common), (b) a mechanical restriction of one or more EOMs, or most commonly, (c) a lesion of cranial nerves III, IV, or VI. Symptoms of nonconcomitancy often include diplopia, nausea, vertigo, headaches, abnormal head posture, or awareness of loss of stereoscopic vision.

Clinical Alert

A supranuclear (above the nucleus of III, IV, or VI) lesion results in restricted pursuit and saccadic eye movements, but the deviation is concomitant.

---

1. Versions
   Guidelines
   a. Purpose. To determine under- or overaction of any EOM.
   b. Equipment. Fixation target (e.g., penlight).
   c. Procedure. The procedure is the same as that described in duction testing (section III,b.), except that neither eye is occluded. In addition to the six diagnostic positions of gaze described in monocular testing, the primary, straight-up, and straight-down positions are also important in binocular assessment. These nine diagnostic positions of gaze are primary position, dextroversion, levoversion, supraversion, dextrosupraversion, levosupraversion, infraversion, dextroinfraversion, and levoinfraversion. A penlight can be used as a fixation target in each of these nine positions for Hirschberg testing, to determine if the strabismic angle increases or decreases in each position of

Table 10-3. Estimation Ranking of Nonconcomitancy Severity

0 = no underaction	0 = no overaction
1− = mild underaction	1+ = mild overaction
2− = moderate underaction	2+ = moderate overaction
3− = marked underaction	3+ = marked overaction
4− = no action	4+ = very marked overaction

gaze. If a strabismus is not manifest, a vertical prism (e.g., 8^Δ base-down) before an eye can be used for dissociation. Since fusion is broken, a manifest change in the deviation is observable. The eyes can make either saccadic or pursuit movements to reach each of the nine positions.

  d. Results. Overactions or underactions may be ranked on a scale of 1 to 4 (see Table 10-3), and they suggest nonconcomitancy. Some examples of underactions follow: If the right eye lags on dextroversion causing an eso deviation, the underacting EOM is the right lateral rectus (RLR). If the left eye lags on levoversion, the underacting EOM is the left lateral rectus (LLR). If the left eye lags on dextroversion causing an exo deviation, the underacting EOM is the left medial rectus (LMR). If the right eye lags on levoversion, the underacting EOM is the right medial rectus (RMR). For the eight cyclovertical muscles, the identification of the underacting muscle is more complicated; other tests, described below, are often necessary.

Clinical Alert

The clinician must be aware of which eye is fixating in order to determine if an eye is underacting or overacting. For example, if there is a greater eso deviation on dextroversion, is the right eye underacting or the left eye overacting? If the left eye is fixating, the right eye is underacting, as might occur with a paretic RLR. If, however, the right eye is fixating, the left eye is overacting. Observation of angle kappa aids in determining the fixating eye.

---

  2. Alternate cover test in diagnostic positions of gaze
      Guidelines
      a. Purpose. Objective quantification of nonconcomitancy.
      b. Equipment. Occluder, detailed fixation target, prisms.
      c. Procedure. The same as previously described for the primary gaze measurement (section II, 4 and 5); however, it is repeated in all other diagnostic positions of gaze. It is very important to keep the measuring prism centered before the eye in all positions of gaze. Unless care is taken, patients sometimes look around the prism rather than through it.
      d. Results. The affected eye with the underacting muscle can be differentiated from the unaffected eye. For example, paresis of the LLR would be expected to result in an eso deviation that is greater when the affected left eye is fixating than when the unaffected right eye is fixating. This procedure also allows the deviation to be measured in all positions of gaze. The ranking of severity of nonconcomitancy may be qualified as follows: $6–10^\Delta$ change in deviation is mild, $11–15^\Delta$ moderate, and greater than 16^Δ marked. This ranking can be applied to the 0 to 4 estimation scale for underaction and overaction severity (see Table 10-3).

Clinical Alert

An uncorrected anisometropia may give a false indication of nonconcomitancy, as if the primary and secondary angles of deviation were different. For example, an emmetropic right eye and a hyperopic left eye will result in a greater eso deviation when the left eye is fixating than when the right eye is fixating.

---

3. Park's three-step test
   Guidelines
   a. Purpose. To determine which cyclovertical EOM is underacting in a vertical nonconcomitant deviation.
   b. Equipment. Occluder, detailed fixation target.
   c. Procedure. Step 1: Observe which eye is more hyperphoric or hypertropic in the primary position of gaze. Step 2: Observe if the hyper deviation increases in either the right or left position of gaze (dextroversion or levoversion). Step 3: Observe if the hyper deviation increases on either right head tilt or left head tilt (Bielschowsky head tilt test). These observations can be made with the alternate cover test (preferred method) or the Hirschberg test (less sensitive).
   d. Results. The recorded results from the three steps can then be related to Table 10-4 to determine the underacting EOM, or the oval patterns may be used (see example in Figure 10-10).

Clinical Alert

The three-step method works only if there is *one* cyclovertical EOM underacting (usually paretic), and it may be unreliable if the paretic condition is of long duration due to a spread of concomitancy.

---

4. Red lens test in DAFs
   Guidelines
   a. Purpose. Estimation of the subjective angle of deviation in the diagnostic positions of gaze.
   b. Equipment. Red lens, penlight or transilluminator, prisms.
   c. Procedure. The same as previously described for the primary gaze measurement (section II, B, 2); however, the deviation is not neutralized with prism. If diplopia is present, the patient is asked to concentrate on one of the lights,

Table 10-4. Park's Three-Step Test Results

Hyper Eye in Primary Gaze	Hyper Increase on Gaze	Hyper Increase on Head Tilt	Underacting EOM
R	R	R	Left inferior oblique
R	R	L	Right inferior rectus
R	L	R	Right superior oblique
R	L	L	Left superior rectus
L	R	R	Right superior rectus
L	R	L	Left superior oblique
L	L	R	Left inferior rectus
L	L	L	Right inferior oblique

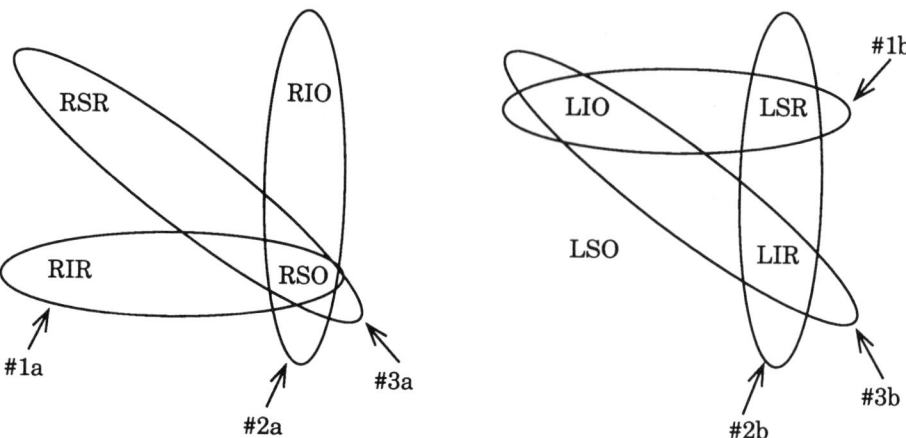

Step 1: Right Hyper can be caused by an underacting RIR, RSO, LIO or LSR (ovals #1a & b)

Step 2: Increased Right Hyper on left gaze can be due to an underacting RSO or LSR (ovals #2a & b)

Step 3: Increased Right Hyper on right head tilt (ovals #3a & b) is due to the underacting RSO because this affected muscle is included in all three ovals

Figure 10-10. Example of the ovals to determine that the isolated right superior oblique muscle is underacting as a result of testing with the three-step method.

noting the relative position of the other light, while the penlight or trans-illuminator is moved into the DAFs. If the separation of the lights changes, the DAF where the separation of the lights is the largest is determined. If diplopia is not present, a small vertical prism (e.g., 6^Δ) may be introduced to make the deviation manifest.

d. Results. If the diplopia is only horizontal, the muscles involved are either the medial or the lateral recti. If the deviation is only vertical or mixed horizontal and vertical, the vertical separation should be concentrated on first to identify the affected cyclovertical EOM. To determine the underacting EOM, the DAF where the image separation is largest (i.e., image projected farthest) must be identified. The eye with the underacting muscle will project the image toward the side where its movement is limited. For example, if the red lens is over the left eye and the red image is projected farther than the white image, the left eye has the underacting muscle. The DAF with the largest separation will identify the muscle that is affected in that eye.

Clinical Alert

This test is affected by the presence of anomalous correspondence (ARC). This procedure can also be performed with the Maddox rod (more dissociative); however, the horizontal and vertical components must be measured separately.

---

5. Two or more affected muscles
Careful analysis is required when more than one EOM is affected, e.g., in paresis. (For more details, refer to the Suggested Readings for information on Hess-Lancaster and other testing methods.) Interpretation of two affected muscles is illustrated in Figure 10-11.

If the RLR causes a moderate noncomitancy, the diagram is:

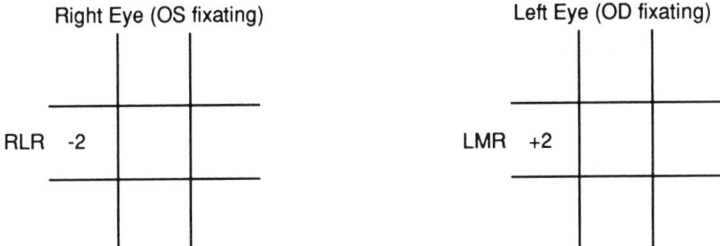

If the RSO causes a marked noncomitancy, the diagram is:

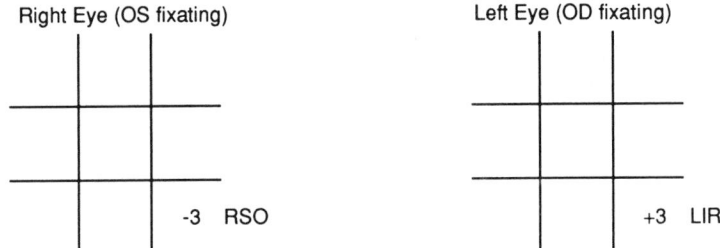

Combining the above examples (paretic RLR and RSO) results are as follows:

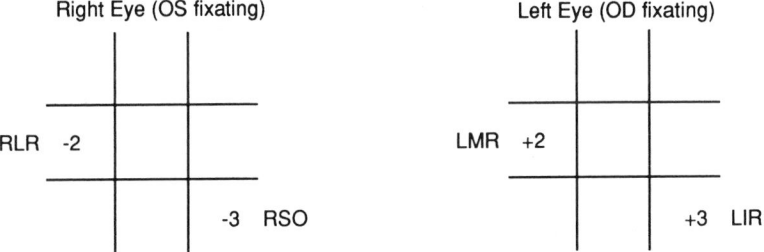

Figure 10-11. Example of underaction of both the right lateral rectus and the right superior oblique in a patient tested objectively (either Hirschberg or alternate cover test) and results assessed with the four-point estimation ranking of the severity of noncomitancy.

D. *Examples of nonconcomitant syndromes*

There are many syndromes that cause nonconcomitancy. Two of the most commonly encountered are Duane's syndrome and Brown's syndrome.

1. Duane's syndrome presents in several varieties; however, the classical pattern is a retraction of the globe in the orbit when the eye adducts, coupled with a simultaneous narrowing of the palpebral fissure. Commonly, there is an associated vertical deviation occurring with adduction. Severe limitation of abduction may also be present; consequently, there is an esotropia on temporal gaze. However, many patients have fusion in the primary position of gaze. A compensatory

head turn will be toward the restricted muscle action., e.g., head turn toward the left if the LLR is restricted.

There are a number of theories concerning the etiology of Duane's syndrome, both structural and innervational. Currently, an innervational disturbance of brain stem origin is the preferred theory, rather than structural muscle anomalies such as fibrosis. Some cases of Duane's syndrome are inherited as an autosomal dominant trait, but many do not have a familial origin.

Surgical treatment is often inefficacious and is only indicated if a significantly large deviation is present in the primary position of gaze. Vision therapy to improve sensory-motor fusion, and possibly prisms, may be beneficial in mild cases.

2. Brown's syndrome (also known as Brown's superior oblique tendon sheath syndrome) is characterized by greatly restricted elevation on adduction due to inferior oblique underaction. This is possibly due to a congenital anomaly of the sheath of the superior oblique tendon. Elevation is less restricted, or possibly normal, on abduction. Occasionally there will be a widening of the palpebral fissure on adduction. Monocular duction testing will reveal a Brown's syndrome restriction, whereas a paretic inferior oblique restriction may be found on versions, but not necessarily on ductions. Forced duction testing (eye moved by forceps on conjunctiva) is indicated for differential diagnosis; the eye with Brown's syndrome will show restriction of passive elevation nasally.

    Surgical treatment for Brown's syndrome is usually not efficacious. Fortunately, resolution of symptoms is often achieved simply by compensatory head posturing.

IV. Adaptive Sensory Conditions in Strabismus

Strabismus is neither a purely motoric nor a purely sensorial anomaly. Rather, it is a sensory-motor problem affecting binocularity. The etiology of a strabismus may be attributable to a primary problem of the sensory system, such as unilateral ptosis in an infant resulting in esotropia. Another example is a unilateral cataract resulting in exotropia in an elderly person. On the other hand, a motor problem will likely cause abnormal adaptations in the sensory system. It is probable that suppression, amblyopia, and anomalous correspondence (ARC) are the results of a manifest motoric deviation of the visual axes (i.e., strabismus).

A. Suppression

1. Characteristics. Suppression can occur when there is a manifest deviation (strabismus). The foveal area will be suppressed first to avoid confusion (superimposition of dissimilar images). The next retinal area of the strabismic eye to be suppressed is that on which the fixated target (seen by the fovea of the nonstrabismic eye) falls, i.e., point zero. (Figure 10-12.) This is done to avoid diplopia. Eventually, the area between point zero and the fovea may be suppressed along with other adjacent portions of the retina. The younger the individual, the more able is the individual to suppress. Most young children can suppress to avoid diplopia, but most adults cannot and must learn to ignore a diplopic image. Although clinicians relate suppression zones to retinal loci, active suppression presumably occurs in the visual cortex.

Clinical Alert

Anisometropia may also cause suppression, but the suppression is usually only foveal. This occurs to avoid confusion of dissimilar image size and/or clarity; diplopia is usually not a factor. Frequently, however, strabismus and anisometropia coexist, resulting in a mixed etiology for the suppression.

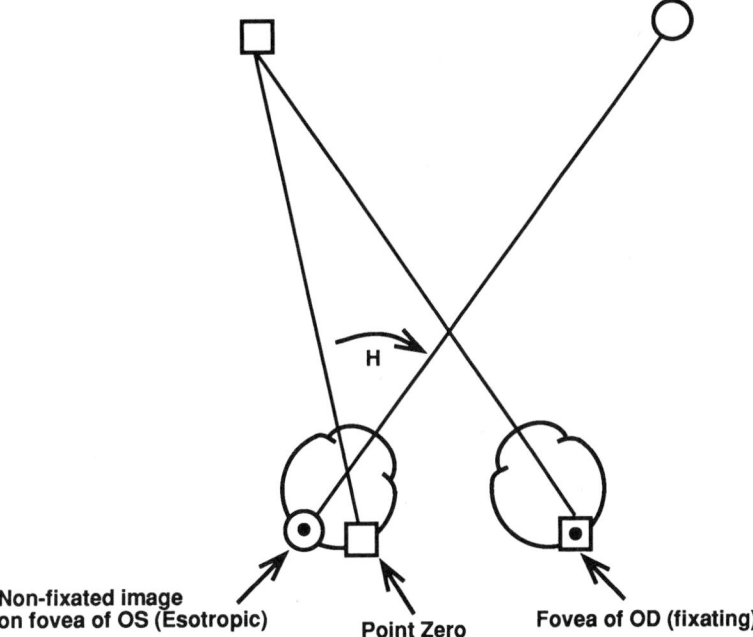

**Non-fixated image
on fovea of OS (Esotropic)**   **Point Zero**   **Fovea of OD (fixating)**

Figure 10-12.   Foveal suppression and suppression of the target-point (zero) in the left esotropic eye.

2.   Testing. The intensity of suppression can be assessed by the "naturalness" of the testing procedure. The more natural the procedure, the more likely that the suppression will be revealed. For example, an individual looking at the Worth four-lights through red and green filters (Figure 10-13) in a well-lighted room (relatively natural) is more likely to have suppression than in a darkened room (relatively unnatural). The size of the suppression zone can be assessed by varying the target size. The Worth four-lights test at far allows for assessment of only a small area of the retina, whereas more periphery can be assessed when testing at near. This is because the retinal image size is much larger when the target is closer to the patient.

Clinical Alert

Because the Worth four-lights test is very dissociative, particularly in a darkened room, a heterophoric individual with otherwise good binocularity may be unable to see four lights (latent deviation becoming manifest). It is likely that five dots will be reported. Professional judgment, therefore, is required when interpreting results of the Worth four-lights test.

There are many vectographic targets that are more "natural," and therefore more sensitive, than the Worth four-lights test for detecting shallow suppression. One example is the Pola-Mirror test.

3.   Pola-mirror test
Guidelines
a.   Purpose. Testing for suppression.
b.   Equipment. Polarizing filters, mirror.
c.   Procedure. The patient wears the crossed-polarizing filters while holding an ordinary flat mirror at a distance of approximately 25 cm. The patient is

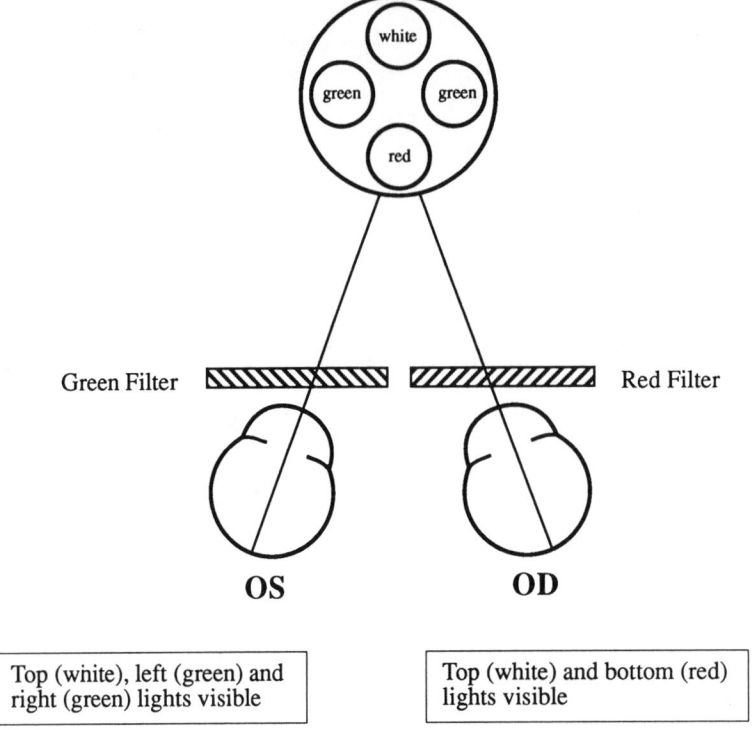

Figure 10-13.   Target and filters used with the Worth four-dot test.

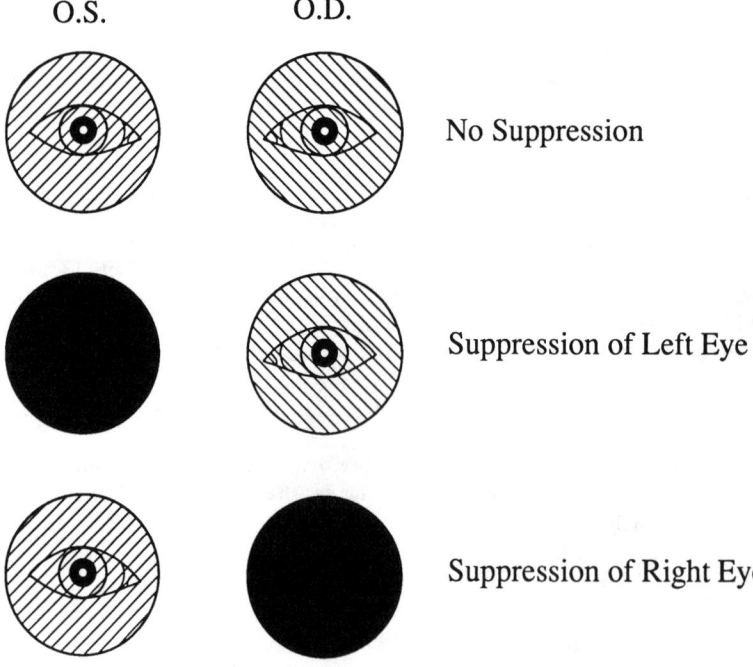

Figure 10-14.   Pola-Mirror test for suppression.

instructed to look into the mirror and report which eye is seen (Figure 10-14). As a confirmation of the response, the patient is instructed to close one eye and report what is seen. (The patient should see the polarizing filter before the closed eye as being black.)

    d. Results. When both eyes are open, no suppression is indicated if both eyes are seen at the same time. However, if only one eye at a time can be seen while the other is not, suppression is present in the eye behind the "black" polarizing filter.

Clinical Alert

This is for near and intermediate distances only. Note that the visual testing distance is double the distance between the patient's eyes and the mirror. For example, when the patient holds the mirror beyond arm's length, the test becomes difficult for the patient, because the eyes are not easily seen by the patient behind the polarizing filters.

B. *Amblyopia*

    1. Characteristics. Functional amblyopia is generally defined as reduced visual acuity due to strabismus and/or ametropia. Eccentric fixation may or may not be present.

        If the fovea remains suppressed for a sufficient time in the early developmental years, amblyopia will result. This is likely to occur in infants and young children, less so in older children, and highly unlikely in teenagers and adults. Suppression has an effect of nonuse of the foveal area. Likewise, deprivation of foveal seeing in infants and young children will result in reduced visual acuity, e.g., uncorrected refractive error, ptosis, and cataracts.

        Eccentric fixation is often associated with strabismic amblyopia. Suppression of the fovea possibly prompts the use of an extrafoveal area for fixation. Acuity is necessarily compromised at this nonfoveal site on the retina. It is held by some authorities that eccentric fixation is the result of sensorial deficiencies, whereas others postulate that it is due to a motoric anomaly. It is plausible to speculate that the problem of eccentric fixation is sensorial in etiology, which results in the manifestation of a motoric defect.

        Visual acuity testing results are affected by contour interaction (crowding phenomenon) in amblyopia with eccentric fixation when testing with the Snellen chart. Clinically, the peripheral vision appears to be unaffected, since suppression tends to affect central vision with only minimal adverse effects on peripheral vision.

    2. Testing

      a. Visual acuity. Snellen acuity testing with the whole chart (symbolized by $\boxed{X}$), single line (symbolized by $\boxminus$), or single letter (symbolized by $\boxdot$) should be done to assess the effect of contour interaction (crowding). For example, the patient looking at a whole Snellen chart with the amblyopic eye will often have several correct calls over a wide range of acuity demands, almost as if guessing. The reliability of the acuity measurement is therefore very poor. Single-line acuity provides more reliability than whole-chart testing. Scoring is done by the 50% threshold as in conventional testing of nonamblyopic eyes. Often the first and last letters on the line will be correctly called, but the letters in between will be missed. This is presumably due to the crowding phenomenon in amblyopia, which is particularly associated with eccentric fixation. Single-letter acuity testing is vitally important, because a favorable prognosis is indicated when acuity is much better than that found with a line of letters.

Psychometric acuity testing, such as the Flom S-Chart or Wesson cards[a] (Figure 10-15), is more reliable than Snellen chart testing in controlling for effects of contour interaction.

Wesson cards

Guidelines

(1) Purpose. To determine a reliable visual acuity in amblyopia.

(2) Equipment. Wesson cards.

(3) Procedure. Each card is numbered and calibrated for a visual acuity at 3 m (10 feet). The patient's estimated visual acuity determined with previous testing (e.g., Snellen) provides a starting point for testing. Ultimately, five data points are graphed, acuities represented by two cards below, two cards above, and the nearest estimated visual acuity card. Initially, the nonamblyopic eye is patched and the patient is instructed to call out the orientation of the tumbling Es in a clockwise fashion starting at the upper left corner. Each of the five cards is tested sequentially from the lowest to the highest visual acuity. The results are recorded and graphed. (Refer to suggested readings for further information.)

(4) Results. A sigmoid (best fit) curve is drawn through the five plotted points. The calculated visual acuity is the point where the curve crosses the 5/8 correct responses column (50%, corrected for guessing).

Clinical Alert

Young children may have difficulty following the directions and responding accurately to this test; therefore, isolated targets such as tumbling Es with contour interaction bars[b] (Figure 10-16), Lighthouse Picture Cards[c] of house, apple, and umbrella (Figure 10-17), or Broken Wheel cards[d] (Figure 10-18) can be used to assess visual acuity.

---

b. Fixation. Another factor to be tested in amblyopia is the status of fixation, which is either *central* or *eccentric*. A direct ophthalmoscope with a grid target can be used to determine whether or not there is eccentric fixation. This ophthalmoscopic procedure is referred to as visuoscopy.

Visuoscopy

Guidelines

(1) Purpose. To determine the direction and magnitude of eccentric fixation.

(2) Equipment. Direct ophthalmoscope with projection grid.

(3) Procedure. Occlude the eye not being tested and begin ophthalmoscopy as usual, focusing on the retina. Once the grid target is clearly focused on the patient's retina, the patient is asked to fixate the center of the target. The clinician then determines if the foveal reflex is in the center of the target (central fixation) or if fixation is extrafoveal (eccentric). The *steadiness* of the fixation should also be assessed (either steady or unsteady). The direction and estimated magnitude of the eccentricity should be assessed. Testing should be repeated several times for each eye, and the time-averaged magnitude recorded. This is necessary when there is either unsteady or wandering fixation.

---

[a]Wesson cards available from Dr. Michael Wesson, 4912 Indian Valley Rd., Birmingham, AL 35244.
[b]Tumbling Es with contour interaction bars available from the Optometry Alumni Association, School of Optometry, University of California at Berkeley, Berkeley, CA 94720.
[c]Lighthouse picture cards available from the Lighthouse Low Vision Services, 111 East 59th St., New York, NY 10022.
[d]Broken Wheel cards available from Bernell Corporation, 750 Lincolnway East, P. O. Box 4737, South Bend, IN 46634.

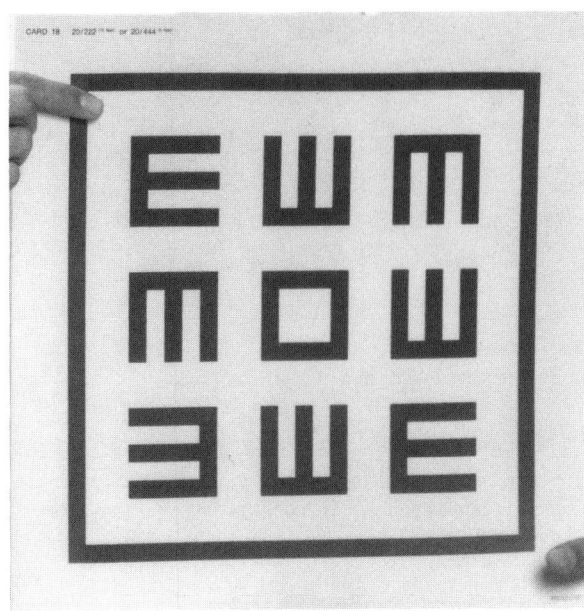

Figure 10-15. Example of a Wesson card for psychometric visual acuity testing.

(4) Results. A diagram of the grid target can be drawn with the relative position of the foveal reflex incorporated. (Figure 10-19.) This will aid in determining the direction and magnitude of eccentricity. To determine the magnitude in prism diopters from the grid markings on the target, the grid can be projected from 1 meter onto a centimeter scale. Each centimeter mark represents one prism diopter; therefore the magnitude in prism diopters from the center of the target to the hashmarks can be determined.

Clinical Alert

This procedure may be invalid if one eye of the patient is not occluded. Also, visuoscopy is very difficult to perform accurately if demarcation of the fovea is not evident.

C. *Anomalous correspondence*

Anomalous "retinal" correspondence (ARC) is the condition in which homologous retinal points (each fovea, for example) do not have the same directional value. This results in the objective horizontal angle of deviation (H) being different from the subjective angle (S).

1. Characteristics. ARC is an antidiplopia mechanism in strabismus; therefore, it is not evident under monocular seeing conditions. The etiology is debatable, but the

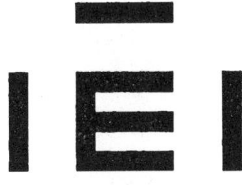

Figure 10-16. Example of a tumbling E with contour interaction bars.

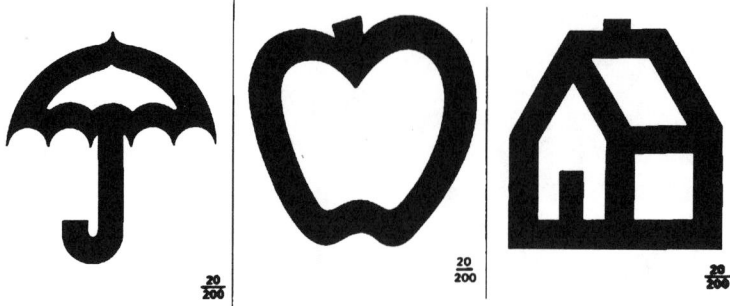

Figure 10-17.   Three lighthouse pictures in the series of acuity demands.

consensus is that ARC is associated with early-onset strabismus of long duration. ARC is classified as either harmonious (subjective angle is 0 in manifest strabismus) or various types of unharmonious in which S is neither zero nor equal to H (see Figure 10-20 for clarification.)

Clinical Alert

ARC is the traditional abbreviation for anomalous correspondence; however, the correspondence actually occurs in the visual cortex. This abbreviation is popularly accepted because clinicians refer to *retinal* (rather than cortical) loci for angular measurements of H, S, and the angle of anomaly (A).

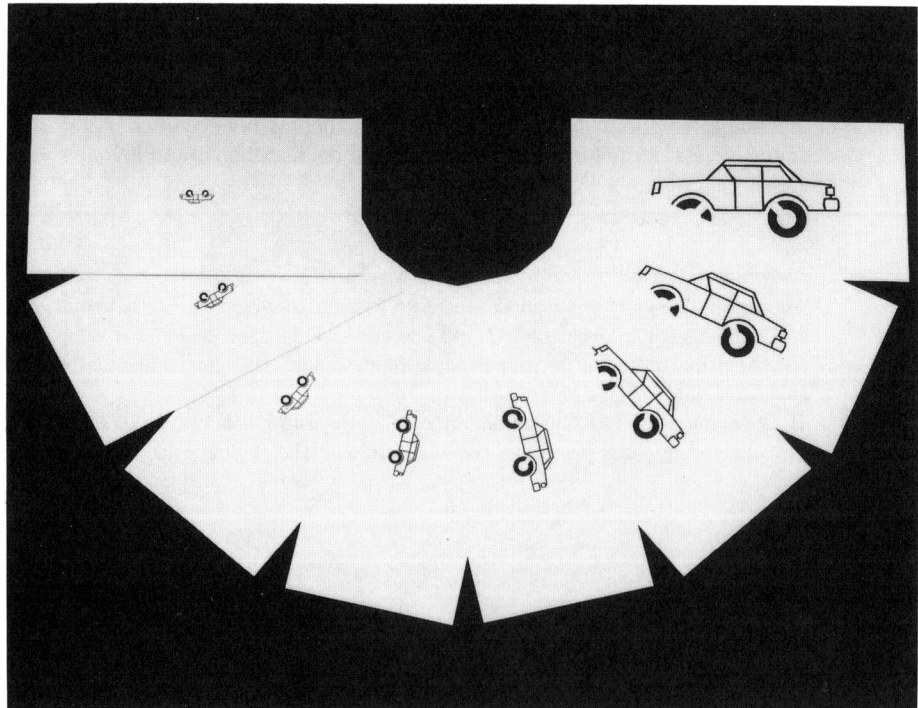

Figure 10-18.   Example of a Broken Wheel acuity test card (photo courtesy Bernell Corp.).

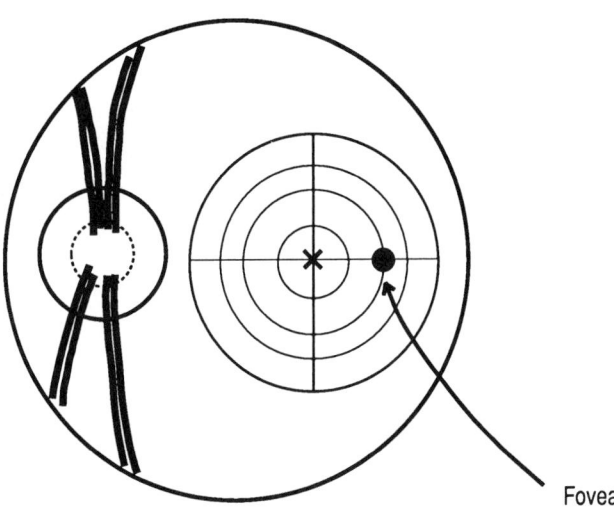

Fovea

OS fundus drawing illustrating 2 △
nasal eccentric fixation

Figure 10-19. Visuoscopy with a direct ophthalmoscope with the projected grid pattern indicating nasal eccentric fixation of 2 prism diopters.

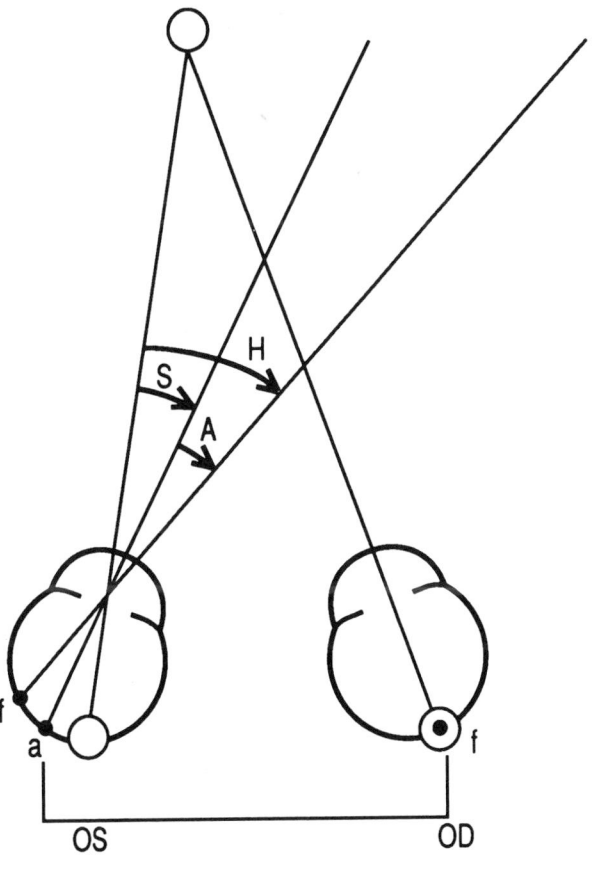

OS   OD

Figure 10-20. Illustration of unharmonious ARC in a patient with esotropia of the left eye showing the relationship of the three angles, horizontal objective angle (H), subjective angle of directionalization (S), and angle of anomaly (A).

2. Testing. ARC is detected by comparing the magnitude of H (e.g., from alternate cover test) with the magnitude of S (e.g., from Maddox rod). Normal retinal correspondence (NRC) is found if H and S are the same in direction and magnitude, angle A being equal to zero. If H and S are significantly different (allowing for clinical measurement error), ARC is suspected and further testing is necessary. Standard tests for ARC include major amblyoscope, Hering-Beilschowsky afterimage, Bagolini striated lenses, Cüppers bifoveal, and Haidinger's brush combined with Brock-Givner afterimage transfer. (Consult the Suggested Readings for further information on ARC testing.) The Hering-Beilschowsky afterimage test can be performed easily in a clinical setting.

Hering-Beilschowsky afterimage test

Guidelines

a. Purpose. To differentiate NRC from ARC, and to measure angle A.

b. Equipment. Masked strobe light (e.g., flash attachment of a camera).

c. Procedure. The nonpreferred eye is occluded and the patient is instructed to fixate the central spot on the strobe light (oriented horizontally). The light is flashed, creating a horizontal afterimage for the preferred eye. The occluder is switched to the preferred eye and the sequence is repeated with the strobe oriented vertically. The patient is then seated 1 m from a centimeter scale and instructed to fixate a central target on the scale, centering the gap in the horizontal afterimage on the target. The position of the vertical afterimage in relation to the gap of the horizontal afterimage is reported and the distance of separation measured in centimeters.

d. Results. Separation of the afterimage centers indicates ARC. Angle A is represented by the magnitude of the separation. If there is coexisting eccentric fixation, this needs to be considered in the measurement of A. If the angle of eccentric fixation (E) is in the same direction as A, the two measurements are added together to determine the true angle of anomaly. If, however, the direction of E is opposite to the direction of A, the magnitude of E is subtracted from A to determine the true A.

Clinical Alert

This test may be too difficult for some patients, especially young children. If the patient is having difficulty seeing the afterimages simultaneously, the patient can blink his or her eyes rapidly or the room lights may be flashed to enhance and sustain the afterimages.

V. **Strabismus Diagnosis and Prognosis**

A. *Diagnosis involves three general considerations: case history, test results of the deviation of the visual axes, and test results of adaptive sensory conditions. Possible permutations of diagnoses are unlimited. No two patients have exactly the same deviation and its variables, adaptive sensory conditions, and case histories. For the sake of brevity, three representative diagnoses are presented with prognostic considerations to follow.*

1. Case 1. The strabismic deviation is a concomitant, constant, alternating (OD dominant) esotropia of 25^Δ at far and 15^Δ at near with a low AC/A ratio (2/1). There is alternate deep suppression, ARC, but no amblyopia. Cosmesis is fair and there is only slight cosmetic concern regarding this patient who is 6 years old. Case history reveals onset of esotropia at birth. No treatment was ever given because of the presumption that the child would "grow out of it." Refractive status is plano, OU. Vision is 6/6 (20/20) in each eye.

2. Case 2. The strabismic deviation is a concomitant, constant, unilateral esotropia of the left eye of 20^Δ at far and 30^Δ at near with a high AC/A ratio (10/1) and fair cosmesis. Vision is 6/6 (20/20) OD and 6/12 (20/40) OS. Suppression is deep OS, but there is NRC. Little, if any, motor fusion range (disparity vergence) can be demonstrated. Case history reveals onset at age 4 in this 6-year-old patient. The mode of onset was intermittent for the first year, but the strabismus became constant afterward. There is some concern over cosmetic appearance. No previous treatment was given, but there is eagerness to begin treatment for strabismus. Refractive status is +2.00 D OU.

3. Case 3. The strabismic deviation is a concomitant, constant, intermittent (10% at far, 20% at near), unilateral exotropia of the left eye of 10^Δ at far and 15^Δ at near with a moderately low AC/A (4/1) and good cosmesis. There is no amblyopia and only shallow intermittent suppression. There is NRC, although intermittent ARC is found when the deviation is manifest. Fusion ranges are present, but limited. Case history reveals onset at age 5 in this 6-year-old patient. The mode was gradual and intermittent, and has become slightly more frequent during the past year. There was no previous treatment. Refractive status is −0.25 D OD and −1.00 D OS. Visual acuity with lenses: OD 6/6 (20/20), OS 6/6 (20/20).

B. *Because of the limitless number of possible diagnoses, there are also unlimited prognoses, since prognosis has to be tailored to the diagnosis of each case. There are, however, some generalizations on prognosis in strabismus which are listed below:*
1. Late is more favorable than early onset.
2. Early is more favorable than late treatment.
3. Exo is more favorable than eso deviation.
4. Small is more favorable than large magnitude.
5. NRC is more favorable than ARC.
6. Intermittent is more favorable than constant strabismus.
7. Good motivation and cooperation are favorable factors.
8. Concomitant is more favorable than nonconcomitant deviations (nonconcomitancy needing further investigations for underlying etiologies to rule out organic causes).

C. *Specific applications of these prognostic factors to each of the above individual cases are as follows:*
1. Case 1. The diagnosis gives a poor prognosis for functional cure with any kind of treatment. This is for several reasons: early onset of esotropia (congenital in this case), fairly large magnitude of eso deviation, constancy of the deviation, and ARC. The prognosis for a cosmetic cure with EOM surgery is fair. Because concern about cosmesis is not great, this treatment option may be delayed until a decision is made otherwise.
2. Case 2. This sample diagnosis gives a fair prognosis for functional cure with functional training, possibly in conjunction with surgery. This is for several reasons: late onset, NRC, refractive status with high AC/A ratio (leverage to reduce eso deviation with plus additions), and high motivation for treatment.
3. Case 3. The diagnosis gives a good prognosis for functional cure with functional training procedures, for several reasons: late onset, exo direction of the deviation, small magnitude, and existing fusion ranges. Refractive status is probably a favorable factor in this case, since myopic anisometropia may have contributed to the problem. (Correction of the ametropia may be beneficial.)

D. *The above examples represent many of the possibilities. Professional judgment is always required to assess the prognosis for functional and/or cosmetic cure. Refer to the Suggested Readings for other sources of information on diagnosis and prognosis in strabismus.*

VI. **Strabismus Management**

 A. *Strabismus with amblyopia*

 The initial stage of treatment for strabismus is to eliminate amblyopia, which requires prescribing the best optical correction, and to establish central fixation. The sequential treatment strategy for amblyopia is outlined below.

 1. Direct patching. Patching of the nonamblyopic eye is the initial treatment of choice. Guidelines take into account the age of the patient, the time of onset, the duration of amblyopia, and the diagnosis of strabismus and/or anisometropia. Direct occlusion
 Guidelines

 a. Purpose. Improvement of visual acuity with monocular therapy, both passive and active treatment.

 b. Equipment. Eyepatch, e.g., bandage patches, spectacle clipons, or novelty occluders such as "pirate" patches.

 c. Procedure. The nonamblyopic eye is occluded and the patient is instructed to wear the patch full-time if there is a constant strabismus. In very young children, the patch should be alternated to prevent *occlusion amblyopia*. For children aged 2–5 years, direct patching should occur 1 day for each year of age, with an interval of 1 day of indirect patching to complete the cycle. For example, a 3-year-old child would wear the patch on the nonamblyopic eye for 3 days, and wear the patch on the amblyopic eye for 1 day. Children under 2 years should have the patch switched between eyes at least each day. If the amblyopia is due to anisometropia and/or intermittent strabismus, patching can be part-time. As a general rule, 2–4 hours of direct patching daily is necessary, including both passive and active therapy. The daily visual requirements must be considered when prescribing occlusion therapy. For example, a child with a deep amblyopia will be unable to achieve in the classroom if the nonamblyopic eye is patched. Vocational considerations, similarly, apply to adults.

 d. Results. Steady improvement of visual acuity is anticipated in most cases, and therapy is continued until there is a plateau in threshold acuity. Direct patching is discontinued either if there is no improvement after 2 months, or if there is a cessation of improvement after 2 months. Poor compliance of patching is the principal reason for lack of success in amblyopia therapy. However, lack of improvement may be due to an embedded eccentric fixation, or to amblyopia of arrest in which the causative onset (untreated unilateral strabismus and/or significant refractive error) is in infancy and of a relatively long duration. In such cases, other recommendations need to be considered. In the case of amblyopia of arrest, the prognosis is poor, and treatment is discontinued. If there is eccentric fixation which may account for the reduced visual acuity, intensive vision therapy in the form of pleoptics is necessary. Referral to a vision therapy specialist is recommended in such cases.

Clinical Alert

Prolonged patching may precipitate a constant strabismus in patients with either a large heterophoria or an intermittent strabismus unless the clinician carefully monitors the patching regimen. This occurs when a latent deviation decompensates due to fusion being broken with occlusion. It is for this reason that full-time patching is recommended only for constant strabismus.

---

 2. Monocular active therapy. The general rule is that all therapy activities should be within the patient's acuity threshold. Recent studies have demonstrated a differ-

Table 10-5. Monocular Therapy Procedures

Resolution activities
    Watching television, increasing distance to threshold limits
    Near-far accommodative rock, book print to calendar (adjust distance)
    Figure-ground activities, e.g., hidden pictures, jumbled pictures
    Car games, e.g., reading street signs or license plates

Spatial activities
    Ball play, throwing and catching
    Pick-up sticks or similar games, e.g., Tinker Toys, Lite-Brite
    Toothpick-in-the-straw or spearing Cheerios
    Coloring books

Combined activities
    Dot-to-dot pictures or tracing
    Michigan Tracking or filling in Os in printed material
    Jigsaw puzzles of appropriate size
    Video games requiring visual-motor integration

ence between anisometropic amblyopia and strabismic amblyopia. Visual resolution activities are particularly effective in treating anisometropic amblyopia, whereas spatially oriented activities are important in strabismic amblyopia. Both types of activities are generally involved in a therapy regimen. Table 10-5 presents some examples of activities in each of these categories.

3. Binocular active therapy. Visual acuity in the amblyopic eye should generally be better than 20/100 (6/30), and preferably approaching 20/40 (6/12), in order to begin binocular training procedures. For the anisometropic amblyope, binocular therapy to emphasize sensory and motor fusion is the same as that described in section VII. In cases of strabismic amblyopia, therapy is directed toward treating the strabismus.

B. *Strabismus with ARC*
1. If prognosis is good
    a. Exotropia. Anomalous correspondence in exotropia does not always mean the prognosis is poor. Even if the exotropia is constant, the ARC may be eliminated. If at least some fusional convergence can be elicited, the angle of anomaly will covary with the objective angle of deviation and diminish as the strabismic angle decreases. Taking this concept to its logical conclusion, the angle of anomaly becomes zero when the eyes can be held in the ortho position. Therefore, ARC can be intermittent in exotropia, only being present when the deviation is manifest.

        The initial thrust in the treatment of exotropia is to reduce the magnitude of the strabismic angle by fusional convergence, rather than directly attacking ARC. If sensory fusion can be achieved with the aid of lenses and/or prisms, motor fusional vergence responses are prompted. Sufficient base-in prism to create "optical orthophoria" is an initial approach. However, a more effective approach is the use of overminus lenses to stimulate accommodative convergence. Sensory fusion may then be possible when the eyes are aligned, thereby eliminating the ARC provided the patient is able to maintain fusion while disparity (fusional) vergences are also in effect.

        From this point on, motor fusional vergence ranges are trained as though the patient were exophoric (to be discussed in section VII).

    b. Esotropia. As opposed to ARC in exotropia, this can be a significantly adverse factor in esotropia. Unless the ARC is intermittent, as in exotropia (rare in esotropia), therapy should be directed toward establishing normal correspondence.

An efficacious approach to disruption of ARC is the use of overcorrecting prisms. This procedure is appropriate in primary eye care practice. However, if this approach is not effective and sensory stimulation regimens may be necessary to eliminate the ARC, referral to a specialist in strabismic vision therapy is recommended.

Overcorrecting prism regimen

Guidelines

(1) Purpose. To eliminate ARC.

(2) Equipment. Fresnel press-on prisms, occluder, loose prisms.

(3) Procedure. Following the alternate cover test with prism neutralization, a Fresnel prism is applied to the spectacle lenses which is large enough to produce a reversal of the eso deviation (creating a small exo deviation). The patient is then monitored every 10 minutes with the alternate cover test to determine if any prism adaptation has occurred. If prism adaptation occurs within 30 minutes, a larger amount of prism is applied and the patient is then monitored again every 10 minutes for a total of 30 minutes. Once the prism can be worn for 30 minutes without prism adaptation, this amount is applied to the habitual spectacle lenses and the following home training program is established: full-time occlusion with one 30-minute session per day of associated viewing through the prism (active eye-hand or visual motor activities are encouraged during this period); return the next day for reassessment of prism adaptation. If there is still no prism adaptation in a 30-minute period, the above program is continued for a 1-week period. If there is prism adaptation, a larger amount of prism is indicated, and the initial steps are repeated. On successive visits to monitor prism adaptation and testing for ARC, the number of 30-minute associated viewing sessions per day may be increased, or the length of the sessions may be increased (with proper monitoring), as indicated.

(4) Results. The amount of prism necessary to produce the desired response may gradually decrease, thereby allowing a reduction in the prism power worn for vision training. A change in correspondence is anticipated following several weeks or months of vision training.

Clinical Alert

The cosmetic appearance of the strabismus will be worse with the overcorrecting prism due to the optical effect of prism on the lenses. This is also due to the increase in the angle when prism adaptation occurs.

---

2. If prognosis is poor. A program of patching to maintain the gains made in amblyopia therapy is recommended. Vision training is usually not recommended when the prognosis for a functional cure is poor. If a cosmetic cure is desired, EOM surgery may be recommended. However, the results of surgery cannot be guaranteed when ARC is present, because the eyes may "drift" back toward the original deviation. Another possible poor outcome is a surgical overcorrection, e.g., consecutive exotropia following surgery for esotropia.

C. *Strabismus without ARC*

1. Esotropia. In the absence of ARC, sensory fusion therapy is initiated at the subjective angle, which is identical to the objective angle. For example, a Wheatstone Mirror Stereoscope[e] can be adjusted to place the images on each fovea by

---

[e]Mirror Stereoscope available from Bernell Corporation, 750 Lincolnway East, P. O. Box 4737, South Bend, IN 46634.

having the patient achieve superimposition of two first-degree targets. If suppression is present, movement of the suppressed image, increasing the illumination to the target, adding color to the target, or having the patient touch the target will help to break suppression. Similar procedures can be prescribed using Brewster stereoscopes. Once superimposition is reliably achieved, second-degree targets are introduced. Motor fusion is begun by developing fusional divergence, starting at the strabismic angle. Once there is sufficient divergence range, fusional convergence is trained. The patient should be able to converge and diverge efficiently.

Out-of-instrument training at the centration point is the next step. The crossing point of the visual axes of an esotrope is calculated as follows: $D = H/IPD$. For example, if H is 15^Δ eso, and the IPD is 6 cm, then D is 2.50 diopters. The 2.50 dioptric distance is equivalent to 40 cm, which represents the centration point when the patient is looking through $+2.50$ diopter addition lenses. For the strabismic patient, this creates an ortho demand in true space. A convenient target is ordinary newsprint. Suppression can be monitored using either polarized or tranaglyphic strips placed on the page as the patient wears the appropriate polarizing or red-green filters. Gradually, base-in and base-out training prisms can be incorporated in this procedure to increase motor fusion ranges. Many other training procedures are possible, some of which will be discussed later.

The patient can be dismissed when there are adequate fusional vergences with clear, comfortable, efficient, binocular vision. Relieving prisms may be necessary, however, if this goal is only partially met. This is the least amount of prism necessary to relieve symptoms and meet the goal of efficient binocular vision. If excessive prism is necessary (larger than 20^Δ), surgery should be considered to reduce the magnitude of the deviation. It is important to evaluate a patient postsurgically for vision therapy in order to stabilize and improve binocularity as quickly as possible, if necessary.

2. Exotropia. Initially, lenses and/or prisms may be prescribed, as discussed in exotropia with ARC, to establish sensory fusion. The emphasis of therapy is motor fusion, specifically convergence, once stable sensory fusion is attained.

Gross convergence activities out-of-instrument (e.g., pencil pushups and Brock string) assist in stimulating the convergence response. Procedures that require sensory fusion (e.g., Allbee 3-Dot Card and Colored Circles), as well as increasing the convergence demand, are incorporated as their convergence ability improves. Finally, targets with stereopsis demands are instituted, both in- and out-of-instrument, e.g., eccentric circles, Vectograms®, Aperture Rule trainer, and Brewster stereoscope cards. (Refer to the Suggested Readings for detailed information and recommended instructions on the procedures listed above.) A home therapy program to maintain the improved abilities is very important, particularly in cases of large heterophoria. In such cases, a prism prescription and/or surgery may also be considered, with the same guidelines as discussed above.

D. *Vertical deviations*

A hyper deviation of only 15^Δ is considered large by clinical standards, whereas a horizontal deviation of 30^Δ is considered large. Such vertical deviations are usually strabismic and practically always have a torsional (cyclo deviation) component. Unfortunately, there is no optical means to compensate for a cyclo deviation; treatment relies either on vision training or on surgical intervention. The prognosis is generally poor for cyclotropia, but not necessarily for cyclophoria. For the vertical component, however, both large amounts of compensating vertical prism and EOM surgery may be attempted.

Vertical deviations can be classified as either primary (present in both the strabismic and horizontal orthoposition alignment) or secondary (present only when the horizontal strabismus is manifest). Secondary vertical deviations occur frequently with large exotropias, but less frequently with esotropias (with the exception of overacting inferior oblique muscles) or small exotropias. Because the vertical deviation is usually not manifest when the eyes are in the orthoposition, vertical prism is not generally required in the treatment plan for secondary vertical deviations. In primary vertical deviations, however, relieving vertical prism in a spectacle correction is the recommended first step, if normal sensory fusion is attained. When the vertical component of the strabismus is neutralized, the horizontal component can be more effectively managed than without this complication.

Keep in mind that vertical prisms may cause lens distortion, increased lens weight, prism adaptation, and poor cosmesis due to the eyes appearing to be vertically displaced.

Whether a horizontal deviation is present or not, horizontal vergence ranges should be expanded. This will stabilize fusion, and the amount of neutralizing vertical prism required may be reduced with time in many cases. Vertical divergence ranges may also be expanded by direct base-up or base-down training; however, the degree of improvement is usually not as significant as with the indirect approach of horizontal vergence training.

Clinical Alert

Many patients with infant-onset strabismus may have a dissociated vertical deviation (DVD). In this condition, each eye exhibits a hyper deviation when occluded. Prisms are not prescribed until normal sensory fusion is present, and then only if a primary vertical deviation remains (usually in the eye showing the largest hyper DVD).

E. *Nonconcomitancy*

The chief concern in recent-onset nonconcomitancy is to determine the etiology. Referral to other health care specialists is often recommended. The initial vision therapy procedure consists of prevention of EOM contracture of the homolateral antagonist or the contralateral synergist. For example, a paretic right lateral rectus muscle may result in contracture of the right medial rectus (homolateral antagonist) and the left medial rectus (contralateral synergist). Contracture can be prevented with alternate patching combined with pursuit and saccadic duction training (monocular "calisthenics").

The next step in binocular training is to reestablish fusion in as many positions of gaze as possible. This may require the regional application of Fresnel prisms on spectacle lenses to compensate for the deviations in the affected positions of gaze. This allows vergence training to expand the fusion ranges. Although patients may complain of the cosmetic effect of the prisms, this treatment is usually accepted when they are informed that these prisms will only be worn temporarily. The majority of newly acquired pareses resolve within a few months of onset, and the optical and training interventions assist the return to the prior binocular status. If, however, the nonconcomitancy does not resolve, a surgical consultation may be indicated. Surgery will not restore function to a paretic muscle; however, a large angle deviation can be reduced to improve cosmesis in most cases. A partial functional restoration can be achieved in many cases.

F. *Infantile strabismus*

Infantile strabismus is more often esotropic than exotropic, and the onset is from birth to 6 months of age. In many cases, either a DVD or bilateral overacting inferior oblique muscles are present. As distressing as these may be cosmetically, the functional prognosis is not significantly affected by their presence. Most patients, especially those with esotropia, have very large angles of deviation that must be closely monitored. Fortunately, the strabismus is usually alternating, and patching to prevent amblyopia is usually not necessary. If the strabismus is unilateral, however, occlusion therapy is necessary to prevent amblyopia. In large deviations, surgical intervention as early as possible is usually recommended. Before surgery, binocular stimulation activities should be attempted to improve the chances of achieving functional binocularity postsurgically. Application of neutralizing Fresnel prisms to ametropic correcting lenses will assist binocular stimulation. A binocular vision therapy specialist can use anaglyphic binocular stimulation activities to promote fusion; a referral may be advised.

Unless binocularity can be achieved before age 2 years and early treatment is given, the prognosis for a functional cure by any treatment means is very poor. Therefore, the earlier the treatment, the better is the prognosis in cases of infantile strabismus.

VII.   Nonstrabismic Vision Therapy

After the major sensorial adaptations in strabismus have been treated and a fair degree of motor fusion established, vision therapy to improve visual skills is begun. This is also the starting point for heterophoric patients and many mild cases of intermittent strabismus. Resources cited in the Suggested Readings provide detailed treatment regimens; however, a brief overview is given for the six principal vergence anomalies: convergence insufficiency, convergence excess, divergence insufficiency, divergence excess, basic exo deviation, and basic eso deviation. Vertical deviations are also discussed.

A.   *Convergence insufficiency (CI)*

Although there are many definitions of this anomaly, the most clinically useful one is as follows: a nearpoint problem of asthenopia and reduced vision efficiency in which the exo deviation at near significantly exceeds the exo (if any) at far, and compensating fusional convergence is insufficient.

Therapy for CI

Guidelines

1. Purpose. To improve fusional convergence at near.
2. Equipment. Pencil, vectographic targets, chiastopic fusion targets.
3. Procedure. Therapy is similar to the motor fusion training outlined above on treatment of exotropia. Three exemplary procedures are discussed. The initial procedure in this therapy sequence is pencil pushups. The patient attempts to maintain bifixation of the pencil tip as it is slowly moved toward the patient from an intermediate distance to a nearpoint position where bifixation is lost. The objective is to improve the nearpoint of convergence. Fusional convergence is being indirectly trained because this is the component that can overcome the exo deviation and allow clear, single, binocular vision as the target is approaching the patient. Direct training of relative fusional convergence can be done with vectographic targets at near, e.g., 40 cm (Figure 10-21). The patient views the targets through crossed-polarizing filters as base-out demands are gradually increased, while maintaining clear, single, binocular vision throughout the procedure. This sets the stage for base-out training in true space (*chiastopic* fusion). Keystone Eccentric Circles are excellent targets for this purpose (see Figure 10-22). The two eccentric circle cards are held at near (e.g., 40 cm), with the right eye seeing the left card and the left eye seeing the one to the right. If the patient can cross-fuse these two cards, one fused image will be perceived as being framed on each side by a card. A stereoscopic floating of a portion of the fused image should also be reported. The relative fusional convergence demand can be increased by slowly increasing the separation of the cards.
4. Results. Fusional convergence is continued, both in-office and out-of-office, until an adequate fusional convergence range is achieved.

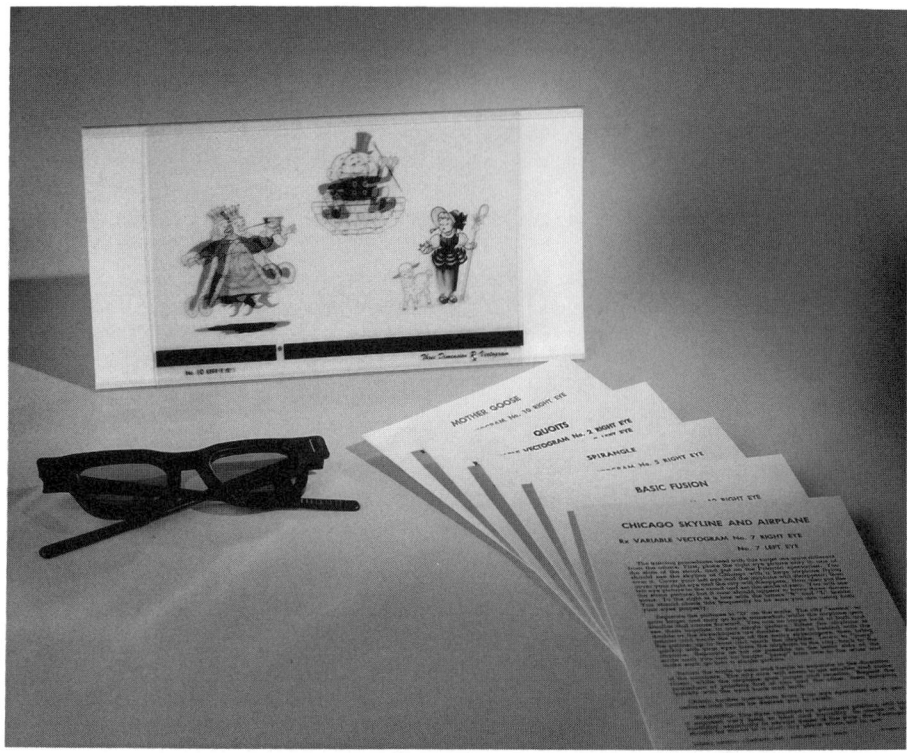

Figure 10-21.   Mother Goose and other Vectograms® (photo courtesy Bernell Corp.).

Clinical Alert

Before vergence training can be effective, therapy must have been completed for other visual skills, when necessary. These include position maintenance (fixations), saccades, pursuits, and accommodation, among other visual skills.

B. *Convergence excess (CE)*

This is a condition in which the eso deviation at near significantly exceeds the eso (if any) at far, and fusional divergence is inadequate to compensate for the excessive convergence at near. Symptoms and signs of asthenopia and vision inefficiency may result from CE.

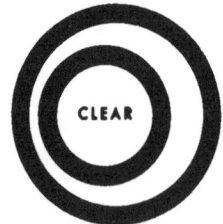 

Figure 10-22.   Keystone Eccentric Circles.   **A   B   B   A**

Therapy for CE
Guidelines

1. Purpose. To improve fusional divergence to overcome any problem caused by the eso deviation at near.
2. Equipment. Similar to that used for treatment of CI.
3. Procedure. Pencil pushups are done initially, although intuition would seemingly contradict this approach for a patient with an eso deviation. The clinical effectiveness of this indirect procedure, however, can be explained. Since the eso deviation increases at closer fixation distances, fusional divergence is necessary to compensate for the increasing eso deviation during pushup training in order to maintain clear, single, binocular vision. Direct training of relative fusional divergence can be done with Vectograms® and true-space fusion targets as in cases of CI, the difference being that base-in rather than base-out training is emphasized. Transparent cards with Keystone Eccentric Circles are used for CE therapy (rather than opaque cards for CI therapy). This procedure is known as *orthopic* fusion. The patient is instructed to look through the transparent cards and view a distant object in order to encourage divergence. When the right eye fixates the right-hand target and the left eye fixates the left-hand target, a fused, composite image should be perceived between the two. Greater base-in demands are effected by increasing the separation between the cards.
4. Results. In-office and out-of-office base-in training is continued until an adequate fusional divergence range is achieved. The goal is to overcome problems at near caused by the convergence excess.

Clinical Alert

Orthopic fusion is very difficult for most CE patients. The clinician may need to use plus addition lenses to help the patient get started on this procedure. Furthermore, the clinician may need to prescribe plus addition lenses (e.g., bifocals) for nearpoint work. This may be necessary for the CE patient if vision training alone is not completely effective in abating the eso problems. It is unwise, however, to rely completely on plus addition lenses in most CE cases, because vision training is the initial treatment of choice. Bifocals should be prescribed, however, only when necessary.

C. *Divergence excess (DE)*

DE can be defined as an exo deviation at far that significantly exceeds the exo deviation (if any) at near, and may cause asthenopia and vision inefficiency at far.

Therapy for DE
Guidelines

1. Purpose. To increase fusional convergence at near.
2. Equipment. Brock string, loose prisms, farpoint chiastopic fusion targets.
3. Procedure. Begin with training at near where the exo deviation is closer to orthophoria, and adequate sensory-motor fusion is expected. If motor fusion ranges are insufficient, training can be performed as in CI, except that push-aways are emphasized rather than pushups. Bifixation can be monitored more precisely with a Brock string than with a pencil target. The patient is asked to fixate a bead on the string while perceiving the diplopic images of the string to intersect exactly at the fixated bead. A slight vergence error (fixation disparity) is indicated if the intersection is slightly in front of the bead (eso), and an exo fixation disparity is indicated if the intersection is slightly behind the bead. The goal of this procedure is to maintain accurate bifixation, without suppression, on each bead as the distance is increased. When this can be achieved at distances of 2–3 m, base-out

prisms are introduced to train fusional convergence. After this procedure is mastered, farpoint chiastopic fusion training can be attempted. The best way to approach this is to have the patient first perform nearpoint chiastopic fusion as in CI therapy. The patient can then progress to chiastopic push-aways and walk-aways. Enlarged eccentric circles are excellent farpoint targets.

4. Results. Adequate base-out ranges at far should be the goal of therapy. As in all vergence training, the forced vergence should include monitoring for suppression, fixation disparity, discomfort, and blurring as the prism demand is increased. Facility of vergence (base-in and base-out demands) should be included in the finishing process of therapy.

Clinical Alert

A temporary eso deviation at near may result from excessive base-out training at far due to prism adaptation, and also due to the high AC/A which produces eso at very near distances in patients with DE. Consequently, some DE patients may require plus addition lenses in the form of bifocals. Not only do the bifocals lenses equalize the exo magnitudes at far and near, but fusional convergence training takes place whenever the patient is clearly viewing objects at near. Nevertheless, it is clinically wise to be conservative with plus addition powers. Pseudo DE should be ruled out (i.e., BX case) by prolonged occlusion and further testing.

D. *Divergence insufficiency (DI)*

DI can be defined as an eso deviation at far that is significantly greater than the eso deviation (if any) at near, and it may cause asthenopia and vision inefficiency at far. This is due to an insufficiency of fusional divergence.

Therapy for DI

Guidelines

1. Purpose. To increase fusional divergence at far.
2. Equipment. Brock string, prisms, TV trainer.
3. Procedure. Training in cases of DI is much the same as in DE. Training begins at near, where the patient can perform more easily, and proceeds to farther distances. On the Brock string procedure, however, base-in prisms are used to create fusional divergence demands. Base-in prisms can also be incorporated with a television trainer, utilizing either polarized or red-green filters to monitor suppression.
4. Results. The purpose of DI therapy is to increase fusional divergence and maintain clear, single, efficient, binocular vision at far. When this is achieved, the patient can be put on a home maintenance program of fusional divergence training.

Clinical Alert

Base-out relieving prisms should be avoided in most cases of DI. This is because an exo deviation at near may be optically created. Furthermore, the base-out prisms in spectacle lenses stimulate fusional convergence at near, thereby working against the farpoint fusional divergence therapy. For similar reasons, bifocals are contraindicated. Treatment of DI generally depends on vision training, and possible surgical intervention in a few DI cases with eso deviations of large magnitude.

E. *Basic exo deviation (BX)*

BX can be defined as a condition in which the exo deviation is approximately the same at all distances. Asthenopia and vision inefficiency may occur at all distances, but generally the problems are more prominent at far than at near.

BX therapy

Guidelines

1. Purpose. To increase fusional convergence at all distances.
2. Equipment. The same as for DE.
3. Procedure. Vision training for BX and DE are essentially the same.
4. Results. The same outcome expected for DE is also expected for BX. An exception, however, is that base-in relieving prisms can be effective in some BX cases, since a nearpoint eso problem is not created with the prisms. Consequently, the clinician has both prisms and training procedures as treatment options for BX patients.

Clinical Alert

As in all vergence training, particularly in patients with exo deviations, adequate base-in and base-out ranges should ultimately be achieved because of the probability of prism adaptation.

F. *Basic eso deviations (BE)*

BE can be defined as a condition in which the eso deviation at near is approximately the same as that at far. Asthenopia and vision inefficiency may be present at all distances, but they are usually more prominent at far.

Vision therapy for BE

Guidelines

1. Purpose. To increase fusional divergence at all fixation distances.
2. Equipment. Same as that for DI cases.
3. Procedure. Same as that for cases of DI, except that base-out relieving prisms are more likely to be prescribed because creating a nearpoint optical exo deviation is not a factor.
4. Results. Once adequate fusional divergence ranges are achieved at all distances, a home maintenance training program can be continued. Convenient targets for orthopic fusion can be prescribed, as in CE training.

Clinical Alert

Full-time wear of base-out prisms may cause a convergence adaptation, thereby causing an eso problem when the spectacles are removed. Esophoric patients, for example, who desire to remove their spectacles may experience esophoric symptoms. This is the reason optical relieving prisms are usually less than satisfactory unless vision training is included.

G. *Vertical deviations*

Unlike horizontal deviations, relatively small vertical deviations can cause significant symptoms. In smaller amounts of vertical deviation when there is hyperphoria, a combination of relieving prism and vision training is usually effective in abating the symptoms and improving vision efficiency.

Vision therapy for hyperphoria

Guidelines

1. Purpose. To relieve symptoms and develop adequate vertical divergence ranges of fusion.

2. Equipment. Loose prism, ordinary equipment used for vision training of horizontal deviations.

3. Procedure. Vision training proceeds as in cases of horizontal deviations, except that compensating vertical prisms (e.g., loose prisms or trial lens prisms) are incorporated in the therapy procedures. The objective is to develop sufficient horizontal ranges while the patient has the benefit of vertical compensation of hyperphoria. Gradually the patient is weaned from the relieving vertical prism until an adequate horizontal fusional range is stabilized. Eventually, vertical prism demand in the opposite direction is introduced as horizontal ranges are tested and trained. For example, if the patient has 5^Δ of left hyperphoria, horizontal vergence training commences with 5^Δ base-down before the left eye. Gradually the prism power is reduced and several prism diopters of base-up can be introduced before the left eye, assuming horizontal fusional vergence ranges remain adequate. Often, permanent relieving prism must be prescribed in spectacle lenses. Fixation disparity testing is a good way for the clinician to arrive at a tentative prism prescription. Generally, the amount of prism that neutralizes the vertical fixation disparity is the recommended power. Conventional clinical wisdom, however, is an even better guideline for prism prescribing. This involves several trials, sometimes requiring the patient to wear the tentative prism (e.g., Fresnel prism) for several hours or days, to determine the most effective prism power that relieves symptoms.

4. Results. Relief of asthenopia and improved vision efficiency are the indicators of effective treatment.

Clinical Alert

Some patients will not want vision training, and prefer the immediate relief afforded by prism compensation. Unfortunately, prism adaptation may occur in some patients; therefore, patients receiving relieving prisms should be followed closely.

VIII. Specialized Vision Therapy

Vision therapy is not necessarily completed just because adequate vergence ranges have been achieved. Vision efficiency problems, such as poor position maintenance, pursuits, saccades, and accommodative skills, may still exist. These visual skills are important for individuals in their educational, occupational, and avocational activities.

A. *Educational vision*

Good oculomotor movements (among many other requisite visual skills) are important for efficiency in classroom activities. For example, poor saccadic eye movements may cause the reader to skip words and lines, thereby losing his or her place. A practical clinical test of saccadic function is the developmental eye movement test (DEM).[f] (Figure 10-23.) Poor saccadic eye movements can usually be treated successfully with vision training. The same is true for pursuits and fixations in most cases. As an example, a brief overview is given for saccadic training. The Suggested Readings contain resources for further information on therapy for oculomotor problems.

---

[f]Developmental Eye Movement Test (DEM) available from Bernell Corporation, 750 Lincolnway East, P. O. Box 4737, South Bend, IN 46634.

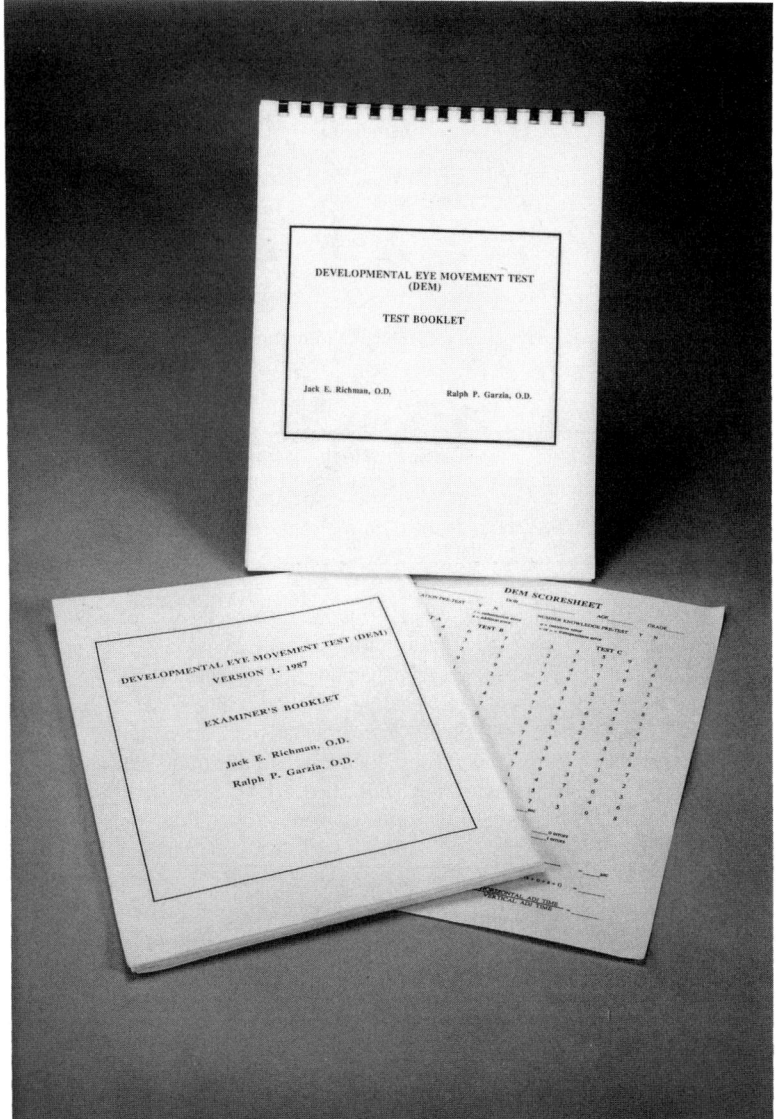

Figure 10-23.   Developmental Eye Movement test (DEM) (photo courtesy Bernell Corp.).

Therapy for saccades
Guidelines
1. Purpose. To improve saccadic function, particularly for fine saccades involved in the act of reading.
2. Equipment. Farpoint Hart Chart or similar custom-made targets (Figure 10-24).
3. Procedure. The patient is instructed to read aloud each letter in the proper sequence, starting with the first row of letters. A more complicated demand is to have the patient read every other letter, and later read every third letter. Incorporating a metronome (or rhythmic hand clapping if a metronome is not available) additionally requires auditory-visual integration and motor planning during the saccadic task.
4. Results. Good saccadic ability is demonstrated when the patient is able to read

O F T D V N P E H C
K A Y B Z R X L E O
W K T E H A M P F B
R X B V T M O F C S
T P A R E V D O T X

Figure 10-24.   Custom-made chart
of letters for saccadic therapy.

the letters quickly and accurately while meeting the auditory demands of a metronome.

Clinical Alert

The above procedure is but one of many effective procedures, and further reading on therapy of eye movement dysfunctions is highly recommended.

Visual perceptual and visual motor skills are also necessary for scholastic achievement. These functions should be tested if the educational history suggests the possibility of a learning problem. Visual perceptual assessment can be made with the Test of Visual Perceptual Skills (TVPS)[g] and visual motor with the Beery Visual-motor Integration Test (VMI).[h] These skills are particularly important in the development of reading readiness in prekindergarten, kindergarten, and first-grade children. From the second grade on, additional testing with The Dyslexia Screener (TDS)[i] is indicated if the educational history suggests a *specific* reading disability. A presumptive dyslexic child should be referred for educational assessment and therapy, but vision therapy may also be necessary when there are *general* reading problems related to visual dysfunctions.

B.   *Occupational vision*

Visual fatigue and asthenopia in the workplace are the subjective reports often attributed to binocular problems, particularly accommodative and vergence dysfunctions. Symptoms and vision inefficiency are exacerbated if there are accompanying ocular problems such as uncorrected hyperopia and astigmatism. Many occupations require precise and efficient binocular vision, e.g., aviators, cartographers, microchip assembly workers, surgeons, and others using binocular instruments. Considerable interest has surrounded the increasing use of computers and video display terminals (VDTs) with respect to visual symptoms. The weight of authority holds that binocular dysfunctions contribute to symptoms of discomfort reported by VDT workers. Vision therapy by means of lenses, prisms, and training should be appropriately prescribed to treat existing binocular problems. Ergonomic factors such as proper lighting and workstation arrangement must also be taken into account. These can be empirically customized to meet the needs of each individual VDT worker.

---

[g]Test of Visual Perceptual Skills (TVPS) available from Psychological and Educational Publications, Inc., 1477 Rollins Rd., Burlingame, CA 94010.

[h]Visual-Motor Integration Test (VMI) available from Modern Curriculum Press, 13900 Prospect Rd., Cleveland, OH 44136.

[i]The Dyslexia Screener (TDS) available from Reading and Perception Therapy Center, 3840 Main St., Culver City, CA 90232.

C. *Avocational vision*

Individuals desire to have at least one hobby that provides pleasure and satisfaction. Avocational interests promote healthful, recreational experiences that may also foster educational and occupational achievements. As in work and study, efficient visual skills are advantageous in most hobbies, ranging from the demands of nearpoint needlework to those of the farpoint firing range. A predominant avocational theme in clinical practice is *sports vision*. Many patients are professional athletes; most, however, are amateurs. Sports vision encompasses two broad areas: (1) prescribing protective eyewear and (2) testing visual functions, treating deficiencies, and enhancing normal skills with vision training. Binocular function is an important component of the latter, which emphasizes improvement of an individual's automaticity, peripheral awareness, and response time.

IX. Comments

The full scope of binocular vision care has much more breadth and depth than can possibly be presented in this overview for the primary eye care practitioner. The Suggested Readings supplement the topics discussed in this chapter. These resources are also applicable to binocular vision specialists who provide secondary and tertiary care. Referral to a specialist is indicated when treatment of a patient's binocular anomalies is beyond the scope of primary care.

Suggested Readings

This sample list is by no means exhaustive; there are many other excellent unlisted citations on testing and therapy for binocular vision problems.

Arthur BW. Long-term stability of alignment in the monofixation syndrome. *J Pediatr Ophthalmol Strabismus* 1989;26:224–331.

Bloch DA. Differences between strabismic and anisometropic amblyopia: Research findings and impact on management. In: Rutstein RP, ed. *Amblyopia. Probl Optom* 1991;3:276–292.

Brownlee GA, Goss DA. Comparisons of commercially available devices for the measurement of fixation disparity and associated phoria. *J Am Optom Assoc* 1988;59:451–460.

Caloroso EE. A sequential strategy for achieving functional binocularity in strabismus. *J Am Optom Assoc* 1988;59:378–387.

Caloroso EE, Rouse MW. *Clinical Management of Strabismus*. Boston: Butterworth, 1993.

Christensen GN, Rouse MW, Adkins DA. Management of infantile-onset esotropia. *J Am Optom Assoc* 1990;61:559–572.

Ciuffreda KJ. Components of clinical near vergence testing. *J Behavioral Optom* 1992;3:3–13.

Ciuffreda KJ, Levi DM, Selenow A. *Amblyopia: Basic and Clinical Aspects*. Boston: Butterworth-Heinemann, 1991.

Coffey B, Reichow AW, Colburn PB, Clark DL. Influence of ocular gaze and head position on 4M heterophoria and fixation disparity. *Optom Vis Sci* 1991;68:893–898.

Cooper J. Orthoptic treatment of vertical deviations. *J Am Optom Assoc* 1988;59:463–468.

Cotter SA. Conventional therapy for amblyopia. In: Rutstein RP, ed. *Amblyopia. Probl Optom.* 1991;3:312–330.

Daum KM. Characteristics of convergence insufficiency. *Am J Optom Physiol Opt* 1988;65:426–438.

Daum KM, Rutstein RP, Cho M, Eskridge JB. Horizontal and vertical vergence training and its effect on vergences and fixation disparity curves. *Am J Optom Physiol Opt* 1988;65:1–7.

Dowley D. Fixation disparity. *Optom Vis Sci* 1989;66:98–105.

Eskridge JB, Perrigin DM, Leach NE. The Hirschberg test, correlation with corneal radius and axial length. *Optom Vis Sci* 1990;67:243–247.

Eskridge JB, Wick B, Perrigin D. The Hirschberg test: A double-masked clinical evaluation. *Am J Optom Physiol Opt* 1988;65:745–750.

Firth AY. Anisometropia: Cause of amblyopia or result of undetectable retinal defect? *Br Orthoptic J* 1989;46:112–116.

Flynn JT. Amblyopia revisited. *J Pediatr Ophthalmol Strabismus* 1991;28:182–201.

Frantz KA. The importance of multiple treatment modalities in a case of divergence excess. *J Am Optom Assoc* 1990;61:457–462.

Freeman RA, Isenberg SJ. The use of part-time occlusion for early onset unilateral exotropia. *J Pediatr Ophthalmol Strabismus* 1989;26:94–96.

Gallaway M, Vaxmonsky T, Scheiman M. Management of intermittent exotropia using a combination of vision therapy and surgery. *J Am Optom Assoc* 1989;60:428–434.

Garzia RP. Management of amblyopia in infants, toddlers, and preschool children. In: Scheiman MM, ed. *Pediatric Optometry. Probl Optom* 1990;2:438–458.

Giangiacoma J. Differential diagnosis and management of childhood strabismus. In: Galin M, Mills KB, Rosen ES, eds. *Strabismus. Semin Ophthalmol* 1988;3:181–184.

Goss DA. *Ocular Accommodation, Convergence, and Fixation Disparity: A Manual of Clinical Analysis.* New York: Professional Press, 1986.

Griffin JR. Binocular Vision Assessment: Ranking Scores of Clinical Findings in Visual Skills Testing. *So Afr Optom* 1989;47:26–29.

Griffin JR, Carlson GP. Duane retraction syndrome and vision therapy: A case report. *J Am Optom Assoc* 1991;62:318–321.

Griffin JR, Grisham JD. *Binocular Anomalies: Diagnosis and Vision Therapy.* 3rd ed. Boston: Butterworth-Heinemann, 1995.

Grisham JD. Visual therapy results for convergence insufficiency. *Am J Optom Physiol Opt* 1988;65:448–454.

Grisham JD, Bowman MC, Owyang LA, Chan CL. Vergence orthoptics: Validity and persistence of the training effect. *Optom Vis Sci* 1991;68:441–451.

Hardesty HH. Management of intermittent exotropia. In: Galin M, Mills KB, Rosen ES, eds. *Strabismus. Semin Ophthalmol* 1988;3:169–174.

Holbach HT, Von Noorden GK, Avilla CW. Changes in esotropia after occlusion therapy in patients with strabismic amblyopia. *J Pediatr Ophthalmol Strabismus* 1991;28:6–9.

Holopigian K, Blake R, Greenwald MJ. Clinical suppression and amblyopia. *Invest Ophthalmol Vis Sci* 1988;29:444–451.

Levi DM. Visual acuity in strabismic and anisometropic amblyopia: A tale of two syndromes. In: Greenwald MJ, ed. *Pediatric Ophthalmology. Ophthalmol Clin No Am* 1990;3:289–301.

London R. Passive treatments for early onset strabismus. In: Scheiman MM, ed. *Pediatric Optometry. Probl Optom* 1990;2:480–495.

London R, Silver JL. Diagnosis of amblyopia: Emphasis on nonacuity factors. In: Rutstein RP, ed. *Amblyopia. Probl Optom* 1991;3:258–275.

Ludwig IH, Parks MM, Getson PR, Kammerman LA. Rate of deterioration in accommodative esotropia correlated to the AC/A relationship. *J Pediatr Ophthalmol Strabismus.* 1988;25:8–12.

Magoon EH. Botulin therapy in pediatric ophthalmology. In: Smolin G, Friedlaender MH, eds. *Pediatric Ophthalmology. Int Ophthalmol Clin* 1989;29:30–32.

Metz HS, Mazow M. Botulinum toxin treatment of acute sixth and third nerve palsy. *Graefes Arch Clin Exp Ophthalmol* 1988;226:141–144.

Miller PJ. Clinico-legal aspects of infantile strabismus. *Optom Vis Sci* 1990;67:148–149.

Molarte AB, Rosenbaum AL. Clinical characteristics and surgical treatment of intermittent esotropia. *J Pediatr Ophthalmol Strabismus* 1991;28:137–141.

Oster JG, Simon JW, Jenkins P. When is it safe to stop patching? *Br J Ophthalmol* 1990;74:709–711.

Pickwell D. *Binocular Vision Anomalies: Investigation and Treatment.* 2nd ed. Boston: Butterworths, 1989.

Pickwell D, Yekta AA. The effect on fixation disparity and associated heterophoria of reading at an abnormally close distance. *Ophthalmic Physiol Opt* 1987;7:345–347.

Press LJ. Strabismus (topical review). *J Optom Vis Dev* 1991;22:5–20.

Press LJ. Topical review of the literature—amblyopia. *J Optom Vis Dev* 1988;19:2–15.

Richman J. Annual review of the literature. *J Optom Vis Dev* 1990;21:5–26.

Rutstein RP. Alternative treatment for amblyopia. In: Rutstein RP, ed. *Amblyopia. Probl Optom* 1991;3:331–354.

Rutstein RP. Evaluation and treatment of incomitant deviations in children. In: Scheiman MM, ed. *Pediatric Optometry. Probl Optom* 1990;2:528–561.

Rutstein RP, Daum KM, Eskridge JB. Clinical characteristics of anomalous correspondence. *Optom Vis Sci* 1989;66:420–425.

Saladin JJ. Interpretation of divergent oculomotor imbalance through control system analysis. *Am J Optom Physiol Opt* 1988;65:439–447.

Saladin JJ, Alspauch DH, Penrod LR. Effect of vision therapy on stereophotogrammetric profiling: A controlled clinical trial. *Am J Optom Physiol Opt* 1988;65:325–330.

Saulles H. Treatment of refractive amblyopia in adults. *J Am Optom Assoc* 1987;58:959–960.

Scheiman M, Ciner E, Gallaway M. Surgical success rates in infantile esotropia. *J Am Optom Assoc* 1989;60:22–31.

Scheiman M, Herzberg H, Frantz K, Margolies M. A normative study of step vergence in elementary school children. *J Am Optom Assoc* 1989;60:276–280.

Scheiman MM, Wick B. Optometric management of infantile esotropia. In: Scheiman MM, ed. *Pediatric Optometry. Probl Optom* 1990;2:459–479.

Schor C. Influence of accommodative and vergence adaptation on binocular motor disorders. *Am J Optom Physiol Opt* 1988;65:464–475.

Scott AB, Magoon EH, McNeer KW, Stager DR. Botulinum treatment of strabismus in children. *Trans Am Ophthalmol Soc* 1989;87:174–184.

Shaw DE, Fielder AR, Minshull C, Rosenthal AR. Amblyopia: Factors influencing age of presentation. *Lancet* 1988;2:207–209.

Somersalo M. Children referred for pleoptic treatment. *Acta Ophthalmol* 1988;66:509–513.

Veronneau-Troutman S. Prism adaptation test (PAT) in the surgical management of acquired esotropia. *Arch Ophthalmol* 1991;109:765–766.

Wick B. Vision therapy for very young children. In: Scheiman MM, ed. *Pediatric Optometry. Probl Optom* 1990;2:354–364.

Yekta AA, Pickwell LD, Jenkins TC. Binocular vision, age and symptoms. *Ophthalmic Physiol Opt* 1989;9:115–120.

Kevin L. Alexander. *The Lippincott Manual of Primary Eye Care*. Copyright © 1995 by J.B. Lippincott Company.

CHAPTER **11**

Pediatric Optometry

Elise Ciner
Maria L. Parisi
Chaya Herzberg

I. When to Examine Children

A. *1st exam—6 months*
   Rationale
   1. Vision system is rapidly developing.
   2. Most components of vision developed by 1 year.
   3. Problems can occur early.
   4. Early detection = better treatment.

B. *2nd exam—2–3 years of age*
   Rationale
   1. Vision problems occur during this time.
   2. Commonly include accommodative esotropia and meridional amblyopia.
   3. Children can begin to communicate.
   4. Easy to examine.
   5. Less fearful than at ages 1–2.

C. *3rd exam—5 years of age*
   Rationale
   1. Ensures child entering kindergarten has optimal vision for learning.
   2. Detects problems before they impact on learning.
   3. May be required in some states or school districts.

D. *Yearly exams—throughout school years*
   Rationale
   1. Vision demands are changing as academic skills increase.
   2. Learning to read in early grades involves primarily large print, which is less visually demanding. Check visual perceptual skills if learning difficulties.
   3. Reading to learn in middle to upper grades involves smaller print, which is more visually demanding. Check visual efficiency skills if learning difficulties (accommodative, binocular, and ocular motor problems become evident due to increased nearpoint demand).
   4. Refractive error changing throughout childhood.

II. General Guidelines for Examining Children

A. *Schedule appointments when child is alert; avoid nap time or late in the evening, unless looking for a visual problem related to fatigue or excessive near work.*

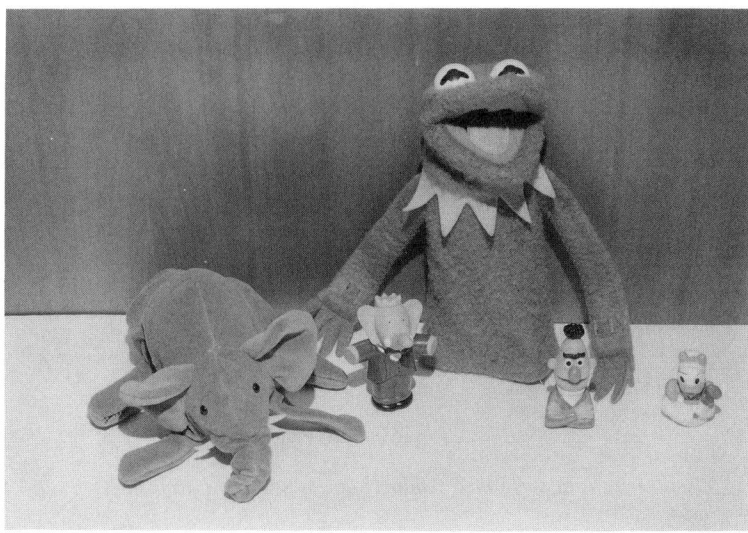

Figure 11-1.   Fixation targets for infants and toddlers (*photo by Ron Davidoff*).

B.   *Work quickly, especially with younger children who fatigue and lose attention; prioritize testing.*
C.   *Refrain from wearing a white lab coat during testing.*
D.   *Engage the child through conversation, jokes to enhance attention and cooperation.*
E.   *Use appropriate fixation targets, e.g., hand or finger puppets, colorful stickers, small pictures to maintain child's attention (Figures 11-1 and 11-2).*
F.   *Use verbal praise, stickers, or prizes to enhance cooperation.*
G.   *Allow infants to have a bottle, cracker, or favorite toy with them during the exam.*
H.   *Have a booster seat or pillows available to enable optimal positioning for young children.*

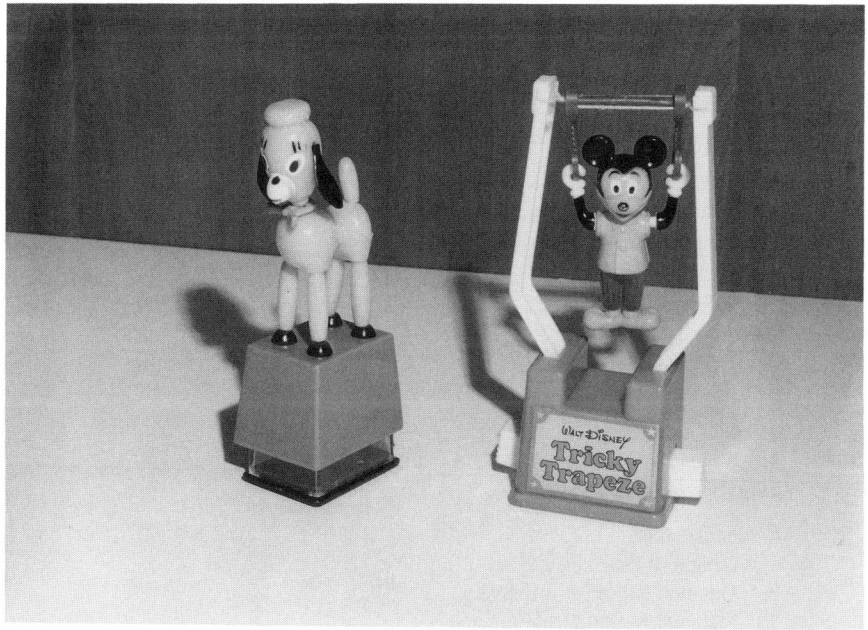

Figure 11-2.   Fixation targets for preschool children (*photo by Ron Davidoff*).

    I.   *Allow infants and young children to sit on their parent's lap or rest over parent's shoulder.*

    J.   *Allow parents to sit in during exam if child needs them.*

    K.   *Dilate children at first visit and every other year thereafter unless following pathology or new signs or symptoms arise.*

    L.   *Dilate at end of exam, defer until second appointment, or have an assistant administer the drops to maintain rapport with child.*

III. Areas to evaluate

    A.   *History/development.*

    B.   *Visual acuity. Contrast sensitivity.*

    C.   *Ocular health*
        1. Posterior segment
        2. Anterior segment

    D.   *Color vision.*

    E.   *Visual fields (not performed routinely unless suspect a problem).*

    F.   *Binocularity.*

    G.   *Accommodation.*

    H.   *Ocular motor system*
        1. Pursuits.
        2. Saccades.
        3. Position maintenance.
        4. Vergence
            a. Motor.
            b. Sensory.

    I.   *Refractive error.*

IV. History. When examining children, a comprehensive history is an invaluable aid in detecting, diagnosing, and managing vision problems. The following information can be elicited through a questionnaire mailed to the parent or filled out prior to the beginning of the exam.

    A.   *Background information*
        1. Child's age (see Table 11-1).
        2. School attending and grade.
        3. Reason for visit.
        4. Natural, foster, adopted.

    B.   *Family vision history*
        1. Nearsightedness/farsightedness/astigmatism.
        2. Amblyopia/strabismus (lazy eye).
        3. Blindness.
        4. Eye disease.

    C.   *Previous eye care*
        1. Glasses.
        2. Patching.
        3. Medication.
        4. Surgery.
        5. Therapy.

    D.   *Pregnancy*
        1. Length of pregnancy.
        2. Duration and type of delivery.
        3. Maternal health during pregnancy.
        4. Birth complications.

Table 11-1. Key Problems to Look for by Age

Birth–2 Years	2–5 Years	5–8 Years	9–18 Years
Common parental concerns			
Eye turning	Eye turning	Routine exam prior to school	Squinting
Tearing	Squinting	Difficulty copying	Blurred vision at near
Squinting	Eye rubbing	Difficulty learning to read	Loses place when reading
Eye rubbing	Photophobia	Letter or word reversals	Headaches with near work
Photophobia	Holds books or objects very close	Loses place when reading	Losing interest in school
Family history of vision problems	Clumsy/bumps into things	Blurred vision	Grades dropping
	Avoids books or fine motor tasks	Rubbing eyes	Double vision
		Intermittent eye turning	Rubbing eyes
			Intermittent eye turning
Common optometric concerns			
Congenital malformations of eye, lid, and adnexa	Moderate refractive errors	Mild to moderate refractive errors	Mild refractive errors
Neurologic disorders, including ptosis and nystagmus	Ocular pathologies	Oculomotor dysfunction	Accommodative dysfunction
Ocular pathologies such as cataracts or retinoblastoma	Neurologic disorders	Significant phorias or tropias	Binocular vision dysfunction
	Amblyopia (strabismic or refractive)	Visual perceptual problems	
	Strabismus (accommodative esotropia/intermittent exotropia)		

E. *Postdelivery period*
    1. Birth weight.
    2. Apgar score.
    3. Number of days in hospital.
    4. Jaundice.
    5. Incubator use.
    6. Infections.
    7. Sucking problems.
    8. Breathing difficulties.
    9. Swallowing difficulties.
    10. Birth defects.

F. *Infancy—toddler period*
    1. Were/are any of the following present—to a significant degree?
        a. Colic.
        b. Excessive restlessness.
        c. Diminished sleep.
        d. Frequent headbanging.
        e. Excessive number of accidents.
        f. Did not enjoy cuddling.
        g. Was not calmed by being held and/or stroked.
    2. Additional questions for preschoolers
        a. What are child's favorite toys, games, songs?
        b. Is there anything the child is frightened of?

G. *Preschool to school-age children. Ask about the following signs and symptoms of a vision problem (depending on the child's age):*
    1. Blurred vision.
    2. Double vision.

     3. Headaches.

     4. Eye turning in or out/lazy eye.

     5. Frequently closes or covers one eye.

     6. Skips lines when reading.

     7. Letter or word reversals.

     8. Eye-hand coordination difficulties.

     9. Moves head excessively while reading.

    10. Eyestrain.

    11. Frequently rubs eyes.

    12. Frequently needs to reread lines.

    13. Difficulty remembering things that were seen.

    14. Difficulty with depth perception.

    15. Uses a finger while reading.

    16. Gets close to reading materials.

    17. Avoids reading.

    18. Excessive time to complete written work.

H. *Academic history. Knowledge of a child's academic performance will often help uncover vision problems. Ask about the following areas:*

     1. Spelling.

     2. Mathematics.

     3. Reading—what level?

     4. Writing.

     5. Behavior.

     6. Has child ever repeated a grade? Why?

     7. Is child in special education or receiving remedial help?

I. *Additional testing*

     1. Neurologic.

     2. Psychological/psychiatric.

     3. Medical.

     4. Educational.

     5. Nutritional.

     6. Lead levels.

     7. Developmental.

     8. Hearing/speech and language.

J. *General development*

     1. Assessed through careful history.

     2. Formally evaluated using a screening test (e.g., Denver developmental screening test [DDST]), which evaluates four areas:

        a. Language.

        b. Social.

        c. Fine motor.

        d. Gross motor.

     3. DDST is a screening only.

     4. Useful in helping practitioners detect abnormalities in development.

     5. DDST may miss mild delays.

V. Visual Acuity

A. *Developmental changes*

     1. Infants have a rapid improvement in visual acuity which approaches adult levels by the end of the first year of life.

     2. The exact values depend on child's age and method used (i.e., visual evoked potentials yield 20/20 visual acuity by 6 months vs. forced choice preferential

looking techniques yield 20/100 visual acuity by 6 months of age and 20/50 by 12 months of age).

3. From birth until age 3 years, testing is done primarily at near, as distant targets fail to hold attention of very young children.
4. Children aged 3 and older can often respond to both near and distance visual acuity tests.
5. Amblyopia can be present as early as 6 months of age.
6. Amblyopia can be effectively treated at any age throughout childhood and beyond.

B. *Clinical presentation of reduced visual acuity*
  1. Reduced visual acuity in infants or toddlers may present as
     a. Poor tracking skills.
     b. Rubbing eyes and redness.
     c. Failure to recognize familiar faces from a distance.
     d. Inattentiveness.
     e. Excessive clumsiness in children as they begin to walk.
     f. Lack of interest in the environment.
     g. Inability to maintain eye contact.
     h. No signs or symptoms if unilateral.
     i. Lack of interest in small, detailed tasks.
     j. No signs or symptoms.
  2. Reduced visual acuity in preschool or school age children may present as
     a. Avoidance of near tasks.
     b. Poor fine-motor coordination or poor athletic performance.
     c. Shyness or reduced physical activity.
     d. Squinting/brow ache.
     e. Headaches.
     f. Holding books or reading material close.
     g. No signs or symptoms.

C. *Diagnostic evaluation: unique tools*
  1. Occlusion
     a. Use appropriate occlusion techniques for monocular visual acuity testing.
     b. Important to prevent peeking, which is especially prevalent in children with amblyopia.
     c. Periodically check for appropriate positioning of occlusion during testing.
     d. General guidelines for the type of occlusion are as follows:
        (1) Birth to age 2—adhesive patch.
        (2) 3–7 years—black patch with elastic.
        (3) 7–10 years—black patch with elastic, or doctor holds occluder.
        (4) 10–18 years—occluder.
        (5) If amblyopia is suspected—use black elastic or adhesive patch regardless of age (Figures 11-3 to 11-5).
  2. Forced choice preferential looking (FPL)
     a. A near visual acuity test used for children from birth to age 5. Also used in physically or mentally impaired older children. Commercially available tools:
     b. PL 20/20 tester (no longer commercially available)
        Unique features
        (1) Portable.
        (2) Internally illuminated, which is good for visually impaired children.
        (3) Central red fixation lights and beeper.
     c. Teller acuity cards (Figures 11-6 and 11-7)
        Unique features
        (1) Portable.
        (2) Allows good eye contact with child.
        (3) Allows easy use of puppets and other attention-enhancing toys.

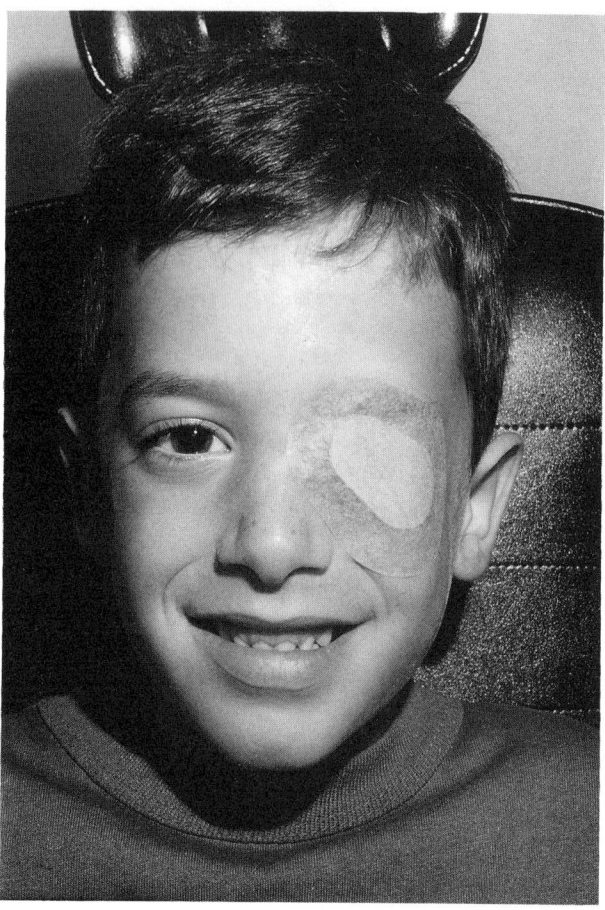

Figure 11-3. Adhesive patching for visual acuity testing (*photo by Ron Davidoff*).

       (4) Can be held vertically or in other positions if necessary (e.g., to test a child with nystagmus).

       (5) Can purchase a half set of cards at less expense. Extensive research on usefulness.

    d. General protocol for FPL

       (1) Place child at appropriate test distance on parent's lap if necessary.

       (2) Present largest grating (examiner should not know which side stripes are on).

       (3) Determine if infant shows a preference for one side.

       (4) Reverse presentation.

       (5) Does infant now look at other side?

       (6) If no looking preference is shown, go to larger target.

       (7) If looking preference is correct, go to smaller stripes.

    e. Modifications to preferential looking

       (1) Use examiner's face, hand puppets, or finger puppets to enhance child's attention.

       (2) Play music behind card to maintain attention.

       (3) Blow bubbles in front of card to enhance attention to stripes.

       (4) Operant preferential looking (OPL)—same as above, but child is rewarded with a cereal or raisin for correctly pointing to the stripes.

       (5) For nonresponsive children—send parents home with copy of stripes and instructions to train the child to point to the stripes for several weeks prior to retesting.

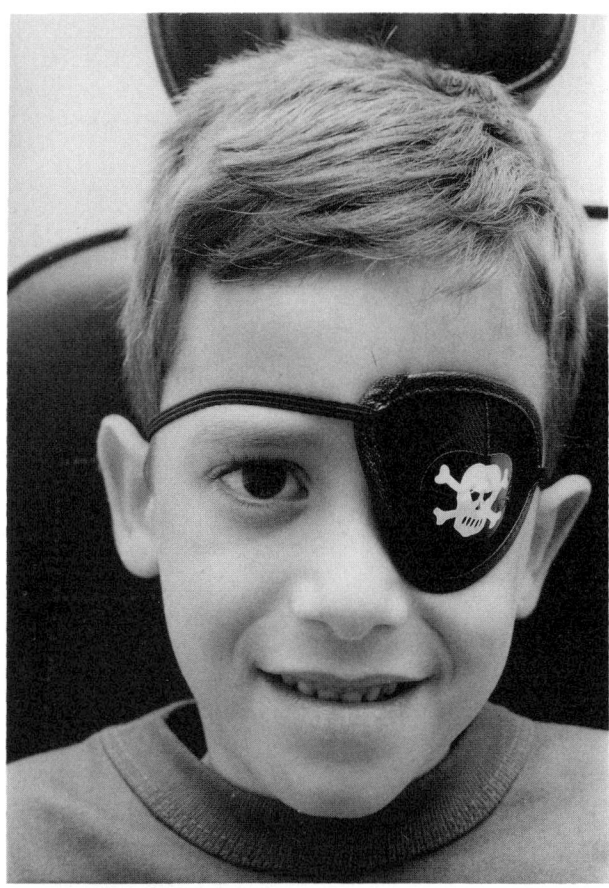

Figure 11-4.   Elastic Patching for visual acuity testing (*photo by Ron Davidoff*).

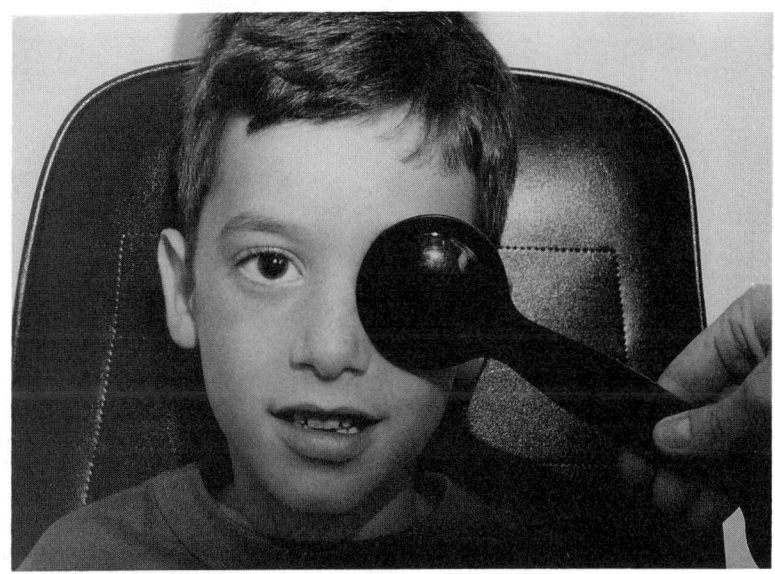

Figure 11-5.   Occluder held by examiner (*photo by Ron Davidoff*).

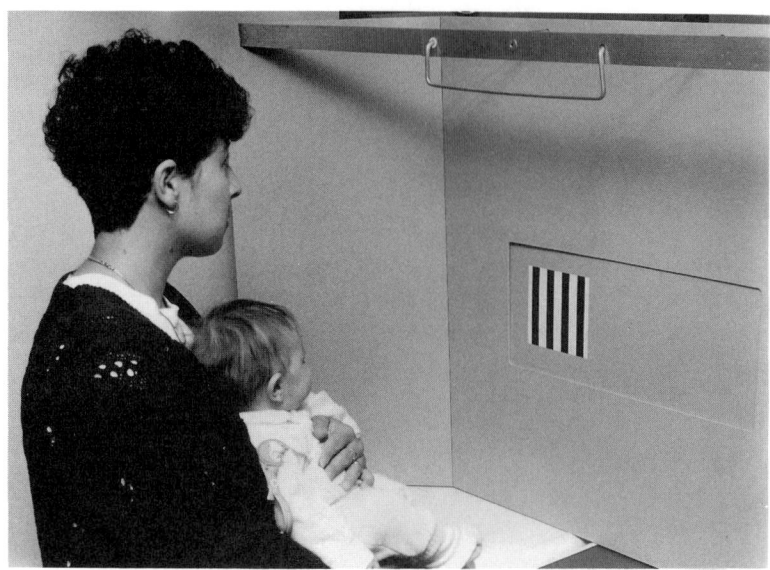

Figure 11-6.   Visual acuity assessment using preferential looking (*photo by Ron Davidoff*).

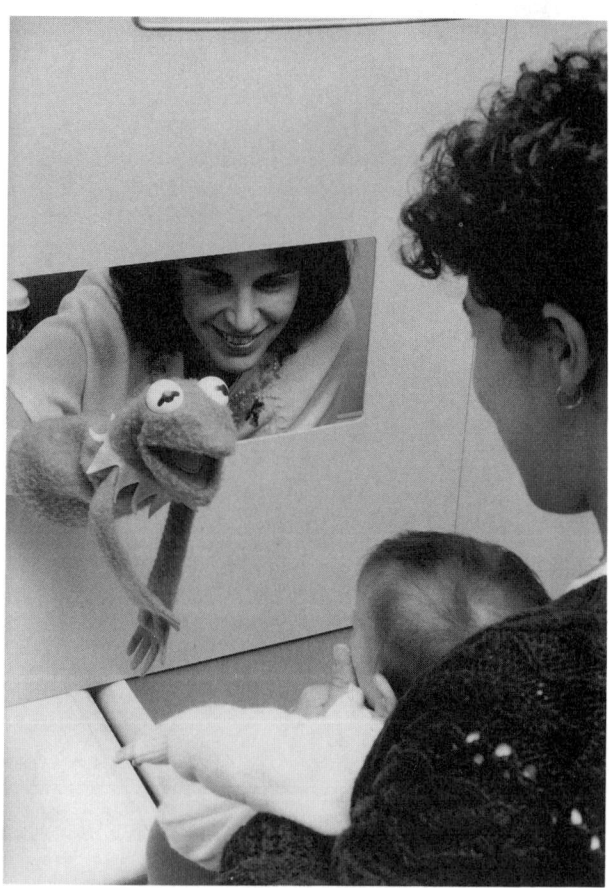

Figure 11-7.   Use of toys to enhance and maintain attention during preferential looking (*photo by Ron Davidoff*).

(6) Children with horizontal nystagmus or strabismus—arrange the striped targets in a vertical presentation and watch for vertical eye movements.

(7) Increase or decrease the standardized test distance.

(8) For children who object to occlusion—send a patch home with parents for several days prior to testing.

f. Interpretation of FPL results

(1) FPL (a grating acuity) is different from Snellen (a recognition acuity task).

(2) FPL results may overestimate actual results obtainable with Snellen optotypes.

(3) FPL may underestimate visual acuity when compared to visual evoked response results.

(4) FPL may not detect strabismic amblyopia.

(5) FPL may underestimate refractive amblyopia when compared to measures of recognition acuity.

(6) FPL may not actually test central vision up to age 2 years.

(7) FPL is currently the clinical method of choice to assess visual acuity in young children.

(8) Normative data available which are useful in detecting vision anomalies.

3. Broken wheel test

a. A distance visual acuity test effective in children beginning at age 3. Also can be used in older children who are physically or mentally impaired or who have difficulty with letters or numbers (Figure 11-8)

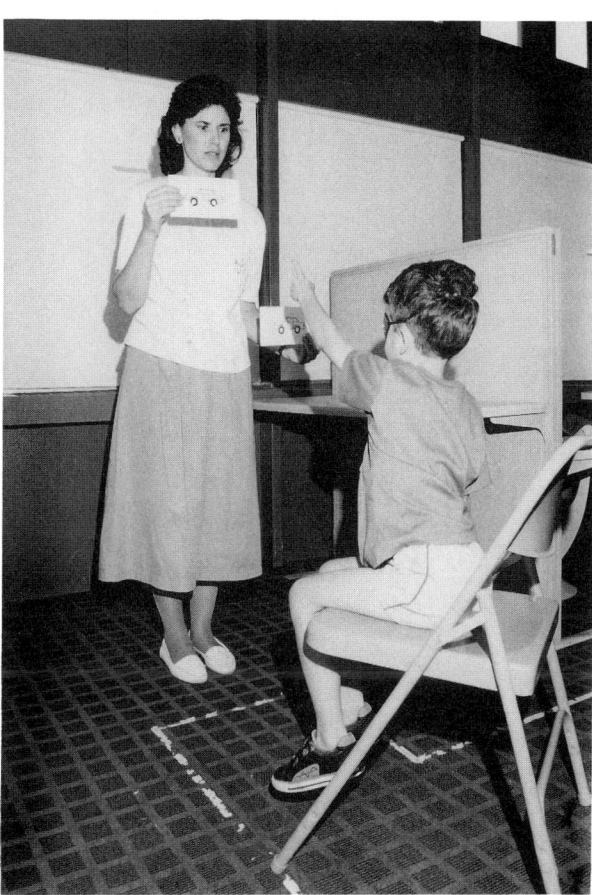

Figure 11-8. Broken wheel test for visual acuity (*photo by Ron Davidoff*).

      b. Unique features
- (1) Inexpensive.
- (2) Portable.
- (3) Correlates well with Snellen acuity.
- (4) No expressive language needed (child just points).

      c. General protocol
- (1) Present demonstration (20/100) targets at 30 cm and ask child to identify the car with the broken wheels. Child must be consistent on 4 of 4 trials to pass this pretest.
- (2) Present 20/100 card at 10 feet and ask child to again identify the car with the broken wheels.
- (3) If child is unable to respond or child has difficulty maintaining attention, present test at 5 feet or closer and recalibrate cards.
- (4) Child must choose correctly on 4 of 4 trials to continue to next lower acuity level.
- (5) Make sure child looks at both cards before choosing.
- (6) Separate cards both horizontally and vertically to allow easy interpretation of the child's pointing response.
- (7) Watch child's eye movements along with pointing response.

4. LEA symbols (1992 version)

      a. Distance and near visual acuity tests that use picture optotypes (Figure 11-9).

      b. Unique features
- (1) Portable.
- (2) Calibrated for 10 or 20 feet.
- (3) Pictures easy to match.
- (4) New optotypes eliminate many problems inherent in older "apple, umbrella, house" cards.
- (5) Puzzle of optotypes available to enhance interest, match cards, or train child for test.
- (6) Crowded and uncrowded test cards available.

      c. General protocol
- (1) Several versions of LEA symbols are available.
- (2) Examiner holds up picture and child must name, identify, or match.
- (3) 3-dimensional puzzle available for matching.

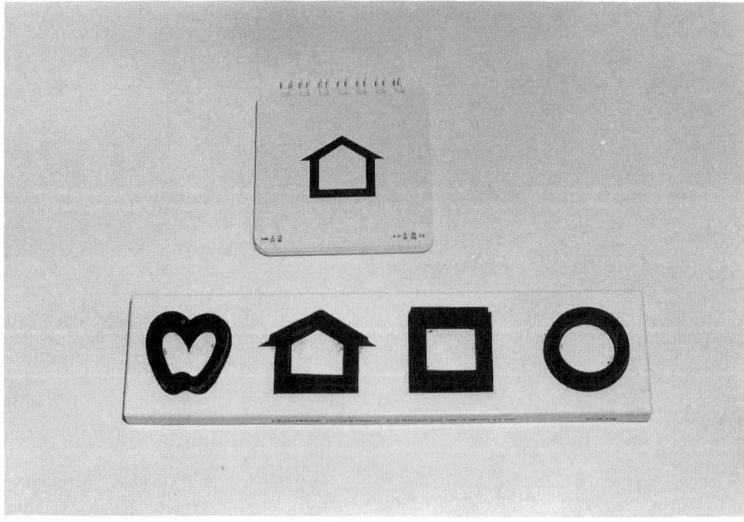

Figure 11-9.   LEA symbols with matching puzzle (*photo by Ron Davidoff*).

5. Tumbling E chart
   a. A near or distance visual acuity test which is most effective in children beginning at age 5. Children with right-left confusion may have difficulty with this test.
   b. Unique features
      (1) Already on many projected charts.
      (2) No expressive language needed.
   c. General protocol
      (1) Present a vertical line of letters from approximately 20/70 to 20/30 and ask the child to identify the direction of each "E."
      (2) Have child use his or her hand or a prototype "E" to show the direction.
      (3) When left–right confusion is evident, ask the child to identify whether the E is up or down or to the side. If confusion continues, use only vertical (up and down) presentation of the E, or use the broken wheel test.
      (4) Isolate the horizontal line of the smallest letter the child was able to read vertically and continue testing.
6. Snellen chart
   a. A near or distance visual acuity test which is most effective in children beginning at age 5, depending on their familiarity with letters.
   b. Unique features. Standard for adult visual acuity.
   c. General protocol
      (1) Procedure is same as for tumbling E.
      (2) Children who know their letters may continue to show difficulty in recalling letter names when they are shown at a distance.
      (3) If this occurs, try giving the child a choice of several letters from which to choose a response.
7. Other unique visual acuity tests
   a. Optokinetic nystagmus drum
      (1) Unique features
         (a) Motion detection task.
         (b) Traditionally used in young children.
         (c) Generally performed at near, as children lose interest at a distance.
         (d) Useful in comparing visual acuity between eyes.
         (e) Testing primarily peripheral retina.
      (2) General protocol
         (a) Child is seated in front of optokinetic nystagmus drum.
         (b) Examiner slowly spins drum in front of child and looks for optokinetic nystagmus.
         (c) Spatial frequency of stripes corresponds to visual acuity.
         (d) Change visual acuity by changing width of stripes or moving further away from child.
   b. Candy bead test
      (1) Unique features
         (a) Resolution task.
         (b) Differs from Snellen or grating acuity.
         (c) No expressive language required.
         (d) Near visual acuity task.
      (2) General protocol
         (a) Child is seated in front of apparatus.
         (b) Child asked to find or point to candy beads of various sizes.
         (c) Size of candy is decreased until threshold is reached.
   c. H.O.T.V. matching method
      (1) A letter matching test for preschool children.
      (2) Unique features
         (a) Uses four optotypes that have the same image when viewed with a mirror or without.

         (b)   Avoids laterality problems in young children.

         (c)   Incorporates crowding bars for amblyopes.

     (3) General protocol

         (a)   Child is shown optotype at a distance.

         (b)   Child must point to identical optotype on card in front of him or her.

  d. Cardiff acuity test cards

     (1) Uses high-frequency, vanishing pictures presented on cards that incorporate principles of preferential looking.

     (2) Unique features

         (a)   Uses a vertical direction of gaze for easier observation of looking responses.

         (b)   Familiar pictures for targets. Useful as a detection and resolution task.

         (c)   Three cards at each acuity level.

     (3) General protocol

         (a)   Examiner presents cards beginning with highest acuity level.

         (b)   Examiner watches for up or down eye movement.

         (c)   After positive responses to two cards at a particular acuity level, the next lower level is presented.

  e. N.V.T.C. (near vision test for children)

     (1) A near vision test for use with young children or older children who experience reading difficulty or delay. The tasks required of children in this test are representative of the reading tasks required of them in educational settings. This helps differentiate between the child's cognitive and visual abilities.

     (2) Unique features

         (a)   Has various types of nearpoint reading tasks.

         (b)   Includes individual letters, words, and short stories.

         (c)   Short stories were written by children.

         (d)   For children aged 3 and older or with special needs.

     (3) General protocol: four parts to test

         (a)   Selected word reading card.

         (b)   Short stories by children.

         (c)   Word matching.

         (d)   Letter matching.

  f. Baily-Hall cereal test

     (1) Forced choice recognition task that measures visual acuity by asking child to point a familiar types of cereal.

     (2) Unique features

         (a)   Uses optotype child is familiar with (Cheerios).

         (b)   Recognition task.

         (c)   Can incorporate operant procedures to enhance attention and provide reinforcement.

     (3) General protocol

         (a)   Child looks at two cards.

         (b)   One card has a cereal picture, other has a square of equal size.

         (c)   Child must point to cereal.

         (d)   Child is given a matching cereal to eat for correct response.

D. *Differential diagnosis and common problems based on age. Reduced acuity in children may indicate*

  1. Malingering.

  2. Pathological/neurological problem.

  3. Refractive error.

4. Accommodative dysfunction.

5. Amblyopia.

E. *Malingerers. Rule out by screening for other causes and by*

1. Isolating single letters of varying sizes on chart.

2. Look for inconsistency in responses.

3. Trial frame plano or low plus and ask child to read chart.

4. Check visual acuity using less obvious methods, i.e., keystone telebinocular cards, Flom chart.

5. Inquire about child's interest or anticipated need for glasses.

6. Inquire if other family members or friends recently received glasses.

7. Check for normal stereopsis findings.

F. *Amblyopia*

1. Definition. Unilateral or bilateral condition in which the best corrected visual acuity is poorer than 20/20 in the absence of any obvious structural or pathologic anomalies.[1]

2. Classification

   a. Strabismic.

   b. Refractive

      (1) Anisometropic.

      (2) Isoametropic.

      (3) Meridional.

   c. Image degradation.

3. Associated findings

   a. Eccentric fixation.

   b. Reduced contrast sensitivity.

   c. Abnormal saccades and pursuits.

   d. Optokinetic asymmetry.

   e. Reduced accommodative responses and vergence (in deep amblyopia).

   f. Subtle afferent pupillary defect.

   g. Crowding phenomenon during visual acuity testing.[1]

4. Diagnostic tests

   a. History.

   b. Cover test.

   c. Ocular health evaluation.

   d. Pupils.

   e. Color vision

      (1) No defect in functional amblyopia.

      (2) May be defect in pathology.

   f. Neutral-density test

      (1) Differentiates functional from organic vision loss.

      (2) Visual acuity decreases with neutral-density filter when pathology present.

      (3) No change in visual acuity with neutral-density filter with functional loss.

   g. Visual evoked potentials.

5. Prognostic tests/factors

   a. History: earlier onset = poorer prognosis.

   b. Visual acuity.

   c. Laser interferometry: pretherapy laser findings predictive of posttherapy visual acuity.

   d. Visuoscopy: eccentric fixation = poorer prognosis.

   e. Age: not a significant factor, amblyopia should be treated at any age.

   f. Motivation: patient and parent must be motivated and willing to comply with treatment.

6. Treatment
   a. Depends on reason and level of vision loss, age of child, and motivation of parent and child.
   b. Daily home and office vision therapy emphasizing the following:
      (1) Accommodation.
      (2) Eye movement and fixation.
      (3) Form recognition/visual memory.
   c. Patching therapy (direct occlusion)
      (1) Primarily home based.
      (2) Begin with 3 to 4 hours.
      (3) Modify when necessary.
      (4) Try to avoid patching during school hours to avoid peer problems.
      (5) Use appropriate occlusion and monitor child to prevent peeking.
      (6) Engage child in activities which are challenging but not frustrating for the child's current level of visual acuity.
      (7) Can be accomplished through penalization therapy of good eye by atropine or overplusing.
   d. Inverse occlusion
      (1) For eccentric fixation.
      (2) Only if direct patching therapy not effective.
      (3) Must be full time.
      (4) Must be done in conjunction with controlled foveal stimulation.
7. Monitoring improvements from amblyopia therapy
   a. Frequency
      (1) In-office therapy—monitor weekly.
      (2) Home-based therapy—monitor monthly.
   b. Clinical tests
      (1) Visual acuity
         (a) Forced choice preferential looking.
         (b) Broken wheel cards.
         (c) Lighthouse cards.
      (2) Visual acuity tests that control for crowding
         (a) Broken wheel cards.
         (b) Wessen cards.
         (c) Flom chart.
      (3) Contrast sensitivity
         (a) Infants—Mr. Happy contrast sensitivity test (Berkley).
         (b) Preschool—lighthouse chart.
         (c) School Age—Vistech contrast sensitivity chart.
      (4) Eccentric fixation
         (a) Visuoscopy.
         (b) Haidinger brush.
   c. Maintenance therapy
      (1) Amblyopia may first occur up until age 7.
      (2) Amblyopia may reoccur until age 9.
      (3) Careful monitoring important.
      (4) Minimal level of maintenance therapy or patching important to prevent regression.
      (5) Level must be determined on an individual basis.

VI. Ocular Health

A. *Developmental changes*
   1. Iris
      a. Amount of iris pigmentation causes variation in eye color.
      b. Infants usually born with "steel" gray eyes due to lack of iris pigmentation.

      c. Iris pigmentation increases over first 6 months with associated darkening of iris color.

      d. Change in iris color usually completed by approximately age 1 year.

2. Pupils

      a. Dilator muscle poorly developed at birth.

      b. Infant's pupils usually miotic.

      c. Normal size and function at 6 months of age.

3. Cornea

      a. Cornea is steep at birth and there is a deep anterior chamber.

      b. Corneal diameter is approximately 10 mm at birth (use to rule out microcornea, macrocornea, congenital glaucoma).

4. Lens. Lens power is greater and compensates for shorter axial length.

5. Sclera

      a. Sclera less rigid at birth.

      b. Sclera is thinner and translucent at birth and may appear blue due to the appearance of the underlying choroidal melanin.

6. Retina

      a. Vessels tortuous at birth.

      b. Retinal hemorrhages may be present at birth, resolving spontaneously without consequence.

      c. Lighter color of retina and optic nerve at birth.

      d. Smaller cup size.

      e. Fovea not fully differentiated until 45 months of age.

      f. At 8 months vasculature complete to nasal ora and temporal equator.

      g. At 9 months vascularized to temporal ora.

      h. Overall axial length of eye is shorter.

7. The premature eye

      a. Decreased corneal diameter (usually <9 mm).

      b. Shorter axial length.

      c. Steeper cornea.

      d. Miotic pupils.

      e. Transient and permanent remnants of tunica vasculosa lentis common.

      f. Transient lenticular opacities.

      g. Incomplete retinal vascularization.

B. *Unique tools and procedures*

1. Posterior segment evaluation

      a. All children should have a dilated fundus examination at their first visit (Table 11-2).

      b. Have a technician or child's parent hold a favorite toy in the diagnostic positions of gaze.

      c. Direct ophthalmoscopy is useful for detection of media opacities as well as initial evaluation of the posterior fundus.

      d. Monocular indirect ophthalmoscopy is advantageous in the younger child and has the following advantages over direct ophthalmoscopy (Figure 11-10):

        (1) Wider field of view.

        (2) Enables more extensive views of the retina than direct.

        (3) Less threatening to child.

        (4) Light is not as bright as a binocular indirect.

        (5) Child's fixation is not essential.

        (6) Provides good view of disc, macula, and posterior pole with minimal cooperation.

        (7) Particularly useful in uncooperative children or those who are tactually defensive.

      e. Binocular indirect ophthalmoscopy should be performed on all children and cooperative younger children.

Table 11-2. Dilation and Cycloplegic Agents for Children

Age	Dilating Agent	Cycloplegic Agent	Precautions
Premature or low-birth-weight infants	1 gtt cyclomydril[a]	1 gtt cyclomydril[a]	Children are often systemically comprised and vital signs must be monitored[b]
Neonate–3 months	1 gtt cyclomydril or 1 gtt 0.5% or 1% mydricyl[c]	1 gtt cyclomydril or 1 gtt 0.5% cyclopentolate[c,d]	
4 months–1 year	1 gtt cyclomydril or 0.5% or 1% mydricyl[d] and 2.5% phenylephrine[c]	1 gtt cyclomydril or 1 gtt 0.5% or 1% cycloplen-tolate[c,d]	Never use > 2.5% phenylephrine or > 1% cyclopentolate
1–18 years	1 gtt 0.5% or 1% mydriacyl[d] and 2.5% phenylephrine[c]	1 gtt 1% cyclopentolate or 1 gtt 1% mydriacyl (repeat in 5–10 minutes)[c]	Beware of system toxic reactions with cyclopentolate, especially in Down's syndrome. Never use > 2.5% phenylephrine or > 1% cyclopentolate

[a]Cyclomydril = 0.2% cyclopentolate and 1% phenylephrine in combination.

[b]Examinations at this stage are usually done to rule out retinopathy of prematurity and should be performed by a pediatric ophthalmologist or retinal specialist.

[c]Generally preceded by 1 drop of a local anesthetic to promote action of drops.

[d]Repeat in 5–10 minutes if necessary.

      f. Any child who cannot be examined with one of the above methods should be referred for an examination under anesthesia if warranted by symptoms.
      g. Dilation and cycloplegia using a "spray" in place of drops has been advocated by some practitioners due to increased ease of application in young children.[2]
      h. NEVER USE *GREATER THAN* 2.5% PHENYLEPHRINE OR 1% CYCLOPENTOLATE IN CHILDREN (see Table 11-2).
      i. BEWARE OF SYSTEMIC TOXIC REACTIONS WITH CYCLOPENTOLATE AND ATROPINE, ESPECIALLY IN DOWN'S SYNDROME PATIENTS.
  2. Anterior segment evaluation
      a. Externally inspect anterior segment in all children.
      b. Check for presence of
         (1) Patent nasolacriminal system.
         (2) Pupillary anomalies.
         (3) Iris color and appearance.
         (4) Intact anterior segment structures: lids, lashes, sclera, vasculature, cornea, anterior chamber, lens.
         (5) Leukocoria.
         (6) Ptosis or other lid anomalies.
      c. Palpate orbital region to detect masses or other abnormalities.
      d. Penlight or transilluminator for gross inspection.
      e. Burton lamp or hand-held magnifier allows for better inspection.
      f. Hand-held slit lamp for infants or less cooperative children.
      g. Standard slit lamp for some cooperative infants and toddlers and older children.
  3. Tonometry
      a. Not routinely performed on young children due to need for cooperation.

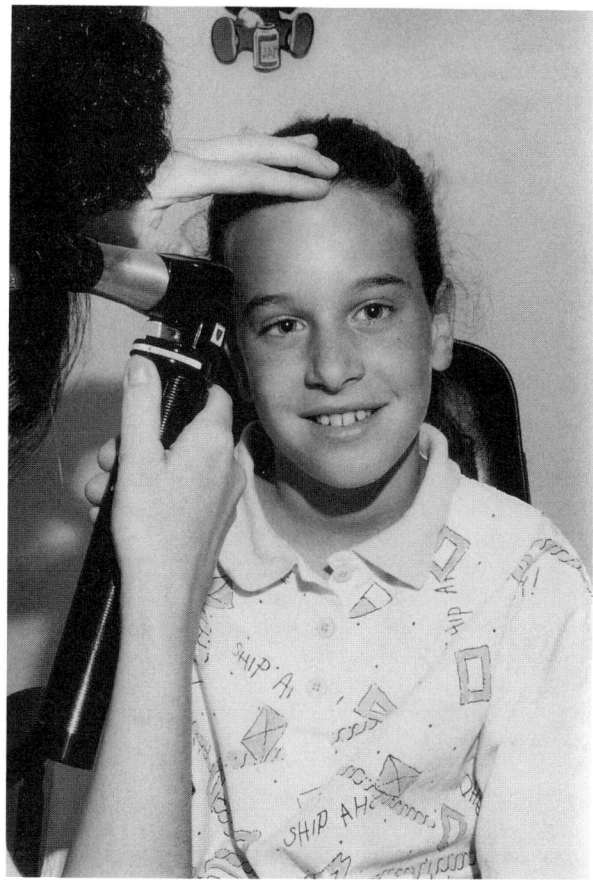

Figure 11-10. Monocular indirect ophthalmoscopy (*photo by Ron Davidoff*).

    b. Portable noncontact tonometry can be performed on infants or cooperative older children.

    c. Portable applanation tonometry (i.e., Goldmann) or digital electronictonometry (Tonopen) can also be performed on cooperative infants and older children.

    d. Monitor for other signs of increased intraocular pressure (IOP):
        (1) Increased corneal diameter.
        (2) Cloudy cornea.
        (3) Large or asymmetric cupping.
        (4) Optic atrophy (often associated with glaucoma).
        (5) Other associated systemic anomalies.

    e. Refer to pediatric ophthalmologist when glaucoma is suspected in children.

C. *Commonly presenting pathologies in children*
    1. Leukocoria
        a. White pupil is the presenting sign in many of the common childhood diseases seen in private practice. In the early stages, these diseases may not produce leukocoria and therefore a thorough anterior and posterior examination is necessary to rule out the presence of these conditions.

        b. Differential diagnosis
            (1) Retinoblastoma.
            (2) Coats' disease.
            (3) Persistent hyperplastic primary vitreous (PHPV).

         (4) *Toxocara canis* granuloma.
         (5) Retinal astrocytoma.
         (6) Coloboma.
         (7) Congenital cataract.
         (8) Retinopathy of prematurity.
         (9) Other rare causes.

2. Retinoblastoma (RB)
   a. Malignant, childhood ocular tumor.
   b. Background information
      (1) Heredity
          (a) Autosomal dominant with 80% penetrance OR
          (b) Sporadic mutation.
          (c) Bilateral cases are usually inherited.
          (d) A few have chromosome 13 deletion and are mildly mentally retarded.[3]
          (e) RB gene has been localized to chromosome 13 and it is now possible to perform genetic testing in some hereditary cases to determine carriers. This will aid in early diagnosis and treatment.[3]
      (2) The following individuals are at a *higher risk* for RB:
          (a) Sibling with RB and a positive family history.
          (b) Parent with unilateral RB and a positive family history.
          (c) Parent with bilateral RB with or without family history.
      (3) The following individuals are at a *lower risk* for RB:
          (a) Sibling with RB and a negative family history.
          (b) Parent with unilateral RB and a negative family history.
          (c) Parent with a sibling with RB.
   c. Characteristics
      (1) Unilateral (70%) or bilateral (30%).
      (2) Single or multiple tumors.
      (3) Whitish-gray, pink, or black lesions.
      (4) Lumpy appearance (due to calcium particles) or can also be smooth with neovascularization on surface with associated hemorrhaging.
      (5) Usually diagnosed before 5 years of age.
      (6) Reports of older children and adults with newly diagnosed active RB.[4]
      (7) Symptoms in older children and adults include pain, floaters, and decreased vision.[4]
      (8) Signs in older children may include atypical inflammation or intraocular hemorrhage.[4]
   d. Clinical presentation
      (1) Early presentation
          (a) Strabismus if macula involved.
          (b) Vision variably affected (no vision loss if macula uninvolved and small tumor).
          (c) Flat, small tumors of posterior pole or periphery.
          (d) Leukocoria visible only in extreme gaze.
      (2) Late presentation
          (a) Blind leukocoric eye.
          (b) Rubeosis with iris color change.
          (c) Enlarged protruding eye.
          (d) Hyphema, hypopyon.
          (e) Orbital cellulitis (due to tumor necrosis).
          (f) Nystagmus (if bilateral decreased vision at an early age).
      (3) Systemic associations
          (a) High risk of secondary systemic malignancy.

         (b) Trilateral RB = bilateral RB with a primary pineal or parasellar mass.

  e. When to examine for RB

     (1) Varying opinions, although generally children at any risk should be examined the first week of life.

     (2) High-risk children should be seen every month beginning the first week of life until 6 months, then every few months until age 3, twice a year until age 6, then yearly.[3]

     (3) Low-risk children should be seen every 4 months until age 1, twice a year until age 5, and then yearly.[3]

     (4) Examination under anesthesia with scleral depression may be necessary unless the child is cooperative, since an inadequate view of the retina could be life-threatening.

     (5) Referral within 24 hours to a pediatric ophthalmologist or retinal specialist, preferably one who specializes in ocular oncology. Delay in treatment results in increased morbidity and mortality.

  f. Management

     (1) Enucleation, especially if unilateral and severe involvement.

     (2) External beam radiotherapy, radioactive episcleral plaque, chemotherapy, laser photocoagulation, or cryotherapy, especially for small tumors.

     (3) Genetic counseling and examination of all available immediate family members to aid in determination of hereditary expression.

3. Coats' disease

  a. Background information

     (1) Retinovascular disease characterized by idiopathic retinal telangiectatic vessels.

     (2) Advanced stage resembles retinoblastoma.

     (3) Nonhereditary.

     (4) Usually unilateral.

     (5) Most frequently seen in males.

     (6) Clinically seen usually during the first two decades of life, but may occur at any age, although the vascular abnormality is thought to be congenital.

  b. Characteristics

     (1) Early stages

        (a) Circinate pattern of yellow exudates and refractile cholesterol around dilated telangiectatic vessels.

        (b) Most commonly in the superior temporal retina.[5]

        (c) Disease progression: extensive exudation and hemorrhage. Vision variably affected depending on whether the exudation is limited to the periphery or involves the posterior pole and macula (cystoid macular edema or macular exudation).

     (2) Late stages

        (a) Exudative retinal detachment with refractile cholesterol particles on the surface.

        (b) Abnormal vascular profusion can cause ischemia and subsequent

           i. Retinal neovascularization.

           ii. Retinal or vitreous hemorrhage.

           iii. Heterochromia secondary to rubeosis.

           iv. Spontaneous hyphema (occasionally).

           v. Neovascular glaucoma.

        (c) Leukocoria may be present secondary to retinal detachment.

        (d) Blindness.

    c. Differential diagnosis
      (1) Fluorescein angiography in mild cases reveals late leakage of fluorescein around vascular abnormalities, arteriovenous collaterals, and capillary dropout.
      (2) Leukocoric stage—ultrasound, CT scan, MRI, cytologic assessment of aspirated subretinal fluid and aqueous tap may be performed to rule out RB.
      (3) Differential diagnosis from RB
        (a) Exudation prominent in Coats'.
        (b) Exudation is refractile in Coats' due to cholesterol crystals while RB shows dull calcium particles.[6]
        (c) Carcinoembryonic antigen may be present in RB.
    d. Management
      (1) Cryotherapy/photocoagulation for mild telangiectasias/exudation.
      (2) Drainage of subretinal exudate for localized retinal detachment.
      (3) Scleral buckle for total retinal detachment.
      (4) Enucleation of blind painful eye secondary to acute congestive glaucoma.
      (5) Treatment of a hopelessly blind eye with total detachment may be a viable option to observation, since observation more frequently leads to a painful glaucomatous eye which requires enucleation and less desirable cosmesis.[7]

4. Persistent hyperplastic primary vitreous (PHPV)
    a. Background information
      (1) Remnant of the primary fetal vitreous.
      (2) Nonhereditary.
      (3) Affects males and females equally.
      (4) Usually unilateral.
      (5) Congenital.
      (6) Affected eye is usually microphthalmic.
      (7) Diagnosed shortly after birth due to microphthalmos.
      (8) Vision is variably affected.
    b. Characteristics
      (1) Leucokoria due either to a retrolental mass with a clear lens or later to a posterior cortical cataract that may develop and progress to a complete, swollen cataractous lens.
      (2) Microphthalmia in typical PHPV.
      (3) Shallow anterior chamber both anatomically and secondary to a swelling cataractous lens.
      (4) Mild cases may present with only a white posterior lenticular opacity and a persistent hyaloid artery.
      (5) Advanced cases show microphthalmia, cataractous lens with visible ciliary processes, and a vascularized retrolental membrane attached to the back of the lens.
      (6) There may be posterior pole involvement in the form of fibrovascular bands on, near, or extending from the disc to the ora.
      (7) This traction may lead to a retinal detachment with associated leukocoria.
      (8) Complications include
        (a) Acute pupil block glaucoma.
        (b) Vitreous hemorrhage.
        (c) Retinal detachment.
        (d) Strabismus.
    c. Differential diagnosis (Table 11-3)
      (1) Advanced leukocoric cases may resemble RB due to cataract or retinal detachment.

Table 11-3. Differential Diagnosis of Leukocoria in Children

Pathology	Age	Unilat vs. Bilat	Anterior Segment Findings	Posterior Segment Findings
Retinoblastoma	Primarily birth–4 years	Either	Rubeosis Enlarged protruding eye Hyphema Hypopyon Orbital cellulitis	Retinal tumors Retinal detachment Retinal hemorrhage
PHPV	Present at birth	Unilateral	Glaucoma Microphthalmos Cataract Shallow anterior chamber	Retrolental membrane Fibrovascular bands Retinal detachment Vitreous hemorrhage Hypoplastic disc
Coats' disease	2–10 years	Unilateral	Rubeosis Spontaneous hyphema Neovascular glaucoma	Telangiectasia of vessels Exudates around normal vessels Refractile bodies Retinal detachment Retinal hemorrhage Vitreous hemorrhage
Toxicaria canis	2–40 years	Either	Uveitis Synechiae Cataract Hypopyon	Retinal detachment Fibrotic traction bands Round raised mass (granuloma) all in posterior pole or periphery
Coloboma	Present at birth	Either	Coloboma of iris or lens	Coloboma of disc, retina, macula Pigmental changes around coloboma Retinal detachment
Astrocytic hamartoma	Congenital	Either	Neurofibroma Exophthalmos Glaucoma Lisch module virus	White oval or lobulated tumors of retina
Cataracts	Congenital—present at birth Acquired—at any age	Either	Lens opacity Anterior synechiae if Axenfeld's anomaly	
Retinopathy of prematurity	Congenital	Either	Narrow angle glaucoma Cataracts Microcornea Pthisis bulbi Band keratopathy	Retinal detachment Vitreous and retinal hemorrhages Fibrovascular proliferation Retinal neovascularization Vascular dilation and tortuosity Arteriovenous shunt

      (2) A-scan shows short anterior-posterior diameter.
      (3) B-scan shows retrolental mass without retinal tumors.
      (4) PHPV eye is usually microphthalmic (RB is not).
      (5) Early diagnosis in PHPV since eye looks "different" at birth.
      (6) Drawn ciliary processes not seen in RB.
  d. Management
      (1) Goal is to prevent glaucoma and avoid enucleation (secondary to painful glaucoma).

        (2) Lens and membrane removal when indicated.

        (3) Early intervention to avoid amblyopia.

        (4) Best correction with direct patching when amblyopia present.

        (5) Postsurgical aphakic correction with patching therapy.

5. *Toxocara canis*

   a. Background information

      (1) Parasitic infection transmitted through dog feces.

      (2) Frequently obtained by eating dirt.

      (3) Granulomas develop throughout the body as the larvae travel through the bloodstream.

   b. Characteristics

      (1) Usually unilateral.

      (2) Any age, although usually seen in ages 2–40.

      (3) Round, raised mass associated with an inflammatory reaction.

      (4) May develop fibrotic traction bands with pigmentary changes.

      (5) The traction bands may lead to a dragged disc and/or retinal detachment.

      (6) Anterior and posterior uveitis with associated posterior synechiae and cataract.

      (7) May present with decreased vision, leucokoria, strabismus (cataract or retinal detachment).

      (8) Vision may range from unaffected with isolated peripheral lesions to severely affected with macular involvement to blindness with retinal detachment.

   c. Differential diagnosis

      (1) Order an enzyme-linked immunosorbent assay (ELISA) for *Toxocara*.

      (2) Severe cellular reaction in *Toxocara* (not present in RB).

      (3) Synechiae and cataract present in *Toxocara* (rare in RB).

   d. Management. Refer to retinal specialist who may, depending on complications

      (1) Administer oral steroids.

      (2) Perform photocoagulation or cryopexy.

      (3) Enucleate if eye is blind and painful.

      (4) Routinely monitor for retinal breaks.

6. Astrocytic hamartoma

   a. Background information

      (1) Autosomal dominant.

      (2) Benign, congenital tumor with slow growth.

      (3) May be associated with

         (a) Café au lait spots.

         (b) Ash leaf spots.

         (c) Shagreen patches.

         (d) Nodular/papular lesions on nose and cheeks (adenoma sebaceum).

         (e) Tuberous sclerosis.

         (f) Neurofibromatosis.

         (g) Seizures.

         (h) Mental retardation.

         (i) Intracranial calcifications.

         (j) Retinitis pigmentosa.

         (k) Other systemic associations such as brain tumors and renal and cardiac abnormalities.

   b. Characteristics

      (1) White, oval tumor or lobulated mulberry-like tumor.

      (2) Often but not always located on or near the disc.

      (3) Vision and fields are variably affected, depending on the location and size of the tumor.

             (4) Papilledema and optic atrophy may occur when associated with brain tumors or hydrocephalus.
- c. Differential diagnosis
  - (1) Systemic involvement common with astrocytic hamartoma and not with early RB.
  - (2) Tumor is nonprogressive and benign.
  - (3) Slow growth of tumor possible, but not rapid as in RB.
- d. Management
  - (1) Rule out RB with retinal specialist.
  - (2) Rule out systemic associations with referral to pediatrician.
  - (3) Examine family members if history not helpful.
  - (4) Genetic counseling.

7. Coloboma
   - a. Background information
     - (1) Faulty fetal fusion of embryonic fissure.
     - (2) Congenital.
     - (3) Autosomal dominant, recessive or no inheritance.
     - (4) Systemic associations include
       - (a) Encephalocele.
       - (b) Cardiac abnormalities.
       - (c) Facial palsies.
       - (d) Chromosome abnormalities.
       - (e) Disorders of the genitourinary and intestinal tracts, musculoskeletal system, nasopharynx, and ear.
       - (f) Ocular associations
         - i. Orbital cysts.
         - ii. Retinal dysplasia.
         - iii. Retinal detachment.
   - b. Characteristics
     - (1) May involve disc, retina, macula, choroid, iris, or lens.
     - (2) Presentation is usually in an inferior location.
     - (3) Disc may appear enlarged.
     - (4) Seen as a lack of tissue in involved area.
     - (5) Retinal and choroidal involvement appears as a yellowish flat or depressed lesion with surrounding pigmentary changes.
     - (6) Retinal detachment is common in disc and retinal colobomas and may cause leukocoria.
     - (7) Vision may be affected if macula is involved.
     - (8) Visual field may be affected due to thinned retinal pigment epithelium.
     - (9) Color vision may be affected.
   - c. Differential diagnosis
     - (1) Leucokoria with retinal detachment may resemble RB.
     - (2) B-scan will not reveal tumor.
     - (3) Retinal lesion is flat or depressed, not elevated as in RB.
   - d. Management[8]
     - (1) Rule out systemic involvement.
     - (2) Protective eyewear to prevent retinal detachment secondary to injury.
     - (3) Education of child and family to signs and symptoms of retinal detachment.
     - (4) Routine eye examinations to monitor for associated retinal changes around the coloboma.

8. Congenital cataract
   - a. Background information
     - (1) Cataracts present within the first year of life.
     - (2) Usually autosomal dominant.
     - (3) May be sporadic.

        (4) May be a result of
- (a) Trauma.
- (b) Radiation.
- (c) Maternal illness, especially during the first trimester.
- (d) Maternal abuse of drugs.

        (5) May be associated with systemic disease:
- (a) Rubella and other infections.
- (b) Hypocalcemia.
- (c) Hypoparathyroidism.
- (d) Hypoglycemia, diabetes mellitus.
- (e) Homocystinuria.
- (f) Alport's syndrome.
- (g) Lowe's syndrome.
- (h) Wilson's disease.
- (i) Galactosemia.
- (j) Others.

b. Characteristics
- (1) May present with obvious leukocoria or varying degrees of opacification.
- (2) Unilateral or bilateral.
- (3) Associated with nystagmus if cataracts are dense and bilateral, if visual acuity is severely affected and opacity is present during the critical period of visual development.
- (4) Associated with amblyopia, especially if unilateral, treatment is delayed, or there is noncompliant aphakic correction and patching therapy.
- (5) May be associated with Axenfeld-Rieger anomaly and glaucoma.

c. Types
- (1) Polar—involves the anterior or posterior capsule centrally and causes minimal or no vision impairment.
- (2) Zonular—involves a zone of the lens (nuclear, lamellar, sutural, spear-like, coralliform, floriform, capsular).
- (3) Total—involves entire lens.

d. Differential diagnosis
- (1) Rare for cataract to be present with RB.
- (2) B-scan to rule out mass.
- (3) Rule out associated ocular disease such as glaucoma, Axenfeld-Rieger anomaly, microphthalmia with PHPV, uveitis with *Toxocara*.

e. Presurgical management
- (1) Estimation of visual function should be determined before and after lens removal.
- (2) Slit lamp examination to determine location and degree of involvement.
- (3) Dilated fundus examination to rule out associated retinal disease and to determine visibility of fundus details, which correlates with patient's visual function.
- (4) Referral to pediatric ophthalmologist for surgical removal of lens within days of diagnosis to enhance visual prognosis and diminish risk of severe amblyopia.
- (5) Referral to pediatrician to rule out associated systemic disease.

f. Postsurgical management
- (1) Unilateral aphakia
  - (a) Contact lens within days after surgery.
  - (b) Aggressive patching/amblyopia therapy.
  - (c) Monitor visual acuity.

(d) Infants should be overcorrected by approximately 2.5 D to account for their close working distance.

    (2) Bilateral aphakia

      (a) Contact lenses within days after surgery.

      (b) Glasses when contact lenses contraindicated due to poor compliance or other considerations.

      (c) Monitor visual acuity.

      (d) Patching/amblyopia therapy if acuities unequal.

      (e) Overcorrect infants by approximately 2.5 D.

      (f) Provide bifocal to preschoolers and older children.

9. Retinopathy of prematurity (ROP)

  a. Background information

    (1) Vasoproliferative disorder that occurs mostly in premature infants and rarely in full-term infants

    (2) Etiology: capillary nonperfusion whereby avascular zone stimulates neovascularization.

    (3) Risk factors include

      (a) Birth weight—lower birth weight = higher risk of ROP.

      (b) Postnatal oxygen exposure contributory but not a necessary factor, since ROP is also seen without oxygen use.

      (c) Prematurity—infants most susceptible to ROP and its later ocular complications include[9]

        i. Infants 1600 g (3.52 lb) or less.

        ii. Infants on 50 days or more of oxygen.

    (4) Examinations are usually performed in the hospital initially.

  b. Characteristics[9]

    (1) Classic lesion is the arteriovenous (AV) shunt clinically seen as a gray-white, pink, or red demarcation line between vascular and avascular retina.

    (2) PLUS disease: posterior pole vascular dilatation and tortuosity which usually indicates progressive ROP.

    (3) Acute mild ROP: flat white demarcation line between vascular and avascular retina.

    (4) Severe ROP: fibrovascular proliferation of AV shunt which becomes elevated and progresses into the vitreous. It may have associated posterior pole vascular dilation and tortuosity (PLUS disease) and can lead to traction, vitreous and retinal hemorrhage, and/or retinal detachment.

    (5) Location of ROP is seen mostly temporal, since temporal retina is not fully vascularized until 9 months of age.

    (6) There are rare reports of isolated nasal involvement as well.

    (7) Regression occurs in 90% of cases.

    (8) Proliferation occurs in 10% of cases, resulting in neovascularization, fibrovascular proliferation, traction, and retinal detachment.

    (9) ROP and non-ROP premature infants have a 55% and 36% respective incidence of future eye problems such as strabismus, amblyopia, refractive anomalies (myopia, astigmatism), decreased vision, and retinal pathology.[10]

    (10) Other complications include[11]

      (a) Narrow-angle glaucoma.

      (b) Nystagmus.

      (c) Cataracts.

      (d) Peripheral retinal breaks.

      (e) Microcornea.

      (f) Band keratopathy.

          (g)   Optic atrophy.

          (h)   Phthisis bulbi.

  c. Differential diagnosis: Based on history of prematurity and/or oxygen use and retinal findings.

  d. Management

    (1) All children with a history of prematurity should be routinely examined at an early age regardless of a history of ROP or oxygen use.

    (2) Clinicians following these patients should be knowledgeable in zones and staging of ROP, which is beyond the scope of this text.

    (3) Examination is usually performed in the hospital when the infant is systemically stable and able to tolerate the exam.

    (4) Dilated fundus exam performed with vital signs closely monitored.

    (5) Repeat exams depend on zone and stage of disease.

    (6) Routine exams after threat of acute disease to monitor vision and rule out common complications.

    (7) Presence of acute ROP warrants consult to retinal specialist.

        (a)   Cryotherapy to avascular zone.

        (b)   Cryotherapy to severe ROP can reduce incidence of complications by 50% as compared to untreated eye.[12]

        (c)   Scleral buckle and/or vitrectomy for retinal detachment.

10.   Common childhood tapetoretinal degenerations

  a. Retinitis pigmentosa

    (1) Background

        (a)   Mostly hereditary, may be sporadic.

        (b)   Autosomal recessive, autosomal dominant, X-linked recessive.

        (c)   Autosomal dominant milder, later onset and slower to progress.

        (d)   Generalized photoreceptor disorder initially affecting rods.

        (e)   Dystrophy of retinal pigment epithelium secondary to loss of photoreceptors.

    (2) Characteristics

        (a)   Onset usually during childhood with dark adaptation difficulties.

        (b)   Visual acuity not affected until 2nd or 3rd decade of life.

        (c)   Salt and pepper appearance to fundus.

        (d)   Narrowing of retinal arterioles.

        (e)   Bone spicules and clumps of pigment in midperipheral retina.

        (f)   Progresses to periphery and posterior pole.

        (g)   Progressive peripheral field loss.

        (h)   Macula typically spared until late in disease process.

        (i)   Early complaints of dark adaptation.

        (j)   Early abnormal ERG precedes retinal changes, abnormal EOG.

  b. Leber's amaurosis

    (1) Background

        (a)   Onset at birth or within first few months of life.

        (b)   Autosomal recessive heredity.

        (c)   Abnormality of photoreceptors, generalized retinal degeneration.

    (2) Characteristics

        (a)   Blindness or reduced vision at birth.

        (b)   Searching nystagmus.

        (c)   Sluggish or absent pupillary light reflexes.

        (d)   Photophobia.

        (e)   Oculodigital reflex.

        (f)   Variable fundus features which may be normal in appearance, especially early in disease process.

        (g)   Eventual pigmentary retinopathy with

            i.   Bone spicules.

       ii. Irregular pigmentation.
      iii. Attenuated arterioles.
      iv. Optic atrophy.
   (h) Keratoconus and keratoglobus with increased age.
   (i) May be associated with mental retardation.
   (j) May be associated with neuromuscular disorders.
   (k) Abnormal ERG.[13]

c. Punctata albescens
  (1) Background
    (a) Retinal disorder due to abnormally slow rhodopsin regeneration.
    (b) Autosomal recessive inheritance.
  (2) Characteristics[14,15]
    (a) Progressive.
    (b) Stationary reaches normal levels after prolonged dark adaptation (DA) test.
    (c) Slightly irregular, punctate white lesions throughout retina.
    (d) Usually not present in posterior pole.
    (e) Moth-eaten appearance to fundus.
    (f) Considered a flecked retina disease.
    (g) May be bone spicules peripherally.
    (h) Arteriole narrowing.
    (i) Abnormal ERG and EOG.

d. Fundus albipunctatus[14,15]
  (1) Background
    (a) Autosomal recessive inheritance.
    (b) A form of congenital stationary night blindness.
    (c) A delay in regeneration of the visual pigments.
    (d) Mimics punctata albescens.
    (e) Considered a flecked retina disease.
  (2) Characteristics
    (a) Stationary disease.
    (b) Congenital night blindness.
    (c) Grayish-white mottling of the fundi that spares the macula.
    (d) May be abnormal dark adaptation.
    (e) Vessels and optic disc normal.
    (f) May be abnormal ERG and EOG.
    (g) Normal visual acuity and fields.

e. Choroideremia
  (1) Background
    (a) X-linked recessive tapetochoroidal dystrophy.
    (b) Unmasking of choroid vessels which leads to complete loss of choroid and retinal pigment epithelium in males.
    (c) Females show minimal fundus changes and no functional vision loss.
  (2) Characteristics[14,16]
    (a) Females show mottling of pigment in fundus only.
    (b) Loss of pigment around disc forms ringlike halo.
    (c) Males develop full-blown disease.
    (d) Choroidal thinning and midperiphery choroidal atrophy by age 10 (disc and macula are spared).
    (e) Marked pigmentary dispersion throughout the fundus.
    (f) Arterioles appear slightly thinner, veins appear normal.
    (g) Visual acuity unaffected until 40–60 years of age.
    (h) Enlarged blind spot and multiple midperiphery scotomas during childhood progress to total field loss.
    (i) Normal color vision.

(j) ERG abnormal in females, absent in males.
(k) Increased incidence of myopia.
(l) Abnormal dark adaptation in males only.
f. Laurence-Moon-Biedl syndrome
(1) Background. Autosomal recessive disorder.
(2) Characteristics[17]
(a) Pigmentary dystrophy.
(b) Poor dark adaptation.
(c) Nystagmus.
(d) Optic atrophy.
(e) Strabismus.
(f) Mental retardation.
(g) Spastic paraplegia.
(h) Hypogenitalism.
(i) Polydactyly.
(j) Obesity.
(k) Short stature.
11. Common childhood macular degenerations
a. Nonprogressive cone dystrophies are discussed in section VII.
b. General features
(1) Often involve an area larger than the macula, although primarily the posterior pole.
(2) Familial, bilateral, and often symmetric.
(3) Progressive loss of visual acuity.
(4) Onset during childhood.
(5) Gradual progression.
(6) Genetic patterns important to diagnosis.
(7) Management
(a) Low vision aids or referral to vision rehabilitation specialist.
(b) Genetic counseling[18,19]
c. Stargardt's disease
(1) Background
(a) Disorder of retinal pigment epithelium.
(b) Onset in children between 6 and 20 years.
(c) Autosomal recessive inheritance.
(d) Causes a loss of photoreceptors and pigment epithelium in perimacular area.
(e) Felt to be a variant of fundus flavimaculatus.
(2) Characteristics
(a) Bilateral and symmetric atrophic macular degeneration.
(b) "Beaten bronze" appearance to macula.
(c) Horizontal, oval area of pigment epithelial atrophy.
(d) May proceed to peripheral involvement.
(e) Peripheral involvement shows round granular black pigmentations surrounded by depigmented areas.
(f) Visual acuity loss may precede fundus changes.
(g) Initially a decreased foveal reflex; followed by a round pigmented macular degeneration.
(h) Progressive loss of central vision.
(i) Visual acuity decreases to 20/200 and equal in two eyes.
(j) Normal peripheral vision and night vision.
(k) Mild color vision defect.
(l) Normal ERG; EOG normal when central involvement only.[18]
d. Best's vitelliform degeneration
(1) Background
(a) Retinal pigment epithelium abnormality.

          (b) Accumulation of lipofuscin granules within the retinal pigment epithelium.

          (c) Onset in children between 3 and 15 years.

          (d) Autosomal dominant inheritance.

     (2) Characteristics[14]

          (a) Appearance may vary.

          (b) Onset usually during 1st or 2nd decade.

          (c) May be mild pigmentary disturbance.

          (d) Can proceed to egg yolk (vitelliform) lesions at macula.

          (e) Vitelliform lesions may be replaced by atrophic scar.

          (f) Usually bilateral, but may be unilateral.

          (g) Variable prognosis, may retain 20/30 to 20/50 visual acuity.

          (h) Mild to moderate reduction in color vision.

          (i) Normal dark adaptation.

          (j) Abnormal EOG, normal ERG.

          (k) Central visual field defects, normal peripheral fields.

          (l) Associated with hyperopia, esotropia, and strabismic amblyopia.

  e. Fundus flavimaculatus

     (1) Background

          (a) Disorder of retinal pigment epithelium.

          (b) Autosomal recessive inheritance.

          (c) Felt to be same entity as Stargardt's disease.

          (d) Vision loss usually begins in first 2 decades.

          (e) Considered a flecked retina disease.

     (2) Characteristics[14]

          (a) Progressive loss of central vision or may retain 20/20 visual acuity.

          (b) Yellowish-white fishtail lesions of variable shape, size, and density in the posterior pole and equator.[18,19]

          (c) Lesions fade with time and new lesions continue to appear.

          (d) Visual acuity ranges from 20/20 to 20/200.

          (e) Acquired color defect.

          (f) Dark adaptation usually normal.

          (g) Photophobia.

          (h) Central scotoma possible.

          (i) Usually abnormal EOG; ERG may be normal.

  f. X-linked retinoschisis

     (1) Background

          (a) X-linked hereditary disease.

          (b) Affects males.

          (c) Splitting of nerve fiber layer of retina.

          (d) May be present at birth.

     (2) Characteristics[14]

          (a) Foveal schisis (may be only finding).

          (b) Spokelike pattern of cystoid macular changes.

          (c) May progress to macular hole, retinal detachments, or vitreous hemorrhages.

          (d) ERG shows reduced B-wave; EOG normal in mild cases.

          (e) Variable visual acuity that decreases over time (may decrease to 20/200).

          (f) Tritan color defect early, deutan defect later.

          (g) Central and peripheral scotomas depending on involvement.

          (h) Reduced dark adaptation.

          (i) May be slow progression.

          (j) Associated with strabismus, nystagmus, or hyperopic astigmatism.

(3) Management
(a) Photocoagulation.
(b) Genetic counseling.
(c) Referral to low vision specialist.
g. Cone dystrophies
(1) Background
(a) Primarily autosomal dominant.
(b) May be autosomal recessive.
(c) Symmetrical.
(d) Sensory retinal involvement of cones.
(e) Eventual complete disappearance of the photoreceptors in macular and paramacular areas and associated degeneration and disappearance of retinal pigment epithelium.
(2) Characteristics
(a) Onset in first two decades of life.
(b) No fundus changes in early stages
(c) Later stages of visual acuity loss
Bull's-eye appearance to macula
Later attenuation of retinal vessels and peripheral pigmentary retinopathy and optic atrophy.
(d) Central dark red area surrounded by a sharply defined ring of depigmentation.
(e) Progressive decrease in visual acuity.
(f) May progress to total achromatopsia and 20/400 visual acuity.
(g) Visual acuity loss followed by progressive color vision defect.
(h) Progresses to central and peripheral visual field loss.
(i) Progresses to total color defect.
(j) Often photophobia and acquired nystagmus.
(k) Abnormal ERG, early normal EOG, late abnormal EOG.
12. Additional selected syndromes
a. Axenfeld-Rieger syndrome[20]
(1) Background
(a) Autosomal dominant heredity.
(b) Incomplete development of aqueous outflow structures.
(c) Defect in tissues derived from cranial neural crest cells.
(d) May be due to developmental arrest during 3rd trimester of gestation.
(2) Characteristics
(a) Bilateral.
(b) 50% of patients develop glaucoma, often during childhood.
(c) Microcornea or megalocornea (more common) may be present.
(d) Corneal opacities.
(e) May be variations in the size and shape of corneal endothelial cells.
(f) Prominent Schwalbe's line.
(g) Iridocorneal adhesions.
(h) Scleral spur obscured by peripheral iris which inserts in posterior trabecular meshwork.
(i) May be stromal thinning, marked iris atrophy, corectopia, or ectropion uveae (may be progressive).
(j) Associated with
   i. Strabismus.
   ii. Limbal dermoids.
   iii. Cataracts.
   iv. Distorted pupil.
   v. Transillumination defects of iris.

      vi. Retinal detachment.
     vii. Macular degeneration.
    viii. Chorioretinal colobomas.
     ix. Choroidal hypoplasia.
      x. Hypoplasia of the optic nerve.
     xi. Developmental defects of teeth and facial bones.
     xii. Maxillary hypoplasia.
    xiii. Hypertelorism.
    xiv. Telecanthus.
     xv. Broad flat nose.[20]

b. Peters' anomaly
  (1) Background
    (a) Autosomal recessive or sporadic inheritance.
    (b) May be changes in Bowman's membrane.
    (c) Abnormality in Descemet's membrane and endothelium.
  (2) Characteristics[21]
    (a) Unilateral or bilateral.
    (b) Central corneal opacity.
    (c) Tissue strands extend from iris to margins of corneal defect.
    (d) Cataracts (may be adhesions between lens cortex and corneal stroma and displacement of the lens).
    (e) Glaucoma.
    (f) May be systemic associations in more severe forms.
    (g) May be elevated IOP.

c. Albinism[14]
  (1) Oculocutaneous albinism
    (a) Background
       i. Autosomal recessive inheritance.
      ii. Tyrosinase negative = pale blue iris, red reflex present, white hair, tyrosinase absent, more severe form resulting in poorer visual acuities.
     iii. Tyrosinase positive = variable iris color, variable hair color which darkens with age, tyrosinase present, less severe form resulting in better visual acuities.
     iv. May be associated Hermansky-Pudlak or Chediak-Higashi syndrome.
    (b) Characteristics
       i. Nystagmus.
      ii. Photophobia.
     iii. 20/100–20/400 visual acuity (may be better).
     iv. Relationship between visual acuity and amount of pigmentation.
      v. With-the-rule astigmatism.
     vi. Typically esotropic.
     vii. Iris transillumination.
    viii. Yellow-white coloration with isolated choroidal vessels.[14]
     ix. Flat red appearance to macula.
      x. Absent foveal reflex.
     xi. Color vision may be normal.
     xii. Normal visual fields.
    xiii. Normal dark adaptation.
  (2) Ocular albinism
    (a) Background
       i. Albinism affects primarily the eye.
      ii. X-linked inheritance.

        (b) Characteristics
- i. Visual acuity 20/60–20/200.
- ii. Patchwork fundus changes showing varying pigmentary deficiencies.
- iii. With-the-rule astigmatism.
- iv. Sector iris transillumination.
- v. Normal color vision.
- vi. Normal visual fields.
- vii. Normal dark adaptation.

(3) X-linked ocular albinism
- (a) Background
  - i. X-linked recessive inheritance.
  - ii. Eye is lacking pigment.
- (b) Characteristics
  - i. Decreased visual acuity.
  - ii. Transillumination of irides.
  - iii. Congenital nystagmus.
  - iv. Photophobia.
  - v. Foveal hypoplasia.
  - vi. Hypopigmentation of the fundus.
  - vii. Normal ERG.

d. Microcornea
- (1) Background
  - (a) Autosomal dominant or recessive and sporadic inheritance.
  - (b) Corneal diameter of 7–10 mm.
- (2) Characteristics
  - (a) Associated with
    - i. Colobomas.
    - ii. Congenital cataract.
    - iii. Nystagmus.
    - iv. Glaucoma.
    - v. Strabismus.
  - (b) Occurs with
    - i. Nanophthalmos.
    - ii. Microphthalmos.

e. Aniridia
- (1) Background
  - (a) Congenital partial absence of iris.
  - (b) May appear complete, but partial iris always present.
  - (c) Autosomal dominant inheritance, may also have sporadic form.
- (2) Characteristics
  - (a) Pendular nystagmus.
  - (b) Photophobia.
  - (c) Macular hypoplasia.
  - (d) Retinal dystrophy.
  - (e) Glaucoma.
  - (f) Polar cataracts.
  - (g) Increased prevalence Wilms' tumor of kidneys (sporadic form).
  - (h) Strabismus.
  - (i) Ectopia lentis.
  - (j) May be associated with genitourinary defects.

VII. Color Vision

A. *Developmental changes*
1. Rods functioning by 4–8 weeks of age.
2. Consistent chromatic discrimination possible by 7 weeks.

3. Presence of two types of cones by 8–10 weeks.
4. Three types of cones functioning at 2 months of age.
5. At 4 and one-half months infants prefer red over blue.
6. The most common X-linked recessive red-green defects occur in 1 in 12 males vs less than 1 in 200 females.
7. 1 in 50,000 males has inherited blue-yellow defect.[22]

B. *Color vision defects*
 1. Acquired
    a. Associated with ocular or systemic anomalies.
    b. Unilateral or bilateral.
    c. Rare unless associated with retinal or optic nerve pathology.
    d. May be difficult to document in children.
    e. Kollner's rule for classification (does not always hold true)
       (1) Blue-yellow defects
          (a) Preretinal media.
          (b) Outer retinal layers, i.e.
             i. Retinitis pigmentosa.
             ii. Papilledema.
             iii. Chorioretinitis.
             iv. Juvenile macular degeneration (as disease progresses).
             v. Congenital glaucoma (exception to rule).
             vi. Juvenile diabetes.
       (2) Red-green defects
          (a) Inner retinal layers.
          (b) Optic nerve pathology.
          (c) Higher visual pathways, i.e.
             i. Leber's optic atrophy.
             ii. Juvenile macular degeneration.
 2. Congenital
    a. Present since birth.
    b. Not associated with disease.
    c. Nonprogressive.
    d. Often hereditary.
    e. Bilateral.
 3. Classification of congenital defects
    a. Red-green defects—anomaly of photopigment in cones
       (1) X-linked → expressed gene is inherited through mother.
       (2) Color vision defects in boys will not be passed to their sons, but all will have daughters who are carriers.
       (3) Boys inherit color blindness from mother who is either color defective or is a carrier.
       (4) Maternal grandfathers of these children are color defective.
       (5) Color-defective mother will have all color-defective sons and all daughters will be carriers.
       (6) If a girl is color defective, her father must also be color defective and her mother is at least a carrier.
    b. Blue-yellow defects
       (1) Tritan defects.
       (2) Autosomal dominant.
       (3) Very rare.
       (4) Often associated with pathology.
    c. Red-green or blue-yellow color defectives can be further classified as either trichromats or dichromats.
 4. Trichromats
    a. 6%–7% of males.

    b. 3 photopigments present.
    c. 1 of photopigments is shifted toward another on wavelength axis.
    d. Normal visual acuity.
    e. Varying degrees of anomalous color desaturation.
    f. Protanomalous trichromacy
      (1) Reds appear dimmer.
      (2) 1%–2% of male population.
      (3) Abnormal luminosity function.
    g. Deuteranomalous trichromacy
      (1) 4%–5% of male population.
      (2) Normal luminosity function.

5. Dichromats
    a. 2% of males.
    b. Normal visual acuity.
    c. 1 of 3 cone photopigments is missing, therefore only 2 photopigments present.
    d. Protanopia
      (1) 1% of male population.
      (2) Only middle wavelength-sensitive pigments are present.
      (3) Lacking erythrolabe.
      (4) Reds appear very dim.
    f. Deuteranopia
      (1) 1% of male population.
      (2) Only long wavelength-sensitive pigments are present.
    g. Tritanopia
      (1) Rarest type of dichromacy.
      (2) Missing cyanolabe.
      (3) Blue appears dimmer.

6. Complete typical achromatopsia[21]
    a. Also known as rod monochromatism.
    b. Extremely rare (3 in 10,000 births).
    c. Only one type of photopigment present in the retina (rods).
    d. Autosomal recessive.
    e. Nonprogressive.
    f. 20/200 range of visual acuity.
    g. Associated signs
      (1) Nystagmus.
      (2) Photophobia.
      (3) Abnormal ERG.
      (4) May have strabismus and astigmatism.
      (5) May have absence of foveal reflex.
      (6) May have pigment stippling.
      (7) Slow pupillary response to light.
      (8) Normal pupillary response to dark adaptation.
      (9) Central scotoma, normal peripheral field.
      (10) Normal ocular examination.
      (11) No color vision present.

7. Incomplete typical achromatopsia[14,23]
    a. Same features as complete, but less severe.
    b. Photophobia and nystagmus may be absent.
    c. Abnormal ERG.

8. Blue cone monochromatism[14]
    a. Known as blue cone monochromacy.
    b. X-linked form.
    c. Nystagmus.

   d. Photophobia.
   e. Reduced visual acuity 20/60–20/200.
   f. May be myopic.
   g. May be some color vision.
   h. Rods and blue cones present.
   i. Normal ocular examination.
  9. Central cone monochromatism[14]
   a. Very rare.
   b. Autosomal recessive.
   c. 20/200 visual acuity.
   d. Nystagmus.
   e. May be some color vision.
   f. Rods and green cones present.
   g. Photophobia.
   h. Abnormal ERG.

C. *Color vision testing*
  1. A concern to parents, especially of preschoolers.
  2. Important to differentiate
   a. Color vision defects.
   b. Color naming abilities.
   c. Color pointing abilities.
  3. The following sequence will help differentiate color vision defects from color identification or naming difficulties.
  4. Color identification or naming is directly related to a child's developmental level and cognitive abilities.
  5. Color naming
   a. For children who can already point to colors.
   b. Brightly colored blocks, beads, or identical shaped objects in primary and pastel colors.
   c. Good illumination.
   d. Examiner points to a block and asks child to name the color.
   e. Begin with primary colors, proceed to pastel colors.
   f. Reassure parent of child's abilities.
   g. Identify colors child is having difficulties with.
   h. Usually develops by approximately age 3 to 4 years.
  6. Color identification (pointing)
   a. Evaluate child's ability to point to various primary and pastel colors.
   b. Brightly colored blocks, beads, or identically shaped objects.
   c. Good illumination.
   d. Ask child to point to each color.
   e. Begin with primary colors, proceed to pastel colors.
   f. Reassure parent of child's abilities.
   g. Identify colors child is having difficulties with.
   h. Usually develops by approximately age 3 to 4 years.
  7. Color vision discrimination
   a. To assess the presence of a color vision defect.
   b. Performed binocularly in children unless pathology is suspected.

D. *Sequence of color vision testing in children (infants–9 years)[21]*
  1. F2 or PACT preferential looking plates (Figure 11-11)
   a. Use initially for screening.
   b. Suitable for all ages.
   c. Forced choice test.
   d. No understanding of task required.

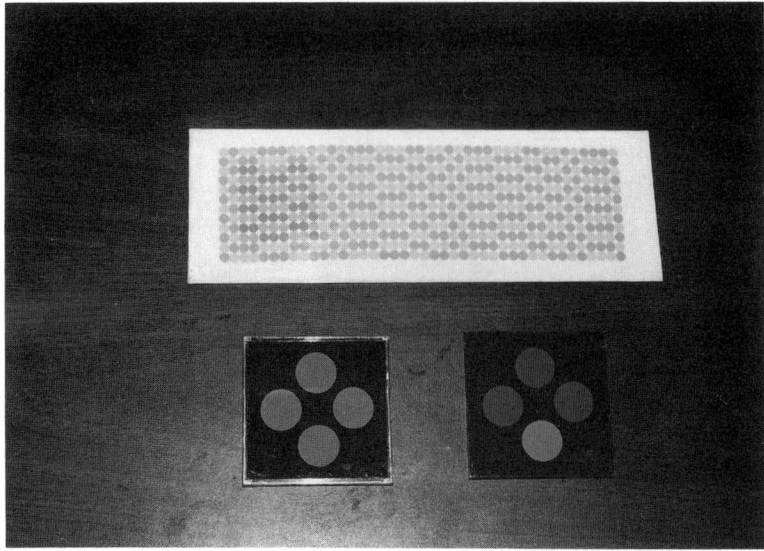

Figure 11-11.   F2 (PACT) plates (top); Berson and Portnoy plates (*photo by Ron Davidoff*).

    e. Detects mild, moderate, or severe red-green defects.

    f. Detects moderate to severe blue-yellow defects.

2. Portnoy plates (Figure 11-11)

    a. Determines severity of problem.

    b. Differentiates mild from moderate and severe color defects.

    c. Differentiates protan, deutan, and tritan.

    d. Munsell colors similar to those used in D15 test for adults.

    e. Forced choice discrimination task using 3 different plates.

    f. Child must identify which 1 of the 4 color circles appears different.

    g. Each plate is presented 6 times.

    h. Child must respond correctly 4 of 6 times to pass each plate.

    i. Standard and desaturated versions.

    j. Moderate defects will fail desaturated test, but pass standard test.

    k. Severe defects will fail standard test.

    l. Requires some level of receptive language skills.

    m. Suitable for children aged 2–3 and older depending on their cognitive skills.

3. Berson test (Figure 11-11)

    a. Used if child is unable to pass Portnoy plates.

    b. Diagnostic for presence of achromatopsia.

    c. Differentiates autosomal recessive complete rod monochromacy and sex-linked blue cone monochromacy.

    d. Forced choice discrimination task.

    e. Same instructional set as Portnoy plates[23]

4. Infant color vision test (Figure 11-12)

    a. Pseudoisochromatic plates.

    b. Child must identify picture.

    c. Identifies mild, moderate, or severe color vision defects.

    d. Identifies deutan vs protan color vision defects.

    e. Useful in children aged 3 and older.

    f. Requires some receptive and expressive language skills.

5. City University color vision test

    a. Screens moderate and severe color vision defects.

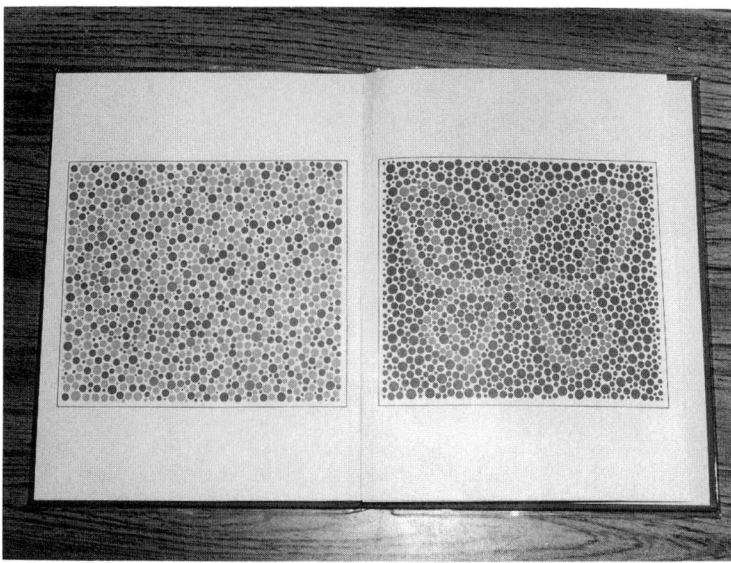

Figure 11-12.   Children's color vision Test (*photo by Ron Davidoff*).

      b.   Differentiates protans, deutans, and tritans.
      c.   Matching task.
      d.   May be useful in preschool and older children.
  6. Nagal Anomaloscope
      a.   Accurate to screen and classify red-green color vision problems.
      b.   May be difficult to administer in children.
      c.   Child must be able to identify when colors are matching.
      d.   Useful in children 3 years and older depending on cognitive skills.
      e.   Requires some knowledge and expertise to administer.
  7. Standard adult pseudoisochromatic plates
      a.   For children 9 years and older.
      b.   May be used in younger responsive children.
      c.   Ask younger children to trace numbers with Q-tip/paintbrush.
  8. D-15 test
      a.   For children 9 years and older.
      b.   Will not detect mild color defects.
      c.   Ask child to pick circle that looks most like the sample.
      d.   Continue by asking which remaining circle looks most like the one just chosen.
      e.   Children often understand task, but may be unable to complete.
      f.   Color circles may be too small for some young children.[23]

VIII. Accommodation

  A. *Developmental changes*
    1. Accommodation in newborns is an all or nothing response, allowing the infant to lock in at approximately 20 cm.
    2. By 3–4 months of age, accommodative responses are more accurate and similar to those seen in an adult.
    3. Clinically timed accommodative facility responses are not adultlike in children and continue to improve during the school years.

4. Testing of binocular accommodative facility is useful only in children over the age of 9 due to large variation in scores of younger children.

B. *Clinical presentation*
   1. Fatigue and rubbing of eyes.
   2. Redness and tearing.
   3. Avoidance of near work.
   4. Reduced acuity.
   5. Blurred vision at distance after extended near work.
   6. Headaches associated with close work.
   7. Asthenopia associated with close work.
   8. Difficulty copying from the board.

C. *General guidelines for accommodative testing*
   1. When testing accommodation, the targets should be 20/30 or one line above the child's best visual acuity and of good quality.
   2. It is helpful to ask children about the details of the target and to change targets periodically to heighten their interest, verify their attention, and maintain their focus.

D. *Diagnostic evaluation: unique tools*
   1. Types
      a. Visual acuity testing.
      b. Monocular accommodative facility testing.
      c. Binocular accommodative facility testing.
      d. Accommodative amplitude.
      e. Monocular estimation method dynamic retinoscopy (MEM).
      f. Negative relative accommodation/positive relative accommodation (NRA/PRA).
      g. Fused cross cylinder.
   2. Visual acuity
      a. Decreased visual acuity at near in the absence of significant refractive error may indicate an ill-sustained or decreased accommodative ability.
      b. Fluctuating distance visual acuity in the absence of significant refractive error may indicate an accommodative spasm.
   3. Monocular accommodative facility testing (Figure 11-13)
      a. For children aged 6 and older (Table 11-4).
      b. Child wears habitual distance Rx.
      c. Present a 20/30 target at 16 inches.
      d. Patch one eye.
      e. Place a +2.00 lens in front of the child's open eye.
      f. Ask the child to begin reading the letters when he or she can first see them clearly.
      g. Next place the −2.00 lens in front of the child's open eye and again ask the child to read the letters when he or she can first see them clearly.
      h. Continue alternating flippers for 1 minute.
      i. Count the number of cycles the child is able to clear in 1 minute.
   4. Binocular accommodative facility testing
      a. Most useful in children aged 9 and older.
      b. Child wears habitual distance Rx.
      c. Present a 20/30 target at 16 inches.
      d. Use an antisuppression target such as the No. 9 vectogram card, near illuminated testing system (NITS) test, or a red/green or polaroid bar reader.
      e. Place the appropriate polaroid or anaglyphic glasses on the child.
      f. Place a +2.00 flipper in front of the child's eyes.

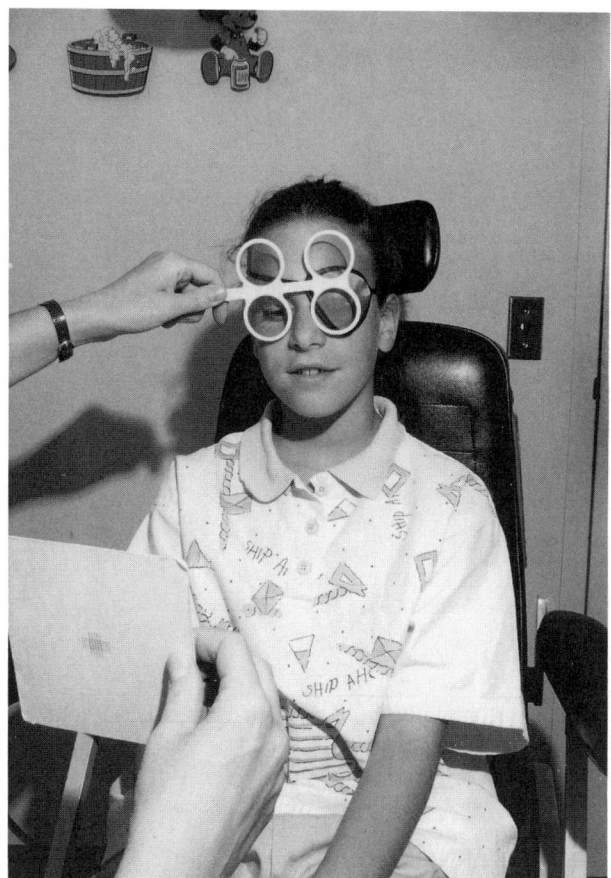

Figure 11-13. Monocular accommodative facility testing (*photo by Ron Davidoff*).

g. Ask the child to begin reading the letters when he or she can first see them clearly.
h. Next place the −2.00 flipper in front of the child's eyes.
i. Ask child to begin reading when the letters are clear and single and no bars are black (if a bar reader is used).
j. Count the number of cycles the child is able to clear in 1 minute.

Table 11-4. Expected Findings for Accommodative Facility Testing for Children

Age	Monocular Facility Norms	Binocular Facility Norms
6 years[a]	5.5 cpm ± 2.5 cpm	3 cpm ± 2.5 cpm
7 years[a]	6.5 cpm ± 2.0 cpm	3.5 cpm ± 2.5 cpm
8–12 years[a]	7 cpm ± 2.5 cpm	5 cpm ± 2.5 cpm
Over 12 years[b]	11 cpm ± 5.0 cpm	8 cpm ± 5.0 cpm

[a]Children called out numbers or letters.

[b]Children stated when letters were clear.

Data from: Scheiman & Wick—Clinical Management of Accommodative, Non-Strabismuic Binocular Vision & Eye Movement Disorders

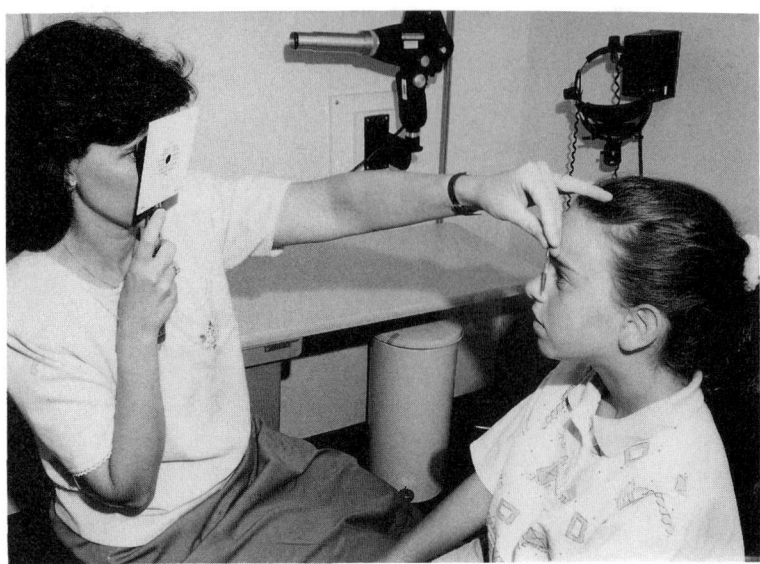

Figure 11-14.   Monocular estimation method (MEM) retinoscopy (*photo by Ron Davidoff*).

5. Accommodative amplitude
    a. The pull away method is most effective for children and eliminates the tendency to over- or underestimate amplitudes.
    b. For children aged 3 years and older.
    c. Child wears habitual distance Rx.
    d. Cover one eye with an occluder or patch.
    e. Hold a detailed picture or 20/30 letter at approximately 2 inches directly before the open eye.
    f. Be sure the child is not able to see the target initially.
    g. Ask the child to identify the target as soon as he or she recognizes it.
    h. Slowly pull the target away until the child can identify it.
    i. Measure the distance from the target to the eye and convert to diopters.
    j. The minimal expected amplitude for children is Hofstetter's formula: 15 − one-quarter of the child's age.
6. Monocular estimate method dynamic retinoscopy (MEM) (Figure 11-14)
    a. This test is appropriate for children 3 years and older.
    b. Child should wear habitual near vision Rx.
    c. Use appropriate graded reading words or pictures held at child's normal working distance.
    d. Ask the child to read the target while scoping each eye from directly behind the reading material.
    e. Look for inequality of accommodative lag between eyes.
    f. Quickly introduce small amounts of plus before one eye to neutralize the lag of accommodation.
    g. Do not leave lens in place for more than a second, as this may change the accommodative response.
7. NRA/PRA
    a. This test is performed in the standard manner administered to adults.
    b. This test is not useful in children who are unable to sit behind a phoropter.
8. Fused cross cylinder
    a. This test is performed in the standard manner administered to adults.
    b. This test is often not useful in children below the age of 8 due to inability to sit behind the phoropter and difficulty understanding the instructional set.

E. *Differential diagnosis of accommodative problems*
1. Accommodative problems typically become manifest during the middle grades of schooling (3rd grade and up).
2. A child may be completely asymptomatic, but show signs such as lack of interest in reading, poor grades, inability to concentrate in school, academic underachieving etc.
3. Academically, a child may have done well in the lower grades, with a pattern of gradually decreasing performance and lack of interest in school.
4. Children may perform better on accommodative testing in the morning when they are alert than in the evening when they are fatigued; therefore, consider time of day testing occurred.
5. Classification of accommodative problems.
   a. Accommodative insufficiency
      (1) Low amplitude.
      (2) Low positive relative accommodation (PRA).
      (3) High MEM retinoscopy findings.
      (4) Low accommodative facility monocularly and binocularly with minus flippers (AFM & B with −).
      (5) High fusional convergence (FCC).
   b. Ill-sustained accommodation
      (1) Amplitude may be normal, but diminishes with time.
      (2) Low PRA.
      (3) High MEM retinoscopy findings.
      (4) Low AFM & B with −.
      (5) High FCC.
   c. Accommodative excess
      (1) Low NRA.
      (2) Low MEM retinoscopy findings.
      (3) Low AFM & B with +.
      (4) Low FCC.
   d. Accommodative infacility
      (1) Low negative relative accommodation (NRA) and PRA.
      (2) Low AFM & B with + and −.

F. *Patient management of accommodative anomalies*
1. Ill-sustained accommodation and accommodative insufficiency
   a. Plus lenses for near and/or
   b. Vision therapy.
2. Accommodative excess: Vision therapy
3. Accommodative infacility: Vision therapy

IX. Ocular Motilities

A. *Pursuits. The ability of the eyes to follow a slow-moving target.*
1. Developmental considerations
   a. At birth—infant pursuit movements are present, but not well developed and may not be full into extreme gaze.
   b. Tracking at birth is typically done using a combination of pursuits and saccades.
   c. Smooth pursuit movements are present in infants by 6–8 weeks of age.
   d. Smooth and steady pursuits in infants are also indicators of good visual acuity.
   e. In school-age children, pursuits should be smooth and steady with accurate fixation and without head movement once the child has been instructed not to move his or her head.
   f. Infants and preschoolers have less steady pursuits than adults.
   g. Pursuits in a child may be influenced by attention, fatigue, and emotional stress.

     h.   Inaccurate and delayed pursuits can be indicators of neurologic disease.

     i.   Jerky pursuits can be associated with "soft signs" of underlying neurologic dysfunction even though radiological lesions are not found.[24]

2. Diagnostic evaluation: unique tools

     a.   Use a target of high interest to the child, such as a detailed picture or letter pasted on tongue depressor or finger puppet.

     b.   A large mirror is useful in infants, inattentive children, or malingerers.[25]

     c.   Move the target at a slow steady speed in the horizontal, vertical, and diagonal directions while keeping the head at rest.

     d.   In infants, it is permissible to gently hold the child's head still while moving the target.

     e.   In older children, inability to perform without head movements is considered abnormal.

     f.   If pursuits are felt to be reduced due to inattention, use a more interesting target; ask the child to actually read the letters or pictures on the tongue depressor as they are moved; turn the tongue depressor to the reverse side, asking the child to state when the target "changes."

     g.   Test with an optokinetic (OKN) drum or tape to look for asymmetries (slow phase of OKN is a pursuit), i.e., a right parietal lobe lesion may cause a reduced OKN response moving the stripes to the patient's right; the patient's pursuits to the right may also be deficient.

     h.   Other methods to test pursuits[24]

         (1) Southern California College of Optometry system.

         (2) Heinsen & Schrock system.

         (3) Eye-Trac.

         (4) Flicker method.

         (5) Afterimages.

3. Clinical presentation of problems[24]

     a.   Poor readers.

     b.   Poor athletic ability.

     c.   Neurological signs and symptoms.

     d.   Vertigo, nausea.

     e.   Asthenopia.

     f.   Poor copying.

4. Differential diagnosis

     a.   Pursuit disorders include

         (1) Abnormalities of initiation.

         (2) Abnormalities of velocity.

         (3) Asymmetric pursuits.

     b.   Initiation abnormalities cause delayed onset of pursuits. Known to occur in cortical lesions and latent nystagmus.[25]

     c.   Velocity abnormalities can be of two types:

         (1) If the pursuit velocity is reduced (the pursuit does not match the velocity of the target), a catch-up saccade is seen. In children this is usually a nonlocalizable lesion, but it can be caused by drugs, medications, anxiety, inattention, and nonspecific disorders of the cerebrum, cerebellum, and brain stem.

         (2) If the pursuit velocity is faster than the velocity of the target, a back-up saccade is seen. This is seen when increased innervation is sent to a paretic muscle that is forced to fixate. Likewise, increased innervation will be sent to the normal yoke muscle causing increased velocity when it is again allowed to fixate.

     d.   Asymmetric pursuits[25]

         (1) Impaired pursuits to the side of the lesion may occur in unilateral lesions of the posterior cerebral hemisphere (also occurs in lesions of the thalamus, midbrain tegmentum, pontine nucleus, and cerebellum).

          (2)   Vertical pursuit disturbance may occur with internuclear ophthalmoplegia.

          (3)   Monocular testing may show asymmetries in latent nystagmus.

     e.   General differential diagnosis. Rule out a neurologic etiology with "soft signs" such as seen with minimal brain dysfunction and "hard signs" seen with other neurologic implications

5. Patient management

     a.   Refer patients with neurologic signs to neurologist.

     b.   Treat amblyopia.

     c.   Pursuit training to prevent contracture with palsies and paresis.

     d.   Pursuit training for enhanced visual efficiency when interfering with learning.

6. Other considerations

     a.   Other influences may affect pursuits; e.g., the clinician may be moving the target too rapidly, causing cogwheeling (saccadic movements).

     b.   Pursuits may be affected by drugs and medications.

     c.   Poor pursuits and OKN inversion can be seen in congenital nystagmus.

     d.   Amblyopia causes monocular pursuit irregularities.

     e.   Poor visual acuity causes jerky and unsteady pursuits.

     f.   Pursuits are sometimes used as a gross indicator for visual acuity when vision cannot be measured.

     g.   Consider remeasuring pursuits after final Rx has been given.

B.   *Saccades*

1. Developmental considerations

     a.   Saccades are the fastest eye movements.

     b.   May be voluntary and produced upon command or involuntary (reflexive) in response to an auditory or visual stimulus.

     c.   Saccades contribute to the fast phase of OKN and vestibular stimulation.

     d.   Present at birth and utilized usually after a few weeks of age.

     e.   Saccades in infants typically show an increased latency.

     f.   Velocity of saccades may be normal in the alert infant, although they may make small saccades before reaching their destination, in contrast to one large smooth saccade seen in older children and adults.

     g.   Saccadic abnormalities may be associated with organic "soft signs" even though the patient may be otherwise neurologically normal.

     h.   Functional saccadic problems may also be secondary to poor vision or poor attention.

     i.   Voluntary saccadic deficiencies may indicate neurologic disease, and may be associated with other signs including pupillary abnormalities, strabismus, optic nerve abnormalities, and delayed development.

     j.   By 8 years of age, saccades should be accurate without secondary head movement. Children should be able to read standard grade level textbooks without using their fingers and without loosing their place.

2. Diagnostic evaluation: unique tools

     a.   Gross saccades

          (1)   Ask the child to look alternately between 2 targets in each field of gaze. The targets may be simple, such as your nose and a penlight or a letter or picture pasted on a tongue depressor. Younger infants respond to illuminated finger puppets or other small toys.

          (2)   Check for fatigue with repetition of saccades (a sign of myasthenia gravis).

          (3)   Evaluate by looking at the fast phase of the OKN response.

     b.   Fine saccades. Developmental eye movement test (DEM)—an oculomotor test that filters out nonocular factors such as attention, word recognition and retrieval, integration time, hesitation, automaticity of speech, and speaking time. It includes normative data for children aged 6–13 years and is used for diagnosis and treatment of learning-related ocular motility disorders.

3. Clinical presentation of problems
   a. Signs and symptoms[24]
      (1) Inefficiency in reading, including word omissions, skipping lines, loss of place, excessive head movement, finger support.
      (2) Poor athletic abilities.
      (3) Sudden difficulty in reading.
      (4) Gaze deficits.
      (5) Diplopia (uncommon).
      (6) Blur (seen with inappropriate saccades).
      (7) General complaints of problems with glasses or eyes.
   b. Saccadic disorders in children include
      (1) Abnormalities of speed.
      (2) Abnormalities of latency.
      (3) Abnormalities of accuracy.
      (4) Inappropriate saccades.
4. Differential diagnosis[25]
   a. When saccadic speed is abnormally SLOW, the differential diagnosis is
      (1) Ocular motor palsies.
      (2) Internuclear palsies (slow adduction present).
      (3) Fatigue.
      (4) Poor attention.
      (5) Drugs, alcohol, or medications.
   b. When saccadic speed starts out FAST, but becomes fatigued or stops (the saccade is actually too small), the differential diagnosis is
      (1) Myasthenia gravis.
      (2) Orbital tumors.
      (3) Stutterers.
   c. When the time to INITIATE the saccade is too slow or too fast, the differential diagnosis is
      (1) Ocular motor apraxia secondary to bilateral cerebral lesions.
      (2) Congenital ocular motor apraxia (associated with blinking followed by head thrusting at the beginning of a saccade to aid the eye movement); improves with age.
      (3) Metabolic and degenerative diseases.
   d. When the saccade is INACCURATE (dysmetria), the following may occur[25,26]
      (1) OVERSHOOTS (hypermetria) and UNDERSHOOTS (hypometria) indicate
         i. Cerebellar disease.
         ii. Less commonly, brain stem disease.
         iii. Drug or medications (anticonvulsants).[26]
      (2) UNDERSHOOTS—may be normal, especially when the target is unpredictable or a large saccade is required, but should disappear with repetition of the same target.
      (3) OVERSHOOTS—may be normal in downward saccades, but should disappear with repetition of the same target.
   e. The following are types of INAPPROPRIATE SACCADES:
      (1) Square-wave jerks are saccades that take the eyes off the target followed by a corrective saccade while the child is trying to maintain fixation. They are a type of saccadic intrusion with a normal interval. They are found in the following[25]:
         (a) Cerebellar disease.
         (b) Cerebral lesions.
         (c) Schizophrenia.
         (d) Strabismus.
         (e) Dyslexia.

        (2) Macrosquare-wave jerks are large square-wave jerks seen in cerebellar disease.

        (3) Ocular flutter (bursts of horizontal saccades).

          (a) Mimic nystagmus.

          (b) Horizontal oscillation around fixation.

          (c) Occur in bursts of 3–4 cycles.

          (d) Rapid and pendular.

          (e) Symptom is blurred vision rather than oscillopsia.

          (f) Associated with
            i. Brain stem.
            ii. Cerebellar dysfunction.

        (4) Opsoclonus saccades are nonrhythmic bursts of multidirectional saccades.

          (a) Mimic nystagmus.

          (b) Conjugate but chaotic.

          (c) May convert from vertical to horizontal at random or occur in any direction.

          (d) Rapid, continuous saccades.

          (e) Persist in sleep.

          (f) Associated with
            i. Myoclonic jerks of the extremities, neck, and trunk.
            ii. Brain stem disorders.
            iii. Cerebellar dysfunction.
            iv. Neonatal encephalitis.
            v. Upper respiratory infections.
            vi. Neuroblastoma (less common).

        (5) Ocular dysmetria

          (a) Mimics nystagmus.

          (b) Saccadic oscillation, not constant.

          (c) May only be evident during ocular motility testing.

          (d) Patient is asked to fixate from a peripheral target to a primary position target.

          (e) Upon refixation, the eyes undershoot or overshoot, followed by to and fro oscillations around the target until fixation is finally accomplished.

          (f) Etiology includes
            i. Cerebellar disease.
            ii. Gaucher's disease.
            iii. Ataxia telangiectasia.
            iv. Brain stem tumors.
            v. Agenesis of the corpus callosum.

   5. Differential diagnosis for saccadic dysfunction: Rule out a neurologic etiology.

   6. Management

     a. Referral for neurologic evaluation.

     b. When functional in nature, saccadic training to improve visual efficiency.

C. *Position maintenance: fixation of a stationary object*

   1. Developmental considerations

     a. Nystagmus may be a sign of or associated with systemic diseases or neurological disorders.

     b. Associated lesions should be assumed in nystagmus until ruled out.

     c. Nystagmus: oscillatory, rhythmic eye movements that are not normally seen in children (Table 11-5).

   2. Diagnostic evaluation: unique tools

     a. Ask child to look binocularly at an appropriate engaging distance target for 5 seconds, then at a near target for 5 seconds (at 40 cm).

Table 11-5. Nystagmus Associated with Decreased Vision

Location	Condition	Additional Ocular Signs and Symptoms	Systemic Associations	Differential Diagnosis	Pertinent Testing
Media opacities	Bilateral corneal scars	Central corneal opacities Glaucoma	Rule out systemic associations with Peters' anomaly	Peters' anomaly Sclerocornea Congenital glaucoma Intrauterine infections	IOP Gonioscopy A & B scan Antibody titer
	Bilateral cataracts	Leukocoria	Dermatological disorders Hypoglycemia Intrauterine infections Hypocalcemia Hypoparathyroidism Homocystinuria Alport's syndrome Lowe's syndrome Wilson's disease Galactosemia Diabetes melitis Others	Rule out associated ocular pathology Rule out other causes of leukocoria	A & B scan DFE, IOP, SLE Blood studies by pediatrician to rule out systemic association
Anterior segment	Bilateral aniridia	Lack of iris tissue Foveal/optic nerve hypoplasia Cataracts/subluxation Photophobia Glaucoma[a] Corneal changes[a] Microcornea	Wilms' tumor Mental retardation Genitourinary abnormalities Craniofacial abnormalities	Axenfeld-Rieger SX Iris coloboma	IOP, gonioscopy Kidney and genitourinary evaluation
Retina	Albinism	Hypopigmented fundus Fair hair and skin[b] Iris transillumination defects Photophobia Foveal hypoplasia Strabismus Color blind (Forsius-Eriksson)	Bleeding disorders Lung disease Infections Malignancies Deafness[c]		Hematology VER, ERG Hair bulb analysis Skin biopsy Pedigree analysis Genetic counseling
	Leber's congenital amaurosis	Decreased pupil responses Photophobia/eye rubbing Normal/mild pigmentary retinopathy/classic RP Vessel narrowing Optic atrophy High hyperopia	Renal anomalies Neurologic abnormalities Mental retardation	Retinitis pigmentosa Other retinal pigmentary disorders	ERG, VER Genetic counseling
	Achromatopsia	Severe photophobia Color blind ↓ pupil reaction or paradoxical response to dark Normal fundus Strabismus Astigmatism Myopia	None	Other cone dystrophies	ERG Color vision test Genetic counseling

(continued)

Table 11-5.   Nystagmus Associated with Decreased Vision—(*Continued*)

Location	Condition	Additional Ocular Signs and Symptoms	Systemic Associations	Differential Diagnosis	Pertinent Testing
Optic nerve	Biateral optic nerve hypo-plasia	Various field defects Double ring signs Small discs Subtle segmental changes Segmental with tilted disc Decreased pupil reaction	Septo-optic dysplasia Endocrine abnormalities Diabetes insipidus Growth/mental retarda-tion Midline brain anomalies Craniopharyngiomas Astrocytomas Cerebral palsy Seizures/epilepsy	Optic atrophy Rule out other causes of decreased vision PHPV Aniridia	Endocrine evaluation MRI VER Photographic techniques Measure C/D ratio
	Congenital optic atrophy	Pale disc (total or temporal) Field defect R/G color defect Normal vessels ↓ or paradoxical pupil reaction	Usually none Less common; muscle rigidity, mental retar-dation, ataxia ↓ bladder control	R/O acquired optic atrophy Compressive lesions Hydrocephaus Metobolic/toxic abnormalities Leber's amaurosis	ERG (normal) CT/MRI Neurologic evaluation

aUsually occur later—1st or 2nd decade of life.

bPresent in tyrosinase-positive individuals.

cPresent in some types.

Abbreviations: IOP, intraocular pressure; DFE, diluted fundus exam; SLE, slit lamp exam; VER, visual evoked response; ERG, electroretinogram; MRI, magnetic resonance imagery; C/D, cup to disc; PHPV, persistent hyperplastic primary vitreous; RP, retinitis pigmentosa; R/O, rule out; R/G, red/green; CT, computed tomography.

   b. An ophthalmoscope can also be used to check for subtle movements while observing the disc.

   c. Repeat monocularly at both distances to detect increases in nystagmus upon occlusion, which would indicate latent nystagmus.

   d. If child is unable to maintain steady fixation, repeat the procedure with the child fixating his or her own thumb (proprioceptive input).

   e. Normally less steady in young children (preschool).

3. Differential diagnosis

   a. Nystagmus.

   b. Monocular decreased vision may cause slow vertical drifts.

   c. Acquired cerebellum lesions cause saccadic intrusions and slow drifts such as ocular dysmetria, flutter, opsoclonus, square-wave jerks.

4. Clinical presentation of problems

   a. Look for nystagmus, saccadic intrusions, drifting or eye movements around the fixation target.

   b. Inability to maintain fixation indicates one of the following:

      (1) Nystagmus.

      (2) Psychological lack of attention.

      (3) Fatigue.

      (4) Drugs, medications.

      (5) Neurologic disease.

5. Diagnostic evaluation of nystagmus

   a. Classification of nystagmus

      (1) Unilateral vs bilateral.

       (2) Amplitude
          (a) Fine = 1 mm.
          (b) Medium = 1–3 mm.
          (c) Large = greater than 3 mm.
       (3) Frequency
          (a) Beats/minute in Hz.
          (b) Hz = 1 cycle/second
              i. Slow = less than 1 Hz.
             ii. Medium = 1–2 Hz.
            iii. Fast = greater than 2 Hz.
       (4) Constant vs intermittent.
       (5) Conjugancy: opposite vs same direction.
       (6) Symmetric—equal amplitude in each eye.
       (7) Type
          (a) Jerky
              i. Slow and fast phases.
             ii. Named after fast phase (right, left, up, down).
          (b) Pendular: equal velocity in each direction.

b. Useful background information in the diagnosis of nystagmus
    (1) Age of onset.
    (2) Head nodding.
    (3) Anomalous head position.
    (4) Drug use of parents.
    (5) Medications such as antiepileptics.
    (6) Head or ocular trauma.
    (7) Neurosurgical intervention.
    (8) Neurologic symptoms or signs.
    (9) Seizures.
    (10) Developmental status.
    (11) Birth history.
       (a) Weight.
       (b) Gestational age.
       (c) Complications.
       (d) Maternal age during pregnancy.
       (e) Apgar score.
    (12) Infections, surgery, hospitalizations.
    (13) Family history of ocular or systemic diseases.
    (14) Allergies.

c. Examination of nystagmus
    (1) Gross observation while playing with child.
    (2) Observe eye movements.
    (3) Note head position.
    (4) Check for head nodding.
    (5) Check convergence with appropriate target.
    (6) Check 9 positions of gaze for change in amplitude, frequency, or direction.
    (7) Check for increase or decrease in nystagmus while child fixates on a distant target.
    (8) Evaluate OKN response.
    (9) Look at nystagmus with magnification, i.e., ophthalmoscope.
    (10) Cover test to evaluate presence of strabismus/latent nystagmus.
    (11) Evaluate confrontation fields.

d. Commonly associated conditions
    (1) Visual deprivation
       (a) Media opacities.
       (b) High refractive error.

(2) Albinism (iris transillumination).

(3) Aniridia.

(4) Achromatopsia.

(5) Optic nerve abnormalities.

(6) Macular disease.

(7) Retinal disease.

6. Types of childhood nystagmus

  a. Congenital nystagmus

    (1) Onset within the first few weeks of life.

    (2) Head nodding common, may be compensatory for the eye movement and may develop later in life.

    (3) Bilateral and grossly symmetric movements.

    (4) Disappears with sleep.

    (5) Usually asymptomatic.

    (6) Commonly associated with latent nystagmus.

    (7) OKN inversion in majority of cases.

      (a) Patient with right jerky nystagmus.

      (b) Moving stripes to left will decrease or reverse the nystagmus.

      (c) In normal patients, moving the stripes to the left will induce a right jerky nystagmus.

    (8) Fixation increases the oscillations.

    (9) Convergence decreases the oscillation (may result in better VA at near).

    (10) May be pendular or jerky.

    (11) Usually horizontal.

    (12) Remains horizontal in all positions of gaze.

    (13) Null point where movement is minimized.

    (14) Head turn to move gaze into the null point and maximize visual acuity.[27]

  b. Latent nystagmus

    (1) Congenital.

    (2) Present only upon occlusion of one eye.

    (3) Usually bilateral.

    (4) A jerk nystagmus which always has the slow phase toward the occluded eye (toward the nose).

    (5) Associated with strabismus, especially congenital esotropia.

    (6) Associated with double hyperphoria.

    (7) Not associated with systemic or neurologic disorders.

    (8) May become manifest by amblyopia, loss of eye, or strabismus.

  c. Acquired nystagmus

    (1) Neurologic signs associated with acquired nystagmus

      (a) Seizures.

      (b) Poor balance and uncoordinated movements.

      (c) Failure to thrive as an infant.

      (d) Poor sucking.

      (e) Breathing abnormalities.

      (f) Large head circumference.

      (g) Delayed developmental milestones.

      (h) Less common in childhood.

        i. Gait irregularities.

        ii. Dizziness.

        iii. Tinnitus.

        iv. Pain, numbness, weakness.

    (2) Pendular nystagmus

      (a) Horizontal.

      (b) Indicative of poor vision.

      (c) Afferent system does not develop according to age norms, resulting in the development of nystagmus.

(d) Onset at 1–3 months of age.

(e) Head nodding common.

(f) Fixation exaggerates the nystagmus.

(g) Disappears with eyes closed and sleep.

(3) Spasmus nutans

    (a) Triad of symptoms

        i. Nystagmus.

        ii. Head nodding.

        iii. Anomalous head position.

    (b) Acquired, horizontal, fine, fast pendular nystagmus.

    (c) Can also be vertical or torsional.

    (d) Asymmetric amplitude between eyes.

    (e) Commonly associated with strabismus.

    (f) Onset is 6 months–3 years.

    (g) Resolves within 1 to 8 years.

    (h) Etiology unknown.

    (i) Associated with hypothalamic gliomas, optic nerve gliomas, chiasm gliomas, and subacute necrotizing encephalitis (SNE).

    (j) All children must have a brain CT or MRI.

    (k) All children must be referred for a neurologic evaluation.

(4) Downbeat nystagmus

    (a) Jerk nystagmus with fast phase down.

    (b) May not be present in primary position and evident only in inferior gaze to the right and left.

    (c) Uncommon.

    (d) Etiology includes congenital lesion of the craniocervical junction affecting the inferior cerebellum and brain stem.

(5) Ocular bobbing

    (a) Intermittent, vertical eye movement.

    (b) Both eyes saccade inferiorly, then slowly return to primary gaze.

    (c) Associated with paralysis of horizontal gaze.

    (d) Etiology is pontine disease.

    (e) Patient is usually comatose.

(6) Nystagmus associated with congenital esotropia

    (a) Large angle alternating esotropia with cross fixation.

    (b) Fine amplitude shimmer.

(7) Nystagmus blockage syndrome

    (a) Congenital nystagmus that decreases as esotropia increases.

    (b) Adducted eye is usually the fixating eye.

    (c) Child develops a face turn toward the adducted eye.

(8) Mimickers of Nystagmus

    (a) Square-wave jerks.

    (b) Opsoclonus.

    (c) Ocular flutter.

    (d) Ocular bobbing.

    (e) Ocular dysmetria.

7. Differential diagnosis for nystagmus

  a. Eye movement recordings may be helpful in obscure cases.

  b. ERG to rule out retinal disorders.

  c. Visual evoked response.

  d. Opsoclonus: order a urinary vanillymandelic acid test and abdominal CT.

  e. CT/MRI—when questionable neurologic implications and when the following are present:

  (1) Optic disc pallor.

  (2) Optic disc edema.

  (3) Afferent pupillary defect.

      f. Endocrine evaluation in optic nerve hypoplasia.

      g. Skin biopsy in albinism.

      h. TORCH studies to rule out intrauterine teratogens (e.g., toxoplasmosis, rubella, cytomegalovirus, herpes).

      i. Red cell galactokinase levels to rule out galactosemia.

      j. Rule out Wilms' tumor in aniridia.

8. Management

    a. Rule out neurologic associations.

    b. Lenses

      (1) Base out prism to produce convergence and dampen nystagmus (questionable results).

      (2) Correct all refractive errors to maximize vision.

      (3) Contact lenses to provide optimal optical correction and dampen nystagmus.

    c. Vision therapy[28]

      (1) Pleoptics to improve foveal fixation.

      (2) Intermittent photic stimulation.

      (3) Auditory biofeedback.

    d. Surgery

      (1) Kestenbaum procedure—moves null point to the primary position to maximize visual acuity in the primary position and eliminate anomalous head position.

      (2) Strabismus surgery for nystagmus blockage syndrome.

X. Vergence

A. Developmental considerations

1. The fusional vergence system is developed in infants by 3–4 months of age.

2. Prior to this time it is normal for the eyes to occasionally "drift" or act independently.

3. By 4 months of age, the eyes should be straight.

4. Stereopsis is present by 4 months of age.

5. "Pseudostrabismus" may be present when there are prominent epicanthal folds.

6. Children may outgrow a "pseudostrabismus" as their facial structures change.

7. Children generally do not outgrow an actual strabismus.

8. The presence of a true congenital strabismus is rare.

9. Esotropia, which is the most common form of congenital strabismus, usually appears between birth and 6 months of age.

10. Accommodative esotropia, another common form of early strabismus, usually appears between 2 and 3 years of age.

11. Intermittent exotropia can appear at any age, even in young infants.

12. Binocular vision problems, such as convergence insufficiency or convergence excess, generally become manifest and interfere with learning after 3rd grade as the reading demand increases.

13. Congenital noncomitant deviations may be isolated or associated with one of the following systemic developmental disorders:

    a. Developmental delay.

    b. Cerebral palsy.

    c. Seizures.

    d. Hydrocephalus.

    e. Hemiplegia.

    f. Mental retardation.

    g. Other.

B. Clinical presentation of problems

1. Signs

    a. Physical appearance of an eye turn.

    b. Redness.

       c. Poor motor coordination.

       d. Poor visual perceptual skills.

       e. Lack of concentration.

       f. Avoidance of close work.

       g. Covering one eye to read.

       h. Squinting one eye in bright sunlight.

2. Symptoms

       a. Diplopia.

       b. Fatigue.

       c. Headaches.

       d. Blur.

C. *Diagnostic evaluation: unique tools*

1. Tests for motor alignment and vergence ability

    a. Observation. Observe head posture before examining the child.

       (1) In waiting room.

       (2) During play.

    b. Hirschberg reflexes

       (1) Used to determine the presence of strabismus.

       (2) Only a gross measurement.

       (3) May miss a small-angle strabismus.

       (4) Hold penlight or illuminated finger puppet at approximately 16 inches, avoid aiming light directly in child's eye to avoid dazzle response.

       (5) Look at child from directly behind the light and observe the placement of the light reflexes on the corneas.

       (6) Compare monocular to binocular placement.

       (7) Reflexes should be slightly nasal on the cornea.

       (8) Any displacement in comparison to monocular viewing represents a strabismus.

       (9) 1 mm displacement = approximately 22 prism diopters of strabismus.

       (10) Nasal displacement = exotropia.

       (11) Temporal displacement = esotropia.

    c. Krimsky test

       (1) Use to measure a strabismus.

       (2) Follow Hirschberg method.

       (3) Slowly introduce neutralizing prism before the strabismic eye (base in for exotropia) until the placement of the reflexes is the same (mirror images).

       (4) This amount of prism equals the magnitude of strabismus.

    d. Cover test

       (1) Provides precise measurements of a tropia or a phoria in children.

       (2) In children below the age of 3, rest your hand on top of the child's head and use your thumb as an occluder.

       (3) Use appropriate fixation target as follows:

          (a) Birth–age 3: small, bright target, preferably illuminated (e.g., finger puppet on a penlight).

          (b) 4–6 years: small "swinging" puppet (photo) or small detailed picture on a tongue depressor.

          (c) 6 and up: use a single isolated letter which is one line above best near visual acuity on the end of a stick or tongue depressor (Figure 11-15).

       (4) Have several different targets available for each age, as children tire of the same target, making continued fixation difficult.

       (5) Use a dynamic cover test to ensure adequate fixation by moving the target periodically and checking to see that the child continues to fixate the target.

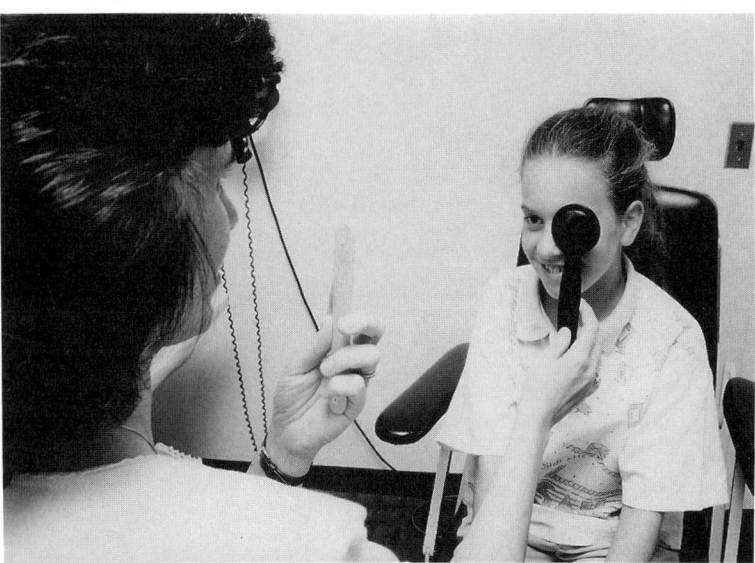

Figure 11-15.   Cover test using appropriate fixation targets for school-age children (small letter or picture on a tongue depressor) (*photo by Ron Davidoff*).

(6)   Use a prolonged occlusion to elicit a possible latent strabismus. This is especially useful if parent reports an eye turn, but none is observed during routine testing (especially in the morning when child is still alert). Cover one eye for approximately 30 minutes using an adhesive patch. Observe position of the covered eye as the occluder is removed.

(7)   Cover testing in 9 positions of gaze should be done whenever a tropia is present to check for comitancy.

e.   Vergences
(1)   Measured in a phoropter in children over the age of 8.
(2)   Prism bar vergences are performed on younger children or when the phoropter yields questionable findings (Figure 11-16).
(3)   Present a 20/30 letter at distance or near.
(4)   Slowly increase base-in or base-out prism one step at a time until child reports constant blur or diplopia, or eye turns in or out.
(5)   Slowly decrease the prism until child reports one target or the eyes appear to pick up fixation.

f.   Motilities
(1)   Observe 9 positions of gaze using interesting target or illuminated finger puppet.
(2)   Look for restrictions of motility.
(3)   Look for subtle deviations in Hirschberg reflex.
(4)   If restrictions are present:
(a)   Hold child's head with both of your hands.
(b)   Rotate the child's head to place the eyes in the action field of the suspected muscle.
(c)   I.e., if a left abduction deficit is suspected, rotate the child to move eyes in left gaze (doll's head maneuver).
(d)   A restriction is present if the child is still unable to move his or her eyes during this procedure.

g.   Additional tests for motor alignment and vergence ability that are not unique to children but that can be used if child understands test are as follows:
(1)   Von Graefe phorias—detects and measures phorias in phoropter.

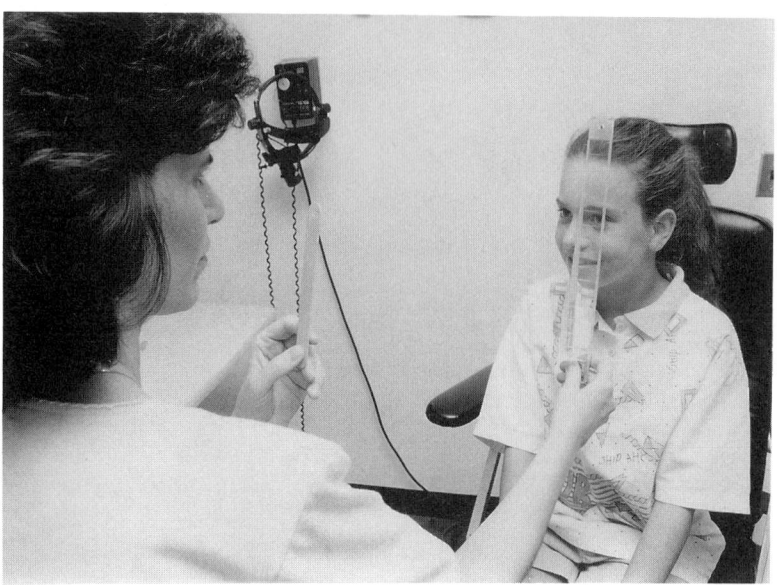

Figure 11-16.   Prism bar vergence testing (*photo by Ron Davidoff*).

        (2)   Modified Thorington—detects and measures phorias in free space.
        (3)   Fixation disparity—detects small ocular misaligments that do not interrupt binocularity.
  2. Tests for sensory fusion
      a. Worth 4 dot and 3 figure flashlight (Figure 11-17)
        (1)   Child wears red/green glasses.
        (2)   Examiner holds flashlight at distance and near.
        (3)   Child reports number of dots or pictures seen (Table 11-6).
      b. 3 bears test
        (1)   Child wears red/green glasses.
        (2)   Examiner must ascertain that child knows names of colors in order to proceed with testing.
        (3)   Examiner holds three 1-inch fuzzy bears in his or her hand.
        (4)   Bears are red, green, and black.
        (5)   Child must be able to pick out red, green, and black bears upon request by examiner.
        (6)   Confusion with identification of colors indicates suppression.

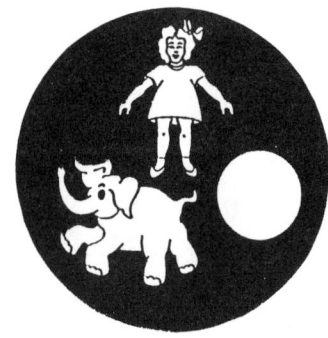

Figure 11-17.   3-Figure flashlight (used with permission of Bernell Co.).

Table 11-6. Interpretation of Worth 4 Dot/3 Figure Flashlight

	Ages	NRC	Suppression	ARC	Diplopia
Worth 4 dot	5 years and older	4 dots with no strabismus present during test	2 red dots or 3 green dots	4 dots with strabismus present during test	5 dots Exo = crossed Eso = uncrossed
3 figure flashlight	2–5 years	3 pictures with no strabismus present during test	2 pictures	3 pictures with strabismus present during test	4 pictures Exo = crossed Eso = uncrossed

3. Tests for stereopsis
    a. There are numerous tests of stereopsis now available. A representative sample is described below.
    b. Lang stereo test
        (1) For children aged 3 and older.
        (2) Uses a process called panography to create a 3-dimensional effect without the use of polaroid glasses.
        (3) Test is presented at 40 cm.
        (4) Child must point to or name pictures seen.
        (5) Can modify test to a matching task by copying and enlarging the sample of each picture on the test brochure.
        (6) Parallax may give false negative results on this test.
        (7) This test may miss a child with a small-angle strabismus.
        (8) Advantages. No need for stereo glasses, which are sometimes difficult to keep on child's face.
    c. Each of the following stereo tests requires the use of polarized glasses. It is sometimes problematic keeping these traditionally black glasses on a young child's face. An alternative is to use inexpensive but colorful children's sunglasses, replacing the regular lenses with polarized lenses. By having several colors with different motifs available, the child can choose which glasses to wear. A mirror is also helpful in encouraging the child to keep the frames on his or her face.
    d. Stereo fly
        (1) Advantages
            (a) Easy to administer.
            (b) No language skills necessary.
            (c) Shows if child has some degree of stereopsis.
        (2) Limitations
            (a) May be difficult to interpret child's responses.
            (b) Misses small-angle strabismus.
            (c) Contour or line stereo test only.
            (d) Monocular cues present.
            (e) Fly = 3000 sec stereopsis.
        (3) General protocol
            (a) Test is performed at 40 cm.
            (b) Child wears polaroid glasses.
            (c) Ask child to "touch" or "grab" the fly's wings.
    e. Random dot E
        (1) Advantages
            (a) Easy to administer.
            (b) No expressive language skills necessary.

           (c)   No monocular cues present.

           (d)   Tests for presence of global stereopsis.

           (e)   Good at detecting small-angle strabismics.

      (2)   Limitations

           (a)   Difficult to measure an actual stereoacuity threshold, as only one level of stereopsis on cards.

           (b)   Although this can be done by increasing the working distance, young children are often less responsive to testing as the distance increases.

      (3)   General protocol

           (a)   Test is administered at 40 cm.

           (b)   Child wears polarized glasses.

           (c)   3 cards

               i.   Blank.

               ii.   Training card with raised E.

               iii.   Stereo E.

           (d)   Holding blank and training card, ask child to point to E or "picture."

           (e)   Consistent responses indicate child understands task.

           (f)   Hold blank and stereo E and ask child to again point to E.

           (g)   4 of 4 correct responses indicates the presence of stereopsis.

   f.   Randot E/stereo butterfly (Figure 11-18)

      (1)   Advantages

           (a)   Can modify testing based on child's cognitive skills and age.

           (b)   Tests both global and local stereopsis.

           (c)   3 different tests in book.

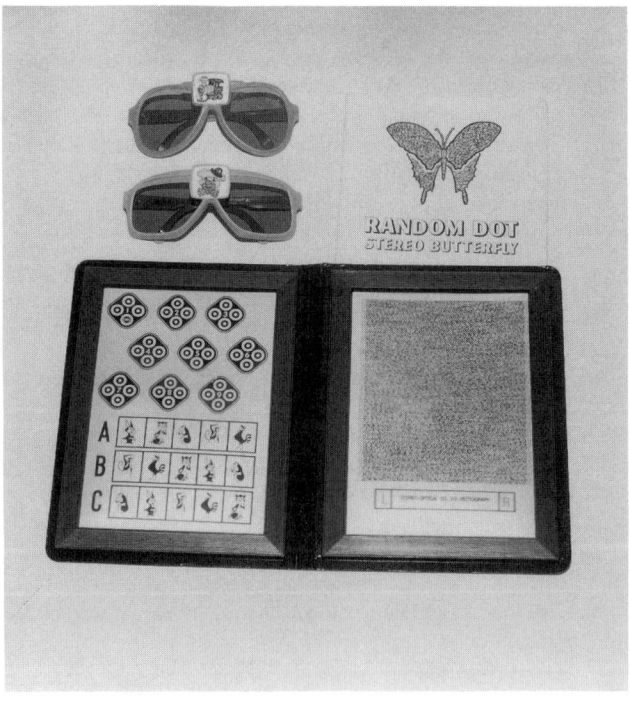

Figure 11-18.   Random dot stereo butterfly test with colorful children's sunglasses in place of traditional black frames (*photo by Ron Davidoff*).

        (d) Test for global stereopsis requires identification or matching of geometric shapes.

        (e) 2 tests for stereoacuity level using either animals or circles.

    (2) Limitations. Difficult to test children under the age of 3.

  g. Stereo butterfly—synthetic optics

    (1) Advantages

        (a) Child takes a more active role in test.

        (b) Tests for global stereopsis.

        (c) Can pick up small-angle strabismics.

    (2) Limitations

        (a) Very young children may not understand task.

        (b) Response may be difficult to interpret.

    (3) General protocol

        (a) Test is performed at 40 cm.

        (b) Tests for presence of stereopsis.

        (c) Uses two pair of glasses, "yes" and "no."

        (d) Child tries on each pair and reports which are "magic."

  h. Goggle-less stereo test

    (1) Advantages

        (a) Similar to Randot E, but does not require glasses.

        (b) Includes several tests for stereopsis.

        (c) Useful in children over the age of 3 years.

    (2) Limitations

        (a) Parallax may limit effectiveness.

        (b) May not detect small-angle strabismics.

    (3) General protocol. Similar to the Randot E.

  i. Preferential looking stereo cards (Figure 11-19).

    (1) Advantages

        (a) Random dot test.

        (b) Uses a happy face target.

        (c) Forced choice or operant preferential looking format.

        (d) Can be administered to all age groups.

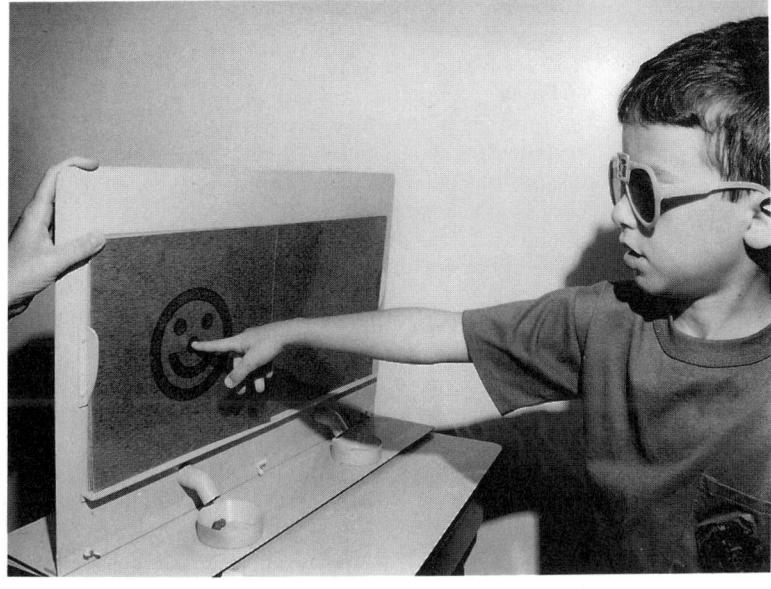

Figure 11-19. Operant or forced choice stereo preferential looking (*photo by Ron Davidoff*).

(2) General protocol
    (a) Child is shown training card with smiley face on one end which is seen without need for binocularity.
    (b) When child demonstrates ability to point to or look at smiley face, test cards are used.
    (c) Child points to or looks at smiley face.
    (d) Either preferential looking or child rewarded with Cheerio.
    (e) Child must pass 6 of 8 trials at each disparity.
j. Other tests for stereopsis
    (1) Frisby test
        (a) True depth perception test.
        (b) Does not require polarized glasses.
        (c) Child must identify a square in 1 of 4 boxes.
        (d) Easily contaminated if child moves due to parallax.
    (2) Stereo butterfly (stereo optical)
        (a) Similar to stereo butterfly above.
        (b) Does not use "yes" and "no" glasses.
    (3) Stereo reindeer (stereo optical)
        (a) Similar to fly.
        (b) Not as frightening to a child.

D. *Differential diagnosis and common problems based on age*
    1. Classification of binocular vision problems
        a. Phoria vs tropia.
        b. Magnitude.
        c. Constant vs intermittent.
        d. Frequency if intermittent.
        e. Unilateral or alternating (tropia).
        f. Comitant vs noncomitant.
        g. Presence of accommodative component.
        h. Periodicity (present at only distance or near).
        i. Time, mode of onset, and course.
        j. Congenital vs acquired (congenital occurs before age 6 months).
        k. Presence of other motor or sensory anomalies, i.e.
            (1) Nystagmus.
            (2) Ptosis.
            (3) Amblyopia.
            (4) Diplopia (rare in congenital strabismus).
            (5) Anomalous vs normal retinal correspondence.
            (6) Suppression.
        l. Associated signs and symptoms.
        m. Binocular vision anomalies in children are generally of two types: functional and organic.
    2. Functional
        a. A result of inborn nature; may or may not be associated with abnormal relationships between accommodation and convergence.
        b. Features
            (1) Generally comitant.
            (2) No other associated neurological signs or symptoms.
            (3) Often long-standing nature.
            (4) Becomes expressed as environmental stresses increase (e.g., computer or near work).
            (5) Progression related to magnitude of environmental stresses.
            (6) May be associated with
                (a) Amblyopia.

   (b) Anomalous head positions.

   (c) Reduced stereopsis.

3. Commonly occurring functional conditions include (the following conditions are most often functional in nature; however, an organic basis for each problem must first be ruled out):

 a. Congenital esotropia

  (1) Onset by 6 months of age.

  (2) Comitant deviation.

  (3) Double hyper component may be present (dissociated vertical deviation).

  (4) Latent nystagmus.

  (5) May be partially accommodative.

  (6) Treatment consists of

   (a) Full correction of any hyperopia to achieve alignment.

   (b) Bifocal if necessary to achieve alignment at near.

   (c) Occlusion therapy if amblyopia is present.

   (d) Prism if residual angle remains.

   (e) Vision therapy.

   (f) Surgery (if above treatment unsuccessful after 6 months).

 b. Accommodative esotropia

  (1) Onset 2–3 years of age.

  (2) Comitant deviation.

  (3) Eso deviation greater at near than distance.

  (4) Secondary to uncorrected hyperopia and/or a high AC/A ratio.

  (5) Treatment consists of

   (a) Correction of hyperopia to obtain ocular alignment.

   (b) Bifocal if additional plus at near eliminates or significantly reduces angle of strabismus.

   (c) Occlusion therapy if amblyopia is present.

   (d) Prism if residual angle remains.

   (e) Vision therapy.

 c. Intermittent exotropia/divergence excess (DE)[29,30]

  (1) Clinical findings

   (a) Exo deviation often greater at distance than near.

   (b) Usually no amblyopia.

   (c) No diplopia awareness (with DE).

  (2) Signs and symptoms

   (a) Primarily a cosmetic problem.

   (b) Eye "wanders" when tired or inattentive.

   (c) No symptoms (with DE).

   (d) Symptoms similar to CI with intermittent exotropia at distance and near.

   (e) Onset may occur at any age.

   (f) Often presents as divergence excess whereby exo is greater at distance than at near.

   (g) Child is usually unaware when eye turns out.

  (3) Treatment

   (a) Minimal occlusion alternate patching to increase diplopia awareness.

   (b) Minus lenses (depends on success with other treatment).

   (c) Vision therapy.

 d. Convergence insufficiency

  (1) Clinical findings

   (a) Exo deviation greater at near than distance.

   (b) Reduced near point of convergence.

           (c) Reduced base out ranges at near.

           (d) Reduced NRA.

           (e) Fails plus on accommodative facility binocularly.

    (2) Signs and symptoms

           (a) Headaches.

           (b) Diplopia.

           (c) Blurred vision.

           (d) Covers one eye to read.

           (e) Avoidance of close work and reading.

           (f) Usually presents during school years.

           (g) Aggravated as child gets older and school demand increases.

           (h) Symptoms worsen toward end of day and dissipate weekends.

    (3) Treatment

           (a) Vision therapy.

           (b) Prism (only when vision therapy (VT) not feasible).

e. Convergence excess

    (1) Clinical findings

           (a) Eso deviation greater at near than distance.

           (b) Reduced base in ranges at near.

           (c) Reduced NRA.

           (d) Fails minus on accommodative facility monocularly.

    (2) Signs and symptoms

           (a) Headaches.

           (b) Diplopia.

           (c) Blurred vision.

           (d) Covers one eye while reading.

           (e) Avoidance of reading and close work.

           (f) Usually presents when child is in school.

           (g) Aggravated as child gets older and school demand increases.

           (h) Symptoms worse toward end of day and after near work.

    (3) Treatment

           (a) Plus lenses for near.

           (b) Vision therapy.

f. Divergence insufficiency[31]

    (1) May present at any age.

    (2) Not associated with learning.

    (3) Diagnosed by

           (a) Greater eso at distance than near.

           (b) Comitant.

           (c) Gradual onset.

           (d) Mild diplopia.

           (e) Symptoms worse with fatigue.

           (f) No papilledema.

           (g) No endpoint nystagmus.

    (4) Must differentiate from

           (a) Divergence paralysis

                i. Sudden onset.

                ii. Marked diplopia.

                iii. Gait disturbances.

                iv. May be papilledema.

           (b) Sixth nerve palsy

                i. Sudden onset.

                ii. Marked diplopia.

                iii. Endpoint nystagmus.

                iv. May be papilledema.

        (5) Treatment consists of
           (a) Plus lenses for distance if hyperopia present.
           (b) Prism.
           (c) Vision therapy.

4. Organic
   a. Disorders associated with neurologic signs and symptoms.
   b. Features
      (1) Often noncomitant.
      (2) Often recent onset.
      (3) May have progressive nature.
      (4) May be other associated signs and symptoms, including
         (a) Diplopia.
         (b) Muscle paresis.
         (c) Nystagmus.
         (d) Saccadic disorders.
         (e) Pupillary anomalies.
         (f) Headaches.
         (g) Dizziness.
         (h) Vomiting.
         (i) Gait disorders.
         (j) Loss of appetite.
         (k) Sudden weight loss or gain.
         (l) Anomalous head positions (unless in association with nystagmus).
      (5) Rarely associated with amblyopia.
      (6) May be associated with developmental delays.
      (7) Measure head circumference, weight, and height.

5. Organic conditions include
   a. Convergence retraction nystagmus
      (1) Disorder of upward voluntary saccades.
      (2) Attempt at upward saccades causes convergent movements and globe retraction.
      (3) May also cause excessive convergence on horizontal saccades resulting in difficulty with reading.
      (4) Etiology is midbrain lesions, e.g., pineal masses, infiltrative masses, neurosyphilis, trauma, multiple sclerosis, stroke.
      (5) Associated neurological signs include
         i. Partial third or fourth nerve palsies.
         ii. Skew deviations.
         iii. Mid-dilated light-near dissociated pupils.
         iv. Lid retraction (usually bilateral and symmetric).
         v. Corectopia.
         vi. Precocious puberty.
         vii. Convergence paresis.
         viii. Papilledema.
      (6) Treatment requires referral to a neurologist.
   b. Divergence paralysis
      (1) Acute onset comitant esotropia.
      (2) Uncrossed diplopia at distance.
      (3) Convergence insufficiency at near.
      (4) Comitant deviation without restrictions.
      (5) Normal horizontal saccades.
      (6) Etiology: benign idiopathic, pseudotumor, cerebellar tumors, intracranial hematoma, head trauma, lumbar puncture, demyelinating disease, viral infections, encephalitis, neurosyphilis, epidural anesthetic blocks.

(7) Must also rule out bilateral sixth nerve palsy or paresis.

(8) Treatment requires referral to a neurologist when associated with other neurologic signs or symptoms.

c. Convergence paralysis

(1) Acute onset exotropia at near.

(2) Comitant deviation without restrictions.

(3) Signs and symptoms of convergence insufficiency.

(4) May have accommodative and pupillary involvement.

(5) Etiology: flu, ischemic infarction, demyelination.

(6) Treatment requires referral to a neurologist.

d. Spasm of the near reflex

(1) Can be functional or organic.

(2) Variable esotropia.

(3) Pupil constriction.

(4) Patient limits abduction by voluntarily converging.

(5) Symptoms include blur and diplopia.

(6) Etiology

(a) Functional causes: psychological, malingerer, or recent increase in near work.

(b) Organic causes: pineal tumor, posterior fossa lesions, internuclear ophthalmoplegia, encephalitis, metabolic disorders, Arnold-Chiari malformation.

(7) Treatment includes

(a) Referral to a neurologist to rule out organic etiology if functional cause is not found.

(b) Treatment for functional cases.

    i. Saccadic training may "break" the spasm.

    ii. OKN or caloric testing may "break" the spasm.

    iii. Plus lenses or cycloplegics.

    iv. Psychological counseling.

e. Third nerve palsies

(1) A paralysis of the third cranial nerve results in impaired innervation of the superior rectus (SR), levator, inferior oblique (IO), inferior rectus (IR), and medial rectus (MR) muscles, pupils, and accommodation.

(2) Congenital (before 6 months) most common

(a) Birth trauma or forceps delivery.

(b) Developmental anomaly.

(c) Intrauterine insults (maternal infections).

(d) Usually isolated.

(e) Rarely associated with neurologic abnormalities (cerebral palsy, mental retardation).

(f) Most have aberrant regeneration and pupil involvement.

(3) Acquired (after 6 months) (in order of decreasing frequency)

(a) Trauma.

(b) Inflammation/infection—most commonly:

    i. Meningitis.

    ii. Orbital cellulitis.

    iii. Upper respiratory infections.

    iv. Mononucleosis.

    v. Sinusitis.

    vi. Chickenpox/mumps.

    vii. Tumors—most commonly:

    Cerebellar astrocytomas.

    Medulloblastomas.

    Brain stem gliomas.

         viii. Aneurysms.
         ix. Ophthalmoplegic migraines.
         x. Other, e.g., myasthenia gravis.
- (4) Signs and symptoms
  - (a) Complete unilateral paralysis
    - i. Exotropia.
    - ii. Hypotropia.
    - iii. Partial or complete ptosis.
    - iv. Limitation of adduction (varying degrees).
    - v. Limitation of elevation or depression (varying degrees).
    - vi. Pupil dilated and nonreactive.
    - vii. Paralysis of accommodation.
    - viii. Aberrant regeneration may occur during recovery: pseudo-Graefe sign—retraction of upper lid in downgaze or adduction (may see contraction of pupil concurrent with the retraction).
  - (b) Incomplete or isolated muscle involvement[32]
    - i. Rare.
    - ii. Isolated superior rectus paresis or isolated inferior rectus paresis is rare and usually congenital.
    - iii. Inferior oblique paresis is rarest (first rule out Brown's syndrome, which is more common).
- (5) Management
  - (a) Immediate CT or MRI unless clearly congenital.
  - (b) Full neurologic examination.
  - (c) Blood work by history (e.g., infection present).
  - (d) After diagnosis and during recovery period
    - i. Prisms (if deviation small).
    - ii. Alternate patching to prevent amblyopia, suppression, and muscle contractures.
    - iii. Surgery if full recovery has not occurred after 6–12 months and deviation is stable over several visits.
- f. Fourth nerve palsy
  - (1) A paresis or paralysis of the trochlear nerve, which solely innervates the superior oblique muscle.
  - (2) Congenital
    - (a) Birth trauma.
    - (b) Developmental abnormalities.
  - (3) Acquired
    - (a) Closed head trauma (most common).
    - (b) Encephalitis.
    - (c) Meningitis.
    - (d) Myasthenia gravis.
    - (e) Hydrocephalus (rare).
    - (f) Aneurysm (rare).
    - (g) Tumor (rare): brain stem gliomas, rhabdomyosarcoma.
  - (4) Signs and symptoms
    - (a) Hypertropia of the involved eye.
    - (b) Motility restriction when looking down and in.
    - (c) The following are present in congenital cases:
      - i. Anomalous head position.
      - ii. The child usually tilts head to side opposite involved eye to decrease deviation.
      - iii. Increased vertical fusional amplitudes (>3 prism diopters).
      - iv. Early photographs show anomalous head posture.
      - v. May decompensate with time.

       (d) The following are present in acute or acquired palsies in older children:

          i. Diplopia.

          ii. Eyestrain.

          iii. Tilting of images.

          iv. Difficulty reading.

(5) Management

    i. Monitor when large fusional amplitudes and photographs reveal long-term anomalous head posture.

    ii. Tensilon test and CT or MRI for a symptomatic child without large fusional amplitudes and no history of trauma.

    iii. Neurologic evaluation and CT or MRI when other neurologic signs or symptoms are present.

g. Sixth nerve palsy

  (1) Inability of the lateral rectus muscle to partially or completely abduct the eye.

  (2) Etiology

      (a) Congenital (rare)—reports of transient paresis at birth that resolves within the first 2 months.[32]

      (b) Acquired[6,32]

         i. Trauma (common).

         ii. Tumors (common)

            Pontine glioma.

            Brain stem glioma.

            Neuroblastoma.

            Posterior fossa tumor.

            Orbital rhabdomyosarcoma.

         iii. Head injury.

         iv. Benign intracranial hypertensions (pseudotumor cerebri).

         v. Hydrocephalus.

         vi. Infection (bacterial meningitis, varicella).

         vii. Vascular (arteriovenous malformation).

         viii. Idiopathic following upper respiratory infection, fever, virus, immunization —resolves within 2–3 months.[33]

  (3) Signs and symptoms

      (a) Unilateral or bilateral.

      (b) Partial or complete.

      (c) Esotropia greater at distance than near.

      (d) Abduction deficit (partial or complete).

      (e) Head turn toward involved eye.

      (f) Doll's maneuver does not eliminate abduction deficit.

      (g) Occlusion does not eliminate abduction deficit.

      (h) Diplopia (reported by child, or child closes or covers one eye or turns head).

      (i) Associated neurologic signs (afferent pupillary defect, papilledema, etc.).

  (4) Differential diagnosis

      (a) Congenital esotropia with cross fixation.

      (b) Duane's retraction syndrome.

      (c) Mobius syndrome.

  (5) Management

      (a) Assume a tumor is present if no history of trauma.

      (b) Neurologic exam.

      (c) CT or MRI.

    (d) Following neurology workup and during recovery period: alternate patching to prevent ARC, suppression, contracture, and amblyopia.

    (e) If no spontaneous recovery after 6 months, consider prism and vision therapy for small deviations, surgery for large deviations.

h. Duane's retraction syndrome
  (1) Features
    (a) Congenital, stable disorder of eye movements.
    (b) Incomitant strabismus.
  (2) Signs and symptoms
    (a) Usually unilateral.
    (b) Left eye more often involved than right.
    (c) Females more often involved than males (varying reports).
    (d) Up or down shooting of the eye on adduction.
    (e) Associated head turn to maintain fusion.
    (f) May be associated with
      i. Coloboma.
      ii. Heterochromia.
      iii. Microphthalmia.
      iv. Esotropia or exotropia.
      v. A and V syndromes.
      vi. Cataracts.
      vii. Malformations of face, limbs, ears, or spinal column.
      viii. Cleft palate.
      ix. Hearing loss.
    (g) May occur in isolation.[32]
  (3) Classification of Duane's retraction syndrome[32]
    (a) Type I
      i. Abduction deficit.
      ii. Normal or slightly limited adduction.
      iii. Globe retraction on adduction.
      iv. Fissure narrowing on adduction.
      v. May have associated esotropia with face turn away from normal eye.
    (b) Type II
      i. Adduction deficit.
      ii. Globe retraction on adduction.
      iii. Normal or slightly limited abduction.
      iv. May have associated exotropia with face turn toward normal eye.
    (c) Type III—combination of I and II
  (4) Management
    (a) Rule out other causes of abduction and adduction deficit.
    (b) Reassure parents of nonprogressive nature.
    (c) Refer to pediatrician to rule out systemic associations.
    (d) Rule out associated ocular conditions.
    (e) Treat amblyopia or refractive error if present.
    (f) Prism.
    (g) Surgery to eliminate grossly anomalous head position or large-angle strabismus.[32]

i. Mobius syndrome
  (1) Features
    (a) A congenital developmental disorder with paresis of the face and lateral recti muscles.
    (b) Affects cranial nerves VI, VII, and XII.

      (2) Signs and symptoms
        (a) Paralysis of unilateral or bilateral abduction.
        (b) Normal vertical gaze and convergence.
        (c) Esotropia common.
        (d) Defects of eye closure.
        (e) Associated with
          i. Paralysis of the face and tongue (variable) resulting in expressionless face and feeding and sucking problems.
          ii. Deformities of the head, extremities, chest and neck, fingers, and toes.
        (f) Usually diagnosed in infancy due to sucking problems and expressionless face.
     (3) Management
        (a) Treat amblyopia.
        (b) Surgery for large-angle esotropia.
  j. Brown's superior oblique tendon sheath syndrome
     (1) Features
        (a) Congenital anomaly of the superior oblique muscle.
        (b) Motility pattern simulates an inferior oblique paresis.
        (c) May be acquired in trauma, inflammation, and metastasis.
        (d) May be familial.
     (2) Signs and symptoms
        (a) Restricted or absent elevation in adduction.
        (b) Simulates an inferior oblique paresis.
        (c) Positive forced duction test.
        (d) Elevation may be normal in primary gaze and abduction.
        (e) Usually unilateral.
        (f) May have a hypo deviation in primary gaze.
        (g) May have diplopia in elevated adduction.
        (h) May have anomalous head position.
          i. Chin elevation to avoid upgaze.
          ii. Face turn away from affected eye to avoid adduction.
        (i) May show widening of palpebral aperture in adduction.
        (j) V syndrome exotropia in upgaze.
        (k) Overaction of the ipsilateral superior oblique muscle usually does not occur.
        (l) May have spontaneous recovery.
     (3) Differential diagnosis
        (a) Overaction ipsilateral superior oblique muscle.
        (b) Inferior oblique paresis (rare).
        (c) Trauma to trochlea.
        (d) Blowout fracture of orbital floor.
     (4) Management
        (a) Often no treatment is necessary if fusion and binocularity are present.
        (b) Prism to correct small hypo deviation in primary position.
        (c) Surgery to correct significant hypo deviations, cosmetic anomalous head postures, or significantly cosmetic deviations in adduction.

E. *General patient management in palsies in children*
  1. Rule out systemic and neurologic disease.
  2. Often no treatment is necessary if fusion and binocularity are present.
  3. Alternate occlusion to prevent diplopia, amblyopia, or contracture.

4.   Vision training or prism for small deviations which are stable or have become more comitant (<30 prism diopters).

5.   Surgery when large-angle strabismus is still present after 6–8 months (>30 prism diopters).

6.   Surgery for ptosis or disfiguring head position.

XI. Refractive Error

A. *Developmental changes—population changes*

1.   Most children are born with a mild to moderate degree of hyperopia (2.0 D = mean, SD = 2.75) (Table 11-7).

2.   A wide range of refractive errors is common, however, with the overall distribution being symmetrical (−6.00 to +10.00).

3.   A high incidence and high magnitudes of astigmatism are common in young children, with much of the astigmatism being against the rule.

4.   This variability in refractive error decreases due to the disappearance of the higher-magnitude refractive errors in the process of emmetropization.

5.   By age 6 there is a leptokurtic distribution which is skewed toward mild hyperopia.

6.   The incidence of astigmatism has also dropped by age 6, from a high of 50% during the first year of life to the 10% incidence found in adults.

7.   There is a shift from against the rule astigmatism toward with the rule astigmatism, while the oblique astigmats tend to remain constant.

8.   By puberty, the curve in spherical refractive error is skewed toward mild myopia and continues in this direction until adulthood when it stabilizes.

B. *Individual changes during the school years*

1.   Children with greater than 1.5 D of hyperopia tend to remain hyperopic.

2.   Children with +0.50 to +1.25 D of hyperopia entering school will tend to become emmetropic.

3.   Children with 0 to +0.50 Diopters of hyperopia tend to become myopic.

4.   Children with myopia will tend to become more myopic.

5.   There is no significant change in the magnitude or incidence of astigmatism.

C. *Clinical presentation of problems—differential diagnosis and common problems by age*

1.   The clinical presentation of a refractive error depends on the type and magnitude of the refractive error and the age of the child.

Table 11-7. Signs and Symptoms of Refractive Error in Preschool Children

Difficulty with depth perception
Eye and coordination difficulties
Confuses likeness and minor differences
Frequently rubs eyes
Blinks excessively
Complains of double vision
Cannot maintain fixation on a task
Frequently closes or covers one eye
Lack of interest in outdoor activities
Gets close to TV or books
Squinting
Lack of interest in near tasks
May be no signs or symptoms

From Ciner EB. Refractive error in young children: Evaluation and prescription. *Pract Optom* 1992;3:182–90.

2. Myopia
   a. Birth to age 5
      (1) Lower-magnitude refractive errors often have no clinical symptoms and do not need correction.
      (2) Higher magnitudes cause children to demonstrate a lack of interest in objects or people at a distance or may cause children to get close to toys, books, or TV.
   b. 5 years and older
      (1) Tend to hold books closer (low to high).
      (2) Squint to see the blackboard (low to moderate).
      (3) Typically fail the school screenings (all magnitudes).
      (4) Demonstrate poor visual acuity at all distances (high magnitudes).
3. Hyperopia
   a. Birth to age 5
      (1) Lower magnitudes often have no clinical symptoms and do not need correction.
      (2) Moderate to high hyperopes often present with an esotropia, commonly between 2 and 3 years of age.
      (3) Moderate to high hyperopes may have a lack of interest in near tasks and demonstrate poor eye-hand coordination and other perceptual skills.
   b. 5 years and older
      (1) Lower magnitudes may be asymptomatic.
      (2) Moderate hyperopes may have a lack of interest in close work, demonstrate poor reading skills, or may have general asthenopic complaints.
      (3) Higher-magnitude hyperopes often demonstrate reduced visual acuity at distance and near.
4. Astigmatism
   a. Birth to age 3. No known symptoms or presentation.
   b. 3 to 5 years
      (1) May demonstrate reduced visual acuity.
      (2) Decreased interest in fine detailed tasks.
   c. 5 years and older
      (1) Reduced visual acuity at distance and near.
      (2) Nearpoint asthenopia due to underlying accommodative problem.
5. Anisometropia
   a. Birth to age 4
      (1) May be no clinical manifestations.
      (2) Decreased stereopsis or other binocular skills.
      (3) Amblyopia.
   b. 4 years and older
      (1) Decreased stereopsis or other binocular skills.
      (2) Amblyopia.
      (3) Nearpoint asthenopia.

D. *Diagnostic evaluation: unique tools*
   1. Types
      a. Mohindra-nearpoint retinoscopy.
      b. Distance retinoscopy.
      c. Cycloplegic refraction.
      d. Photorefraction.
      e. Autorefraction.
   2. Nearpoint retinoscopy (Mohindra) is useful in children between birth and 3 years of age and can be used in older children when necessary. Important points:
      a. Fixation target is retinoscope beam.
      b. 50 cm working distance from child.

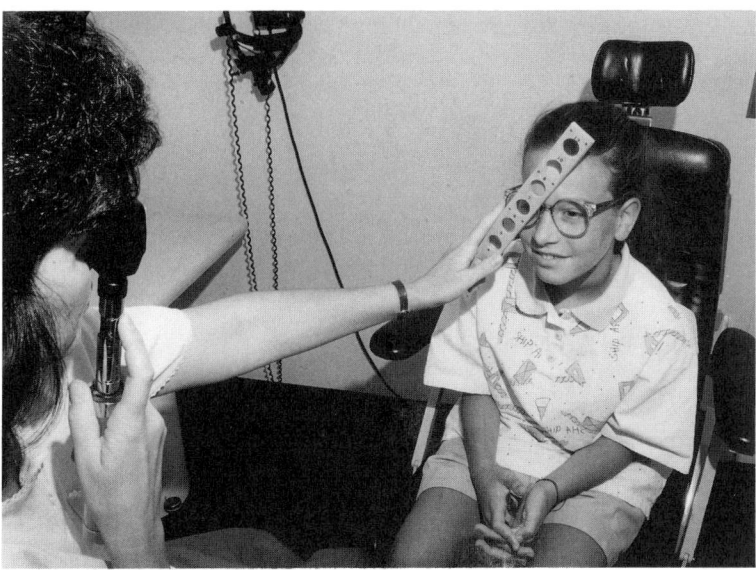

Figure 11-20. Lens rack refraction on school-age children using colorful fogging lenses (*photo by Ron Davidoff*).

    c. Room lights should be off, with no extraneous sources of light which may distract child.

    d. Retinscope beam should be low.

    e. Use a lens rack or loose lenses to measure—a blackened lens rack is desirable to minimize distractions to child.

    f. Use sound effects to maintain child's attention and aid child in localizing light.

    g. Subtract 1.25 from gross findings in each meridian for refractive error.[34]

3. Distance retinoscopy can generally be done on children aged 3 and up. Prior to this age, children are unable to maintain attention on distance tasks for any prolonged period of time.

    a. Fixation target

      (1) 3–10 years

        i. TV/VCR with cartoons, Sesame Street, children's programs.

        ii. Slide projector with children's pictures set on timer.

        iii. "Switch" toy with lights, sounds, or music.

        iv. Remote control toy, e.g., "barking dog"/blinking lights.

      (2) 10–18 years

        i. Use a large nonaccommodative target.

        ii. 20/200 E, large picture or muscle light.

    b. Fogging lenses (Figure 11-20)

      (1) Desirable in order to control accommodation.

      (2) Especially important when strabismus, "pseudomyopia," or latent hyperopia is suspected or present.

      (3) Older children (8 years and older)—use phoropter and dial in either the retinoscopy lens or a designated working distance lens.

      (4) Younger children—use a lens rack as phoropter is undesirable due to attentional issues and cooperation.

      (5) Use "refracting glasses" in attractive frames with the retinoscopy working distance and a lens rack.

      (6) Allows for effective control of accommodation and allows the examiner

to maintain eye contact with the child as well as monitor the child's fixation on the distance target.

4. Cycloplegic refraction is useful at any age in certain circumstances, but especially in the following:
   a. Fluctuating reflexes.
   b. Inability to maintain child's attention.
   c. Uncooperative children.
   d. Strabismus, especially esotropia.
   e. Suspected latent hyperopia.
   f. Amblyopia.
   g. Anisometropia.
   h. High lag of accommodation.
   i. Measurement of questionable significant refractive error using other methods.

5. Photorefraction is primarily an instrument to screen for the presence of refractive errors.[35]
   a. Can detect as little as 0.5D of ametropia.
   b. Cannot quantify refractive errors greater than 6 D.
   c. Useful in large screenings.
   d. Noninvasive, child sits far from camera.
   e. Quick and easy to administer.
   f. Easy to interpret results.
   g. Some units require "film" development which can be time consuming.
   h. Some units are computerized and not easily transportable.

6. Autorefraction is useful in children from approximately 3 years of age.
   a. Autorefractor with attractive children's fixation target is most desirable.
   b. Used primarily to confirm retinoscopy findings.
   c. Less effective for screening very young children.
   d. Useful to verify significant refractive errors.

7. Keratoscope is useful to confirm the presence of significant astigmatism in young or uncooperative children (Figure 11-21).
   a. Internally illuminated placedo disc.
   b. Pattern of disc is reflected off the cornea.

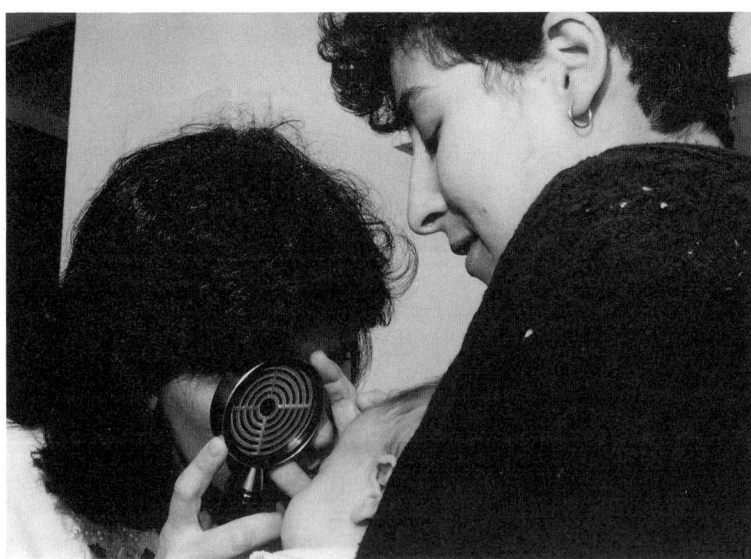

Figure 11-21.   Keratoscope used to measure cylinder on an infant (*photo by Ron Davidoff*).

Table 11-8. Guidelines for Prescribing Refractive Error in Children

Refractive Error	Concern for Amplyopia	Effect on Binocularity	Interference with Learning	Consider Prescribing
Myopia	>5 D	Undercorrect eso Fully correct exo[a]	Depends on child's age	>5 D all ages > 3 D > 1 yr >1 D > 3 yr
Hyperopia	>2 D	Undercorrect exo Fully correct eso[a]	>2.5 D school age	>2.0 D depending on age
Astigmatism	>1.25 D	Depends on other factors	Depends on visual acuity	>1.25 D
Anisometropia	>1.0 D	Monitor stereopsis	>1 diopter	>1 D

[a]To maximize binocularity. From Ciner EB. Refractive error in young children: Evaluation and prescription. *Pract Optom* 1992;3:182–90.

      c.   Pattern elongated when cylinder is present.
      d.   Cylinder axis is along elongated meridian.
      e.   Detects approximately 1.50 D or greater.

  E. *Management (Table 11-8)*

    1. Myopia

      a. All ages

        (1) Full correction for exo deviations.

        (2) Modify correction for eso deviations.

      b. Birth–1 year of age. Correct when 5 D or greater.

      c. 1–3 years of age. Correct when 3 D or greater.

      d. 3–5 years of age. Correct when 1 D or greater.

      e. 5–18 years of age

        (1) Correct myopia to obtain visual acuity of 20/20 without overminusing child (maximum plus to maximum visual acuity).

        (2) Monitor simultaneously for accommodative or binocular dysfunction.

        (3) When nearpoint esophoria, accommodative spasm, or latent hyperopia is present or suspected, treat the underlying problem first before correcting myopia.

    2. Hyperopia

      a. All ages

        (1) Correct any hyperopia when an esotropia is present; however, base correction on child's AC/A ratio and monitor for optically induced consecutive exo deviations.[36]

        (2) Consider a cycloplegic refraction whenever hyperopia and esotropia are present.

      b. Birth–5 years of age

        (1) Correct when greater than 2.5 D and no binocular dysfunction and hyperopia is stable over several visits.

        (2) Correct lesser amounts when a significant esophoria or esotropia is present.

        (3) Undercorrect amounts greater than 2 D when an exophoria or exotropia is present.

      c. 5–18 years of age

        (1) Consider correcting when greater than 1.0 D and no binocular dysfunction.

        (2)   Correct lesser amounts when any esophoria or esotropia is present or patient experiences accommodative insufficiency or ill-sustained accommodation.

3. Latent hyperopia

   a. In general, hyperopia that becomes manifest only through cycloplegic refraction should follow the above guidelines for correcting.

   b. Rule out eso deviations and accommodative dysfunction.

   c. Up to 1.00 D of latent hyperopia in the absence of binocular or accommodative dysfunction does not need correction.

4. Astigmatism

   a. Birth–2 years of age

      (1) Do not correct astigmatism.

      (2) Monitor every 3–6 months.

      (3) Monitor visual acuity using preferential looking.

      (4) Monitor oblique and with the rule more closely.

   b. 2–5 years of age

      (1) Correct when astigmatism exceeds 1.25 D and is stable over several visits.

      (2) Correct when visual acuity is below normal for age.

      (3) Provide full astigmatism correction when prescribing.

   c. 5–18 years of age

      (1) Correct when astigmatism exceeds 1.25 D.

      (2) Correct lower amounts when improves visual acuity.

      (3) Prescribe full astigmatic correction when prescribing.

      (4) Low degrees of against the rule astigmatism, test for underlying accommodative dysfunction before prescribing. Treat accommodative problem first before prescribing.

5. Anisometropia

   a. All ages

      (1) Monitor binocularity.

      (2) Monitor visual acuity, especially in hyperopia, antimetropia, or cylindrical anisometropia.

      (3) Consider correcting when magnitude exceeds 1 D.

   b. Birth–4 years of age

      (1) Monitor over several visits before correction.

      (2) Correct when visual acuity or binocularity is compromised.

      (3) Consider contact lenses when magnitude exceeds 3 D.

   c. 4–18 years of age

      (1) Correct when visual acuity or binocularity is compromised.

      (2) Consider contact lenses when magnitude exceeds 3 D.[37]

Suggested Readings

Harley R. *Pediatric Ophthalmology.* Philadelphia: W.B. Saunders, 1983.

Isenberg SI. *The Eye in Infancy.* Chicago: Year Book Medical Publishers, Inc., 1989.

Press L, Moore B. *Clinical Pediatric Optometry.* Boston: Butterworth-Heinemann, 1993.

Rosenbloom A, Morgan M. *Principles and Practice of Pediatric Optometry.* Philadelphia: J.B. Lippincott, 1990.

Rosner J, Rosner J. *Pediatric Optometry.* 2nd ed. Boston: Butterworths, 1990.

Scheiman M. *Problems in Optometry—Pediatric Optometry.* Volume 2, No. 3. Philadelphia: J.B. Lippincott, 1990.

Scheiman M, Wick B. *Clinical Management of Binocular Vision.* Philadelphia: J. B. Lippincott, 1993.

References

1. Ciuffreda KJ, Levi DM, Selenow A. *Amblyopia: Basic and Clinical Aspects.* Boston: Butterworth-Heinemann, 1991:10–17.

2. Bartlett JD, Wesson MD, Swiatocha J, Woolley T. Efficacy of a pediatric cyloplegic administered as a spray. *Optom. Vis. Sci.* 1992;69;12s:101.

3. Stevens JC, Lane C. Retinoblastoma, Focal Points 1990. *Clinical Modules for Ophthalmologists.* Vol 8, Module 1:1–12.

4. Shields CL, Shields JA, Pankajkumar S. Retinoblastoma in older children. *Ophthalmology* 1991;98:395–399.

5. Sheary JE, Wayne RP. Coats' disease. *J Am Optom Assoc* 1989;60:293–294.

6. Harley RD. *Pediatric Ophthalmology: The Differential Diagnosis of Retinoblastoma.* Philadelphia: W.B. Saunders, 1983:1144–1156.

7. Silodor SW, Augsburger JJ, Shields JA, Tasman W. Natural history and management of advanced Coats' disease. *Ophthalmic Surg* 1988;19:89–93.

8. Alexander LJ. *Primary Care of the Posterior Segment.* East Norwalk: Appleton & Lange, 1989:32.

9. Flynn JT. Treatment of retinopathy of prematurity. In: Eichenbaum JW, Mamelok A, Mihl RN, Orellana J. *Retinopathy of Prematurity* Chicago: Year Book Medical Publishers, Inc., 1990;81–117,154.

10. Cats BP, Tan KEWP. Premature with and without regressed retinopathy of prematurity: Comparison of long term (6–10 years) ophthalmological morbidity. *J Pediatr Ophthalmol Strabismus* 1989;26:271–275.

11. Hunter DG, Mukai S. Retinopathy of prematurity: Pathogenesis, diagnosis, and treatment. In: Jakobiec FA, Azar D. eds. *Int Ophthalmol Clin* Boston: Little, Brown & Co., 1992;32:178–179.

12. Spencer R. The Cryo-ROP study: A national cooperative study of retinopathy of prematurity. In: Eichenbaum JW, Mamelok A, Mihl RN, Orellana J. *Retinopathy of Prematurity* Chicago: Year Book Medical Publishers, Inc., 1990:154.

13. Quinn G. Vitreous and retina. In: Isenberg SI, ed. *The Eye in Infancy.* Chicago: Year Book Medical Publishers, Inc. 1989:340–341.

14. Krill AE. *Hereditary Retinal and Choroidal Diseases.* New York: Harper & Row, 1977;359–375, 665–702, 749–787.

15. Carr RE. Primary retinal degenerations. In: Tasman W, Jaeger EA, eds. *Duane's Clinical Ophthalmology.* Philadelphia: Harper & Row, 1984;(3)24:1–19.

16. McCulloch C, Arshinoff S. Choroideremia and gyrate atrophy. In: Tasman W, Jaeger EA, eds. *Duane's Clinical Ophthalmology.* Philadelphia: Harper & Row, 1984;(3)25:1–20.

17. DiGeorge AM. Ocular changes in endocrine disease. In: Harley RD, ed. *Pediatric Ophthalmology* Philadelphia: W.B. Saunders, 1983:977,1010,1051.

18. Cavender JC, Everett AL. Hereditary macular dystrophies. In: Tasman W, Jaeger EA, eds. *Duane's Clinical Ophthalmology.* Philadelphia: Harper & Row, 1984;(3)9:1–29.

19. Moore BD. Diseases of the posterior segment and neuro-ophthalmic disorders. In: Press L, Moore B, eds. *Clinical Pediatric Optometry.* Boston: Butterworth-Heinemann, 1993:147–189.

20. Shields MB, Buckley E, Klintworth GK, Thresher R. Axenfeld-Rieger Syndrome. A spectrum of developmental disorders. *Surv Ophthalmol* 1985;29:387–409.

21. Laibson PR, Waring GO. Diseases of the cornea. In: Harley RD, ed. *Pediatric Ophthalmology.* Philadelphia: W.B. Saunders, 1983:477–482.

22. Adams AJ, Haegerstrom-Portnoy G. Color deficiency. In: Amos JF, ed. *Diagnosis and Management in Vision Care.* Boston: Butterworths, 1987:671–711.

23. Haegerstrom-Portnoy G. Color vision. In: Rosenbloom A, Morgan M, eds. *Principles and Practice of Pediatric Optometry.* Philadelphia: J.B. Lippincott, 1990:449–466.

24. Griffin JR. *Binocular Anomalies: Procedures for Vision Therapy.* 2nd ed. Chicago: Professional Press, Inc., 1982:362–368.

25. Leigh JR, Zee DS. *The Neurology of Eye Movements.* 2nd ed. Philadelphia: F.A. Davis Company, 1991:79–139.

26. Glaser JS. *Neurophthalmology.* 2nd ed. Philadelphia: J.B. Lippincott, 1990:299–323.

27. Burde RM, Savino P, Trobe JD. *Clinical Decisions in Neuro-Ophthalmology.* St. Louis: CV Mosb 1985:201.

28. Grisham D. Management of nystagmus in young children. In: Scheiman M, ed. *Problems in Optometry-Pediatric Optometry.* Philadelphia: J.B. Lippincott, 1990:519–523.

29. Cooper J. Intermittent exotropia of the divergence excess type. *J Am Optom Assoc* 1977;48:1261–1273

30. Kran BS, Duckman R. Divergence excess exotropia. *J Am Optom Assoc* 1987;58:921–929.

31. Scheiman M, Gallaway M, Ciner E. Divergence insufficiency: Characteristics, diagnosis, and treatment. *J Am Optom Assoc* 1986;63:425–431.

32. VonNoorden GK. *Binocular Vision and Ocular Motility.* 4th ed. St. Louis: CV Mosby, 1990:366–426.

33. Miller NR. Solitary ocular-motor nerve palsy in childhood. *Am J Ophthalmol* 1977;83:106–111.

34. Mohindra I. A non-cycloplegic refraction technique for infants and young children. *J Am Optom Assoc* 1977;48:518–523.

35. Duckman R. Using photorefraction to evaluate refractive error, ocular alignment and accommodation in infants, toddlers and multiply handicapped children. In: Scheiman M, ed. *Problems in Optometry—Pediatric Optometry.* Philadelphia: J.B. Lippincott, 1990:333–353.

36. Ciner EB, Herzberg H. Optometric management of optically induced consecutive exotropia. *J Am Optom Assoc* 1992;63:266–271.

37. Ciner EB. Management of refractive error in infants, toddlers, and preschool children. In: Scheiman M, ed. *Problems in Optometry—Pediatric Optometry.* Philadelphia: J.B. Lippincott, 1990:394–419.

APPENDIX 1

Tools and Resources

Visual Acuity Testing

Adhesive Eye Patches/Elastic band eye patches/Occluders	Bernell Co., U.S. (1-800-348-2225)
	750 Lincolnway East
	P.O. Box 4637
	South Bend, Indiana 46634-4637
	U.S. Optical Co. (1-800-227-2252)
	P.O. Box 4637
	South Bend, Indiana 46634-4637
OKN Drums	Bernell Co.
Broken Wheel Cards	Bernell Co.
LEA symbols	Precision Vision (1-407-352-1200)
	Kathleen Appleby
	7512 Dr. Phillips Boulevard
	Orlando, Florida 32819
PL 20/20 Tester	(not commercially available—can purchase used)
Teller Acuity Cards	VisTech Consultants Incorp. (513-454-1399)
	4162 Little York Road
	Dayton, Ohio 45414-5829

Cardiff Test	Keeler Instruments Co. (special order) (1-800-523-5620)
	456 Parkway
	Broomall, Pennsylvania 19008
N.V.T.C. Test of Children	Gayle Lamb
	Faculty of Special Education & Disability Studies
	Victoria College—Burwood Campus
	221 Burwood Highway, Burwood 3125
	Victoria, Australia
Baily Hall Cereal Test/	
Mr. Happy Contrast Sensitivity	(510-642-0229)
	Berkeley College of Optometry
	360 Minor Hall
	Berkeley, California 94720
H.O.T.V. Test	Good-lite Co., (1-800-362-3860)
	1540 Hannah Avenue
	Forest Park, Illinois 60130
Constrast Sensitivity Charts	Stereo Optical Co. (1-800-322-9500)
	3539 North Kenton Avenue
	Chicago, Illinois 60641
Psychometric Acuity Cards	OEP Foundation (800-424-8070)
	2912 S. Daimler Street
	Santa Ana, California 92205

Ocular Health Assessment:

Monocular Indirect Ophthalmoscope	Lombart Instruments (1-800-566-2278)
	5358 Robin Hood Road
	Norfolk, Virginia 23513
Pulsair Portable Non-Contact	
Tonometer	Keeler Instruments Co. (1-800-523-5620)
	456 Parkway
	Broomall, Pennsylvania 19008
Tonopen	Lombart Instruments
Proton Tonometer	Tomey Technology, Inc. (617-864-6488)
	325 Vassar Street
	Cambridge, Massachusetts 02139
Hand-held slit lamps, Burton Lamps	Lombart Instruments/Western Optical/U.S. Optical

Color Vision Testing:

F2 Plates/Berson Plates/Portnoy Plates	Berkeley College of Optometry
Pediatric Color Vision Test	U.S. Optical Co.
D-15 Color Vision Test	Bernell Co.

Accommodative Testing:

Accommodative Flippers:	Bernell Co./Pacific Prisms
	P.O. Box 554
	Forest Grove, Oregon 97116
MEM Cards	Bernell Co./Pacific Prisms
NITS/#9 Vectographic Card	Bernell Co.

Ocular Motilities:

Developmental Eye Movement Test   Bernell Co.

Stereopsis/Binocular Vision Testing:

Lang Stereo Test   Western Optical Co.
                                              1200 Mercer Street
                                              Seattle, Washington   98109

Reindeer, Randot E, Random Dot E,
    Stereo Butterfly, Preferential
    Looking Stereo   Stereo Optical Co. or Bernell Co.
Random Dot Butterfly   Bernell Co.
Goggle-less Stereo Test   Bernell Co.
Horizontal Prism Bars   Pacific Prisms
Red/green or polaroid bar reader   Bernell Co./GTVT
                                              18807 10th Pl. W.
                                              Lynnwood, Washington   98036

3 Bears Test   Red, Green & Black 1 inch bears
                                              A.C. Moore Crafts, Broomall, Pennsylvania 19008
3-Figure Flashlight   Bernell Co.

Refraction

Autorefractors   Canon Co. (516-488-6700)
                                              One Canon Plaza
                                              Lake Success, New York   11042
                                          Humphries Co.
                                          Topcon Instrument Corporation (201-261-9450)
                                              65 West Century Road
                                              Paramus, New Jersey   07652
                                          Tomey Technology, Inc.
Keratoscope   Welch Allyn, Inc. (1-800-535-6663)
                                              Ophthalmic Instruments Product Manager
                                              4341 State Street Road
                                              Skaneateles Falls, New York   13153
Lens Racks   U.S. Optical Co.; Bernell Co.;
Photorefraction   Clement Clarke Co. (1-800-848-8923)
                                              3128-D East 17th Avenue
                                              Columbus, Ohio   43219
                                          Tomey Technology, Inc.
                                          MTI Photorefractor (1-800-277-1710)
                                              1710 Adams Street
                                              Cedar Falls, Iowa   50613
Clown Bubble Blower   Kapable Kids Inc. (800-356-1564)
                                              P.O. Box 250
                                              Bohemia, New York   11716

CHAPTER **12**

Low Vision

William L. Brown

I. Definitions

A. *Low vision*

1. Low vision is a term used to describe a patient who has reduced visual acuity or reduced visual field even with regular spectacle correction.

   a. "Regular spectacle correction" is defined as the distance refractive correction or a multifocal with a 4.00D add maximum.

   b. More specifically, low vision exists if the vision best corrected with regular lenses in the better eye is no better than 20/70 but better than light projection, or if the maximum diameter of the visual field in the eye with the larger field does not exceed 30°.

   c. Functionally, however, a patient is low vision if the vision, even if better than 20/70, is poor enough with regular lenses that it hinders or prevents him or her from accomplishing tasks which he or she desires to do.

   d. Low vision implies that some useful vision is available, so a person with functional blindness is not generally included within the definition of low vision (see section I.B.2 for definition of functional blindness).

   e. Low vision is synonymous with partially sighted.

   f. Low vision is sometimes used synonymously with visually impaired, but visually impaired can also include a person who is functionally blind (see section I.B.2).

2. Low vision can be either congenital (i.e., present at birth) or adventitious (i.e., acquired at some time after birth).

B. *Blindness*

1. Legal blindness

   a. A patient is legally blind if the visual acuity best corrected with regular lenses in the better eye is no better than 20/200, or if the maximum diameter of the visual field in the eye with the larger field does not exceed 20°.

      (1) Either the acuity or the field criterion must be met, not necessarily both.

      (2) Since the next line smaller than 20/200 is 20/100 in most projected visual acuity charts, the practical definition as applied clinically is that the patient is legally blind if the vision is poorer than 20/100.

      (3) The visual field should be plotted using a 3-mm white target at 30 cm or a 10-mm white target at 1 m.

   b. A person can be low vision and not legally blind.

   c. An optometrist may certify a patient as being legally blind by writing a short note to that effect.

      (1) Certification by an optometrist must be renewed each year.

      (2) Certification by an M.D. does not require renewal.

    d. Benefits obtainable due to legal blindness include:

      (1) Additional personal income tax exemption for the legally blind person may be taken on Federal tax return if income tax is paid personally or jointly with spouse.

      (2) Free postal service is available for those who are blind.

      (3) The Talking Book program is offered through the Library of Congress (administered through local branch libraries) for those who cannot read regular print (includes low-vision patients who are not legally blind).

      (4) Free use of 411 information may be available from the telephone company in some areas.

      (5) In areas with public transportation, it may be possible to obtain a special user's card qualifying the person for a special rate.

      (6) Fire departments in some areas keep a computerized record of persons with disabilities (through a form which the individual completes), so they are aware of special needs should a fire occur in the residence.

      (7) Subscription to Radio Reading Service which is available in some cities.

        (a) Volunteers read portions of newspapers, magazines, books, recipes, and other materials of interest.

        (b) The individual receives the programs on a special receiver which is provided free or for a nominal charge.

2. Functional blindness

    a. A person is functionally blind if the best corrected visual acuity in the better eye is no better than light projection.

    b. It includes total blindness, light perception, and light projection.

3. Total blindness exists when neither eye detects the presence of light visually.

C. *Disorder, impairment, disability, handicap*

1. A disorder is a physical abnormality, such as a change in the peripheral retinal pigment epithelium (RPE).

2. An impairment is the reduction in some measurable test.

    a. Such tests might include visual acuity, contrast sensitivity, visual field, ocular motility.

    b. The American Medical Association has prepared a guide for objectively determining a percentage of permanent visual impairment and its effect on the ability to perform activities of daily living (ADL).[1]

      (1) Corrected visual acuities for distance and near, visual field diameters, and ocular motility with the absence of diplopia are the variables used.

      (2) Extensive tables are used in the determination.

3. A disability is the reduction in one's ability to perform a task, such as reading.

4. A handicap is the impact of the inability to perform a task on one's daily living routine, thus limiting social functioning.

    a. If the individual loses a job or is unable to continue a hobby or other normal daily activity due to the inability to perform a task, then a handicap exists.

    b. If the individual never relied on a particular ability to do a task, a handicap would not exist from that disability.

5. Consider the example of RPE degeneration as a disorder.

    a. Visual field loss is an example of impairment as a result of the disorder.

    b. The inability to drive due to peripheral field loss is an example of disability.

    c. The loss of a job as a truck driver due to the driving disability is an example of handicap.

6. "Person-first" terminology, such as referring to a patient as a "person with a disability" rather than a "disabled person," should be used.

D. *Low vision evaluation*

1. A low vision evaluation is designed to identify the needs and quantify the visual capabilities of the patient and to determine ways to either assist the patient in meeting reachable goals or in reassessing unrealistic goals.

2. The emphasis of a low vision examination is on functional evaluation following medical assessments.

E. *Low vision devices (LV aids). A low vision device is anything which is used by the patient to enhance the use of vision to perform a task.*
1. Optical aids are those which provide magnification through the use of lenses, mirrors, prisms, or electronics (e.g., the closed-circuit television).
2. Nonoptical aids are those which enhance visual performance through means other than those listed above.
   a. Illumination, filters, visors, large-print materials are examples.
   b. Electronic magnification is sometimes considered nonoptical.

II. Statistics

A. *Need for low-vision care*
1. Current statistics for the number of people with low vision are not available.
   a. According to Kirchner,[2] the most recent statistics which are national in scope are from the 1970s.
   b. The following estimates have been compiled by Kirchner.
2. The percentage of people in the United States who have severe visual impairment, defined as an inability to read newspaper print with current glasses, is estimated to be 6.6% (Kirchner,[2] p. 20).
   a. 1% for those under age 45.
   b. 6% for those aged 45–64.
   c. 44.5% for those aged 65 and older.
      (1) In 1977 it was estimated that this represented 990,000 persons 65 years old and older who could not read newsprint.
      (2) By the year 2000, it is estimated that this number will increase 78% to 1,760,000 due to the aging of the population in the United States (Kirchner, p. 52).
   d. In every age group poorer people have higher rates of visual impairment.
   e. It is apparent that the demand for low vision services will increase as the population ages in the United States.

B. *Most common causes of legal blindness*
The most common causes of legal blindness are (as of the 1970s)[3]:
1. For all age groups together: 1) glaucoma, 2) age-related macular degeneration, 3) cataract, 4) optic nerve atrophy, 5) diabetic retinopathy.
2. For those under age 20: 1) cataract, 2) optic nerve atrophy, 3) retinopathy of prematurity.

III. Psychological Adjustment

A. *Livneh and Evans[4] have suggested that there are 12 stages which a person may undergo in adjusting to a disability of recent onset.*
B. *These have been combined into the following 10:*
1. *Shock* is the stage in which there is psychological numbness from the trauma of the physical change.
2. *Anxiety* is the panic-stricken reaction as initial recognition of the traumatic event begins.
3. *Bargaining* is an attempt to recover from the disabling condition through making deals with God or with doctors, for example, and results in consultations with multiple doctors.
4. *Denial* is a defensive retreat from the painful and unpleasant implications of the disability and includes setting unrealistic goals in the face of changed abilities.
5. *Mourning/depression* is the grief response as the personal implications of the disability become realized.

6. *Withdrawal* is the "throwing in the towel" response which includes resignation from social interactions.
7. *Anger* is bitterness and hostility.
   a. It may be self-directed or directed externally at others.
   b. The optometrist and/or staff may be the object of such anger and must recognize it as one of the stages of adjustment.
8. *Acknowledgment* is the objective, intellectual recognition that it is possible and necessary to change one's self-concept and plans for the future to account for the disability.
9. *Acceptance* is the subjective, emotional recognition of the factors discussed under acknowledgment.
10. *Adjustment/adaptation* is the final phase in which the individual is willing to work on new skills and strategies to accomplish plans and goals, some or all of which may have been revised.

C. *The optometrist and staff must recognize that patients presenting with low vision may be in any of these stages of adjustment and that patient behavior will be influenced accordingly.*
D. *It is important that the optometric staff react appropriately to individuals in the various stages of adjustment with the intent of assisting the patient to move on to the next stage.*
E. *Some patients spend longer periods of time than others in one or more of the stages.*
F. *It is unlikely that a patient will be successful in the use of low vision devices until he or she has reached the stage of adjustment/adaptation.*
   1. Patients in earlier stages should be encouraged to seek other resources, such as counseling, to speed their adjustment.
   2. Since it takes time to move through the stages to adjustment, a patient with recent vision loss is much less likely to benefit from low vision devices than one with a more long-standing loss.
   3. Patients with congenital vision loss generally adapt more quickly and easily to low vision devices than patients with adventitious loss.

IV. Comprehensive Approach to Low Vision Services

A. *Effective low vision care encompasses a number of services in addition to the prescription of optical devices.*
   1. A variety of nonoptical devices can assist the patient.
      a. These include kitchen and daily living adaptive aids, computer hardware and software, large-print materials, marking devices, reading guides.
      b. Overlooking the usefulness of these devices or not educating the patient on their availability is a great disservice.
   2. Patients must be trained in the proper use of optical and nonoptical devices in order for them to use the aids successfully.
   3. Some patients require services provided by other disciplines.
      a. Psychological counseling seeks to aid the patient (and the family) in accepting and adapting to the visual impairments.
      b. Rehabilitation teachers assist the patient in relearning skills needed for activities of daily living (ADL).
         (1) ADL skills include such areas as personal hygiene, clothing care, and kitchen skills.
         (2) Communication skills are taught to enhance the patient's ability to receive and convey information through optical aids, nonoptical aids, electronic devices such as closed-circuit televisions and computer systems, and braille, depending on the patient's needs.
         (3) Rehabilitation teachers may visit a patient in his or her home to assist in adapting the kitchen or other areas using techniques such as labeling appliances with common settings, labeling cupboards, and improving lighting.

c.   Orientation and mobility instructors (also referred to as "O and M" or peri-patologists) teach skills such as developing strategies for getting to a desired destination and using a cane.
d.   Vocational counseling provides guidance in career opportunities and direction in preparing for a vocation.
e.   Special education teachers instruct partially sighted students using methods adapted to the capabilities of the students.
    (1)   The student may spend the entire school day with the special education teacher.
    (2)   The student may spend part of the day in the regular classroom and part of the day with the special education teacher.
    (3)   Itinerant teachers travel from school to school, meeting periodically with students who spend the majority of their time in the regular classroom.
f.   Genetic counselors investigate the hereditary nature of the ocular condition and advise the patient regarding risks to their own children.

B.   *These services are vital to the successful adaptation of some low vision patients, especially those who have suffered a recent or severe visual loss.*
C.   *If a practitioner does not have the inclination or facilities to provide comprehensive care, the patient should be referred to a colleague or other agencies or disciplines where care can be given beyond that available from the primary eye care office.*

V.   Magnification

A.   *Most low vision patients have reduced macular function which requires them to use the peripheral retina for viewing.*
    1.   Since the capability to resolve detail is reduced in the peripheral retina, the size of the retinal image must be increased if it is to be resolved.
    2.   Most low vision devices provide an enlarged retinal image through the use of one of the following types of magnification:
        a.   Angular magnification.
        b.   Relative distance magnification.
        c.   Transverse magnification.
        d.   Relative size magnification.

B.   Angular magnification, M_A, *is the ratio of the angle* ω' *subtended by the image seen through a lens to the angle* ω *subtended by the object viewed without the lens (Figure 12-1).*
    1.   The entrance pupil of the eye is used as the reference point for the angles.
    2.   Mathematically this ratio is $M_A = \tan \omega' / \tan \omega$.
    3.   When the task being viewed is at the primary focal point of the lens, $M_A = 1 + hF$, where h is the distance from the lens to the entrance pupil of the eye and F is the equivalent power of the lens.
    4.   Angular magnification is very important in increasing retinal image size of a near object when the lens is farther from the eye (h is large).

C.   Relative distance magnification, M_D, *is the change in angle subtended by an object when it is moved from one distance from the eye,* q_1, *to a second distance,* q_2 *(Figure 12-2):* $M_D = q_1 / q_2$.
    1.   When the object is moved closer, relative distance magnification increases, increasing retinal image size.
    2.   When the object is moved farther away, relative distance magnification decreases.
    3.   The major effect of a high-plus lens held close to the eye is an increase in relative distance magnification.
        a.   The plus lens allows the object to be brought closer to the eye and yet be seen in focus.

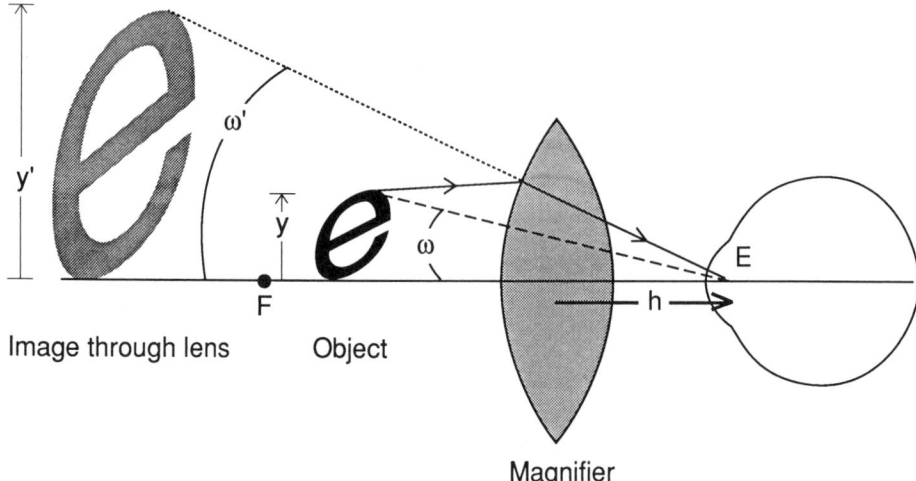

Figure 12-1. Angular magnification M_A through a magnifier compares the angle ω' subtended at the entrance pupil E of the eye by the image seen through the magnifier to the angle ω subtended by the object viewed without the magnifier. (Used by permission Brown WL. The optics of distance and near low vision devices. *Practical Optom* 1991;2:44–54)

      b.   The decreased distance from the eye to the object increases the retinal image size.

   D.   Relative magnification, M_R, *is the combination of angular magnification and relative distance magnification, the two most important types of magnification with most optical devices:* $M_R = (M_A)(M_D)$.

      1.   The angle subtended by the image seen through the magnifier with the object at a distance q_1 from the entrance pupil of the eye is compared to the angle subtended by the object alone (magnifier removed) when it is moved to a second distance $q_2 = d$, where d is a special reference distance (Figure 12-3).

      2.   Relative magnification is frequently used to label magnifiers with an assumed reference distance of $d = 25$ cm.

      3.   Two special cases of relative magnification, rated and conventional magnification, are commonly used to label magnifiers.

         a.   *Rated magnification* applies when the object is placed at the primary focal point of the magnifying lens or system of lenses.

            (1)   Rays emerging from the magnifier are parallel, the image formed by the magnifier is at infinity, and zero accommodation is required to view the image clearly.

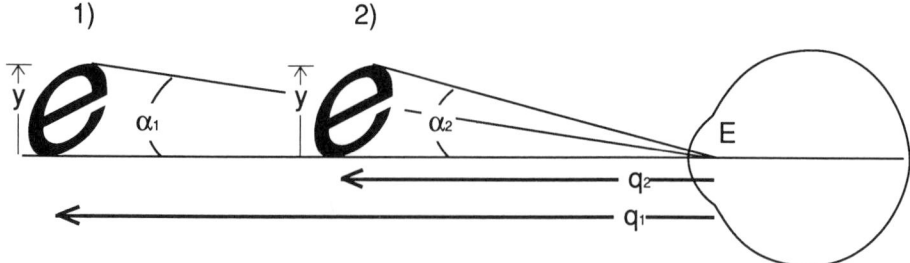

Figure 12-2. Relative distance magnification M_D occurs when the same object is moved from viewing distance q_1 to a new distance q_2. $M_D = \tan \alpha' / \tan \alpha = q_1/q_2$. (Used by permission Brown WL. The optics of distance and near low vision devices. *Practical Optom* 1991;2:44–54)

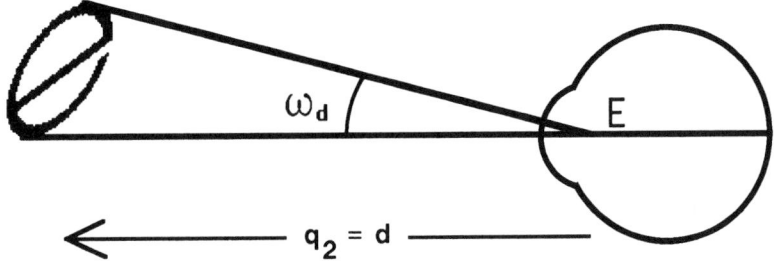

Figure 12-3.   Relative magnification compares the angle ω′ subtended by the image seen through the magnifier (Figure 12-1) to the angle ω_d subtended by the object when the object is moved to a reference distance d and viewed without the magnifier.

(2) Angular magnification becomes $M_A = 1 + hF$.
(3) If the object (such as a page of print) is kept at the focal point and the eye is moved away from the lens, "h" is increased.
  (a) Angular magnification increases.
  (b) However, relative distance magnification decreases at the same rate.
  (c) The net result is that the relative magnification M_R remains unchanged, independent of the distance between the eye and the magnifier.
(4) Relative magnification as rated magnification reduces to $M_R = M_{rated} = dF$, where d is the reference distance.
  (a) The reference distance is usually 25 cm or 0.25 m, in which case $M_{rated} = 0.25F = F/4$.
  (b) 25 cm was chosen years ago rather arbitrarily by manufacturers of magnifiers as the "least distance of distinct vision," supposedly the closest distance that an "average" patient would be able to read comfortably without optical assistance.
  (c) A magnifier marked with a rated magnification of 4× should have an equivalent power of $F = 4(4) = +16D$.
  (d) The rated magnification of 4× with a reference distance of 25 cm means that if the page is at the focal point of the magnifier, no matter how far the eye is from the magnifier, the retinal image with the magnifier is four times larger than the retinal image with the object viewed at 25 cm without the magnifier.
(5) Constant relative magnification with changing viewing distance means that the retinal image size remains unchanged when the eye is moved away from a magnifier with the page kept at its focal point.
  (a) If the patient can read a particular size print with the eye close to the magnifier, then the same size can be read with the eye farther from the magnifier.
  (b) However, the field of view through a magnifier decreases as the eye moves farther from it.
b. *Conventional magnification* is a second special case of relative magnification.
  (1) Conventional magnification applies with the magnifier held as close as possible to the eye (h approximately zero) and the page moved inside the focal point of the magnifier so a virtual image is formed at the reference distance d.
  (2) In this case, relative magnification as conventional magnification reduces to $M_R = M_{conv} = dF + 1$.
  (3) If d is 25 cm, $M_{conv} = 0.25F + 1 = F/4 + 1$.
    (a) A magnifier marked with a conventional magnification of 4× has

an equivalent power of $F = +12D$, which is less dioptric power than if it is marked with a rated magnification of $4\times$.

(b) Since the image is at 25 cm in this case, the eye must accommodate 4D, contributing an extra 4D of plus power.

(c) The extra plus power from the eye accounts for the increase in magnification in this situation.

(d) The conventional magnification in this $4\times$ magnifier means that the retinal image size (with the magnifier close to the eye, and the page held so the eye views the image through the magnifier at 25 cm from the eye) is four times larger than the retinal image when the magnifier is removed and the object is moved to 25 cm.

4. Magnification is a confusing topic, as illustrated by the previous discussion.

   a. The same magnifier has different magnifications depending upon how it is used.

   b. The magnification label on a magnifier is misleading because unless the magnifier is used under the conditions assumed by the label, the magnification effect will be different.

E. Transverse magnification, M_{TR}, *compares the size of an enlarged image, y', to the object size, y (Figure 12-4).*

1. The enlargement may be accomplished through electronics, such as with a closed-circuit television, or by a projection system, such as with an overhead projector.

2. Sometimes electronic and projection magnification are considered separately, but they will be considered together in this chapter.

3. Transverse magnification is easily calculated once the sizes of the image on the screen and the original object have been measured: $M_{TR} = y'/y$.

F. Relative size magnification, M_S, *is produced nonoptically by substituting material of larger size, y_2, for the original material having size y_1.*

1. Relative size magnification is given by $M_S = y_2/y_1$.

2. Large-print books are an example of relative size magnification.

G. Total magnification, M_{TOT}, *is the product of all types of magnification affecting the situation under consideration:* $M_{TOT} = (M_A)(M_D)(M_{TR})(M_S)$.

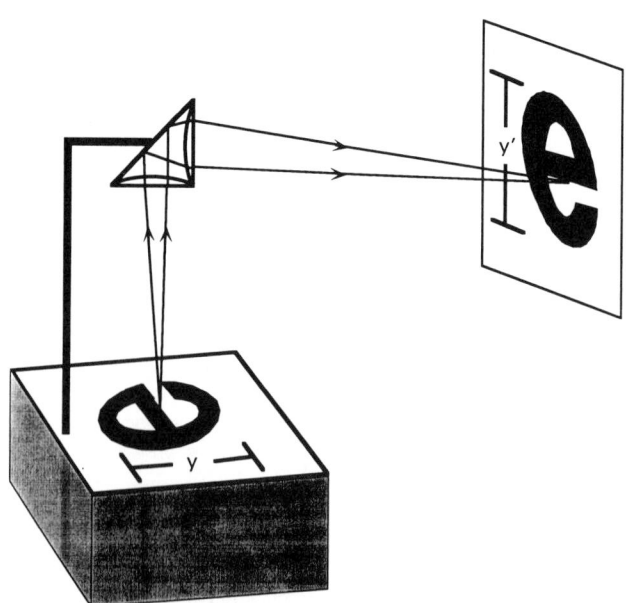

Figure 12-4.   Devices such as the overhead projector provide transverse magnification M_{TR} by creating an enlarged image (height y') of the object (height y). $M_{TR} = y'/y$.

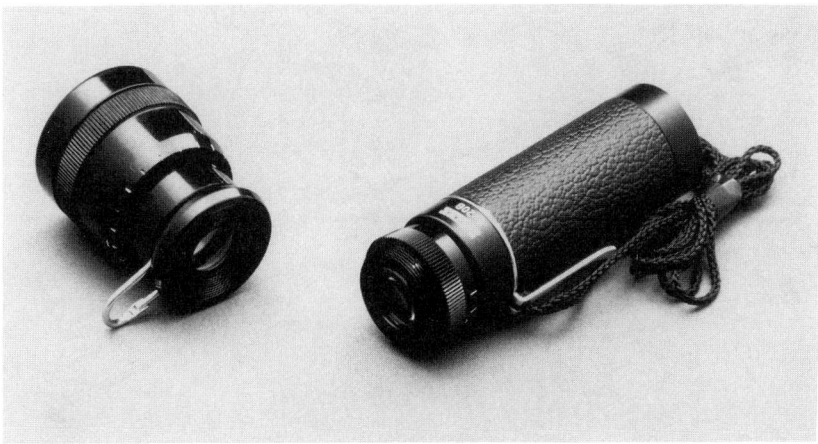

Figure 12-5. Galilean telescope (left) and Keplerian telescope (right).

VI. Optics of Low Vision Devices

A. *Low vision optical devices can be divided into three groups according to the distance at which they are used: distance, intermediate, and near.*

B. *Distance magnification is obtained through telescopes.*

1. A telescope consists of a plus objective and a higher-powered eyepiece separated by an airspace.

2. Telescopes are either Galilean or Keplerian in form (Figure 12-5).

a. A Keplerian telescope has a positive eyepiece, while a Galilean telescope has a negative eyepiece (Figures 12-6 and 12-7).

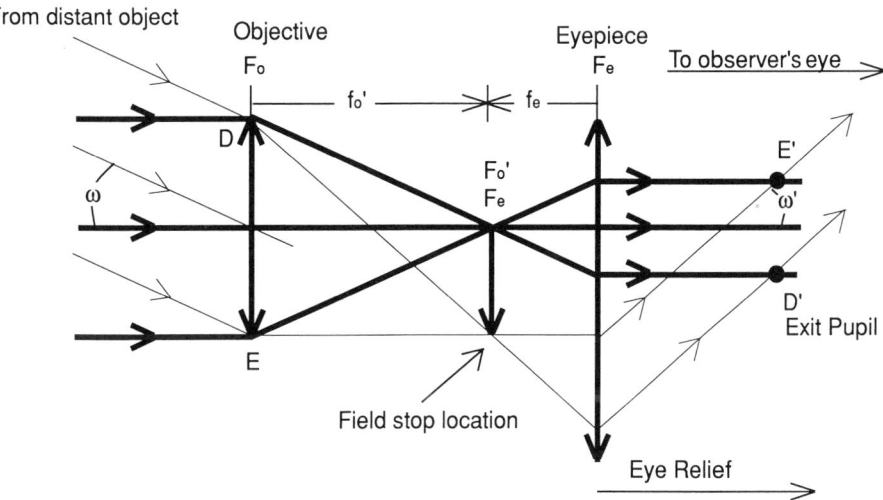

Figure 12-6. Keplerian telescope (without prism) in afocal setting. Two pencils of parallel rays from distant objects, one on axis and one off axis, enter the objective and are imaged in its secondary focal plane F_o', which is also the primary focal plane F_e of the eyepiece. Parallel rays emerge from the eyepiece. The angle subtended by the object points is ω while the angle subtended by the image is ω'. (Used by permission Brown WL. The optics of distance and near low vision devices. *Practical Optom* 1991;2:44–54)

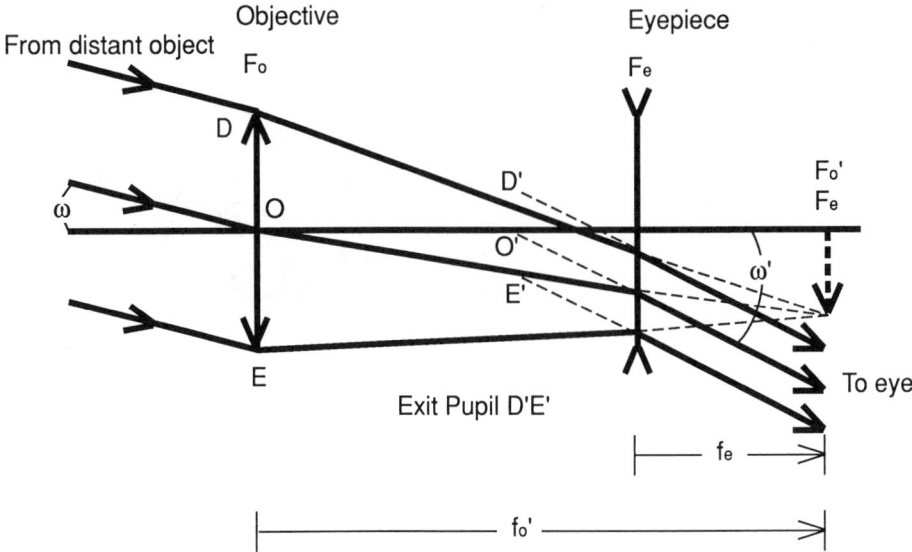

Figure 12-7.   Galilean telescope in afocal setting. A pencil of parallel rays from an off axis object subtending an angle ω is converged by the objective toward a potential image at its secondary focal plane F_o'. But the minus eyepiece, having its primary focal plane F_e at F_o', is interposed in the converging pencil so parallel image rays emerge, the image subtending an angle of ω'. (Used by permission Brown WL. The optics of distance and near low vision devices. *Practical Optom* 1991;2:44–54)

   b.   When the telescope is in the standard afocal setting, parallel rays from a distant object emerge parallel from the eyepiece (zero vergence in; zero vergence out).
      (1)   The secondary focal point of the objective and primary focal point of the eyepiece are coincident.
      (2)   The objective forms a real image of the distant object at its secondary focal point.
      (3)   The separation between the objective and eyepiece for the afocal Keplerian telescope is the sum of the magnitudes of the focal lengths of the two lenses: separation $= |f_o'| + |f_e'|$.
      (4)   For an afocal Galilean telescope, the separation is the difference between the magnitudes of the two focal lengths: separation $= |f_o'| - |f_e'|$.
3.   The diameter of the objective of the telescope is the entrance pupil of the telescope.
   a.   The entrance pupil of a telescope limits the diameter of the bundle of rays from an object point on the axis (Figures 12-6 and 12-7).
   b.   A Keplerian telescope with a larger objective will have a brighter image than one with a smaller objective, other factors being constant.
   c.   The brightness of the image in a Galilean telescope is dependent on the diameter of the entrance pupil of the patient's eye, not the objective diameter, as will be explained later.
4.   The image of the objective formed by the eyepiece is the exit pupil.
   a.   The exit pupil can be seen through the telescope as a small disc of light when the telescope is held up to a light at arm's length.
   b.   All rays which enter the telescope through the entrance pupil will emerge from the telescope from or through the exit pupil.
   c.   The exit pupil of a Keplerian telescope is a disc located behind the eyepiece as a real image of the objective.

      d.   The exit pupil of a Galilean telescope is a virtual image of the objective, located between the objective and the eyepiece.

      e.   *The position of the exit pupil is a quick way of determining the type of telescope.*

          (1)   If a clearly focused exit pupil is located outside the eyepiece, the telescope is Keplerian.

          (2)   If not, the telescope is Galilean.

5.   To achieve the largest field of view through the telescope, the patient must place his or her entrance pupil in coincidence with the exit pupil of the telescope.

      a.   With a Keplerian telescope this is possible as long as the distance from the eyepiece to the exit pupil (the eye relief) is long enough.

          (1)   Many hand-held telescopes have rubber eye cups that hold the telescope at the proper distance from the eye to achieve this coincidence when no glasses are worn.

          (2)   If the telescope is used over glasses, the telescope is too far from the eye for this coincidence to occur, and the field of view is decreased.

          (3)   If the patient has unsteady hands, a hand-held Keplerian telescope is difficult to use because this coincidence cannot be maintained.

      b.   With a Galilean telescope it is impossible to place the entrance pupil of the eye at the exit pupil, since the exit pupil is inside the telescope.

          (1)   The field of view through a Galilean telescope is smaller than for a Keplerian telescope with similar lens powers and diameters.

          (2)   The largest possible field of view with the Galilean telescope is with the telescope as close as possible to the eye.

6.   Telescopes enlarge the retinal image of a distant object through angular magnification.

      a. δ' is the angle subtended by the image seen through the telescope, and δ is the angle subtended by the object viewed without the telescope (Figures 12-6 and 12-7).

      b.   The angular magnification is sometimes termed the *power* of the telescope.

      c.   The angular magnification of an afocal telescope is the ratio of the eyepiece power to objective power:

$$M_A = -F_e/F_o,$$

where F_e is the eyepiece power and F_o is the objective power.

          (1)   The eyepiece power is greater than the objective to produce magnification.

          (2)   If the objective and eyepiece are both plus lenses, as in the Keplerian telescope, angular magnification is negative.

               (a)   The image is inverted compared to the object.

               (b)   One or more prisms are placed inside a Keplerian telescope which serve to rotate the image 180° both vertically and horizontally through internal reflections.

               (c)   The prism causes the final image to be seen erect through the Keplerian telescope.

               (d)   If the prism is not made precisely, it will decrease the image clarity.

               (e)   The prism may come loose if the telescope is dropped, causing a rattling inside the telescope.

          (3)   The eyepiece in a Galilean telescope is a minus lens, so the angular magnification is positive.

               (a)   The image is upright in a Galilean telescope.

               (b)   No prism is needed inside a Galilean telescope, so it is lighter and generally less expensive than a Keplerian telescope.

      d.   The angular magnification is also given by the ratio of the entrance pupil diameter D to the exit pupil diameter D': $M_A = D/D'$.

          (1)   A convenient clinical method to estimate the power of a telescope is to

measure the object diameter D and measure the exit pupil diameter while holding the telescope at arm's length up to a light.

(2) For a Keplerian telescope, the exit pupil is readily accessible for measurement outside the eyepiece, but for a Galilean telescope the exit pupil diameter can only be estimated by holding a millimeter ruler up against the eyepiece as close to the internal exit pupil as possible.

(3) For example, if the objective diameter is 20 mm, and the exit pupil diameter (not the eyepiece diameter!) is 2.5 mm, the angular magnification is $20/2.5 = 8\times$.

e.   Telescopes are denoted by two numbers, such as 8×20.

(1) The first number is the angular magnification (or power), $8\times$ in this case.

(2) The second number is the objective diameter in millimeters, so $D = 20$ mm in this case.

f.   The field of view through a Keplerian telescope is determined by the diameter of the field stop located inside the telescope near the image formed by the objective.

(1) A typical field stop is a piece of black metal with a hole in the middle to transmit light.

(2) The size of the hole determines the extent of the image that will be seen through the eyepiece, thus determining the field of view.

(3) The hole in the field stop is usually made small enough to exclude peripheral areas of the field of view that would be degraded by aberrations.

(4) The better the optical quality of the telescope, the larger the hole in the field stop can be made, and the larger the field of view becomes.

(5) Since the objective diameter does not affect the field of view in a Keplerian telescope, the relative size of the field of view through two Keplerian telescopes cannot be judged on the basis of the objective diameter.

g.   When a Galilean telescope is used with the eye, the objective acts as the field stop, not as the entrance pupil.

(1) When a pencil of rays from a distant axial object point passes through and emerges from the Galilean telescope, the entrance pupil of the eye limits the diameter even further, so the objective of the telescope is not the entrance pupil for the telescope-eye system.

(2) Instead the objective is the field stop, determining the field of view through the telescope.

(3) The image brightness in a Galilean telescope is determined by the diameter of the patient's entrance pupil, while the field of view is determined by the diameter of the objective.

(a) The field of view also depends upon how close the telescope is held to the eye.

(b) Maximum field of view through a Galilean telescope occurs when the telescope is as close as possible to the eye.

h.   If an uncorrected myope or hyperope uses a telescope, it must be modified to provide the necessary vergence to correct the observer's eye.

(1) The separation between objective and eyepiece can be changed in a focusable telescope.

(a) A myope decreases the separation.

(b) A hyperope increases the separation.

(c) These changes in separation apply whether the telescope is Galilean or Keplerian.

(2) The separation cannot be changed in a fixed-focus telescope, but the patient's correction is sometimes incorporated into the eyepiece of spectacle telescopes.

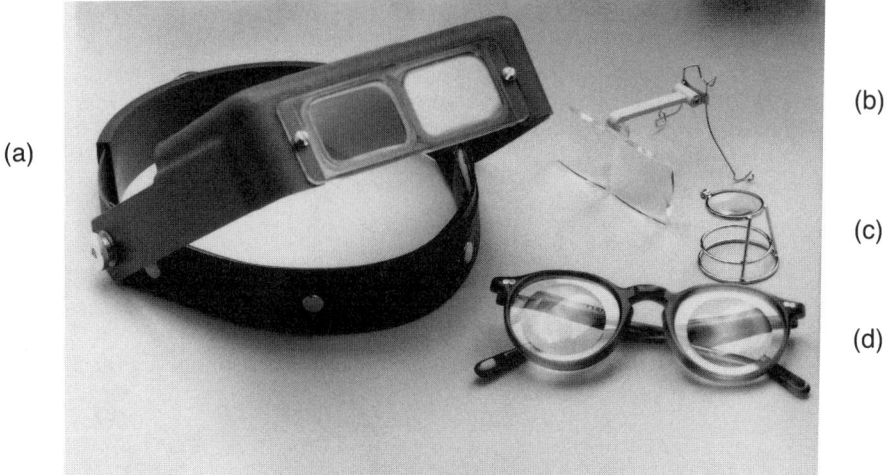

Figure 12-8.   Spectacle plane magnifiers (from left in clockwise order): (a) head-borne loupe with headband; (b) loupe which attaches to spectacles by means of a clip which attaches to the frame top and eyewires; (c) loupe with a metal attachment which slips over the top of the spectacle frame; (d) high-plus lenticular spectacle lenses.

   C. *Near magnification is derived optically from spectacle magnifiers, hand magnifiers, and stand magnifiers which make use of angular magnification and relative distance magnification.*

      1. Spectacle plane devices include single-vision lenses, multifocals, clipon devices, and head-borne devices worn very near the spectacle plane (Figure 12-8).

      2. Hand magnifiers are lenses held in front of the eyes with one hand (Figure 12-9).

        a. Folding pocket magnifiers fold into a case for storage.

          (1) They may consist of two or three lenses which can be used in combinations for different powers.

          (2) These are small enough to be carried in a pocket or purse for spotting.

          (3) Though the small field of view prevents most patients from using them for long-term reading, others prefer multilens pocket magnifiers for their flexibility and use them for most work.

        b. Some hand magnifiers are self illuminated, although the light is often inadequate, especially when batteries begin to weaken.

        c. Inexpensive hand magnifiers are equiconvex, with spherical surfaces.

          (1) Optics are adequate in low powers.

          (2) In higher powers, aberrations reduce the optically useful field of view.

        d. Aspheric lenses provide wider useful fields of view in higher powers.

          (1) One surface is much more curved than the other.

          (2) The more curved surface should be toward the patient when the lens is used at arm's length and away from the patient when used close to the spectacle plane.

          (3) Aspheric lenses are more expensive.

      3. Stand magnifiers are lenses mounted in a stand that holds the lenses at a fixed distance from the page (Figure 12-10).

        a. Most stand magnifiers are fixed focus; a few focusable stand magnifiers allow the distance from the page to the lens to be changed.

        b. Self-illuminated stand magnifiers are available.

          (1) The light may be powered by battery or electric cord.

          (2) Tungsten or halogen models can be obtained, some with variable illumination.

(a)   (b)   (c)

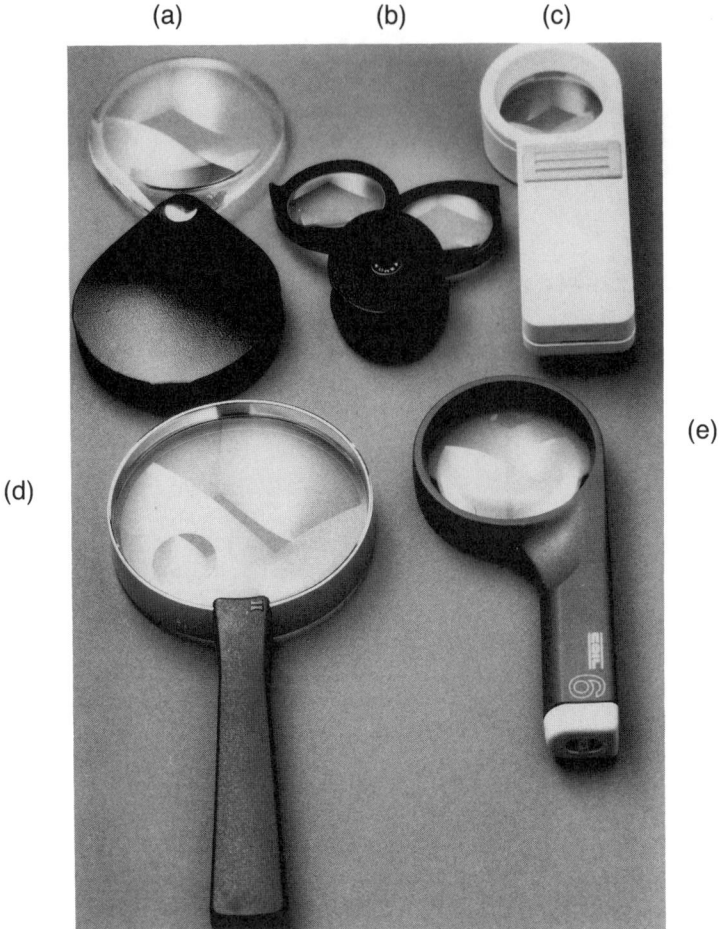

(d)

(e)

Figure 12-9.   Hand magnifiers. (a) Folding pocket magnifier, single lens; (b) folding pocket magnifier, double lens; (c) self-illuminated hand magnifier; (d) hand magnifier with a small, higher-powered insert; (e) high-powered aspheric hand magnifier.

           (3)   The halogen models are very useful for many elderly patients, who require increased amounts of well-directed illumination.

    D.   *As discussed in section V, the use of magnification as a label for a magnifying lens is misleading because the amount of magnification benefiting the patient depends on how it is used.*

        1.   A more useful means of identifying magnifying systems is through the *equivalent power.*

        2.   The important principle is that *lenses or lens systems with the same equivalent power form retinal images with the same size.*

        3.   In low vision the lens system may be an add in the spectacle plane (a single lens), a magnifier with the page at the focal plane so no accommodation is needed (a single lens), or more commonly, a magnifier used with an add or accommodation (a lens system).

        4.   When a patient is able to read a certain print size with a particular lens or lens system, he or she should also be able to read the same size print with any other system having the same equivalent power.

           a.   Field of view, depth of field, and working distance will be different for different systems having the same equivalent power, however.

(a)   (b)   (c)

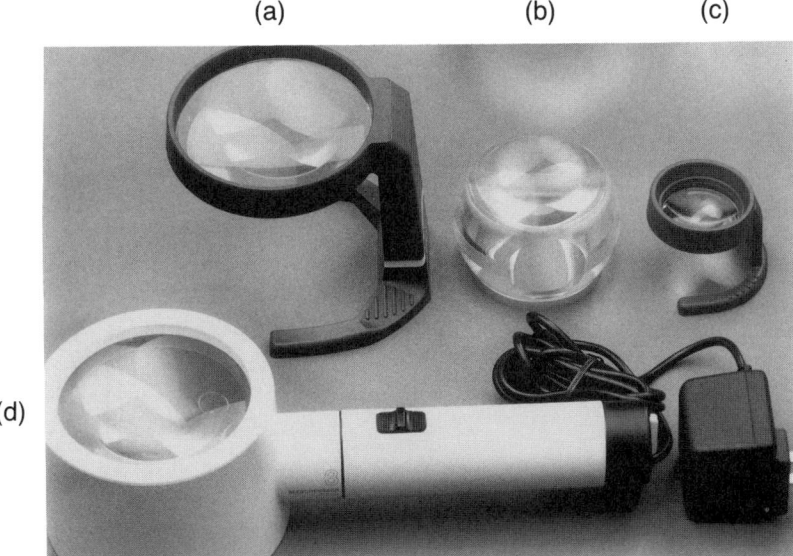

(d)

Figure 12-10. Stand magnifiers. (a) Stand magnifier with a tiltable lens and base open on one side to allow access to material being viewed; (b) stand magnifier with a solid translucent base to allow even illumination; (c) higher-powered stand magnifier similar to (a) but with smaller diameter typical of higher-power lenses; (d) self-illuminated stand magnifier with a halogen bulb powered by an electric cord handle.

      b.   The patient may prefer one lens type because of one or more of these other variables.

   5.   The usefulness of the equivalent power approach hinges on one's ability to determine the equivalent power of a system so that systems can be compared.

   6.   A magnifier having its own equivalent power of F_m may be used with an add in the spectacle plane F_A.

      a.   The separation between the spectacle plane and the magnifier is denoted by t.

      b.   The equivalent power of the general system is $F_{eq} = F_m + F_A - tF_mF_A$.

E.   *The power of the add in the spectacle plane, F_A, is any power in the spectacle plane in excess of the distance prescription:* $F_A = F_L + F_{acc} - F_{Rx}$.

   1. F_L is the total power in the spectacle lens through which the patient views.

   2. F_{acc} is the amount of accommodation used by the patient.

   3. F_{Rx} is the lens necessary to correct the patient's ametropia.

   4.   For example, consider a 4.00D myope who has no lens in the lens plane and uses no accommodation.

      a.   The total add in the spectacle plane is $F_A = 0 + 0 - (-4.00D) = +4.00D$.

      b.   The uncorrected myopia acts as a +4.00D add.

F.   *The add in the spectacle plane, F_A, can either add or subtract from the power of a magnifier, depending on the separation between them. Consider a +20D hand magnifier used by the uncorrected 4.00D myope (a total add of +4.00D in the spectacle plane).*

   1.   If the hand magnifier is held at the spectacle plane ($t = 0$), then the equivalent power of the system is $F_{eq} = +20D + 4D = +24D$ (Figure 12-11a).

   2.   If the hand magnifier is held 5 cm from the spectacle plane, the equivalent power is $F_{eq} = +20D + 4D - (0.05m)(+20D)(+4D) = +20D$ (Figure 12-11b).

      a.   5 cm is the focal length of the magnifier, and the equivalent power has been reduced 4.00D from the maximum +24D.

      b.   The 4.00D reduction in power is equal to the power of the add in the spectacle plane.

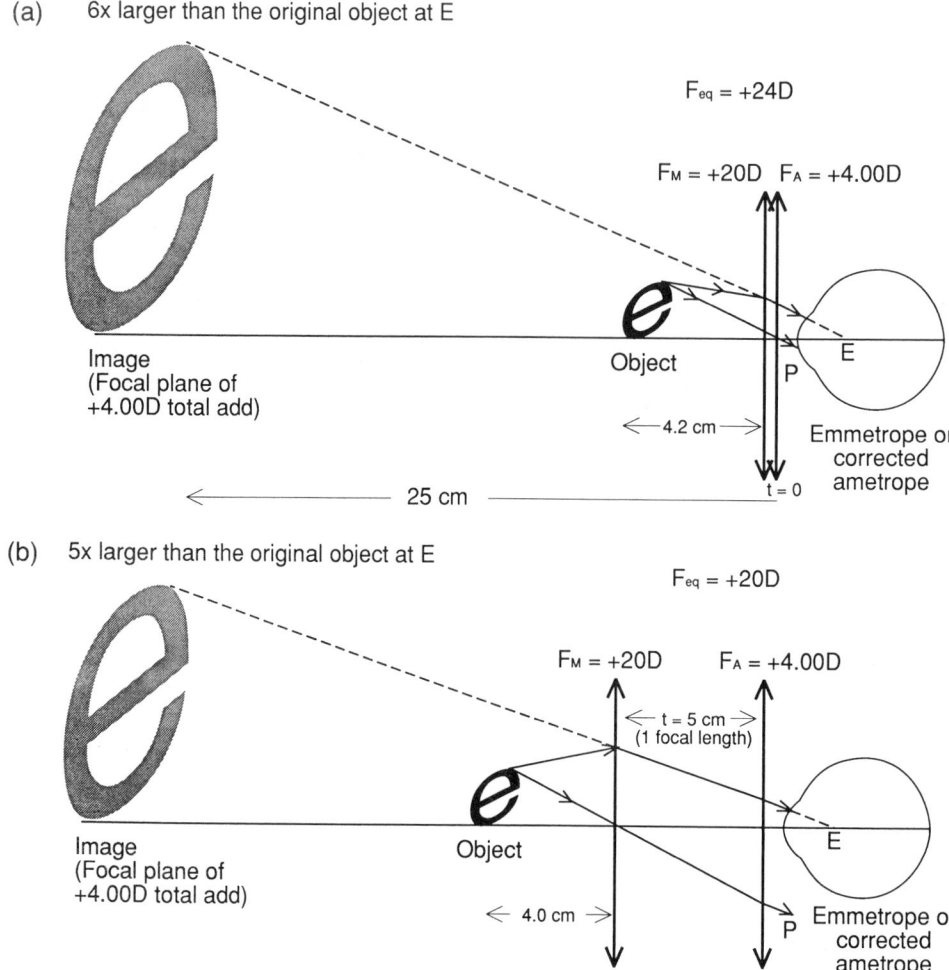

(a) 6x larger than the original object at E

$F_{eq} = +24D$

$F_M = +20D$ $F_A = +4.00D$

Image
(Focal plane of
+4.00D total add)

Object

E

P

4.2 cm

Emmetrope or
corrected
ametrope

$t = 0$

25 cm

(b) 5x larger than the original object at E

$F_{eq} = +20D$

$F_M = +20D$ $F_A = +4.00D$

$t = 5$ cm
(1 focal length)

Image
(Focal plane of
+4.00D total add)

Object

e

E

4.0 cm

Emmetrope or
corrected
ametrope

P

25 cm

Figure 12-11. +20D hand magnifier used at increasing distances *t* from a +4D total add results in decreasing equivalent powers. (a) Hand magnifier at spectacle plane (*t* = 0), so maximum F_{eq} = +24D; (b) hand magnifier at one focal length from add, 5 cm, so F_{eq} decreases by one unit of add to F_{eq} = +20D; (c) hand magnifier at two focal lengths from add, 10 cm, so add decreases two units of add from the maximum F_{eq} to F_{eq} = +16D. (Used by permission Brown WL. The optics of distance and near low vision devices. *Practical Optom* 1991;2:44–54)

    c.   If the separation is one focal length of the magnifier, the equivalent power is reduced from the maximum by one unit of "add" power, in this case 4.00D.

    d.   When the separation is one focal length, the equivalent power is that of the magnifier itself (+20D).

        (1)   The equivalent power at this separation is the same as if the magnifier were used by itself with an add of zero in the spectacle plane.

        (2)   If an add of zero were used, the page would be moved to the focal point of the magnifier so parallel rays emerge from its upper surface.

  3.   If the hand magnifier is held 2 focal lengths away, 10 cm, the equivalent power reduces another 4.00D: F_{eq} = +20D +4D − (0.10m)(+20D)(+4D) = +16D (Figure 12-11c).

  4.   In summary, when a magnifier is used with an add, the separation between the two determines the resultant equivalent power, which in turn determines the increase in the size of the retinal image.

  5.   For each interval of separation equal to a focal length of the magnifier, the equivalent power decreases from the maximum by a unit of add power.

(c)   4x larger than the original object at E $F_{eq} = +16D$

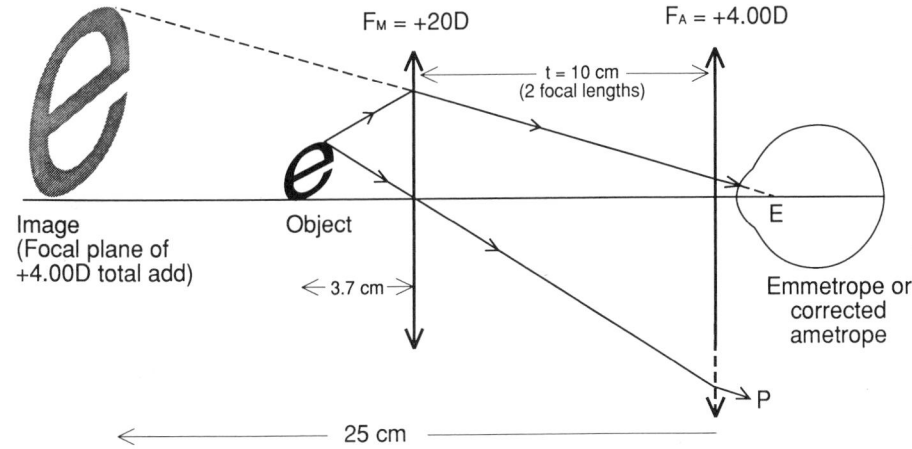

Figure 12-11.   (*Continued*)

G. *Stand magnifiers consist of a plus lens suspended from the page at a fixed distance.*

1. Although a few stand magnifiers are focusable and allow the separation between the len and page to be changed, most stand magnifiers are fixed focus.

2. The distance from the page to the lens in fixed focus stand magnifiers is less than the focal length of the lens.

 a. Rays emerging from the upper surface of the magnifier diverge from a virtual image below the lens.

 b. The amount of divergence is quite variable, up to as much as $-7.00 - -8.00D$.

 c. To see through the magnifier clearly, the patient must have a total add (i.e., add power, accommodation, or uncorrected myopia) sufficient to compensate for this divergence.

 d. If the equivalent power of a stand magnifier is $+20.00D$ and the page is 3.33 cm from the lens, the emerging rays have a vergence of $(1/-0.033m) + 20D = -10D$ (Figure 12-12).

  (1) The image seen through the magnifier is $1/-10D = -0.1m$ or 10 cm below the magnifier.

  (2) If the patient holds the magnifier at the spectacle plane, an add of $+10D$ must be used.

   (a) The equivalent power of the system is $+20D +10D = +30D$.

   (b) Since the magnifier is held closer than its 5 cm focal length, the add contributes extra power to the system.

  (3) If the stand magnifier is held 15 cm from the eye, the image from the stand magnifier is 25 cm from the eye so an add of $+4.00D$ must be used (Figure 12-12).

   (a) The equivalent power of the system is $F_{eq} = +20D + 4D - (0.15m)(+20D)(+4D) = +12D$.

   (b) Since the separation is 3 focal lengths of the magnifier, the equivalent power is reduced 3 add units (3 units of $4.00D$) from its maximum of $+24D$.

   (c) Just as in the hand magnifier, the add subtracts from the equivalent power of the magnifier once the separation exceeds 1 focal length of the magnifier.

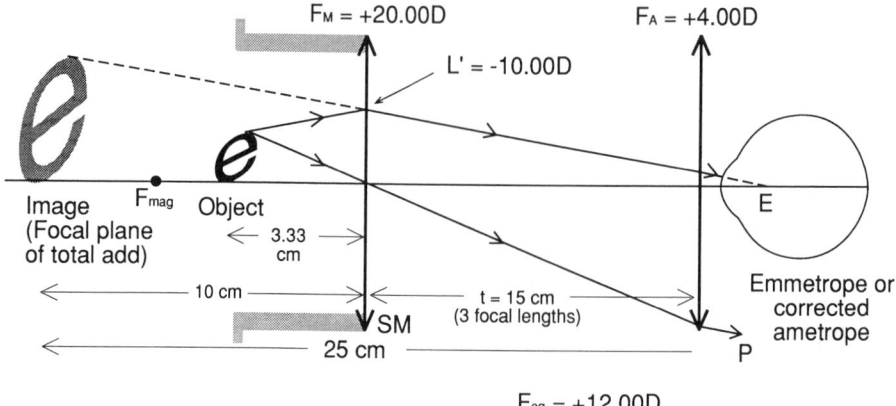

$F_M = +20.00D$ $F_A = +4.00D$

$L' = -10.00D$

Image F_{mag} Object
(Focal plane   ← 3.33 →
of total add)   cm

E

Emmetrope or
corrected
ametrope

←————— 10 cm —————→←— t = 15 cm —→
                                (3 focal lengths)

SM

P

←——————— 25 cm ———————→

$F_{eq} = +12.00D$

Figure 12-12.   +20.00D stand magnifier used with a +4.00D total add. Object is inside the primary focal plane of the stand magnifier, so an enlarged virtual image is viewed through the stand magnifier, requiring the total add of +4.00D to focus when the spectacle plane is 15 cm from the stand magnifier. (Used by permission Brown WL. The optics of distance and near low vision devices. *Practical Optom* 1991;2:44–54)

    e. The equivalent power of a stand magnifier is given by $F_{eq} = (F_{TR})(F_A)$
       (1) F_{TR} is the transverse magnification of the magnifier and F_A is the power of the add.
       (2) Mattingly International includes an excellent summary of optical properties of magnifiers in its catalog (see Appendix 1).
  3. If a patient reports the page is clearer when the stand magnifier is lifted off the page, rays emerging from the stand magnifier are too divergent when the stand magnifier rests on the page.
    a. If the patient has a bifocal, be sure it is being used.
    b. If the page is clearer with the stand magnifier off the page and a bifocal in use, the stand magnifier must be moved farther from the bifocal or the power of the bifocal increased.

  H. *Telemicroscopes (reading telescopes) are telescopes that are modified to view near objects.*
    1. Telemicroscopes can be focused for near or intermediate distances.
    2. If an afocal telescope is used to view a near object, the vergence of the rays from the near object is amplified by the telescope.
      a. A clinical approximation for the amplification is $L' \approx M^2L$, where L is the vergence entering the afocal telescope, M is the angular magnification of the telescope, and L' is the vergence emerging from the eyepiece.
      b. Consider an afocal 4× telescope used to view a book located 40 cm from the objective.
       (1) The vergence emerging from the telescope is approximately $(4)^2(-2.50D) = -40D$.
       (2) The patient must accommodate 40D to view the image clearly, certainly out of the question.
       (3) The approximation is actually quite poor in many situations, but it does serve to emphasize that patients cannot be expected to use an afocal telescope for near work.
    3. If the telescope is focusable, the telescope can be lengthened to focus on a near object.
      a. The separation between the objective and eyepiece is increased to compensate for the increased divergence entering the telescope.

b. The telescope is lengthened for a near object whether the telescope is Galilean or Keplerian.

c. Keplerian focusable telescopes generally have a larger range of focus than Galilean.

    (1) Keplerian telescopes may be focusable to as close as 12".

    (2) Galilean telescopes may be focusable to only 3'–8'.

    (3) Often the range of focusability is designed to correct for ametropia and is quite limited in focusing for a near task.

4. Another way of focusing the telescope for near is to use a reading cap over the objective (Figure 12-13).

a. The reading cap is a plus lens placed in front of the objective to neutralize the divergence of rays from the near object.

b. The reading cap acts much as a bifocal add.

c. The power of the reading cap, F_{RC}, is determined by the distance from the objective to the near task.

    (1) The focal length of the reading cap is made equal to the working distance.

    (2) For example, consider a 4× afocal telescope used to view a near task 20 cm from the objective (Figure 12-13).

        (a) The focal length of the reading cap is 20 cm.

        (b) The power of the reading cap is $F_{RC} = 1/0.20$ m $= +5.00$D.

        (c) Parallel rays emerge from the reading cap to enter the objective of the telescope so the telescope will focus for the near object just as it is for a distant object.

d. The equivalent power of a telescope with a reading cap is $F_{eq} = (M_A)_{TS}(F_{RC})$.

    (1) $(M_A)_{TS}$ is the power (angular magnification) of the telescope.

    (2) In the example of the 4× telescope with a +5.00D reading cap, the equivalent power is $(4×)(+5.00$D$) = +20$D.

        (a) The patient using this telemicroscope is able to read the same size print as would be read with a +20D add.

        (b) The working distance is 20 cm for the telemicroscope, whereas it would be only 5 cm for the add.

        (c) One of the major advantages of a telemicroscope is the increased working distance.

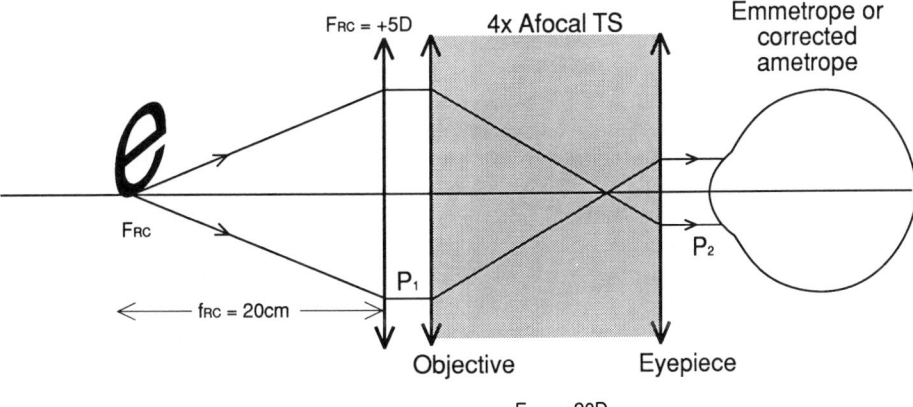

Figure 12-13.   Afocal telescope with a reading cap (F_{RC}): Object e is placed at the focal plane (F_{RC}) of the reading cap. Reading cap neutralizes the divergence of rays from the object so parallel rays enter the objective of the afocal telescope, affording a clear image. (Used by permission Brown WL. The optics of distance and near low vision devices. *Practical Optom* 1991;2:44–54)

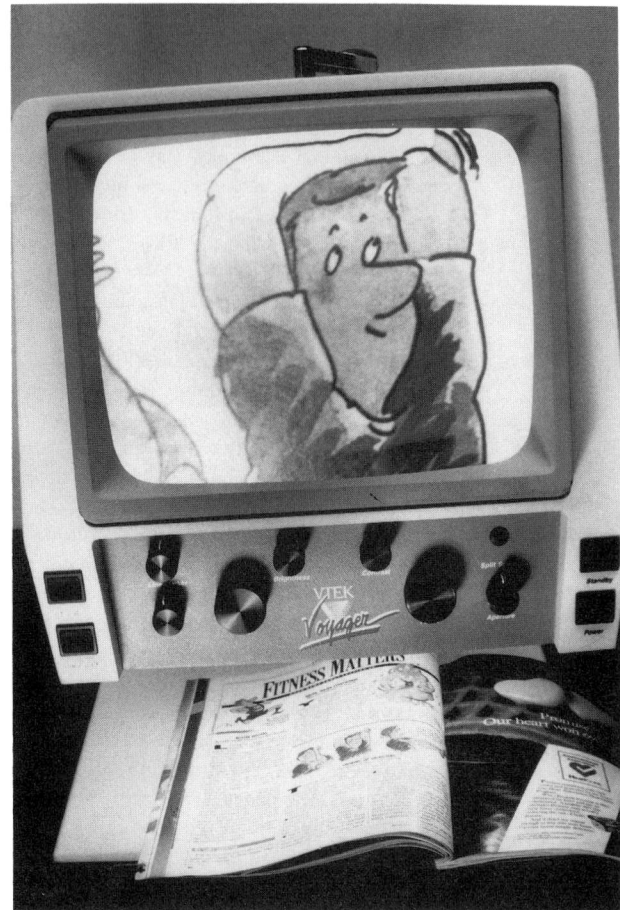

Figure 12-14. Closed circuit television. The picture in the magazine on the stand is imaged onto the screen by a camera hidden under the unit. Knobs control magnification, focus, screen brightness, screen contrast, and reverse contrast.

I.   *Several devices make use of transverse (or lateral) magnification, M_{TR}, to increase the size of the task viewed by the patient.*
  1.   The *closed-circuit television,* one of the most commonly used of these devices, produces transverse magnification electronically.
       a.   The camera focuses on the page of print and transmits an enlarged image that appears on the screen viewed by the patient (Figure 12-14).
       b.   Many closed-circuit televisions permit the magnification to be changed so the maximum amount of information can be placed on the screen with sufficient size to be readable.
       c.   The transverse magnification is easily determined by measuring the size of the image on the screen and comparing it to the size of the object.
  2.   Computer hardware and software are available to enlarge the size of print on the computer screen above the normal size.
  3.   Overhead projectors provide transverse magnification of the transparency.
  4.   The increased image size allows an increased, more comfortable viewing distance to be used.
  5.   A total add in the spectacle plane must be used to view the screen clearly.
  6.   In order to compare the retinal image size from these devices with that from other aids such as hand and stand magnifiers, an equivalent power can be assigned.
       a.   The equivalent power is $F_{eq} = (F_A)(M_{TR})$.

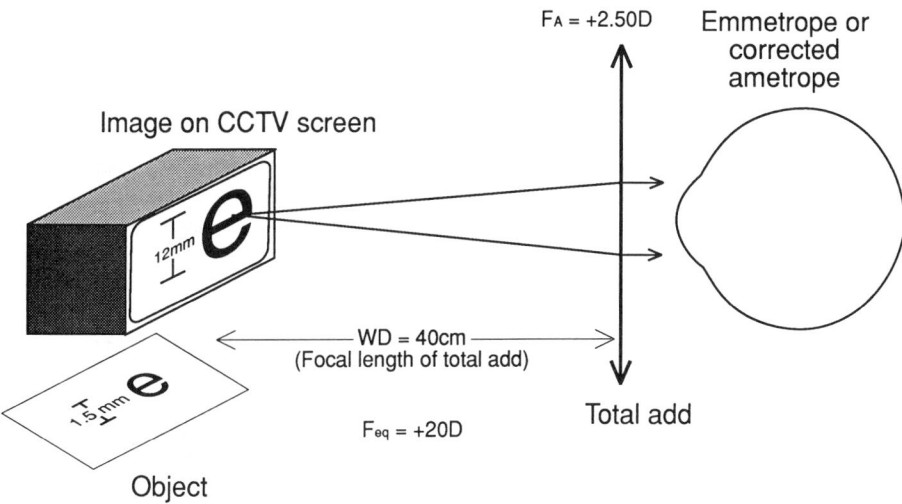

Figure 12-15.   Closed circuit television. Image on the screen (height y') is viewed through a total add having a power equal to 1/WD. I.e., $F_A = 1/.40m = +2.50D$ in this case. The enlarged image of the screen provides transverse magnification (y'/y) while the viewing distance WD provides relative distance magnification. (Used by permission Brown WL. The optics of distance and near low vision devices. *Practical Optom* 1991;2:44–54)

b.   Consider a patient viewing a closed-circuit television at a distance of 40 cm from the screen (Figure 12-15).
   (1)   The small letter "e" on the page is 1.5 mm high while the image of the "e" on the screen measures 12 mm.
   (2)   The transverse magnification is 12 mm/1.5 mm = 8×.
   (3)   The total add to view the screen clearly is 1/0.40 m = +2.50D.
   (4)   The equivalent power is $F_{eq} = (+2.50D)(8\times) = +20D$.
   (5)   The retinal image in this case is the same as if the patient viewed the page with the 4× telescope and +5.00D reading cap at a distance of 20 cm.

VII.   Advantages and Disadvantages of Various Devices

A.   *In the previous discussion it was noted that a particular equivalent power, +20D for example, can be obtained with a number of different systems.*

B.   *Although the patient can be expected to have the same single-letter acuity with all systems having equal equivalent power, other characteristics will usually make one of the forms preferable to another.*

C.   *Some of the most important characteristics of spectacle plane devices, including high plus reading lenses, bifocals, and clipon devices follow.*
   1.   Advantages of spectacle plane devices
      a.   Both hands are free to manipulate working material.
      b.   Wide field of view is obtained with the lens in spectacle plane.
      c.   High adds provide magnification for patients in a familiar form.
   2.   Disadvantages
      a.   The working distance from spectacle plane to the page is short.
      b.   High-plus single-vision lenses may cause disorientation.
      c.   Proper illumination is difficult to orient properly due to the short working distance.
      d.   The page must be held steadily at the focal point of the lens.

D. *Some of the most important characteristics of hand magnifiers follow.*
    1. Advantages of hand magnifiers
        a. The working distance is variable.
            (1) For low powers the distance can truly be changed from spectacle plane to arm's length.
            (2) For high powers, however, a longer working distance results in a severely restricted field of view and considerable distortion.
        b. The magnifier can be moved closer or farther from the page to focus the image.
    2. Disadvantages
        a. One hand holds the magnifier, so only one hand is free to manipulate the material.
        b. Field of view is reduced at longer working distances.
        c. Patients with unsteady hands have difficulty keeping focus.
        d. Reflections from the lens surfaces can be bothersome.

E. *Some of the most important characteristics of stand magnifiers follow.*
    1. Advantages of stand magnifiers
        a. The working distance is variable, although as for hand magnifiers, this is true primarily for lower-power stand magnifiers.
        b. The stand stabilizes the magnifier, so the patient is not required to keep it in focus.
    2. Disadvantages
        a. One hand must move the magnifier.
        b. A patient with a particular spectacle add must use the stand magnifier at a specific working distance.
        c. Reflections of light sources from the upper surfaces can be distracting.
        d. Stand magnifiers can be bulky and inconvenient to take from place to place.

F. *Some of the most important characteristics of telemicroscopes follow.*
    1. Advantages of telemicroscopes
        a. Working distance is increased.
        b. Both hands are free if it is spectacle mounted.
    2. Disadvantages
        a. Field of view is smaller than most other types of magnification.
        b. Depth of field is smaller than most other types of magnification, so accuracy of focus is critical.

G. *Some of the most important characteristics of closed-circuit television systems follow.*
    1. Advantages of closed circuit televisions
        a. Magnification can be changed over a wide range.
        b. Image moves across the screen, minimizing the need for scanning eye movements.
        c. A more normal working distance can be used.
        d. Contrast can be reversed (to white letters on black background) to reduce glare.
        e. Larger areas are more easily viewed together as a unit, such as a photograph.
        f. The screen can be viewed binocularly.
    2. Disadvantages
        a. The size and weight of the closed-circuit television prohibit it from being taken wherever the patient may want to use it.
        b. Closed-circuit televisions are expensive.

VIII. Patient Education at Initial Contact

A. *The eventual success of a low vision evaluation can depend upon proper explanation of the services to the patient at the first contact, through a primary care visit, or during the initial telephone call.*

B. *The patient must be educated to have realistic expectations.*

1. Lost vision will not be restored, but efforts will be made to help the patient use the remaining vision most effectively.
2. If the patient expectations are unrealistic, no amount of improvement short of totally restoring the vision will be satisfactory and the evaluation is doomed to failure.

C. *The patient should bring materials and a list of goals.*

1. Without specific goals, such as reading mail or reading prices in a store, the evaluation is directionless.
2. Special materials that the patient wants to be able to see or read at home or on the job should be included in the testing, since it is difficult to duplicate special print sizes, contrasts, and other variables in the office setting.

D. *The patient should also bring glasses and low-vision devices that are currently used.*

IX. Low Vision Evaluation

A. *Case history. In addition to the ocular and medical history gathered in a typical primary care history, several other areas must be explored to gain an understanding of how the patient's vision is being used.*

1. The duration and course of the reduced vision
    a. When did vision impairment first begin?
    b. Has the vision remained reduced at a constant level, has it decreased in the last 6–12 months, or has it fluctuated?
2. Family history of the same diagnosis (if known) or loss of vision
3. The educational background of the patient
    a. School for the visually impaired or traditional school
    b. Regular classroom, special resource room, or itinerant teacher
    c. Last grade completed
4. Social environment
    a. Living alone or with someone?
    b. Group of supportive family and friends?
5. Occupation
    a. Visual demands and difficulties, including print sizes and working distances
    b. Attitudes of employer in adapting to patient's needs
    c. Mode of transportation to work
6. Hobbies and other interests
    a. Visual demands, working distances
    b. Illumination
7. Mobility/transportation
    a. Need to travel down the street or across town?
    b. Means of transportation
        (1) Bus or taxi
        (2) Friends or relatives
        (3) Drives (date of driver license expiration)
8. Illumination
    a. Best time of day for outdoor vision: daylight, dusk, night
    b. Best type of day for vision: sunny, cloudy
    c. Wear tint or sunglasses? If so, are they dark enough?
    d. Best type of indoor illumination
        (1) Tungsten, fluorescent, halogen
        (2) Overhead or task specific
9. Previous rehabilitation experiences
    a. Low-vision examination: date and results
    b. Rehabilitation training, orientation/mobility training, or other training
    c. Experience with low vision devices: types and amount of success

Table 12-1. Factors Contributing to the Prognosis for Success in a Low Vision Evaluation (adapted from Mehr EB, Freid AN. *Low Vision Care.* Chicago: Professional Press. 1975:8–10)

Visual acuity	Location of scotomas	Education and intelligence
Onset and duration	Etiology	Self image
Motivation	Stability of visual condition	Independence
Flexibility	Age	Color vision retained

10. Goals
    a. Distance needs: driving, seeing bus signs, seeing street information signs while walking, viewing the blackboard, etc.
    b. Intermediate needs: seeing computer screen, reading meters on the job, cooking on the stove, etc.
    c. Near needs: reading, writing, recipes, etc.
    d. Goals should be quantified as much as possible as to size of detail and working distance.
11. A thorough case history gives the examiner insight into a number of factors that contribute to the prognosis for success in the low vision evaluation (Table 12-1).

B. *Distance visual acuity*
    1. Projected charts should not be used.
        a. The number of letters in the lines larger than 20/100 is limited to two or less.
        b. The increments in size between the larger lines are too large.
            (1) For example, the 20/200 line is twice as large as the next lower 20/100 line.
            (2) Patients with 20/120, 20/160, or 20/200 vision will all be recorded as having 20/200.
            (3) Documenting slight increases in performance during refraction for a patient whose vision is between 20/200 and 20/100 is difficult.
        c. The largest letter is usually 20/200 or 20/400.
            (1) If the vision is poorer than 20/400, the only way to measure vision is to move the patient closer to the screen or resort to finger counting.
            (2) Although these may be satisfactory for patients correctable to 20/20, they are not workable for a patient who must be refracted at a 20/200 or 20/400 level.
        d. The illumination level in the room usually cannot be varied without affecting the contrast of the image on the screen.
        e. Projected charts are usually minified or magnified optically to accommodate the length of the room.
            (1) The size of the letters is recorded in "reduced Snellen."
            (2) For example, if the distance from patient to screen is 15 feet (0.75 of 20 feet), the size of the letters on the line denoted as 20/20 is reduced to subtend 5′ arc at the 15-foot distance rather than at 20-foot distance.
            (3) If the patient must be walked to the chart to take an acuity, the acuity cannot be recorded to a Snellen acuity directly because of this size difference.
    2. Specially designed cardboard or rear-illuminated charts should be used (Figure 12-16).
        a. The top line is usually at least a 125-foot size (i.e., subtends 5′ arc at 125 feet).
        b. The larger lines on the chart should have several letters on the line.
        c. The spacing between the letters on each line and the spacing between lines should be proportional to the size of the letters to minimize influences of the crowding phenomenon.

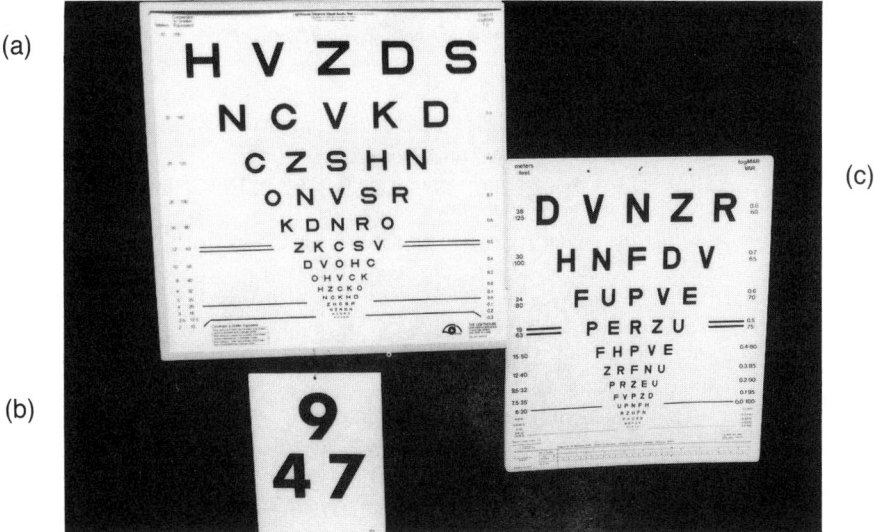

Figure 12-16. Distance visual acuity charts. (a) Lighthouse visual acuity test—rear-illuminated translucent chart, designed for 4 m; (b) Designs for Vision distance chart—numbers; (c) Bailey-Lovie distance chart.

      d.   The letters should be approximately equal in their recognizability.
          (1)   The Sloan letters are 10 letters that satisfy this criterion.
          (2)   The Sloan letters are C, D, H, K, N, O, R, S, V, Z, (Fig. 12-16a).
  3.   These charts are movable, so that by placing the chart closer, the effect of larger lines is created.
      a.   If a chart designed for 20 feet is placed at 10 feet, and the patient reads the line labeled "100," the Snellen acuity becomes 10/100.
          (1)   Since it is designed for 20 feet, the line labeled "100" is 44 mm high and subtends 25′ arc at 20 feet.
          (2)   When the chart is used at 10 feet, the "100" line subtends 50′.
          (3)   The 10/100 acuity can be converted to the conventional 20/? notation by multiplying both numerator and denominator by 2: (10)(2)/(100)(2) = 20/200.
          (4)   It is preferable to record the acuity as 10/100, since this preserves information about the test distance.
      b.   Some newer charts are calibrated to be used at other distances, such as 4 m.
          (1)   The line labeled "100" subtends the requisite 25′ arc when the chart is at 4 m, much like a projected chart calibrated for a short room.
          (2)   When the "100" line is read with the chart at 4 m, the acuity is recorded as 20/100, not 13.7/100 (13.7 feet is the equivalent of 4 m).
          (3)   If the chart is moved to 2 m and the "100" line is read, the acuity is recorded as 20/200.
          (4)   There is no simple way of including the test distance in the acuity with these charts, so the distance should be recorded beside the acuity.
  4.   The logMAR notation is not commonly used clinically to denote visual acuities, but charts designed along logMAR principles have some unique advantages.
      a.   LogMAR stands for *log*arithm of the *M*inimum *A*ngle of *R*esolution.
      b.   The MAR is the angle (in minutes) subtended by the detail in the smallest letter seen.
      c.   For a 20/20 letter, the detail subtends 1′, so the logMAR is log(1) = 0.0.
      d.   For 20/200, detail subtends 10′ and logMAR = 1.0.

      e.   LogMAR charts are designed so the size of the letters in each line is 0.1 log unit smaller than the line above it and 0.1 log unit larger than the line below it.

         (1) 0.1 log unit equals 1.26.

         (2) 0.3 log units equals 2.0, with the result that each line is two times larger than the line three lines below it.

         (3) If the chart is moved closer by a factor of two, the patient should read three lines farther down on the chart.

5.   Some of the distance charts used in low vision are listed below with some comments.

      a.   The Bailey-Lovie chart is a logMAR chart with excellent design qualities and a largest line of "125."

      b.   The New York Lighthouse logMAR distance chart is very similar to the Bailey-Lovie chart.

      c.   The Feinbloom (Designs for Vision) distance chart is a number chart.

         (1) It is several pages in a flip chart format.

         (2) The largest number is "700."

         (3) The largest optotypes have only one number on a page, while for smaller numbers, several lines of numbers are on the same page.

6.   While distance visual acuities are taken other important observations can be made.

      a.   Note whether normal room illumination or some modification is more comfortable for the patient.

      b.   Note whether the patient uses eccentric viewing or head turning to compensate for a scotoma.

         (1) Note whether eccentric viewing is stable or searching.

         (2) Stable eccentric viewing indicates good adaptation to the scotoma and an improved prognosis for success with low-vision aids.

      c.   If the patient consistently misses the middles or one end of several rows, a troublesome scotoma is probably present.

C. Near visual acuity

1.   The emphasis in low vision for near visual acuities (NVA) is on functional abilities rather than single-letter acuities.

2.   Single-letter acuities do not indicate a patient's ability to put letters together to read words, sentences, or paragraphs.

3.   Low vision charts must have large letters as well as small.

4.   NVA are measured at a variety of distances, depending on patient abilities, so the notation used must be flexible.

      a.   Reduced Snellen "20/_" notation is not useful because it does not allow the working distance to be included without potential for confusion.

         (1) If a reduced Snellen chart is designed for 40 cm (16 inches), the "100" line is recorded as 20/100 if the chart is held at 40 cm.

         (2) If the "100" line is read with the chart held at 20 cm, the acuity could be written as "20/100 @ 20 cm," meaning the 20/100 line on the chart was read at 8 inches and the true NVA is 20/200 taken at 20 cm.

         (3) Alternatively, the NVA could be recorded as "20/200 @ 20 cm," meaning the true NVA is 20/200 with the measurement taken at 8 inches.

         (4) This confusion is relieved by using alternative notations.

      b.   M or metric notation is convenient because it allows variable testing distances to be incorporated into the NVA.

         (1) The M number labeling a line of letters denotes the distance in meters at which the lower case letters (without ascenders or descenders) subtend 5' arc, similar to the denominator in a true Snellen fraction.

         (2) 2M letters subtend 5' at 2 m, while 0.5M letters subtend 5' at 0.5 m or 50 cm.

(3) If a 2M letter is read at a test distance of 40 cm, the acuity is recorded by putting the test distance in meters in the numerator and the M size in the denominator.

    (a) The Snellen fraction is 0.40/2M.

    (b) This fraction can be converted to "20/?" notation by multiplying numerator and denominator by 50: $[(0.40)/2](50/50) = 20/100$.

    (c) The factor of 50 is found by determining what number must be multiplied by 0.40 to obtain 20: $20/0.40 = 50$.

(4) An alternative is to simply record 2M @ 40 cm.

c. Point notation is used by printers to specify type sizes.

    (1) One point (pt) equals $\frac{1}{72}$ inch.

    (2) The point size actually indicates the height of the metal slug which carries the letters.

    (3) For 8-pt print, the slug is $\frac{8}{72}$ inch high, while the size of the lower-case letters (without ascenders and descenders) is approximately half the height of the slug.

    (4) NVA is recorded with the point size and working distance: 8 pt @ 25 cm.

d. Some near charts are designed using the logMAR principle.

    (1) The logMAR notation itself is used more for research than for clinical recording.

    (2) These charts are also marked with other notations, such as point size, which are more commonly used for noting acuities clinically.

e. Other notations, such as Jaeger, AMA notation (Snellen based on 14 inches), and decimal notations are not recommended for use in low vision.

5. The following approximate size relationships exist between the various near acuity notations.

a. 1.5 mm = 20/50 (for 40 cm) = 1M = 8–9 pt

b. The overall size of a 20/50 lower-case reduced Snellen letter designed for 40 cm is approximately 1.5 mm.

c. Transitions between units can be made approximately using these relationships.

d. For instance, 2M print is approximately 3 mm high (lower case).

e. If a lower-case letter is measured to be 2.5 mm high, it is approximately $(2.5/1.5)(1M) = 1.7M$ or $1.7(8 pt) = 14$ pt.

6. Certain NVA charts are more commonly used.

a. The Sloan/New York Lighthouse near system consists of a single-letter chart (Figure 12-17a) and a series of continuous text cards (Figure 12-17c,d).

    (1) The single-letter chart is used first to screen the patient's acuity.

    (2) The continuous-text cards consist of paragraphs of various m sizes.

    (3) The continuous-text card slightly larger than the single-letter acuity card is presented, and testing is continued to determine continuous-text acuity.

b. The Bailey-Lovie chart consists of unrelated words, with several words for each size (Figure 12-17b).

    (1) The chart has a logMAR design.

    (2) Each line has a variety of short and long words.

    (3) Acuity notation is in logMAR when used at 25 cm and in N notation (point size with Times Roman print).

7. Two important levels of performance should be noted.

a. The threshold level at which letters and short words are first read, no matter how slowly.

b. The level at which reading is more fluent.

8. Aided visual acuities at near through a bifocal must be taken at the focal distance of the add, which is less than the conventional 40 cm for any add greater than 2.50D.

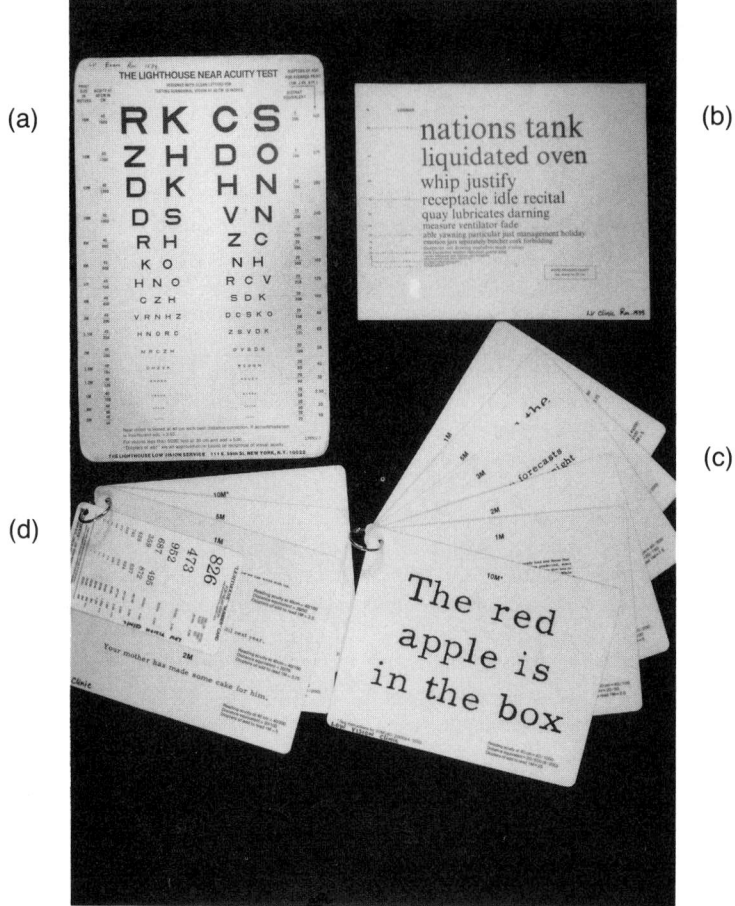

Figure 12-17. Near visual acuity charts. (a) Lighthouse near acuity test: single letters; (b) Bailey-Lovie near charts with unrelated words; (c) Sloan reading cards with paragraphs for adults; (d) Lighthouse "Game" card with numbers and Sloan reading cards with sentences for children.

9.   The following observations should be made during NVA.
    a.   The optimum illumination
        (1)   Intensity
            (a)   Bright or dim.
            (b)   Overhead lights alone or task-specific lamps.
        (2)   Type of lighting
            (a)   Tungsten.
            (b)   Fluorescent.
            (c)   Halogen.
            (d)   Other.
    b.   Effect of yellow "contrast-enhancing" filter
    c.   Effect of a typoscope
        (1)   A typoscope is a piece of opaque material with a slit in it which isolates a single line (see Figure 12-18c).
        (2)   The typoscope helps the patient keep the place on the line and reduces glare from the surrounding white page.
    d.   Effects of scotomas
        (1)   Scotomas may cause the words at the beginning, center, or end of the line to be difficult.

        (2) Longer words may be missed because letters at the beginning, middle, or end of the word are missed.

        (3) The position of the missed letters gives clues to the location of a scotoma.

    e. The direction of any head turn or eccentric viewing should be noted, as it gives an indication of how the patient is compensating for the vision loss.

D. *Entrance tests*

    1. Binocularity

        a. Many low-vision patients have binocularity or the capacity for binocularity, depending on the extent of the vision loss and the amount of eccentric viewing used.

        b. If the scotomas are positioned differently in each eye, binocularity may be impossible.

        c. If a patient is binocular, the patient may be more uncomfortable if a device allows the use of only one eye.

        d. Tests for binocularity include

           (1) Cover test.

           (2) Worth 4-dot test.

           (3) Stereopsis (for lesser impairments).

           (4) Awareness of diplopia with a 10 prism diopter vertical prism held in front of one eye.

    2. Ocular motilities

        a. Note nystagmus and any variation in its amplitude with eye position, including a null point.

        b. Note any restrictions in field of gaze that may affect performance with a device. For example, a high-add bifocal is inappropriate for a patient with restricted gaze inferiorly.

    3. Color vision testing, apart from diagnostic implications, can give important information about how well a person can perform a task which is color dependent.

E. *Visual fields*

    1. Visual field testing is important to determine the size, position, and density of scotomas.

    2. Initial screening tests are often sufficient to give useful information with a minimum of time and patient fatigue.

        a. Confrontations done carefully give important information about peripheral function.

        b. Amsler grid testing is useful to determine loss of function in the central visual field.

           (1) Using the red grid to change contrast or lowering illumination through rheostats or through newer crossed polaroid techniques may help make the test more sensitive.

           (2) The random dot test in the Amsler grid book is sometimes helpful in eliciting a scotoma when the more regular line grids fail.

           (3) Using a grid with an X centered on the fixation point assists the patient having a central scotoma in maintaining straight ahead gaze.

           (4) The Amsler grid is a convenient way to educate the patient about the functional effects of a scotoma.

    3. Tangent screen testing will sometimes elicit a scotoma when the Amsler grid fails.

        a. The tangent screen is performed at 1 m so a small scotoma represents a larger area than on the Amsler grid performed at 13 inches.

        b. An X made with tape and centered on the fixation point of the tangent screen can assist a patient with a central scotoma in maintaining straight ahead gaze.

        c. The position of the physiologic blind spot (PBS) can be a clue to eccentric viewing.

           (1) If the PBS is at its expected position, the patient is viewing straight ahead.

(2) If the PBS is shifted, the patient is eccentrically viewing in the direction of the shift and all scotomas are shifted as well.
4. Goldmann perimetry can quantify peripheral fields to follow up on confrontations.
5. Automated perimetry can also be used, although poor fixation due to a central scotoma can cause difficulty.

F. *Refraction is a very important element in the low-vision evaluation.*
1. Inaccurate correction of refractive error means that extra magnification is required to resolve the blurred retinal image.
2. To avoid missing uncorrected refractive error, keratometry and retinoscopy should be performed to provide guidance for the refraction.
   a. Keratometry gives clues to astigmatism and corneal regularity.
   b. It may be necessary to do retinoscopy at an unusually close working distance in order for the reflex to be bright enough to interpret.
      (1) This is termed radical retinoscopy.
      (2) The prescription is determined by subtracting the working distance lens for the short working distance from the neutralizing lens.
   c. If retinoscopy is not possible, consider doing direct ophthalmoscopy briefly to obtain the correcting lens which allows a clear view of the patient's retina.
      (1) Subtracting the observer's uncorrected refractive error from the ophthalmoscopy lens yields an approximation of the patient's correction.
      (2) This is an alternative starting point for refraction in the absence of retinoscopy.
3. The trial frame is the method of choice for refracting a low-vision patient.
   a. The patient has greater freedom to use eccentric viewing or a head turn with the trial frame than with a phoropter.
   b. The examiner can see the patient's eyes more easily to monitor visual responses during testing.
   c. Vertex distance is more easily controlled and measured.
   d. The trial frame must be properly adjusted.
      (1) Make the vertex distance as short as possible.
      (2) Place proper pantoscopic tilt between temples and front.
      (3) Adjust temple length and turn the adjusting screw so that sufficient tension keeps the temples from lengthening during the examination.
      (4) Adjust the nose pad to rest at the top of the bridge of the nose as comfortably as possible.
   e. When lens changes are made, keep the highest-power sphere in the rear cell.
   f. Rest the handles of cylinder lenses against the lens holders of the frame before adjusting the axis screw for proper orientation; this will prevent the lenses from rotating out of position.
   g. When lens choices are given to the patient, offer the lenses in front of the frame, and put only those lenses into the frame which will be used for further testing.
   h. Fan at least two or three lenses in one hand for quick alternation during testing.
4. Place the distance acuity chart at 10 feet or closer so that the patient can read near the middle of the chart.
5. Begin the refraction by finding the optimum sphere.
   a. Begin with the retinoscopy finding or with the patient's current prescription if available.
   b. If no starting point is available, use several intervals of sphere, both plus and minus, to determine the best sphere.
      (1) Use large intervals of lens change at first to get initial changes in vision, then decrease the interval as vision improves.

(2)   Patients with poorer vision will require larger intervals initially, up to ±4.00D.

(3)   Use the bracketing technique.

    (a)   For each interval of lens power, find the more plus lens and the more minus lens that first begins to degrade vision.

    (b)   Cut the lens interval in half, from ±2.00D to ±1.00D, for example, and test around the midpoint of the interval tested previously.

    (c)   Gradually decrease the power interval to the smallest detectable by the patient.

(4)   If no change in vision is detected with sphere change, test as high as ±20.00D to avoid overlooking very high refractive error.

6. Next determine the cylinder axis and power.

    a.   A hand-held Jackson crossed cylinder held in front of the trial frame is used in the same way as the crossed cylinder in the phoropter.

        (1)   A ±0.50D, ±1.00D, or ±2.00D interval Jackson crossed cylinder is more useful for low-vision patients than the ±0.25D or ±0.37D used for the fully sighted.

        (2)   The changes made in cylinder power during testing should be of the same magnitude as the Jackson crossed cylinder.

    b.   A second method for determining cylinder axis and power is the stenopeic slit.

        (1)   Remove all cylinder from the trial frame.

        (2)   Fog the patient with plus before placing the slit in the trial frame.

        (3)   Rotate the slit to find the orientation which provides clearest vision.

            (a)   Test with spheres to find the sphere which makes the chart as clear as possible.

            (b)   The meridian of the slit is the minus cylinder axis.

            (c)   The power in the meridian of the slit is the power in the trial frame.

        (4)   Rotate the slit 90° away to the other principal meridian and again use spheres or minus cylinders with the axis parallel to the original slit position to make the chart as clear as possible.

        (5)   Write the prescription from the two sphere powers or the sphere and cylinder.

7. Refine the sphere after the cylinder power and axis have been found.

8. Refraction can be done using Halberg clips over the patient's glasses, with the total power measured in the lensometer.

G. *The plus buildup follows the refraction.*

1. The necessary add power should be estimated before the plus buildup using one of several methods.

    a.   The reciprocal of the best corrected distance visual acuity is an estimation of the add necessary to read 1M print.

        (1)   For example, if the best corrected visual acuity is 20/200, the estimated add is (200/20) = +10D.

        (2)   The +10D add would be used at a working distance of 10 cm.

    b.   The reciprocal of a near acuity Snellen fraction taken at 40 cm can be used in the same way.

    c.   If the size of the detail in the patient's goal is not 1M, the necessary add, A, is found from the add for 1M, A_{1M}, using $A = A_{1M}(1M/\text{size of goal})$.

        (1)   The patient with 20/200 wants to read 2M print.

        (2)   The add for 1M was found earlier to be +10D.

        (3)   The add for 2M is A = +10D (1M/2M) = +5.0D.

    d.   If the near acuity is taken at some distance other than 40 cm, the estimated add can be found from the following: $A = A_{NVA}$ (NVA/goal size).

        (1) A_{NVA} is the add necessary to focus on the near visual acuity plane.

(2) If the patient can read 3M at 30 cm, what add is required to read 1M?

    (a) The add for NVA is $1/0.30m = +3.33D$.

    (b) The add for 1M is $A = +3.33D$ (3M/1M) $= +10D$.

    (c) 1M would be read with a $+10D$ add at 10 cm.

e. To minimize calculations, some NVA cards list next to each visual acuity line the estimated add that is necessary to read 1M if the patient reads that particular visual acuity line at 40 cm.

f. The estimated add is only a guideline and must be refined through testing with the plus buildup.

2. Begin the plus buildup with the estimated add over the distance correction and place the test material at the focal distance of the add.

a. Allow the patient to change the distance to obtain best performance.

b. Determine the acuity and reading ability and increase or decrease the add according to the patient's response, changing the working distance accordingly.

c. Be sure to keep the test material at the working distance.

(1) A very common reason for performance that is poorer than expected is that the patient has slowly moved the material out to a more accustomed distance.

(2) Beginning with the material very close to the nose and pushing it out to the clearest distance is sometimes more successful in establishing the proper distance than pulling the material in.

d. Be sure to adjust the lighting to ensure that the page is optimally illuminated each time the add is changed.

e. Near testing can be done in a trial frame or with Halberg clips over the patient's distance glasses.

(1) If the add powers are high, low powers of cylinder can be eliminated without significant loss of acuity for reading.

(2) High add powers can be tested more conveniently using laboratory-fabricated high-plus glasses which are available from several sources in 2.00–4.00D steps.

f. As the add increases, it is a good opportunity to educate the patient to the side effects of higher magnification:

(1) Shorter working distance.

(2) Smaller number of words visible at one time.

(3) Decreased depth of field.

g. Once the goal reading performance is achieved on a reading chart, the material provided by the patient should be used to ensure that it too can be read.

(1) The reduced contrast of newspapers, dot-matrix computer printouts, labels, and other materials often causes difficulty even when print of equal size on a high-contrast acuity chart is read.

(2) The patient's motivation and confidence are increased when it can be demonstrated that his or her own material can be read.

H. *Once an accurate refraction for distance and near has been done, testing with telescopes follows if the patient's goals are primarily for distance.*

1. Determine the magnification necessary for the goal.

a. Put the goal acuity and the patient's best corrected distance acuity in the same form of a Snellen fraction.

(1) If the patient's distance acuity is 10/80 and the goal acuity is 20/40, convert the visual acuity from 10/80 to 20/160.

(2) If the goal acuity is uncertain, use 20/40 or 20/50 as a tentative one.

b. To find the required power, divide the denominator of the visual acuity by the denominator of the goal: $160/40 = 4\times$.

2. Begin with a hand-held telescope having the estimated power.
   a. Focus it for the chart before handing it to the patient.
   b. Explain the parts of the telescope to the patient, including which end to hold toward the eye and how to focus it.
   c. Have the patient look at the chart and then lift the telescope to look through it without changing eye direction.
   d. Determine the visual acuity through the telescope.
   e. Modify the power of the telescope as necessary.
   f. If the patient does not achieve an acuity close to the expected, change to another telescope to make it easier for the patient.
      (1) Galilean telescopes are easier to manipulate because of the internal exit pupil.
         (a) A wider beam of rays emerges from the eyepiece.
         (b) Although the field of view may not be as large as for a Keplerian telescope, the patient has a greater chance of seeing something through the Galilean telescope to get an initial orientation.
      (2) Lower-power telescopes may be used at first to increase the field of view, making them easier to use.
      (3) If the patient has difficulty finding letters on the chart at first, stand near the chart and have the patient find you, look at your face, etc.
   g. If the patient does not read within a line or two of the expected visual acuity, telescopic magnification may not be useful due to scotoma position, media opacities, poor eye-hand coordination, etc.
   h. Once hand-held telescopes have been tested, consider spectacle-mounted telescopes.
   i. If fixed-focus telescopes are tested, place a trial lens over the objective as a reading cap to neutralize the vergence of rays from the chart.
      (1) For instance, if the chart is at 4 m, the vergence from the chart at the eye is $-0.25D$, so a $+0.25D$ lens over the objective will focus the telescope for the chart.
      (2) If this is not done, the chart may be blurred through the telescope because of vergence amplification.

I. *Testing to find the most appropriate form of near optical device is done logically based on the add found during the plus buildup.*
   1. The add which enables the patient to read the goal size print represents the equivalent power that any system, whether it is a hand magnifier, stand magnifier, or any other system, must have to allow the patient to read the goal material.
   2. Test other systems that may be more useful for the patient.
      a. Use systems for which the equivalent power is close to the add of the plus buildup.
      b. Use systems with advantages appreciated or required by the patient.
         (1) If a longer working distance is required, consider hand and stand magnifiers.
         (2) If a longer working distance is needed with both hands free, consider a telemicroscope.
         (3) If the patient has difficulty keeping a magnifier steady, consider a stand magnifier.
         (4) If the patient has much near work to do and an equivalent power of greater than $+20D$ is needed, consider a closed-circuit television or enlarging computer software or hardware.

J. *When a device is selected as potentially useful, it is often helpful to loan it to the patient to use in the home/school/work environment.*

K. *At a second visit the effectiveness of the loaned aid is evaluated and adjustments made if necessary.*

X. Glare control

A. *Many low vision patients are bothered by glare, particularly those who have cloudy media, decreased pigmentation, or retinal pigment epithelium degeneration.*

B. *Quality sunglasses used with fully sighted patients can be helpful for low vision patients, but there are also other more specialized filters that can be used.*

   1. NoIR® sunglasses by Recreational Innovations are fitover goggle-type lenses designed to be worn over existing glasses.
      a. NoIRs are available in amber and gray-green.
      b. They provide good absorption of infrared and ultraviolet light.
      c. Transmissions as low as 1% are available for the particularly sensitive patient.
      d. It is not possible to order a patient's Rx made into one of these lenses.
   2. Corning's Glare Control lenses are photochromic glass lenses that selectively absorb the short end of the visible spectrum.
      a. The 450 absorbs wavelengths shorter than 450 nm, the CPF-511 absorbs shorter than 511 nm, the CPF-527 absorbs shorter than 527 nm, and the CPF-550 absorbs shorter than 550 nm.
      b. The reduction in the blue end of the spectrum is sometimes beneficial for low vision patients.
      c. These lenses are available in single-vision, bifocal, and trifocal prescription lens forms.
   3. Younger PLS (Protective Lens Series) lenses are plastic lenses that have spectral transmissions similar to the Corning Glare Control lenses.
      a. The 530, 540, and 550 lenses are labeled with the cutoff wavelength below which light is absorbed.
      b. These lenses have the tint in the matrix, not on the surface.
      c. PLS lenses are available in prescription forms.
   4. Different densities of tints may be necessary for indoors and outdoors.

C. *Other means of blocking out the sun and bright lights, such as visors, caps, and sideshields, should be considered.*

XI. Nonoptical Devices

A. *Nonoptical devices are those which assist the patient in ways other than providing optical magnification.*

B. *The judicious use of nonoptical aids can augment the effect of magnification and may reduce the amount of magnification that is necessary.*

C. *The effect of various types and levels of lighting should be tested.*

   1. The patient may find tungsten, fluorescent, or halogen to be preferable.
   2. The patient must understand that optimal lighting is necessary for magnification to be useful.
   3. The use of a penlight in dimly illuminated environments, such as restaurants, or a halogen flashlight to search a closet shelf are useful adaptations.

D. *The typoscope is a piece of opaque material with a rectangular slit in it cut to the size of one or two lines of print (Figure 12-18c).*

   1. A typoscope serves two purposes.
      a. It helps the patient keep his or her place on the page while reading by isolating one or two lines of print.
      b. It also decreases the glare from the page by covering much of the white surrounding the line being read.
   2. A typoscope can be ordered from low-vision suppliers or can be made from cardboard, plastic, x-ray material, etc.
   3. A variety of sizes of typoscopes for different materials can be helpful.

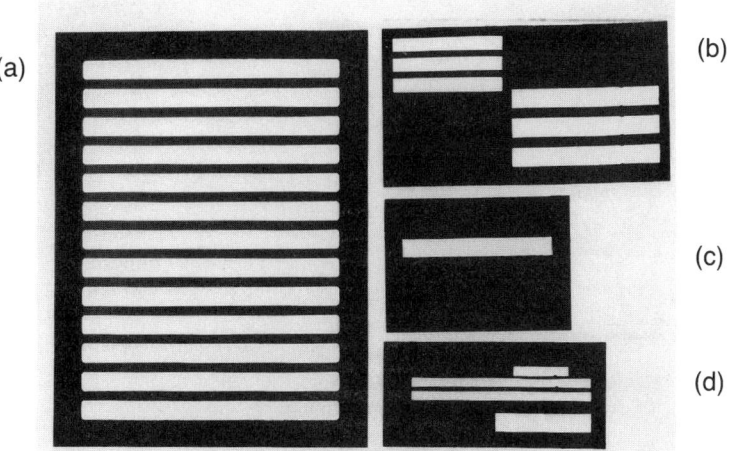

Figure 12-18.   Stencils. (a) Letter stencil; (b) envelope address stencil; (c) typoscope; (d) check stencil.

E. *A number of guides that are more task specific are available.*
    1. A letter writing guide is a 8.5 × 11 inch sheet of black material with many parallel slits cut out to provide a high-contrast visual and tactile guide for writing straight lines (Figure 12-18a).
    2. Envelope stencils (Figure 12-18b) and check stencils (Figure 12-18d) are similar guides with slits cut in specific areas where information must be provided.
    3. A signature guide is a small typoscope that is used to outline with high contrast the position where a signature is required.
        a. If a signature is requested, the requesting party is asked to position the signature guide where the signature is to be placed.
        b. The guide can be carried in the wallet or purse to be readily available.

F. *Materials that provide relative size magnification reduce the amount of optical magnification that is required.*
    1. Large-print books and magazines, large-print checks, marking pens for writing, and large-font printers are examples.
    2. The use of relative size magnification allows the working distance to be increased to provide a more normal working space.
    3. It is sometimes more tolerable for a patient to begin using a lower-power magnifier with large print to develop the necessary hand-eye coordination.
    4. Once the patient has developed some skill with this combination, it may be possible to increase the power of the magnifier in order to read smaller print.

G. *Reading stands and clipboards are very helpful to support material in a more convenient position that improves posture and reduces fatigue while using magnifiers, especially high-powered units.*

XII. Visual Field Enhancement

A. *Patients with peripheral visual field loss have different functional problems than those with central field loss.*
    1. Central field loss, caused by diseases such as macular degeneration, requires magnification to improve performance.
    2. Peripheral field loss, as occurs in retinitis pigmentosa (RP), causes the patient difficulty in orientation.
        a. In advanced RP the visual acuity may remain very good, as macular function is retained, so details can be seen.

      b.   However, the severely constricted peripheral field makes it very difficult to know where to look in order to find the detailed information that is desired.

      c.   For instance, if a person with RP is walking down the street, reading a warning or information sign is not a problem if the sign can be found.

B. *Visual field enhancement techniques are designed to help the patient become more aware of relationships or occurrences in the peripheral visual field.*

C. *Minification is sometimes useful to increase the information available to the remaining retina.*

   1. Minification is only useful if the patient has good central acuity.

   2. A minus lens is occasionally helpful for near work.

   3. A reverse telescope provides minification for distance.

      a.   A hand-held telescope can be used momentarily in reverse to obtain orientation to a new environment, allowing action to be taken on the basis of the information obtained.

      b.   A telescope can be mounted in reverse in a spectacle lens as well for more convenience.

   4. The Amorphic lens by Designs for Vision is a spectacle-mounted reverse telescope that minifies in the horizontal meridian but not in the vertical.

      a.   Minification in all meridians results in distortion of depth, making objects appear farther away than they really are.

      b.   Most patients have more problem with loss of information from the horizontal meridian, so that is the direction of minification in the amorphic lens.

      c.   A cylindrical lens system is used to provide zero power in the vertical.

      d.   The vertical meridian is left unchanged, so perception is linked to reality in that dimension.

D. *Prisms and partially silvered mirrors can assist in obtaining information from the periphery by reducing the amplitude of eye rotations that are necessary.*

   1. These devices can be useful in diseases such as RP, with losses in many directions of the peripheral field, and also in hemianopias.

   2. Partially silvered mirrors attached to the nasal eyewire are angled approximately 45° to the frontal plane.

      a.   A reflected image of the temporal field is seen through the mirror.

      b.   A transmitted image of the normal straight ahead visual field is seen simultaneously through the mirror.

      c.   The view of the peripheral field is superimposed on the normal view, so the patient is aware of events in the periphery without large eye excursions.

   3. Fresnel prisms mounted with the base toward the blind field also enhance the acquisition of information in that field.

      a.   The prism is mounted toward the periphery of the lens, so the eye does not look through it in normal straight ahead gaze.

      b.   When the eye rotates to look through the prism, the images of objects in the peripheral field are displaced inward toward the center of the field.

         (1) The images are displaced toward the apex of the prism.

         (2) The eye movements necessary to see the activity in the peripheral field are reduced.

      c.   Prisms can be mounted temporally and nasally for horizontal fields and superiorly and inferiorly for vertical fields.

      d.   When the prisms are mounted in yoked fashion before both eyes, the patient must learn to compensate for the scotoma at the apex of the prism.

      e. $15^\triangle$–$30^\triangle$ prisms are most useful.

      f.   A central field diameter of less than 10°–20° is usually necessary in RP for the prism to be useful.

g. Some patients find the prism to be very useful, while others do not, so patient selection, education, and training are very important.

h. Prism often serves to train the patient to develop peripheral scanning eye movements which eventually render the prism less useful.

XIII. Training

A. *The successful utilization of low vision devices by most low-vision patients is greatly enhanced by training.*

B. *Adaptive training in the use of the device is imperative.*

1. Patients with 20/100 or better visual acuity and good peripheral vision usually require little training other than instruction in the proper use and care of the devices they use.

2. The patient must understand completely how the device is to be used and what level of performance to expect.

3. Training for telescopes should include the following:
    a. Focusing and aiming.
    b. Spotting and tracking stationary and moving objects while patient is stationary or moving.
    c. Scanning systematically, not randomly.
    d. Using the telescope with or without glasses.
    e. Cleaning and caring for the telescope.

4. Training for near devices should include the following:
    a. Proper distance from page to magnifier.
    b. Proper distance from magnifier to eye.
    c. Proper orientation of magnifier.
        (1) More curved surface of aspheric magnifier toward eye.
        (2) Stand magnifier resting on page.
    d. Proper use of glasses with magnifier: with or without glasses, through the distance or near part of bifocal.
    e. Keeping one's place on a line.
    f. Finding the beginning of the next line.
    g. Proper illumination.
    h. Size print to be read.
    i. Care and cleaning of the magnifier.

C. *For patients with central scotomas, training in eccentric viewing can be profitable, before or while magnifiers are being used.*

1. Instruct the patient regarding the size and position of the scotoma.

2. Determine the best position for eccentric viewing and be sure the patient understands the concept.
    a. Generally, moving the scotoma above or below the task is more successful than moving it to the side.
    b. Training materials with reading exercises have been developed to assist the patient in developing skill with eccentric viewing.[5-7]

D. *Training patients with constricted visual fields centers around orientation and mobility instruction for distance, supplemented with enhancement devices.*

1. Scanning is essential.

2. Training for reading includes techniques to find the beginning of the next line, often the most difficult task.

3. The closed-circuit television is the device of choice for reading.
    a. Reverse contrast reduces glare, a common problem for these patients.
    b. The restricted field can be aimed in one place, with the print moving across the field of view.

XIV.   Verification of Low Vision Devices

A.   *For telescopes, the power (angular magnification) and any correction for ametropia added to the eyepiece (if any) can be verified.*

   1.   The angular magnification of a telescope can be measured several ways, all of which are easier for lower-power than for higher-power telescopes.
      a.   Entrance pupil/exit pupil diameter method
         (1)   Measure the objective diameter and the exit pupil diameter (a contact lens measuring magnifier can assist in measuring the exit pupil).
            (a)   For Galilean telescopes, the exit pupil diameter is estimated with the ruler as close to the eyepiece as possible.
            (b)   Be sure not to mistake the eyepiece diameter for the exit pupil diameter.
         (2)   Divide the objective diameter by the eyepiece diameter to obtain the angular magnification.
      b.   Biocular comparison method
         (1)   With both eyes open, hold the telescope in front of one eye while viewing a distant object with a repeated pattern, such as a concrete block wall or brick wall.
         (2)   A magnified image will be seen with the eye with the telescope and an unmagnified image with the naked eye.
         (3)   Count the number of normal-size elements (e.g., bricks) seen with the naked eye without the telescope which fit within one magnified element seen through the telescope.
         (4)   The ratio of the number of elements seen with the naked eye to the corresponding number seen with the telescope is the angular magnification.
         (5)   For example, if four bricks seen with the naked eye fit into the image of one brick seen simultaneously with the telescope, the angular magnification is 4×.
      c.   Lensometer method
         (1)   Bailey[8] has developed a method for measuring the angular magnification using a lensometer.
         (2)   The change in vergence emerging from the rear of the telescope is measured when the vergence entering is changed using a trial lens.
         (3)   The resulting vergence amplification allows the angular magnification to be found using a chart developed by Bailey.
   2.   A correcting lens for ametropia, usually incorporated only into spectacle-mounted telescopes, can be verified using the lensometer.
      a.   If the telescope is variable focus, change the tube length so the telescope is focused for distance.
         (1)   This can be difficult if the correcting power is high.
         (2)   Fixed-focus telescopes should already be focused for distance, unless they are designed for near.
         (3)   If a fixed-focus telescope is designed for near, place a minus lens over the objective to neutralize the reading cap part of the telescope.
         (4)   For example, if the reading telescope is focused for 20 cm, use a −5.00D trial lens against the objective while using the lensometer.
      b.   Place the telescope into the lensometer with the eyepiece centered on the lens stop.
      c.   Carefully orient the tube of the telescope so it is parallel to the axis of the lensometer; a slight tilt will cause significant errors in cylinder.
      d.   Measure the correcting power in the eyepiece as for any spectacle lens.
         (1)   The mires will be minified due to the reverse position of the telescope.

(2)   If the cylinder power is significantly in error, be sure the tube of the telescope is parallel to the lensometer axis.

B.   *For nearpoint magnifiers the equivalent power is more important than the vertex powers of the magnifier.*
   1.   The power of the magnifier, F_m, in the equations discussed in Sec. VI for the equivalent power of the system is the equivalent power of the magnifier.
   2.   For a thin lens the equivalent power and the vertex powers of the lens are equal, but most magnifiers are not thin lenses.
   3.   Since the lensometer measures vertex powers, it does not accurately measure equivalent power, but it can provide a good approximation in certain situations.
      a.   For lower-power equiconvex magnifiers (less than $+10-+12D$), the vertex power is approximately equal to the equivalent power.
         (1)   Place the lens in the lensometer and measure the vertex power with either of the two identical surfaces against the lens stop.
            (a)   Some magnifiers are so large that they cannot be centered in the lensometer, and measurements are taken through the periphery of the lens.
            (b)   The large amounts of prism induced in the periphery may displace the mires so they are not visible.
            (c)   If so, use a trial lens prism over the magnifier to bring the mires into view.
         (2)   The lens thickness is small enough compared to the focal length of the magnifier to cause little difference in the powers.
         (3)   An error of 0.50D or less in measuring low-power magnifiers is generally insignificant.
      b.   For plano convex magnifiers or biconvex magnifiers in which one surface is close to plano, the vertex power measured with the more curved surface against the lens stop of the lensometer is very close, if not identical, to the equivalent power.
         (1)   Place the magnifier in the lensometer with the more curved surface against the lens stop.
         (2)   Use an auxiliary prism if necessary to center the mires.
   4.   Bailey has described a triangulation technique for measuring the equivalent power of any plus lens.
      a.   This is useful for very high-plus lenses and for lenses such as stand magnifiers that do not fit into the lensometer.
      b.   Locate across the room (5–6 m away) a bright object such as two penlights or the edges of a window.
         (1)   The separation between the penlights or the width of the window is y.
         (2)   The distance from the magnifier to the object (i.e., penlights) is l.
      c.   Measure the size y' of the image formed by the magnifier using a contact lens measuring magnifier or a transparent ruler.
         (1)   The distant object will form a real inverted image at the focal point of the lens.
         (2)   A piece of transparent tape on the ruler serves as a convenient screen for focusing the image.
         (3)   The image must be clearly in focus on the ruler for the size to be measured.
      d.   Calculate the equivalent power of the magnifier, F_m: $F_m = y/(y'l)$
   5.   The vergence of light emerging from the upper surface of a stand magnifier can be measured using trial lenses.
      a.   Place the stand magnifier on a page containing small letters.
      b.   With the eye close to the upper surface of the stand magnifier, place plus trial

lenses on the upper surface while viewing the page through both the stand magnifier and the trial lens.

    (1) Begin with a lens which is enough plus to blur the image.

    (2) Wear your distance correction for ametropia.

c. Gradually reduce the plus power from too much plus to the first lens that clears the image of the page.

d. The power of the trial lens is the magnitude necessary to neutralize the vergence emerging from the upper surface of the stand magnifier.

    (1) For example, assume a +5.00D trial lens is in place when the page is first seen clearly.

    (2) The vergence from the upper surface is −5.00D.

    (3) The virtual image formed by the magnifier is located $1/-5.00D = -0.2m = -20$ cm on the other side of the stand magnifier.

    (4) A +5.00D add is the highest add that can be used with this stand magnifier.

e. The sensitivity in detecting blur in the image can be increased by viewing the image through a telescope that has been focused for distance.

C. *Labels on magnifiers can be misleading.*

    1. Magnification may be intended as rated or conventional magnification, but it is usually difficult to know which is meant unless one is intimately aware of the manufacturer's policies.

    2. Even if the type of magnification is known, the equivalent power of the lens itself is often less than that which is calculated from the magnification.

    3. The American National Standards Institute has published a standard for low-vision aids.

        a. The standard is ANSI Z80.9-1986.

        b. The standard is primarily definitions and methods for measuring power.

        c. Revisions for Z80.9 are currently proposed that set tolerances for equivalent power, angular magnification, etc.

References

1. The visual system. In: *Guides to the Evaluation of Permanent Impairment.* 3rd ed. American Medical Association, 1990:161–172.

2. Kirchner C, Lowman C. Sources of variation in the estimated prevalence of visual loss. In: Kirchner C, ed. *Data on Blindness and Visual Impairment in the U.S.* 2nd ed. New York: American Foundation for the Blind, 1988:4–6.

3. *Vision Problems in the U.S.* National Society to Prevent Blindness, 1980:3–19.

4. Livneh H, Evans J. Adjusting to disability: Behavioral correlates and intervention strategies. *Personnel and Guidance Journal* 1984(Feb):363–365.

5. Freeman FT, Jose RT. The art and practice of low vision. Boston: Butterworth-Heinemann, 1991.

6. Watson G, Berg RV. Near training techniques. In: Jose RT, ed. *Understanding Low Vision.* New York: American Foundation for the Blind, 1983:317–362.

7. Quillman RD. *Low Vision Training Manual.* Kalamazoo: Department of Blind Rehabilitation, College of Health and Human Services, Western University, no date.

8. Bailey IL. New method for determining the magnifying power of telescopes. *Am J Optom Physiol Optics* 1978;55:203–207.

APPENDIX **1**

Selected Sources for Low Vision Devices and Services

Source	Service
Alcom Corporation 1590 Oakland Road, Suite B112 San Jose, CA 95131 (408)453-8251 FAX:(408)453-8255	Speech synthesizers
Al Squared 1463 Hearst Drive Atlanta, GA 30319 (404)233-7065	Large print computer software
Access Unlimited SPEECH Enterprises 3535 Briarpark Drive, Suite 102 Houston, TX 77042 (800)531-5314 (713)461-0006	Speech synthesizers Large print computer software
Adhoc Reading Systems, Inc. 28 Brunswick Woods Drive East Brunswick, NJ 08816 (201)254-7300 FAX:(201)254-7310	Scanner Speech synthesizers
American Bible Society Grand Central Terminal P.O. Box 5656 New York, NY 10017 (215)581-7400	Large print and cassette Bible
American Foundation for the Blind 15 West 16th Street New York, NY 10011 (800)232-5463 (212)620-2171 (201)862-8838	Adaptive products for inde- pendent living
American Printing House for the Blind P.O. Box 6085, Department 0086 Louisville, KY 40206-0085 (502)895-2405	Speech synthesizers
Arkenstone, Inc. 1185 Bordeaux Drive, Suite D Sunnyvale, CA 94089 (800)444-4443 (408)752-2200 FAX:(408)745-6739	Scanner Speech synthesizers

Source	Service
Beecher Research Company 906 Morse Avenue Schaumburg, IL 60193 (708)893-0187	Spectacle plane telescopes
Bible Alliance, Inc. P.O. Box 621 Bradenton, FL 34206 (813)748-3031	Bible on cassette
BIT Corporation 52 Roland Street Boston, MA 02129 (617)666-2488	Adaptive products
Bernell Corporation 750 Lincolnway East South Bend, IN 46634 (800)348-2225	Optical low vision devices
Bossert Specialties, Inc. Magnificantion Center P.O. Box 15441 Phoenix, AZ 85060 (602)956-6637	Optical, nonoptical, electronic low vision devices
Braille Institute of America 741 North Vermont Avenue Los Angeles, CA 90029 (213)663-1111	Nonoptical low vision devices
Choice Magazine Listening P.O. Box 10 Port Washington, NY 11050 (516)883-8280	Recorded periodicals
Deluxe Check Printer, Inc. P.O. Box 64399 1020 West County Road F Shoreview, MN 55126 (800)328-9546 (612)483-7111	Large print checks
Designs or Vision, Inc. 760 Koehler Avenue Ronkonkoma, NY 11779 (800)345-4009 (516)585-3300	Spectacle mounted micro- scopes, telescopes
EZ-Reader, Inc. 1408 North Westshore Blvd, Suite 506 Tampa, FL 33607 (813)328-1222	Hand-held close-circuit TV system
Electronic Visual Aid Specialists P.O. Box 371 16 David Avenue Westerly, RI 02891 (800)872-3827 (401)596-3155	Optical and electronic low vision devices

Source	Service
Eschenback Optik of America 904 Ethan Allen Highway Ridgefield, CT 06877 (203)438-7471	Optical low vision devices
G.K. Hall and Company 70 Lincoln Street Boston, MA 02111 (617)423-3990	Large print and audio books
HumanWare, Inc. 6245 King Road Loomis, CA 95650 (800)722-3393 (916)652-7253	Synthetic speech, closed- circuit TV
Independent Living Aids, Inc. 27 East Mall Plainview, NY 11803 (516)752-8080	Nonoptical low vision devices
Keeler Instruments, Inc. 456 Parkway Broomall, PA 19008 (800)523-5620 (215)353-4350	Hand-held and spectacle- mounted low vision devices
Low Vision Devices, Inc. 540 East Horatio Avenue Maitland, FL 32751 (407)628-3133	Low vision devices
M-Tech Optics Corporation P.O. Box 12110 Birmingham, MI 48012 (313)531-3577	Spectacle telescope
Mattingly International 938-K Andreasen Drive Escondido, CA 92029 (800)826-4200 FAX:(800)368-4111	Optical and nonoptical devices Excellent optical summary
Maxi Aids 42 Executive Boulevard Farmingdale, NY 11735 (800)522-6294 (516)752-0521	Nonoptical low vision devices
McLeod Optical, Inc. 100 Jefferson Park Road Warwick, RI 02888 (401)467-3000	Optical low vision devices
Meditec, Inc. 9485 East Orchard Drive Englewood, CO 80111 (303)771-4863	Syringe adaptations for low vision

Source	Service
Mons International 6595 Roswell Road N.E., Rm 224 Atlanta, GA 30328 (800)541-7903 (404)344-8805	Optical, nonoptical, and electronic low vision devices
National Association for the Visually Handicapped 22 West 21st Street New York, NY 10010 (212)889-3141 (415)221-3201 (CA)	Optical and nonoptical low vision devices
National Library Service for the Blind Library of Congress 1291 Taylor Street, N.W. Washington, DC 20542 (202)707-5100	Recorded books and periodicals
New York Lighthouse for the Blind 36-20 Northern Boulevard Long Island City, NY 11101 (800)453-4923 (718)937-9338	Optical and nonoptical devices Testing charts and materials (very helpful catalog)
Ocutech, Inc. P.O. Box 625 Chapel Hill, NC 27515 (919)967-6460	Spectacle telescope
Opteq Vision Systems 17355 Mierow Lane Brookfield, WI 53045 (414)784-4979	Closed-circuit TV
Phillip Barton Vision Systems 3911 York Lane Bowie, MD 20715 (301)285-1135	Optical and nonoptical devices
Reader's Digest/Large Print Edition Box 241 Mount Morris, IL 61054	Large-print *Reader's Digest*
RX Lenses/Low Vision Aids 1379 Progresso Drive Fort Lauderdale, FL 33304 (800)336-6622 (800)621-6386(FL) (305)764-3313	Optical devices and lamps
S. Walters, Inc. 30423 Canwood Street, Suite 126 Agoura Hills, CA 91301 (800)9-WALTER (818)706-2202	Optical low vision devices
Selsi Importing Company P.O. Box 497 40 Veterans Boulevard Carlstadt, NJ 07072 (201)935-0388 (212)473-4451	Optical low vision devices

Source	Service
Strieter Laboratories, Inc. 222 Vandalia Street Collinsville, IL 62234 (800)851-4557 (618)345-5814	Optical and electronic low vision devices
TeleSensory Corporation P.O. Box 7455 455 North Bernardo Mountain View, CA 94039-7455 (800)227-8418 (800)345-2256(VTEK) (415)960-0920	Closed-circuit TV
The New York Times/Large Print Weekly 229 West 43rd Street New York, NY 10036 (212)556-1234	Large-print *New York Times*
Vis/Aids, Inc. 102-09 Jamaica Avenue Richmond Hill, NY 11418 (718)847-4734 FAX:(718)441-2550	Nonoptical low vision devices

Index

N

O